Disorders of the Cervical Spine

Diagnosis and Medical Management

John H. Bland, M.D.

Professor of Medicine
Rheumatology and Clinical Immunology
Department of Medicine
University of Vermont College of Medicine
Burlington, Vermont

Chapters 2 and 3 written in collaboration with

Professor Dallas Richard Boushey

Assistant Professor of Anatomy and Neurobiology
Section of Gross Anatomy
Department of Anatomy and Neurobiology
University of Vermont College of Medicine
Burlington, Vermont

1987

W.B. Saunders Company

Philadelphia   London   Toronto   Sydney   Tokyo   Hong Kong

W. B. Saunders Company: West Washington Square
                           Philadelphia, PA   19105

Library of Congress Cataloging-in-Publication Data

Bland, John H. (John Hardesty), 1917–

Disorders of the cervical spine.

1. Vertebrae, Cervical—Diseases. 2. Vertebrae, Cervical—
   Wounds and injuries. I. Title. [DNLM: 1. Cervical
   Vertebrae.   2. Spinal Diseases—diagnosis. 3. Spinal
   Diseases—therapy. 4. Spinal Injuries—diagnosis. 5. Spinal
   Injuries—therapy. WE 725 B642d]

RC936.B5 1987   616.7′3   86–10241

ISBN 0–7216–1187–7

Editor: Carol Trumbold
Developmental Editor: Carole Caro Wonsiewicz
Designer: Patti Maddaloni
Production Manager: Bob Butler
Manuscript Editor: Martha Tanner
Illustration Coordinator: Peg Shaw
Indexer: George Vilk

Disorders of the Cervical Spine: Diagnosis and Medical Management   ISBN 0–7216–1187–7

Last digit is the print number: 9   8   7   6   5   4   3   2   1

To Libits, John, Perry, Beth, and Linda—
my best friends.

Foreword

According to Webster, a foreword is defined as ". . . likely to be of interest but not necessarily essential for the understanding of the text of a book and commonly written by someone other than the author of the book." I can assure readers of the nonessentiality but would suggest that another uniform characteristic is that of admiration of the author of the foreword for the author of the text. Everyone who shares my pleasure and privilege of knowing Dr. John Bland would readily agree that he is greatly admired as a very effective teacher, a careful and thorough clinical investigator, a compassionate and problem-oriented physician, an esteemed rheumatologist, and a gentleman with intellectual honesty above reproach.

It is I who am honored by the opportunity to introduce Dr. Bland's monograph to both those who have and those who have not known him either personally, professionally, or by reputation. My introduction via this foreword begins with an admonition to all readers: Be certain to READ THE PREFACE!

Dr. Bland is a graduate of Earlham College and of Jefferson Medical College. Like many of his contemporaries, he entered rheumatology quite indirectly but, nonetheless, quite advantageously. After initially finding that an early interest in surgery was attributable to an admired mentor rather than the specialty itself, he switched to internal medicine and found an interest in functions of electrolytes at a time when metabolism was only an emerging aspect of internal medicine. He was the first to show the metabolic consequences of solute overload in tube-fed, comatose, surgical patients; of very high urinary specific gravity; and of hyperchloremia and hyperchloruria. At that time, chloride, calcium, and phosphorus were the only electrolytes for which measurement methods were available (chloride by the old Volhard method!). He was writing a monograph on clinical and metabolic regulation of water, electrolyte, calories, and hydration when he went to the University of Vermont as a Fellow in Cardiology, but both this and his former interest soon became "too ordinary" to satisfy an apparently innate desire to explore medical subjects of lesser general knowledge and attraction.

Fortunately, his Dean at that time, Dr. William Brown, recognized Dr. Bland's special talents and recommended him to Dr. Walter Bauer, with a suggestion that Dr. Bland's prior interest in electrolytes and metabolism might help him explore some of the dilemmas of proteoglycan and collagen tissue functions. Thus, Dr. Bland became the first Fellow of the New England Arthritis and Rheumatism Foundation. Dr. Bland especially admired Dr. Bauer's approach to the early beginnings of rheumatology as a medical specialty and found Dr. Bauer to be "the greatest scholar I'd ever known. He really turned me around." Thereafter, Dr. Bland's interest in rheumatology became sustained. Following his experience at Massachusetts General and New England Center Hospitals, he also studied in Manchester, England, and at the National Institutes of Health.

Before embarking on this postgraduate training period, Dr. Bland was already Instructor in Medicine at the University of Vermont, but it may be noteworthy that he had no sooner entered into rheumatology when he was promoted to Assistant Professor. Subsequently he advanced in academic rank to Professor. He has authored more than 100 publications, including 8 other books. Those who never have undertaken, let alone achieved, completion of a medical textbook that is both scholarly and clinically useful to students, established investigators, and clinicians can never really know the magnitude of such an undertaking.

As Dr. Bland notes, the cervical spine has been, until only the past two or three decades, a neglected and thus poorly understood aspect of not only rheumatology but also orthopedics, neurology, neurosurgery, and even anatomy and pathology. He has no equal in conquering its fascinations and complexities and is uniquely qualified to author an up-to-date, comprehensive, indeed encyclopedic text on the subject. He has made the subject more interesting and understandable by use of clinical case presentations based on the physiology of muscles, bone, and joints. These are further supplemented by new radiologic, anatomic, and histologic data such as the existence and detailed structure and function of cervical menisci. Also, there is a special chapter on rheumatologic neurology. Whether clinical observations are simple or complex, they are the keystone to improved understanding and advancements of clinical significance when expertly acquired and utilized. Dr. Bland's book will be welcomed, appreciated, and used because of the wealth of information and experience it contains. It is certain to be a classic medical contribution for which he surely will be remembered.

In addition to all of his scientific achievements, Dr. Bland is an accomplished, world-champion, cross-country skier. As a result of this avocation, and in keeping with his past record of attention to fields of medicine that generally are overlooked in their formative years, he now is promoting the concept that the emerging specialty of sports medicine should be more properly a primary concern of rheumatologists than of orthopedists. (We should not overlook the fact that rheumatology itself evolved from orthopedics.) Thus, Dr. Bland continues to be a leader in the evolution of specialties.

Since many of us are prone to read last sentences of a publication first, I conclude as I began, by urging—indeed insisting—that everyone *read the preface*; it is the *real*, personal introduction to Dr. Bland and his valuable text.

Howard F. Polley, M.D., Sc.D., FACP
Professor of Medicine
Indiana University School of Medicine

Emeritus Professor of Medicine
Mayo Medical School

Emeritus Senior Consultant in Rheumatology
Mayo Clinic and Foundation

Preface

This preface is different: it is to introduce you to me, to acquaint us, you and me, author and reader. To write at all is to reveal oneself in some degree. So this preface is, in a sense, autobiographical. It is warm, kindly, conversational, informative, egotistic, friendly—a glimpse at my personality, intellectual processes, humor, and the very personal story of my long interest in, enthusiasm for, and study of pain in the neck.

Now in my sixty-ninth year, I need not stand up and be counted. In fact, I hope to be overlooked. Yet I long to tell the fascinating and neglected story of how and why the neck hurts. This book is an attempt to do that.

The cervical spine is everyone's business, since osteoarthritis is universal after age 50. One of 10 people in the United States in 1986 is over age 65; by the year 2000 that figure will be 1 in 5 people. Thus, we all have osteoarthritis, and all doctors will see it in their patients as well as in themselves!

The reason and justification for this book is that although there are twelve other related publications on the market, none is presented from the medical point of view; virtually all are surgical, neurosurgical, or orthopedic surgical, and basic physiology and pathophysiology of the cervical spine are not included. Surely 90% of the diagnosis and management of cervical spine disorders is medical—hence the need. Cervical spine syndromes are extremely common and are probably the fourth most common cause of pain. At any given time, 9% of men and 12% of women have neck pain, with or without arm and hand pain; 35% of the population can remember having had neck pain at some time. With the enormous increase in knowledge of the cell biology of osteoarthritis, there has been little application of this new knowledge, conceptual and practical, to disorders of the cervical spine. Cervical spondylosis as formulated by Brain and Wilkinson is universal in humans—hence its clinical importance.

I am doing more work now than ever. My job is increasingly fun, exciting, and satisfying. The best is still ahead. My only interest in retiring is at 9 PM. I could not stop practicing and teaching medicine. I am finally getting the hang of it! It is an article of faith with me that if I have studied the clinical aspects of an area in medicine for 30 years, become conversant with the gross pathologic and histologic characteristics of the cells and tissues involved, and am knowledgeable about the pertinent radiology, I am apt to know more about it than someone who has not. These things I have done with the cervical spine. Such confidence is hard-won.

During my fellowship in rheumatology in 1950 at the Massachusetts General Hospital, Drs. Walter Bauer and Hans Waine turned my interest, enthusiasm, and fascination happily and permanently to the field of rheumatology. I became a student of the cervical spine in 1955, when I studied a Vermont farmer, a Mr. Russell Olmstead, who had rheumatoid arthritis with subluxation of the atlas on the axis and gross compression of the spinal cord.

I failed to appreciate and identify the lesion itself or to comprehend the pathophysiologic mechanisms by which it occurred. In 1957–58, I had an honorary research fellowship at the University of Manchester in England where Professors of Rheumatology J.H. Kellgren and James Sharp taught me the clinical characteristics and the radiologic identifying features. Professor John Ball, a superb pathologist, taught me the pathophysiologic characteristics of rheumatoid arthritis of the cervical spine and how to remove a whole human cervical spine intact at postmortem examination. Relatively little attention was paid at that time to the cervical spine generally or to rheumatoid arthritis of the cervical spine specifically. This initiated in me a broader, long-range fascination for all aspects of the cervical spine, that cylindric, anatomic wonder connecting the skull and thorax.

This book represents a 30-year experience and study of the cervical spine and its diseases and disorders. Over this period, my colleagues and I have removed at postmortem examination 16 whole human cervical spines from patients with rheumatoid arthritis. We studied them anatomically, radiographically, pathologically, and clinically. In addition, we collected and studied 130 more whole human cervical spines from postmortem material and from our University of Vermont anatomic laboratory and photographed, radiographed, and dissected them to study anatomy and histopathology of cervical spine disease. Initially there was little available detailed histologic study of the tissues in the cervical spine. Cervical spine radiology (plain films only then) has since become more appreciated and sophisticated. Today we have far more knowledge of the normal cervical spine, its anatomy, radiology, biomechanics, and pathology.

Many heroes have shaped my life, my standards, and my way of thinking. Most pertinent in the current context is Dr. Ernest Amory Codman (1869–1940) of Boston, who was an innovative, independent thinker. He was a largely unsung American surgeon, who made major contributions to many fields in the science of medicine. He practiced a high level of medical biologic science long before there was much science at all. Codman studied the shoulder as I have studied the cervical spine. His book, *The Shoulder*, published at his own expense in 1934, has yet to be equaled, let alone surpassed. He came to know more about that remarkable structure than anyone in the world. I got my idea to study the cervical spine from him.

I never knew or even met Ernest, yet I am on a first-name basis with him. We are good friends. One can have close, even dear, friends one has never met—friends who are long dead. He educates me and always has. I continue to follow his example. He would approve and be gratified by my work on the cervical spine. He showed me how to do it.

This book is designed with a broad and comprehensive approach to any disorder of the cervical spine, from simple pain in the neck to neck pain arising from structures other than the cervical spine. The approach is practical and problem-oriented. Tables are designed for rapid and precise diagnosis, using historical data and physical signs that have a high degree of reproducibility. Historical data and clinical signs are presented as reflections of the underlying pathophysiology in each disorder, clinically relating what we have learned of the cell biology, biomechanics, and pathophysiology of the tissues that make up the cervical spine.

Clinical experience remains the key to real understanding of why the patient comes to the doctor and what can rationally be done about his or her clinical problem. The book is a culmination of a career of clinical study, representing 42 years of daily effort to be a better and better clinician. Chapter

4, *Clinical Methods* is designed to present historical and physical methods of data collection, evaluation, and assessment that lead to an accurate diagnosis.

The book is written for all clinicians who want to understand clinical concepts as reflections of normal physiology, cell biology, pathophysiology, anatomy, and biomechanics and to base their treatment and management on these concepts. Accurate diagnosis, relief of pain, and restoration of function are the most important obligations, main objectives, and crowning achievements of every physician. Arranged in problem-oriented format, this book should be a ready reference for house staff, interns, residents, fellows, and students. Primary care physicians, internists, rheumatologists, neurologists, neurosurgeons, orthopedic surgeons, physiatrists, physical therapists, and occupational therapists will find the book addressed to them.

I believe the final structural arrangement is simple and clear—triple-distilled, with no loss of flavor. There, my neck is out!

JOHN H. BLAND

Acknowledgments

It requires many people to complete a book, both those presently extant and many who no longer answer the roll call. Those listed here have supplied support and help from the beginning to completion. This work was done standing on the shoulders of those long past as well as present, who were or are students of the cervical spine and from whose work and writing I have drawn freely: Sir Charles Bell (1830), James Parkinson (1830), C. A. Key (1838), W. R. Gowers (1892), Alexander E. Garrod (1900), J. Taylor (1901), J. Collier (1901), P. Bailey (1911), L. Casamajor (1911), George R. Elliott (1926), Byron Stookey (1928), C. A. Elsberg (1928), R. Andrae (1929), O. A. Beadle (1931), Max Minor Peet (1932), Dean H. Echols (1932), P. C. Bucy (1944), H.Chanault (1944), R. G. Spurling (1944), W. B. Scoville (1944), F. K. Bradford (1945), J. W. D. Bull (1948), Lord Russell Brain (1948), Lawrence Kaplan (1950), Foster Kennedy (1950), Ragnar Frykholm (1951), G. Tondury (1967), Marcia Wilkinson (1952), C. P. Symonds (1952), E. L. Compere (1959), J. H. Kellgren (1960), John Ball (1960), Sajida Abdullah (1960), Ruth E. M. Bowden (1960), William Hardesty (1963), E. P. Holt (1964), R. T. W. Bailey (1965), J. L. James (1965), I. C. Isdale (1965), J. T. Hughes (1966), P. O. Yates (1966), Bernard Smith (1968), William Martel (1970), Lennart Holt (1971), Detlef von Torklus (1972), J. William Fielding (1974), Ruth Jackson (1977), Yves Dirheimer (1977), Eurig Jeffreys (1980).

Blake and Sheila Lawrence, dear friends and loyal supporters in this literary, scientific enterprise. They teach us how to live life. Many people are intelligent. Few are wise. They are both.

Mary C. Skovira, who believes that things do come to those who wait, but only things left by those who hustle. For her constant loyalty, consummate skill in turning out reams of handwritten manuscript in a short time, devotion to job and project, her wit and warm humor, personal friendship, and her sense of organization and its application.

Professor Dallas R. Boushey, anatomist, friend, and teacher, who always knew we would finish it—just did not know when! For his depth of knowledge and deep interest in anatomy of the cervical spine (as well as the rest of the body) and the education he provided me day-to-day in studying the neck.

Wing Woon, photographer and friend of many years, for his scientific, creative, and artistic approach to photographic illustration, always ready and willing, superb humor—at 11AM on any given day, "No hurry really, just want the slides by noon!"

Gary Nelson, creative and innovative artist and illustrator, for his constant willingness and prompt focus of personal interpretation on the specific illustration, and for his ability to transfer content instantly and intact from the drawing board to the mind of the reader—he was given many a sow's ear and delivered many a silk purse.

Leon Sokoloff, superb pathologist and friend of many years, for his original, creative, and innovative interest and studies in osteoarthritis long before the subject had any perceptible popularity. For his educating me in the cell biology of osteoarthritis in all species, for teaching me how to study whole cervical spines by doing a number of the studies himself, and for our long and durable friendship. It is always there and needs no particular tending.

Lent C. Johnson, pathologist (without peer in bone pathology), Armed Forces Institute of Pathology, long-time educator of orthopedic surgeons and rheumatologists in bone and joint pathology, for his preparation and study of two whole human cervical spines, increasing my knowledge enormously, showing that the joints of Luschka developed severe and proliferative synovitis, with spread of granuloma to vertebra and intervertebral disc, and that the rheumatoid granuloma can arise de novo in bone in the cervical spine.

Aubrey J. Hough, pathologist, friend, and educator, for his good humor and scientific sophistication. For his preparation of four whole human cervical spines, demonstrating that ligamentum flavum, anterior and posterior longitudinal ligaments, and periosteum are involved in osteoarthritis and that there is active, proliferative synovitis in osteoarthritis in the cervical spine, the zygapophyseal joints, and the Luschka joints.

My colleagues in rheumatology: Sheldon M. Cooper, Marshall G. London, Thomas W. Martenis, Richard L. Lipson, and Edward S. Leib, University of Vermont rheumatologists, and Philip H. Davis, orthopedic surgeon, who have participated directly and indirectly in the cervical spine study over many years, for their continued interest, enthusiasm, support, criticism, and compliments.

Frederick W. Van Buskirk (deceased), A. Bradley Soule (deceased), and John P. Tampas, University of Vermont radiologists, for their many hours of reading cervical spine x-ray films and cineradiograms, for educating me in the fine details of film reading, and for the clear demonstration of the problems of observer error.

Professor J. H. Kellgren, Department of Rheumatology, University of Manchester, England, for his inspiration communicated as a teacher and great modern clinician, for his educating me in detailed historical elicitation and physical examination, establishing in my mind the necessity for the maintenance of optimum clinical competence to practice clinical medicine to the hilt, and especially for the deep insights into the epidemiology of rheumatic disease. Professor Kellgren was brought up by the last great clinical investigator (the patient was the assay animal), Sir Thomas Lewis, and demonstrated to the current medical world what a great clinician is. Professor Kellgren first showed me the detailed and complex anatomy, giving me great respect for the complicated articular system of the cervical spine, and taught me the mechanism of atlantoaxial subluxation.

Professor James Sharp, superb clinician, Department of Rheumatology, University of Manchester, England, for his teaching me clinical skills and showing me the epidemiology of rheumatoid arthritis of the cervical spine and the results of optimum management as well as the clinical events occurring in the natural history of the disease in the cervical spine.

Professor John Ball, outstanding pathologist, creative and innovative investigator, for many hours of discussion of the cell biology and pathologic characteristics of both rheumatoid arthritis and osteoarthritis, for showing me the gross pathology of osteoarthritis of the hip, the knee, and the lumbar and cervical portions of the spine, and particularly for teaching me how to remove intact the whole human cervical spine for optimum study, forming the foundation of the present radiologic and pathologic investigations.

Eric G. L. Bywaters, professor of rheumatology, Hammersmith Hospital and the Taplow Red Cross Children's Rheumatologic Hospital, the model of the generalist and specialist with research and clinical productivity almost unparalleled in rheumatology, for his research work on the spine, studies of bursae of the body, for the mentor role he plays and example he sets as the ideal rheumatologist, clinician, educator, and researcher, and especially for his recent demonstration of rheumatoid arthritis of the costovertebral and costo-transverse joints.

Carole Caro Wonsiewicz for her interest, enthusiasm, sensitive judgment, advice, good humor, and criticism in shepherding the book from early manu-script to the finished product.

Contents

Part I ○ SCIENTIFIC FOUNDATION AND DIAGNOSTIC METHODS

Chapter 1

Introduction: "Pain in the Neck"

Pain in the neck is such an everyday event that it has come to be used to describe a situation, certain people, an unpleasant job to be done, or an institution! At any specific time as much as 12% of the adult female population and 9% of the adult male population experience pain in the neck, with or without associated arm pain, and 35% of people can recall an episode.[1] Hult,[2] in a most important epidemiologic clinical study of cervical spine pain, reported a history of stiff neck and arm pain in 80% of a population of male industrial and forest workers. In a second study, the same author modified the figure to 51% in a series of 1193 male workers, but only 5.4% had experienced any work loss as a consequence of the pain.[3] Interestingly, in another important epidemiologic study of neck pain, nearly 70% of a series of adults who had visited their doctors were well or improving within 1 month.[4]

Though precise epidemiologic data of acute and chronic neck pain are not available, it is probable that at one time or another all of us suffer mild to moderate pain in the neck, sometimes recurrent, amounting to a transient annoyance. Still, with that degree of morbidity in the population, a small, very significant percentage of people regard their symptoms as important enough to seek medical attention or feel that the pain impairs their work capability. The overall consequent morbidity is of enormous importance.

An epidemiologic problem is that systematic collection of information has not been done, and until two to three decades ago, much illness that we now know to be caused by cervical spine disease or disorder, such as shoulder pain, disc disease, and "arthritis" of the arm, shoulder, and spine, was regarded as having its primary source elsewhere. Nowadays the cervical spine is recognized as the pathologic site for a large proportion of shoulder, elbow, hand, and wrist disorders. Most people who develop pain in the neck do not seek medical attention, regard it as a necessary evil, and await its disappearance—and properly so. Neck pain commonly appears abruptly after some unusual motion of the neck or prolonged effort at a given job (painting a ceiling) or with unusual use of the arm, forearm, and hand. A common assumption is that one "was caught in a draft" or "had a virus" or "had a wry neck." The pain is usually in the middle of the back of the neck, and cervical spine motion, particularly extension and lateral flexion, increases the pain. If it is unusually intense, is associated with paresthesia, or lasts more than days to a week, the person generally seeks medical attention. The informed doctor recognizes that the differential diagnosis is indeed an extensive one, requiring considerable knowledge of potential mechanisms. Possible diagnoses are the cardiovascular diseases, including myocardial infarction and aortic dissection, meningitis, cervical osteoarthritis, hypertension, temporal arteritis, polymyalgia rheumatica, a spectrum of neurologic diseases and syndromes, various metabolic bone diseases, primary and metastatic cancer, infection, lymphoma, and myeloma. In the ideal circumstance, a complete clinical study and a management program follow. Of importance to the reader is that even when symptoms and signs have persisted for many years, treatment and management are very effective, and the prognosis, by and large, is very good.[5]

The neck is the most mobile segment of the spine. Through this cylinder connecting the head to the thorax pass many delicate and vital structures—the carotid and vertebral arteries, the spinal cord, and the spinal nerves—all of which require the greatest protection and yet have the least. The head, a 15- to 17-lb ball, is perched precariously on top of the extremely flexible 6-in neck, made up of 7 delicate vertebrae in a limber chain held together by 14 zygapophyseal joints, 5 intervertebral discs, 12 joints of Luschka, and a system of ligaments and muscles allowing enormous maneuverability and range of motion—mobility at the expense of stability. The neck conveys structures to and from the head and trunk, the movable segments being placed between two heavy objects. It enables the head to be positioned to receive from the environment all needed sensory information except touch. The cervical spine is a common target for disease and trauma, because it is subjected to marked stress and strain during ordinary daily activities. Even in daily conversation we all exhibit individual gestural patterns, moving the head and neck much more than most of us are aware. Anyone who has suffered the very common, acute, painful stiff neck (spasmodic torticollis) can testify to how thoroughly disabling this simple syndrome can be.

Normal function of the cervical spine demands that all movements be performed without injury to the spinal cord and the millions of nerve fibers passing through it, such as the intervertebral foramina and the foramina transversaria, as well as the vascular supply to the cervical cord, all cervical tissue, and the entire brain. The spinal cord has an amazing capacity to adapt itself to marked alteration in the length of the cervical spinal canal. Flexion of the neck lengthens the spinal canal, and extension shortens it. There is considerable variation in individual thickness of the cervical spinal cord and in diameters of the spinal canal. A perfect anatomy from a functional point of view is seldom provided. In the past two decades, the vast number of cervical clinical syndromes have been appreciated, recognized, and often successfully treated. Only a little less common in clinical practice than backache, pain in the neck is just that to most doctors.

PHYLOGENETIC IMPLICATIONS

During early man's evolutionary process of becoming permanently biped and erect in posture, the cervical spine was well protected by forwardly hunched shoulders, a semierect posture, and enormous posterior cervical muscles holding the head up against the heavier pull of gravity. When arms and hands replaced forelegs and paws, and a stable, permanently erect posture appeared, man's neck was out! The gigantic antigravity muscles atrophied, their job now being only to balance the heavy head on the top of the neck (Fig. 1–1).

Phylogenetically the atlas is not the first cervical vertebra but is the fifth or sixth of the primary

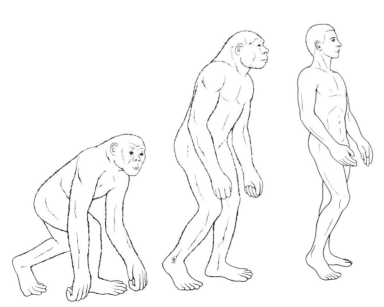

Figure 1–1. Early primate; early Hominidae; modern man. Evolutionary progression to erect posture is depicted with loss of forwardly hunched shoulders, atrophy of the massive posterior cervical musculature opposing the pull of gravity, and finally, an erect posture with the head balanced on the atlas and cervical spine below.

vertebral chain in vertebrate evolution. In mammals the base of the occipital bone is formed by fusion of the first three or four primary vertebral formations, anlagen, called occipital vertebrae in the spondylocranium. Thus, other vertebrates (reptiles and amphibians and those lower in the phylogenetic scale) have four or five more cervical vertebrae than mammals and do not have the marvelous adaptation of the odontoid peg and the ringed atlas, the odontoid peg having once been the body of the atlas. This important development, as valuable in survival as the opposable thumb, allows the head to turn to extreme degrees, subserving and extending the senses of sight, hearing, and smell, and the perception of direction. The head and atlas turn on the odontoid peg like a wheel in eccentric location on an axle (Fig. 1–2). Comparative anatomy shows the tendencies of progression and regression, that is, more and more cervical segments are incorporated within the skull, and the tail regresses, with individual vertebral segments moving cranially. With the great increase in mobility and loss of stability of the cervical spine and shoulder, both structure and function of the cervical spine changed tremendously; large ribless zones were required to make room for the great nerve plexuses supplying the enormously freed-up shoulders, arms, hands, hips, legs, and feet, with various bony rotations and muscle and joint realignments (Fig. 1–3). Figure 1–4 illustrates the shoulder and scapula in semierect and quadriped animals.

The joints of Luschka (uncovertebral joints) appear in the phylogenetic series after the development of the mammalian occiput-atlas-axis complex and are of extreme importance clinically. They are true joints but are absent at birth, appearing at about age 10 to 14 years. They are fissures or clefts that arise secondarily and superoposterolat-

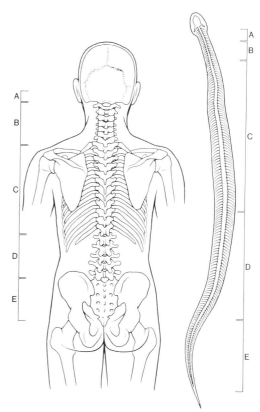

Figure 1–3. Man and snake. Zone **A** in the reptile represents the upper five vertebrae that became the occipital bone, or spondyloforamen, in man; compare with Zone **A** in man. **B** represents the cervical ribbed zone that evolved into a ribless zone in man. The modern cervical spine evolved to accommodate the cervical and brachial plexuses, permitting the great increase in neural traffic consequent to the operation of upper extremities. Zone **B** remains "ribbed" in the modern reptile. Zones **C, D,** and **E** are ribbed in the reptile having no extremities. In man, zone **C** is ribbed thorax, zone **D** is ribless, and the pelvis and lower extremities evolved. Thus, ribless zones had great survival value and became permanent in mammals.

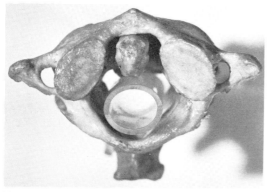

Figure 1–2. Top view of the atlas, showing atlanto-occipital facets: the anterior arch of the atlas articulating with the odontoid process; the foramina transversaria, through which the vertebral artery runs; and the spinal cord, represented by a piece of plastic tubing occupying the cervical canal.

erally in the normal anulus fibrocartilage of the intervertebral discs; they are not primarily peculiarities of the cervical discs. The initial posterolateral cleft develops a synovial lining and a fibrocartilage, which metamorphoses to hyaline cartilage, meniscus-like folds, and a joint capsule. Still, there is no real difference between these "joints" and a true joint. The latter is a primary structure that appears prenatally, and the Luschka joints are secondary fissures in originally normal discs (Fig. 1–5). This process of fissuring and transformation to true joints is a functional adaptation of the intervertebral disc at a moment when the uncinate processes (analogue of costovertebral articulation) are raised to attain their maximum height.[6] The clefts promote the gliding and rotation of adjacent vertebral bodies required in the

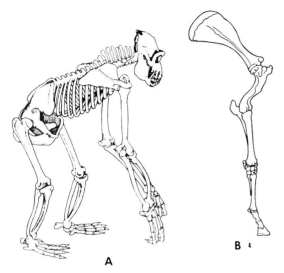

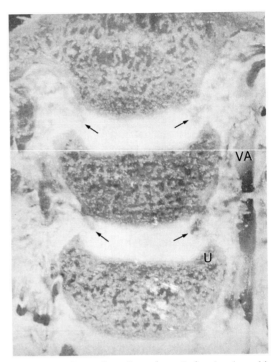

Figure 1–4. *A,* Gorilla skeleton. This semierect mammal has partial weight-bearing forelegs, and its scapulae are situated in the posterior lateral thorax. The glenohumeral joint is weight-bearing, and all muscles of the shoulder girdle serve different functions from those of the corresponding muscles in man, whose posture is fully erect. When the scapula migrates to a completely dorsal position in the thorax, and the humerus rotates about 60 degrees during evolutionary development, the glenohumeral joint is no longer weight-bearing and has greatly increased mobility. *B,* The foreleg of the horse shows the completely lateral position of the scapula on the thorax. The glenohumeral joint is all weight-bearing. The supraspinatus muscle swings and accelerates the foreleg as a pendulum, quite a different function from that in man. (From Codman EA: The Shoulder. Boston: Thomas Todd Co Printers, 1934.)

Figure 1–5. Coronal section of cervical spine in a 14-year-old girl. **U** is the well-developed uncinate process, and **VA** is the vertebral artery. The arrows point to the early developing Luschka joints at C3–C4 and C4–C5 as clefts in the posterolateral anulus, later to evolve into the Luschka joints having the same components as any other diarthrodial joint. (From Hall MC: Luschka's Joint, 1965. Courtesy of Charles C Thomas, Publisher, Springfield, Illinois.)

extensive movements of the cervical spine. They are surely produced by the shearing stress during movement, with loosening of the texture of the anulus fibrosus and splitting of their peripheral lamellae. These joints are just inside the uncinate processes, phylogenetic homologues of the ribs and old costovertebral articulations. Other names for the Luschka joints are uncovertebral articulations, neurocentral joints, and intervertebral half-joints.[7] The clefts tend to spread through the whole disc with age, with a transverse fissure finally separating the cervical disc into two parts. These uncovertebral articulations undergo all pathologic changes that occur in diarthrodial joints, with pannus, erosion, eburnation, osteophytosis, and remodeling.[3–10]

NECK PAIN IN PRACTICE

Cases of cervical pain occur in practice only slightly less frequently than cases of low back pain. A major difference is that cervical pain is far less disabling, seldom compromising work capacity. The cervical syndromes seem not to be real occupational diseases caused by special strains imposed by work, as is back pain. Simple stiff neck, benign torticollis, is a common disorder. Working individuals between ages 25 and 29 years have a 25% to 30% incidence of one or more attacks of stiff neck; for those over 45 years of age this figure rises to 50%. The episodes last from 1 to 4 days and seldom require medical care; the symptoms of patients doing very light work do not differ from those of patients doing heavy work. Brachial neuralgia (cervicobrachialgia) occurs later than stiff neck, with a 5% to 10% incidence in the 25- to 29-year age group and a 25% to 40% incidence after 45 years. The same tendency is seen for low back pain (lumbago) and sciatica; stiff neck and low back pain come first, and brachial neuralgia and sciatica occur later, with no real difference in the symptoms of patients doing light work and those doing heavy work.[11]

Overall, 45% of working men have had at least one attack of stiff neck; 23% have had at least one attack of brachial neuralgia, and 51% have experienced both of these symptoms. The incidence of brachial neuralgia is about three times higher in those who have had a stiff neck, suggesting common factors in pathogenesis, as expected.

Radiographic evidence of cervical spondylosis (osteoarthritis) rises with age to become almost universal at about age 50 regardless of symptoms; patients with symptoms have a 10% higher incidence of radiographic changes. There are, of course, many cases of cervical osteoarthritis in which the patient has no symptoms, but severe radiographic changes are evident. Similarly, other patients have severe symptoms, yet little or no radiographic change occurs. The localization of cervical intervertebral disc osteoarthritis is primarily at the C5–C6 and C6–C7 levels, with the clinical syndromes emanating mostly from the C6–C7 level.[12]

Thus, cervical pain and cervicobrachial and cervicocephalic syndromes are extremely common in all occupational groups, with stiff neck coming first and headache and brachialgia occurring later. The symptoms are radiating pain and segmental paresthesia of the neck, arm, and fingers, head-ache, pseudoangina, and shoulder pain of various types. Symptoms are often mild, but some are severely disabling, presenting difficult diagnostic and therapeutic problems.[2, 3, 10]

PAIN-SENSITIVE STRUCTURES IN THE NECK

The normal cervical spine is the most complicated articular system in the body, containing 37 separate joints. Most structures in the neck are sensitive to pain, some more than others, and a knowledge of the dermatome, sclerotome, and myotome patterns of pain distribution is necessary in clinical diagnosis (see Tables 2–1, 2–2, and 2–3). Differentiation is required to identify and separate neural, vascular, muscular, ligamentous, joint, and bone pain; cord pain and peripheral nerve pain need specific recognition. Figure 1–6 illustrates the dermal segmentation of the nerve fibers that carry the senses of heat, cold, vibration, pain, and touch to the spinal cord root. In other words, it shows where we feel pain sensation carried by a given nerve fiber.

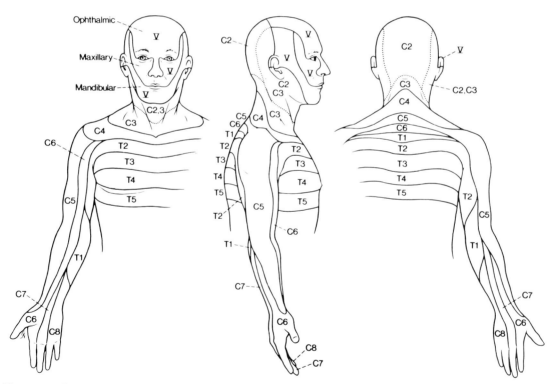

Figure 1–6. Dermatome distribution. Dermatome segmentation from C1 through T5. The nerve fibers carry to the spinal cord root the senses of pain, heat, cold, vibration, and touch felt by the head, neck, arm, hand, and upper thoracic area. Segmentation of sclerotomes and myotomes is similar, but the perceptive sensation is quite different, and the overlap is over much larger areas than that perceived in the dermatome distribution. Pain arising from structures deep to the deep fascia (myotomes and sclerotomes) do not precisely follow the dermatome distribution. The **V** refers to the trigeminal nerve. An exception to conventional dermatome patterns is that C1 is perceived anteriorly in the head, forehead, and retro-orbital and anterofrontal areas of the head. (From Bland JH, Nakano KK: Neck pain. *In* Kelley, Harris, Ruddy, et al (eds): Textbook of Rheumatology. Philadelphia: W. B. Saunders Co, 1981.)

A single cervical spinal posterior root innervates not only its corresponding segmental cutaneous area (dermatome) but also its corresponding sclerotome and myotome—muscles, bones, joints, ligaments, and even viscera, all of which may be remote from the corresponding dermatome. For example, the seventh cervical root supplies the cutaneous area extending down the upper arm usually to the middle finger, but it also supplies several muscles—pectoralis major, triceps, serratus anterior, and latissimus dorsi. So, pain caused by this C7-irritated spinal root can radiate widely to the chest anteriorly and posteriorly, simulating pain of cardiac origin. Ligament, tendon, capsule, or muscle that is primarily irritated may also be perceived as pain throughout the somite distribution. These anatomic facts should be memorized and used clinically; thus cervicobrachialgia cannot occur from the structures above the C5 level and cervicocephalalgia cannot occur from structures below the C4 level.

Lewis[13] showed that pain arising from structures below the deep fascia (ligament, tendon, capsule, bone) has certain characteristics that differ from pain arising from other sites, either deep fascia or more superficial. The cervical spine is no exception. Though segmental, the pain does not precisely follow the dermatome distribution; it also includes sclerotome, myotome, and dermatome distribution patterns. For example, Kellgren[14] showed that injection of highly irritating 6% saline solution in 0.05- to 0.1-ml doses into muscle, tendon, ligament, or joint capsule results in very severe pain lasting approximately 5 minutes. Never perceived at the site of the structure injected, the area of pain is poorly localized and disproportionately large in size. There is tenderness in the tissues at the site of the pain. The pain is not blocked by administering a local anesthetic to the site of pain perception, and there is tenderness in all muscles supplied by the same sensory segment. Injection of 0.1 ml of 6% saline solution into the rhomboid muscles results in severe pain in a wide area of the anterior and posterior shoulder, roughly following the deep segmental sensory distribution of the fifth cervical root; injection of 0.1 ml of 6% saline solution in the periosteum of the humerus near the capsule insertion causes diffuse severe pain in the same area. Injection into the interspinous ligament, a broad, tough membrane between the posterior arch of the atlas and the spinous process of the axis, results in severe unilateral or bilateral, retro-orbital and temple pain. When the interspinous ligament between C4 and C5 is severely irritated, pain is perceived in the upper thoracic spine and well into both proximal arms; irritation of the C7–T1 level is perceived in the midthoracic spine, all posterior, the medial forearm, and the ulnar side of the hand.

Visceral pain of deep structures is often not clinically separable from somatic pain of deep structures. Pain arising in the gallbladder or cardiac tissues can be precisely mimicked by pain arising from ligamentous and joint structures at the T4–T5 and T5–T6 levels in the thoracic spine; esophageal pain may be indistinguishable from cervical spine, ligamentous, or joint capsular pain.[14] It is not always possible to distinguish between pain arising from posterior nerve root compression (when there are no objective sensory or motor components) and deep-structure pain in the neck. Systematic active, passive, and against-resistance movements of the neck allow the clinician fairly precise identification of the pain-sensitive structure or structures. Expert neurologic examination seeking sensory or motor deficits often aids in this clinical differentiation (see Chapter 4, *Clinical Methods*).

Defining the area of pain does not allow precise identification of the structure involved, but the larger the volume of tissue the lesion occupies, the larger the area of pain. There may be skipped areas. For example, assume that severe pain felt in the fifth finger alone is due to a small ligamentous or neural lesion at the C8–T1 level; if the lesion gradually or abruptly becomes much larger, the whole medial arm, forearm, ring and little fingers, and the upper thoracic spine become severely painful. Structures of the same embryologic orgin, that is, all structures ultimately derived from the original, segmented, undifferentiated cellular mass of mesenchyme, refer pain to part or all of the same area. The early dermatome, myotome, and sclerotome are programmed and destined genetically to differentiate and become a number of different structures, all of which may be perceived in pain syndromes of the cervical spine.

The clinical axiom is that historical elicitation of onset, site, duration, distribution, severity, and character of pain and detailed neurologic and rheumatologic examination permit quite precise identification of the pain-sensitive structure or structures. Appropriate diagnostic and therapeutic measures can be based on the pathophysiology involved; even the cell biology of the area is clinically reflected. Etiology and pathogenesis of pain in the neck can usually be accurately formulated.

NECK PAIN ARISING FROM STRUCTURES OUTSIDE THE NECK

Many clinical conditions arising outside the cervical spine but perceived in or about the neck mimic cervical nerve root irritation and muscle, ligament, bone, and joint disorders or even esophageal or vascular disorders of the cervical spine (Table 1–1). These conditions are usually simple to indict or eliminate as pathogenic in cervical syndromes. Disorders of somatic or visceral structures having cervical nerve root innervation (same

Table 1–1. OTHER POTENTIAL CAUSES OF NECK PAIN

Anatomic Location	Disorder	Innervation
Acromioclavicular joint	Trauma, arthritis	C4
Heart	Coronary artery disease	C3, C4, C5, C6
Apex of lung	Pancoast's tumor or bronchogenic carcinoma	C3, C4, C5
Diaphragm muscle	Spasm, hiccups, trauma	C3, C4, C5
Gallbladder	Cholecystitis, biliary calculi	C4, C5, C6
Spinal cord	Tumor, trauma, arthritis	Highly variable
Temporomandibular joint	Arthritis	C7, T1
Upper thoracic spine and proximal arm and shoulder	Fibrositis and fibromyalgia syndromes	C5–T3
Aorta	Aneurysm	C5, C6, C7
Pancreas	Pancreatitis, malignancy	Indeterminate
Other somatic and visceral structures	Disorders of any somatic or visceral structures having cervical nerve root innervation; peripheral neuropathy	Highly variable
Peripheral nerves	Neuropathy—all branches of the brachial plexus	C5–T1
Distal esophagus	Hiatal hernia	C3, C4, C5
Left upper abdominal quadrant	Gastric ulcer	C3, C4, C5, C6
Cervical spine	"Whiplash" syndrome	? C1–T1—highly variable
—	Depression	—
—	Malingering	—
—	Hysteria	—
—	Psychoneurosis	—

embryologic origin) cause pain felt in the neck. Such areas of pain are not tender on deep palpation, but superficial tenderness may be present. These areas constitute reflexly referred pain along the segmental distribution of the nerve roots. Areas of superficial peripheral tenderness are due to reflex or direct sympathetic irritation secondary to vasomotor changes. The painful areas have no associated muscle spasm but may be described as causing a burning sensation or cramping, often accompanied by nausea, vomiting, and pallor.

Peripheral neuritis may result in pain both proximal and distal to the irritative site. Muscle spasm and tenderness of the painful areas do not occur. Spinal cord disease, usually poorly localized and ill-defined, may cause pain in the neck; hyperreflexia, hypertonia, and spasticity are usually present. Immobilization does not relieve it. Deep tenderness and localized muscle spasm are absent, and local anesthetics in the painful area provide no relief. Paralysis or weakness of muscle below the level of the lesion in the cord and a positive Babinski's sign are helpful in diagnosis. Brain lesions (especially recent trauma or tumor) may produce cervical spine pain mimicking nerve root irritation; clinical examination is usually not very helpful, but images produced by means of computed tomography, electroencephalography, or angiography often clarify the issue. Immobilization, traction, and local anesthesia do not relieve the symptoms.

Differential diagnosis is easy if one is aware that compression or irritation of cervical nerve roots with radiation of pain is associated with deep tenderness at the site of pain. Segmental areas of deep tenderness, not painful until palpated, are evidence of nerve root involvement. A 1% injection of lidocaine (Xylocaine) in the area in question results in transient reproduction of the radicular pain pattern followed by relief from pain for days, weeks, or months. Application of a local anesthetic to a painful but nontender area results in fleeting (duration of anesthesia), if any, relief of pain and no reproduction of the radicular pattern. Then, one looks elsewhere for the lesion causing the pain. Visceral or somatic structures having the same segmental nerve supply are the usual cause of pain.

Neck pain is very common in malingerers, depressed patients, those seeking compensation, hysterical and psychoneurotic patients, and automobile crash victims having sustained so-called whiplash. The differential diagnostic points are applicable. These patients derive no relief from administration of a local anesthetic to the painful area. Absence of muscle spasm, the assumption of an antalgic position, and the feigning of limitation of motion should arouse serious suspicion.

Posture, including that of the cervical spine, is a somatic depiction of emotional and general psychologic state. We stand, sit, and move according to how we feel about ourselves, others, and the world at large—consciously or subconsciously depicting our basic attitude and emotional selves. The fatigued, dejected, depressed person is in flexion, especially in the cervical spine. The tense, hyperkinetic person is erect or in some degree of extension. The rest are somewhere in between!

References

1. Lawrence JS: Disc degeneration. Its frequency and relationship to symptoms. Ann Rheum Dis 28:121, 1969.
2. Hult L: The Munkford investigation. Acta Orthop Scand (suppl) 16:1, 1954.
3. Hult L: Cervical, dorsal and lumbar spinal syndromes. Acta Orthop Scand (suppl) 17:1, 1954.
4. British Association of Physical Medicine: Pain in the neck and arm. A multicentre trial of the effects of physical therapy. Brit Med J 1:253, 1966.
5. Lees F, Turner JWA: Natural history and prognosis of cervical spondylosis. Brit Med J 2:1607, 1963.
6. Hall MC: Luschka's Joint. Springfield, Illinois: Charles C Thomas Publisher, 1965.
7. Hadley LA: Anatomico-roentgenographic Studies of the Spine. Springfield, Illinois: Charles C Thomas Publisher, 1964.
8. Cave AJE, Griffith JD, Whitely MM: Osteoarthritis deformans of the Luschka joints. Lancet 1:176, 1955.
9. Tondury G: Morphology of the cervical spine. *In* Jung A, Kahn P, Matert F, et al (eds): The Cervical Spine. Bern: Hans Huber, 1974, p 14–35.
10. Schmorl G, Junghanns H: The Human Spine in Health and Disease. New York: Grune & Stratton, 1959.
11. Hult L: Frequency of symptoms for different age groups and professions. *In* Hirsch C, Zotterman Y (eds): Cervical Pain. Proceedings of the International Symposium, vol 19. Wenner-Gren Center, Stockholm, Sweden: Pergamon Press, 1971.
12. Hirsch G, Schajowicz F, Galante J: Structural changes in the cervical spine. A study on autopsy specimens in different age groups. Acta Orthop Scand (suppl) 37:109, 1967.
13. Lewis T: Pain. New York: Macmillan Publishing Co, 1942.
14. Kellgren JH: On the distribution of pain arising from deep somatic structures with charts of segmental pain areas. Clin Sci 4:35, 1939.

Chapter 2

Anatomy and Biomechanics

written in collaboration with
Professor Dallas Richard Boushey

The anatomy of the cervical spine has characteristics quite different from those of the thoracic or lumbar spine, though the embryologic development of all three spinal sections is quite similar. Interposed between the relatively immobile thoracic spine and the head, the cervical spine has a great range of motion in all directions. The neck, in subserving all the special sense organs—sight, hearing, smell, and taste—requires this extensive mobility. The head is held in place by supporting ligamentous, capsular, muscular, and cartilaginous structures. The very specialized atlas and axis are strikingly different from the other five cervical vertebrae. The cervical muscles have three basic functions, to move the head and neck by gross and fine adjustments, to suspend and move the entire shoulder girdle, and to suspend, fix, and elevate the thoracic inlet. The vertebral canal has its widest diameter in the cervical spine (compared with the thoracic and lumbar portions of the spinal canal). The meninges enclose the spinal cord, the tough dura mater is firmly attached at and about the foramen magnum and normally hangs like a bag, with only loose attachment to the rigid, bony canal. The vertebral arteries encased in the bony foramina transversaria are constantly subjected to the push and pull of the extensive movement of the cervical spine. These critical vessels supply not only the entire contents of the posterior cranial fossa but also the vertebrae, meninges, spinal cord, all zygapophyseal joints, posterior root ganglia, and all cervical nerve roots.

Study of motor mechanisms of the cervical spine discloses how the spine's various anatomic structures function. Functional anatomy, by definition here, is the interpretation of physical properties of anatomic structures according to their functional purpose. For example, the functional anatomy of the ligamenta flava shows these paired ligaments to be highly elastic, allowing separation of the laminae and the spinous processes in flexion, a return to original shape and size in neutral position, and a buckling and folding into the spinal canal in extension (Fig. 2–1).

The term biomechanics, introduced by Brieg,[1, 2] is the study of changes in the form of anatomic structures occurring during movement of the body; thus biomechanics is closely related to functional anatomy. In the present context a good example is the biomechanical change in the form and position of the brainstem and spinal cord during movements of the head and neck. Certain neurologic diseases are readily understood using knowledge of biomechanics of the central and peripheral nervous systems. The state of equilibrium existing between change of structural form and preservation of optimum function may become precarious if impaired by arthritis, trauma, advancing age, and by unfortunate and unnecessary immobilization. An example is the cervical spinal cord, which normally changes its length by about 25% during flexion and extension of the cervical spine. Important changes occur in the form of the nerve tracts in the cord, arteries, and veins, and in the vertebral artery and its relationship to cord blood supply and the anterior and posterior nerve roots.

Before approaching functional pathology, a thorough review of anatomy, functional anatomy, and biomechanics is a sine qua non of clinical assessment. Study and management of disorders of the cervical spine and optimum clinical application are based on physiology, biochemistry, immunology (currently), functional anatomy, and biomechanics.

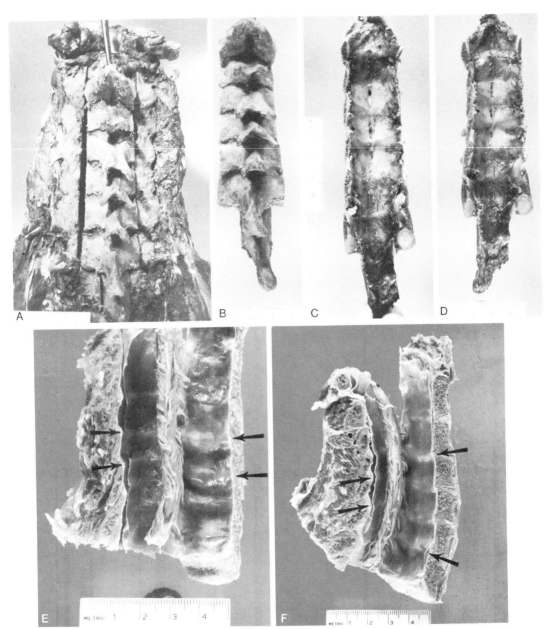

Figure 2–1. *A,* In this specimen, posterior view of a whole human cervical spine, laminae and spinous processes have been removed intact at the junction with the transverse processes and the pedicles, preserving all ligamenta flava. Note bifid spinous processes. *B,* Posterior view of the laminae and ligamenta flava from the specimen pictured in *A.* Part *C* shows the specimen stretched, and part *D* shows it unstretched. Note the remarkable elasticity. *E,* A split, sagittal section of cervical spine showing on the left the bulging of ligamenta flava into the spinal canal from posteriorly in extension (arrows). The right side shows nodular spondylotic bars (osteoarthritis) (arrows) protruding into the spinal cord. The spinal cord in the middle is viewed laterally, showing anterior and posterior rootlets. *F,* Another split, sagittal section of a cervical spine with even more gross ligamenta flava bulging and hypertrophy posteriorly (arrows on left) and massive, nodular, osteoarthritic bars anteriorly both at disc and midvertebral levels (arrows on right), compressing the spinal cord and the roots.

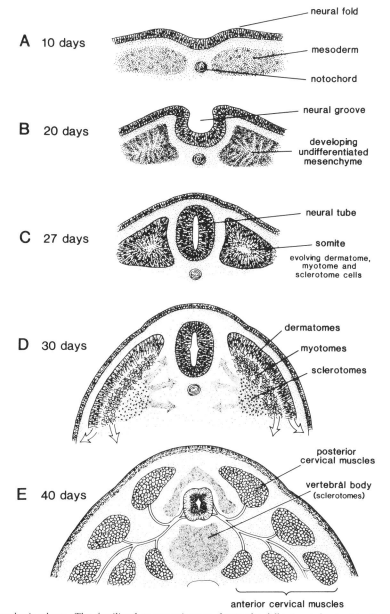

Figure 2–2. Embryologic phase. The fertilized ovum migrates down the fallopian tube in 6 to 7 days and becomes implanted in the uterine cavity. It rapidly passes through the hollow-ball morula stage to the blastocyst stage, and the embryonic disc forms on one side and thickens into two distinct layers of cells, the endoderm and the ectoderm, a bilaminar embryonic structure. At 3 weeks the ectodermal cells (programmed to do so) sink into the dorsal surface of the caudal end of the embryo, separating the two layers to become the mesoderm, which coalesces into the notochord—a semirigid, axial rod. The neural plate, forming simultaneously, begins to fold on itself to become the neural tube, forerunner to the spinal cord and brain. While these events occur, the mesoderm condenses into somites, and at 4 weeks the embryo is fully segmented and poised for a basic metamorphosis into a vertebrate fetus. The primitive, undifferentiated mesenchymal cells of the somites (again programmed to do so) transform to three basic cell types with specific, predestined structure and function: the dermatome (skin), the myotome (muscle), and the sclerotome (bone). These cells migrate to develop into skin, muscle, and bone. *A,* Illustration of the early infolding of the neural plate, dorsal to the notocord, which will become the neural tube. Mesoderm has formed but has not yet segmented into somites. *B,* The neural groove has folded in, and the differentiation into dermatome, myotome, and sclerotome cells is occurring at the same time segmentation or somite formation develops. *C,* The neural tube has closed, and segmentation and cell differentiation into somites has taken place. Cells migrating laterally away from the midline become the branchial arches, the pronephros, and the limb buds. *D,* Dermatome, myotome, and sclerotome cells have differentiated histologically and morphologically and have begun to migrate toward their skin, muscle, and bone sites (indicated by the arrows), taking their nerve supply with them. *E,* Sclerotome cells have formed the early vertebrae, and myotome cells have migrated to specific muscle sites, as have the dermatomal cells to their functional sites. The chondrification and ossification stages thus follow in order.

EMBRYOLOGIC DEVELOPMENT OF THE CERVICAL SPINE

A brief review of the embryology of the axial skeleton provides a proper background for later consideration of congenital and developmental anomalies occurring clinically at various periods throughout an individual's life. Development of the axial skeleton occurs in four distinct but overlapping stages: (1) formation of the notochord; (2) mesenchymal stage, the laying down of mesenchymal and cartilaginous precursors; (3) cartilaginous stage or chondrification; and (4) ossification and growth of the vertebrae (Fig. 2–2).

Notochord Formation. On approximately the 15th day after fertilization of the egg, the notochord appears and extends cephalically from the primitive node. The notochord is a flexible, non-segmented rod with a well-defined sheath, extending forward in the midline over the pharynx, and terminating just before the primitive pituitary gland. The notochord constitutes the framework around which the vertebral column, the basiocciput, and basisphenoid are formed. In normal development the notochord is completely surrounded by and absorbed by the developing spinal column, with the remnants of notochord appearing only as the nucleus pulposus of the intervertebral discs and the apical and alar ligaments of the axis.

Mesenchymal Stages. The mesenchymal stages proceed by rapid segmentation of all the mesodermal cells on each side of the notochord, starting in what is to be the occipital region after about 21 days. This proceeds rapidly caudally, and by the 30th day the process is completed when 42 to 44 pairs of undifferentiated, segmented, primitive mesenchyme, the somites are fully formed. Of great clinical relevance is that the segmental and root innervations of the upper limbs, head, and neck are established at this point. Corresponding to each neuromere or spinal cord segment is a territory of skin (dermatome), muscle (myotome), and skeleton (sclerotome). Note that these cells, though not yet migrated, have the coded information to separate into dermatomes, myotomes, and sclerotomes and migrate to become these structures. The somites are separated from each other by intersegmental septa. There are four occipital somites. The first three disappear at about the 20-somite stage, and the fourth ultimately becomes the occipital bone. There are 8 cervical, 12 thoracic, 5 lumbar, 5 sacral, and 8 to 10 coccygeal somites—7 or 8 of the latter begin to regress on approximately the 40th day after fertilization of the egg.

The somite differentiation into dermatome, myotome, and sclerotome begins in the cervical region. The cells destined to be sclerotomes (skeleton) migrate medially to the notochord; first, the perichordal sheath constitutes a complete but transient septum dividing the mesenchymal provertebral bodies into right and left halves, which later fuse.[3]

At this point, each sclerotome differentiates into loosely packed, cranially situated cells and a dense, cellular caudal half. The dark caudal part grows dorsally around the neural tube, and lateral costal processes extend into the intersegmental septa. It is probable that the costal processes, neural arch and its processes, intervertebral discs, and anterior and posterior longitudinal ligaments are all derived from this region. Note that at the time these bony developments are going on, myotome cells are migrating out to become the muscles that develop out of a given somite level, giving a much broader distribution of both motor and sensory structures than is sufficiently realized clinically.

Of great importance clinically is that each sclerotome, dermatome, and myotome cell migration has taken its nerve supply with it. This embryologic fact allows understanding of how a disease at a given level in the cervical spine could have a widespread distribution of symptoms and signs (Fig. 2–3). For example, inflammation with swelling of a C7 zygapophyseal joint or a posterior nerve root compression could be perceived as pain or paresthesia in the anterior and posterior chest, the shoulder, and down the arm. The myotome, sclerotome, and dermatome distribution patterns from C1 through T1 are shown in Tables 2–1, 2–2, and 2–3. The cranial nerve control of voluntary muscles is also shown (Table 2–3, C1, C2, and C3), suggesting that these nerves arose from even more ancient somites with their own sclerotome, dermatome, and myotome distributions.

Chondrification. Chondrification begins on about the 40th to 45th day, when the embryo is 9 to 10 mm in length. The anteroposterior perichordal septum breaks down in the vertebral body, and cartilage cells develop surrounding the notochord. These centers of chondrification appear on both halves of the body and the neural arch. They soon fuse with the arch in the cervical region before fusion occurs in the posterior arch further down in the axial skeleton. The cartilages of the neural arch send out transverse processes but do not fuse in the midline posteriorly until the 4th month. Remember that all muscle groups, the vertebral body, neural arches, ribs, transverse processes, costotransverse bars, and the arterial supplies to the vertebrae are clearly recognizable at this point—a 60- to 65-day human fetus. The neural canal is open posteriorly; ligaments are readily recognizable, and the collagen fibers of the intervertebral disc are concentrically and obliquely arranged. The zygapophyseal joints are also seen. During this phase of cartilage development the notochord is displaced or pushed out of the vertebral body into the intervertebral disc, or it degenerates.

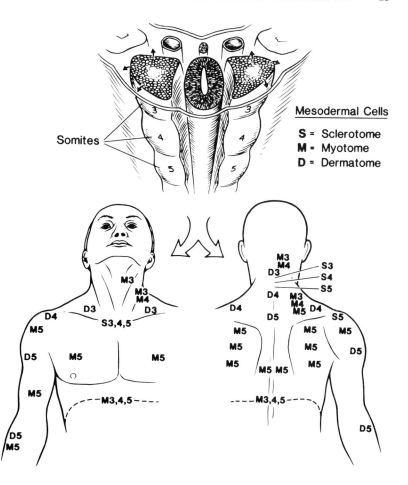

Figure 2–3. *Top,* A cross-section illustrating the notocord, the neural tube, and somites 3, 4, and 5. The small arrows pointing in different directions and away from the paired somites indicate the differentiation and migration of sclerotomal (S), myotomal (M), and dermatomal (D) cells. *Bottom,* The middle arrows depict migration to specific areas on the human figure. On the left (anterior view) M3 and M4 are muscles deriving from myotomes of somites 3 and 4 for the anterior cervical spine. D5 and M5 are the result of dermatome and myotome migration from somite 5. M3, 4, 5 represents the diaphragm muscle, which is derived from myotome cell migration from somites 3, 4, and 5. On the right (posterior view) S3, S4, and S5 represent the migration of sclerotome cells from somites 3, 4, and 5 respectively. M5 represents scapular muscles, and M3 and M4 are suprascapular muscles. D5 is from dermatomal cells that migrated from somite 5.

Ossification. Prior to real bone formation of the vertebral body, streams of vessels enter the cartilage from blood lakes, and calcification begins. The sites of ossification centers appear, usually two on either side of a sagittal plane and two anteriorly and posteriorly in the midline. Ossification centers are present in all the cervical bodies by the 4th month, and ossification of neural arches begins in the upper cervical region in the 2nd month and extends caudally until the 4th month.

At the time of puberty, the upper and lower surfaces of the bodies of the vertebrae and the tips of spinal and transverse processes are still cartilage.

At each point of transition during these four stages in the formation of the axial skeleton (in this context the cervical spine), abnormalities or defects in development may result in skeletal anomalies—some without any symptoms and of no clinical consequence, others predisposing one to mechanical or neurologic disorders later.

The occipital bone (phylogenetically) in mammals is the homologue of cervical vertebrae in reptiles that have no extremities and have ribs at the base of the skull. Though there are four occipital somites in the human embryo, the first three disappear and the fourth persists, developing into the occipital bone. The squamous portion above the superior nuchal line is in membrane and ossifies from two centers, appearing on either side of the midline at the 50th to 60th day. Normally this unites with the remainder of the bone preformed in cartilage. It may remain permanently separated, and in that case it is known as an interparietal bone. The basilar plate is the old body of the vertebra and the hypochordal bow of an upper cervical vertebra. The lateral or condylar part represents the neural arches of the "old" vertebrae. The hypoglossal foramen may be subdivided and is in series with the intervertebral foramina of the cervical vertebrae. The posterior margin of the foramen magnum is formed by an element called the tectal plate, derived from two rapidly diffusing centers of chondrification. Small wormian bones may appear in the posterior margin of the foramen magnum in the 4th month, fusing with the rest of the tectal plate before birth, and are called the "bones of Keckering."

Text continued on page 36

Table 2–1. MYOTOME DISTRIBUTION PATTERNS

Muscle	C1	C2	C3	C4	C5	C6	C7	C8	T1
Sternocleidomastoid-Trapezius		■	■	■					
Rectus capitis posterior major	■								
Rectus capitis posterior minor	■								
Obliquus capitis superior	■								
Obliquus capitis inferior	■								
Geniohyoid	■								
Thyrohyoid	■								
Rectus capitis lateralis	■	■							
Rectus capitis anterior	■	■							
Sternohyoid	■	■	■						
Sternothyroid	■	■	■						
Omohyoid	■	■	■						
Longus capitis	■	■	■	■					
Semispinalis capitis	■	■	■	■	■				
Levator scapulae			■	■	■				
Longus colli		■	■	■	■	■	■		
Anterior intertransversarii		■	■	■					
Posterior intertransversarii		■	■	■					
Diaphragm			■	■	■	■			
Splenius capitis			■	■	■	■	■		
Scalenus medius			■	■	■	■	■	■	
Interspinales			■	■	■	■	■	■	■
Multifidus			■	■	■	■	■	■	■
Scalenus anterior					■	■	■	■	
Semispinalis cervicis					■	■	■	■	■
Rhomboids-Major & Minor					■				
Supraspinatus					■	■			
Infraspinatus					■	■			

Teres major
Deltoid
Teres minor
Subscapularis
Brachioradialis
Biceps brachii
Coracobrachialis
Supinator
Pectoralis major (clavicular portion)
Scalenus posterior
Serratus anterior

Extensor carpi radialis longus
Flexor carpi radialis
Pronator teres
Pectoralis minor
Latissimus dorsi
Triceps brachii
Longissimus capitis-cervicis

Anconeus
Abductor pollicis longus
Extensor pollicis brevis
Extensor carpi radialis brevis
Extensor indicis proprius
Extensor carpi ulnaris
Extensor digitorum
Palmaris longus
Flexor carpi ulnaris
Extensor pollicis longus
Extensor digiti minimi
Pectoralis major (sternal portion)
Flexor digitorum superficialis
Iliocostalis cervicis

Flexor pollicis longus
Flexor pollicis brevis
Flexor digitorum profundus
Adductor pollicis
Flexor digiti minimi
Opponens pollicis
Pronator quadratus
Palmaris brevis
Abductor digiti minimi
Palmar and dorsal interossei
Lumbricals
Abductor pollicis brevis
Opponens digiti minimi

Table 2-2. SCLEROTOME DISTRIBUTION PATTERNS

	C1	C2	C3	C4	C5	C6
SCLEROTOME	Area vertebrae and periosteum	Area vertebrae and periosteum	Area vertebrae and periosteum	Area vertebrae and periosteum	Area vertebrae and periosteum	Area vertebrae and periosteum
JOINTS	Atlanto-occipital, Median atlantoaxial, Lateral atlantoaxial	Median atlantoaxial, Lateral atlantoaxial, Intervertebral	Intervertebral, Luschka, Sternoclavicular, Zygapophyseal	Intervertebral, Luschka, Sternoclavicular, Zygapophyseal	Acromioclavicular, Glenohumeral Luschka, Intervertebral, Elbow, Zygapophyseal, Sternoclavicular	Glenohumeral, Intervertebral, Luschka, Elbow, Zygapophyseal
LIGAMENTS	Alar, Apical dental ligament, Cruciform, Accessory atlantoaxial, Articular capsules, Nuchal ligament, Ant. atlanto-occipital memb., Post. atlanto-occipital memb.	Anterior longitudinal, Atlantoaxial memb., Atlantoaxial, Capsular, Cruciform, Nuchal	Anterior longitudinal, Posterior longitudinal, Capsular, Nuchal	Anterior longitudinal, Posterior longitudinal, Capsular, Ligamentum flavum, Nuchal	Anterior longitudinal, Posterior longitudinal, Capsular, Nuchal, Ligamentum flavum	Anterior longitudinal, Posterior longitudinal, Capsular, Nuchal, Ligamentum flavum
DERMATOME	Posterior scalp	Posterior scalp, Anterolateral neck, Posterior to external ear, Anterior to external ear, Inferior to external ear	Back of neck, Anterolateral neck, Posterior scalp, Region of clavicle	Summit of shoulder, Region of clavicle, Anterolateral neck	Anterior aspect of shoulder, arm and forearm to wrist, lateral to ventral axial line, Small area back of neck	Anterior and posterior areas of upper arm, forearm lateral to ventral axial line. Anterior and posterior areas of thumb. Small area back of neck and shoulder at this level.

16

	C7	C8	T1
SCLEROTOME (JOINTS)	**SCLEROTOME** Area vertebrae and periosteum Elbow Luschka Intervertebral Zygapophyseal	**SCLEROTOME** Area vertebrae and periosteum Intervertebral Luschka Zygapophyseal Elbow Wrist Hand	**SCLEROTOME** Area vertebrae and periosteum Intervertebral Zygapophyseal Costovertebral Elbows Wrist Hand
LIGAMENTS	Anterior longitudinal Posterior longitudinal Nuchal Ligamentum flavum	Supraspinous Interspinous Anterior Longitudinal Posterior Longitudinal	Anterior longitudinal Posterior longitudinal Supraspinous Interspinous Ligamentum flavum
DERMATOME	**DERMATOME** Dorsum of arm and forearm Dorsal and palmar aspects of 2nd and 3rd digits Small area back of neck and shoulder at this level	**DERMATOME** Ulnar aspect of arm, forearm and palmar and dorsal aspect of 4th and 5th digits. Small area back of neck and shoulder at this level	**DERMATOME** Anterior aspect of thorax below clavicle. Antero-medial aspects of arm and forearm to wrist. Small area of back at this level

Table 2–3. DERMATOME, MYOTOME, SCLEROTOME DISTRIBUTION FOR C_1

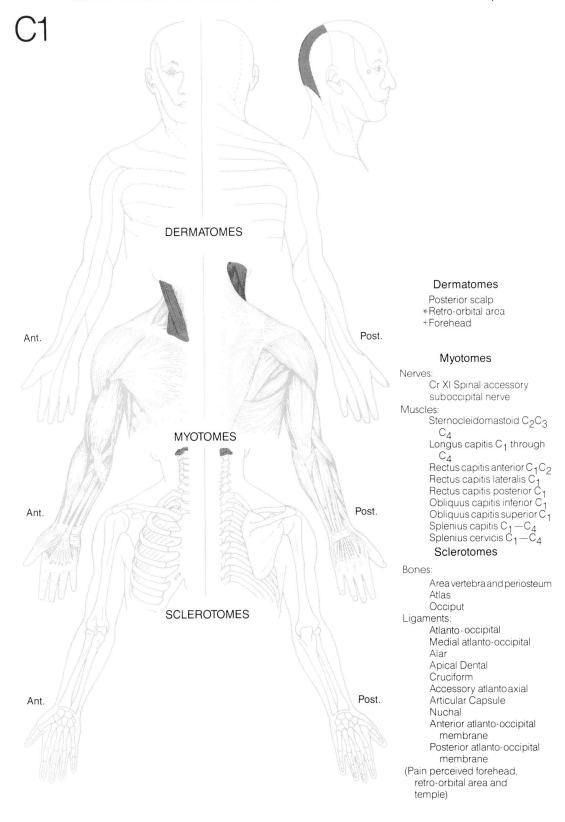

C1

DERMATOMES

Ant.   Post.

MYOTOMES

Ant.   Post.

SCLEROTOMES

Ant.   Post.

Dermatomes

Posterior scalp
＊Retro-orbital area
＋Forehead

Myotomes

Nerves:
　　Cr XI Spinal accessory
　　suboccipital nerve
Muscles:
　　Sternocleidomastoid C_2C_3
　　　C_4
　　Longus capitis C_1 through
　　　C_4
　　Rectus capitis anterior C_1C_2
　　Rectus capitis lateralis C_1
　　Rectus capitis posterior C_1
　　Obliquus capitis inferior C_1
　　Obliquus capitis superior C_1
　　Splenius capitis C_1-C_4
　　Splenius cervicis C_1-C_4

Sclerotomes

Bones:
　　Area vertebra and periosteum
　　Atlas
　　Occiput
Ligaments:
　　Atlanto-occipital
　　Medial atlanto-occipital
　　Alar
　　Apical Dental
　　Cruciform
　　Accessory atlantoaxial
　　Articular Capsule
　　Nuchal
　　Anterior atlanto-occipital
　　　membrane
　　Posterior atlanto-occipital
　　　membrane
(Pain perceived forehead,
　retro-orbital area and
　temple)

Table 2–3. NEUROLOGIC ASSESSMENT: MOTOR FUNCTION, REFLEX, AND OTHER CLINICAL EXAMINATIONS FOR C_1

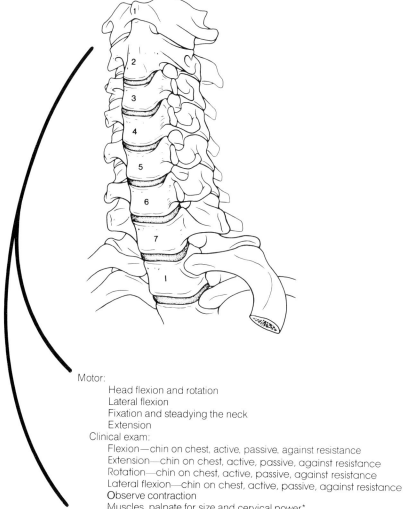

Motor:
      Head flexion and rotation
      Lateral flexion
      Fixation and steadying the neck
      Extension
Clinical exam:
      Flexion—chin on chest, active, passive, against resistance
      Extension—chin on chest, active, passive, against resistance
      Rotation—chin on chest, active, passive, against resistance
      Lateral flexion—chin on chest, active, passive, against resistance
      Observe contraction
      Muscles, palpate for size and cervical power*
Reflexes:
      Jaw jerk—5th cranial nerve (separate lesion above and below foramen magnum)
      Head retraction reflex—5th cranial nerve
      Sensory
      Posterior scalp
      Forehead
      8 cervical nerves; one appraises only weakness of movements, not individual muscles
      *Note: all cervical muscles supplied by branches of all 8 cervical nerves

Table continued on following page

Table 2—3. DERMATOME, MYOTOME, SCLEROTOME DISTRIBUTION FOR C_2

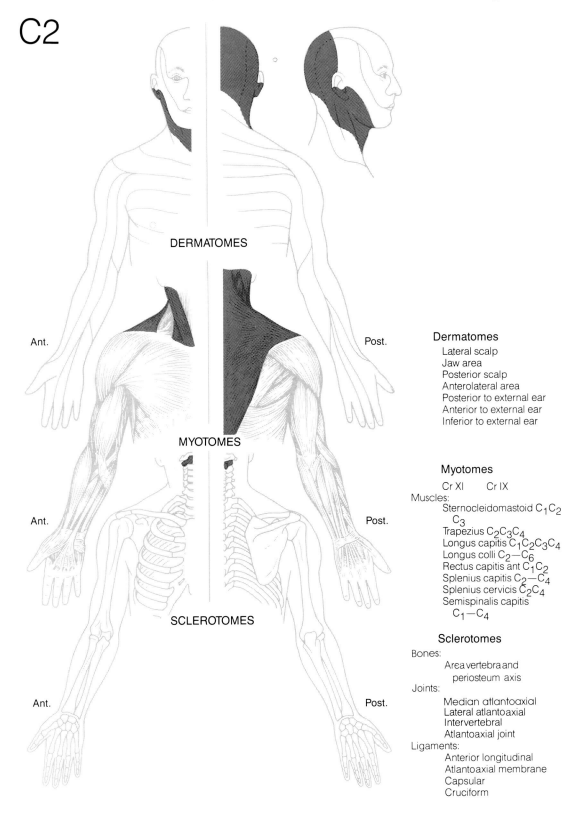

C2

DERMATOMES

Ant.   Post.

MYOTOMES

Ant.   Post.

SCLEROTOMES

Ant.   Post.

Dermatomes
Lateral scalp
Jaw area
Posterior scalp
Anterolateral area
Posterior to external ear
Anterior to external ear
Inferior to external ear

Myotomes
Cr XI   Cr IX
Muscles:
Sternocleidomastoid C_1C_2
C_3
Trapezius $C_2C_3C_4$
Longus capitis $C_1C_2C_3C_4$
Longus colli C_2-C_6
Rectus capitis ant C_1C_2
Splenius capitis C_2-C_4
Splenius cervicis C_2C_4
Semispinalis capitis
C_1-C_4

Sclerotomes
Bones:
Area vertebra and
periosteum axis
Joints:
Median atlantoaxial
Lateral atlantoaxial
Intervertebral
Atlantoaxial joint
Ligaments:
Anterior longitudinal
Atlantoaxial membrane
Capsular
Cruciform

Table 2–3. NEUROLOGIC ASSESSMENT: MOTOR FUNCTION, REFLEX, AND OTHER CLINICAL EXAMINATIONS FOR C_2

C2

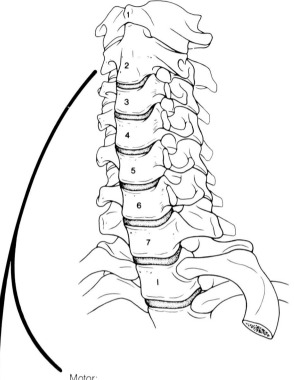

Motor:
　　Trapezius: extension & pull to one side (Cr XI)
　　Sternocleidomastoid-Flex and rotate (Cr XI)
　　Head flexion and rotation
　　Lateral flexion
　　Fixation and steadying neck
　　Extension
Clinical exam*:
　　Extend neck
　　Draw to one side
　　Flexion
　　Extension
　　Lateral flexion
　　Rotation
　　Shrug
　　　Active
　　　Passive
　　　Against resistance
　　Observe muscle contraction
　　Palpate for size and power, tone, volume, contour, compare with opposite side may be slight scapular droop and winging
　　Trapezius function
　　Torticollis present
Reflexes:
　　Sternocleidomastoid reflex—tap muscle at its clavicular end, muscle contracts. (Innervated Cr XI and C_1, C_2C_3)
Sensory:
　　Posterior scalp
　　Anterolateral neck
　　Posterior anterior & inferior external ear
*Note: All cervical muscles supplied by branches of all 8 cervical nerves

Table continued on following page

Table 2–3. DERMATOME, MYOTOME, SCLEROTOME DISTRIBUTION FOR C_3

C3

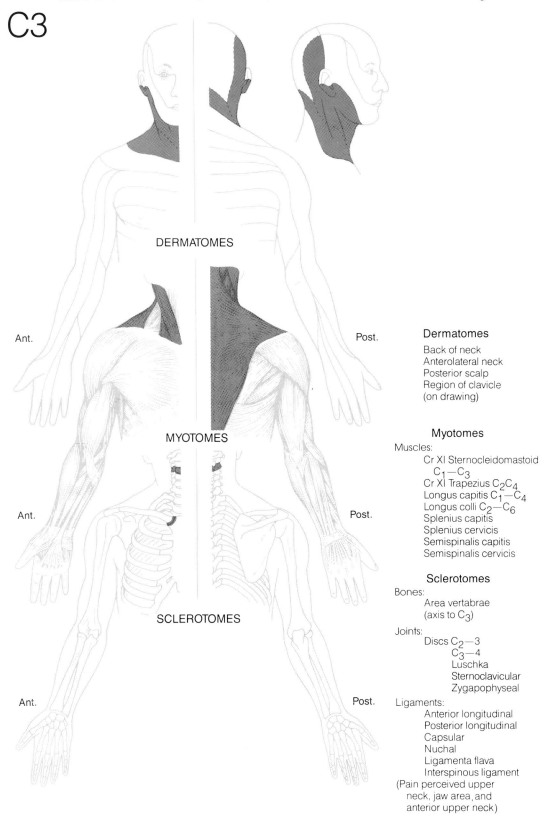

DERMATOMES

Ant.   Post.

MYOTOMES

Ant.   Post.

SCLEROTOMES

Ant.   Post.

Dermatomes
Back of neck
Anterolateral neck
Posterior scalp
Region of clavicle
(on drawing)

Myotomes
Muscles:
    Cr XI Sternocleidomastoid
        C_1—C_3
    Cr XI Trapezius C_2C_4
    Longus capitis C_1—C_4
    Longus colli C_2—C_6
    Splenius capitis
    Splenius cervicis
    Semispinalis capitis
    Semispinalis cervicis

Sclerotomes
Bones:
    Area vertabrae
    (axis to C_3)

Joints:
    Discs C_2—3
        C_3—4
    Luschka
    Sternoclavicular
    Zygapophyseal

Ligaments:
    Anterior longitudinal
    Posterior longitudinal
    Capsular
    Nuchal
    Ligamenta flava
    Interspinous ligament
(Pain perceived upper
    neck, jaw area, and
    anterior upper neck)

Table 2–3. NEUROLOGIC ASSESSMENT: MOTOR FUNCTION, REFLEX, AND OTHER CLINICAL EXAMINATIONS FOR C_3

C3

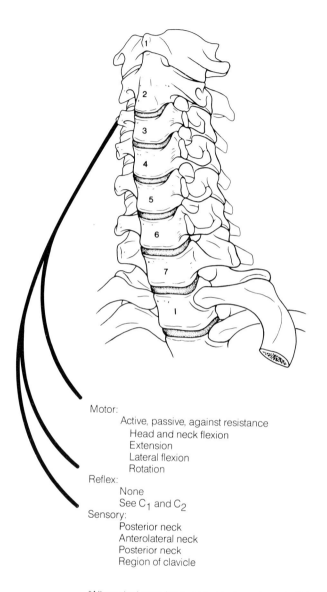

Motor:
  Active, passive, against resistance
    Head and neck flexion
    Extension
    Lateral flexion
    Rotation
Reflex:
  None
  See C_1 and C_2
Sensory:
  Posterior neck
  Anterolateral neck
  Posterior neck
  Region of clavicle

*All cervical muscles supplied by branches of all 8 cervical nerves; one appraises only weakness of movements, not individual muscles.

Table continued on following page

Table 2–3. DERMATOME, MYOTOME, SCLEROTOME DISTRIBUTION FOR C_4

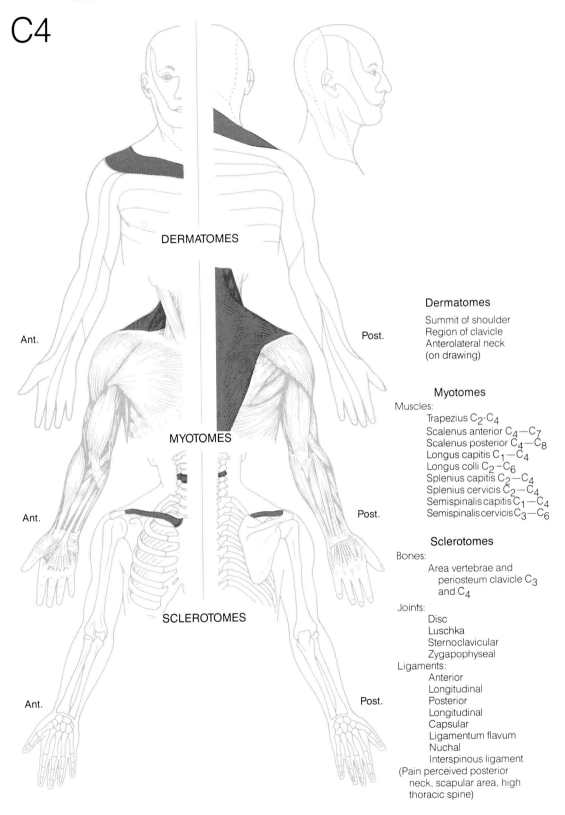

C4

DERMATOMES

Ant.   Post.

MYOTOMES

Ant.   Post.

SCLEROTOMES

Ant.   Post.

Dermatomes

Summit of shoulder
Region of clavicle
Anterolateral neck
(on drawing)

Myotomes

Muscles:
Trapezius C_2-C_4
Scalenus anterior C_4—C_7
Scalenus posterior C_4—C_8
Longus capitis C_1—C_4
Longus colli C_2—C_6
Splenius capitis C_2—C_4
Splenius cervicis C_2—C_4
Semispinalis capitis C_1—C_4
Semispinalis cervicis C_3—C_6

Sclerotomes

Bones:
Area vertebrae and
periosteum clavicle C_3
and C_4

Joints:
Disc
Luschka
Sternoclavicular
Zygapophyseal
Ligaments:
Anterior
Longitudinal
Posterior
Longitudinal
Capsular
Ligamentum flavum
Nuchal
Interspinous ligament
(Pain perceived posterior
neck, scapular area, high
thoracic spine)

Table 2–3.   NEUROLOGIC ASSESSMENT: MOTOR FUNCTION, REFLEX, AND OTHER CLINICAL EXAMINATIONS FOR C_4

C4

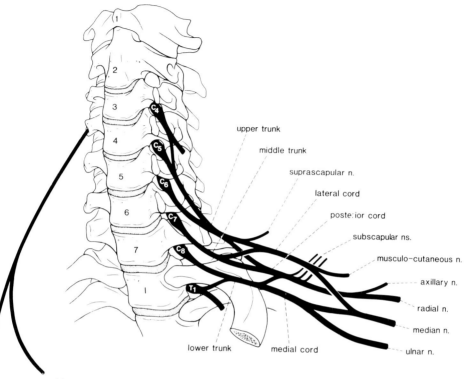

upper trunk

middle trunk

suprascapular n.

lateral cord

poste:ior cord

subscapular ns.

musculo–cutaneous n.

axillary n.

radial n.

median n.

ulnar n.

lower trunk   medial cord

Motor:
Active, passive, against resistance
Head and neck flexion
Extension
Lateral flexion
Rotation
Clinical examination:
Test fixation head and neck (scalenes)
Flexion, tilt and rotation, elevation of
upper thorax
Inspiration (elevation of abdomen-diaphragm
C_3, $C_4 C_5$ phrenic nerve)
Active, passive, against resistance
Flexion
Extension
Lateral flexion
Rotation
Reflex:
Scapulohumeral reflex - tap vertebral border scapula at tip of spine or at its base near inferior angle: response is retraction of clavicle. Rhomboid muscles, dorsal scapular nerve C_4, C_5. May also see elevation scapula and external rotation of humerus
Sensory:
Summit of shoulder
Clavicular region
Anterolateral nerve
Note: All cervical muscles supplied by branches of all 8 cervical nerves; one appraises only weakness of movement, not individual muscles.

Table continued on following page

Table 2–3. DERMATOME, MYOTOME, SCLEROTOME DISTRIBUTION FOR C_5

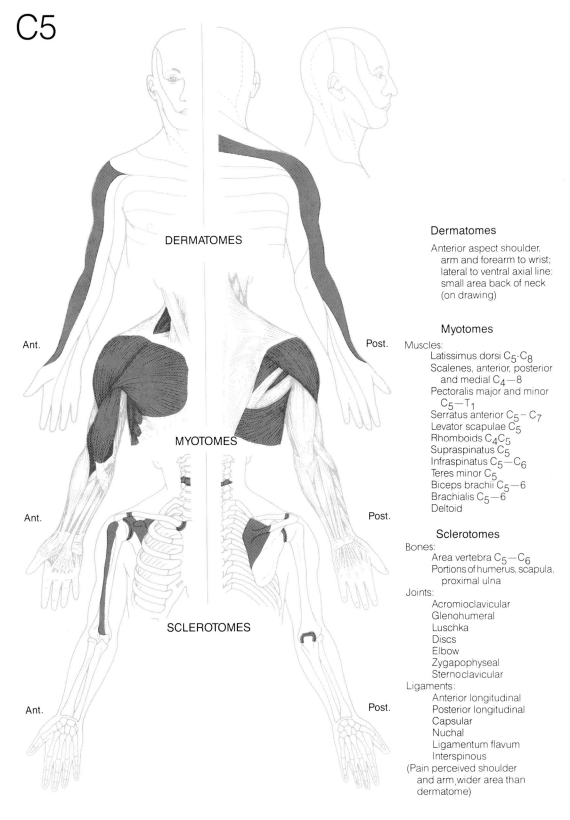

C5

DERMATOMES

Ant.   Post.

MYOTOMES

Ant.   Post.

SCLEROTOMES

Ant.   Post.

Dermatomes

Anterior aspect shoulder,
  arm and forearm to wrist;
  lateral to ventral axial line:
  small area back of neck
  (on drawing)

Myotomes

Muscles:
  Latissimus dorsi C_5-C_8
  Scalenes, anterior, posterior
    and medial C_4—8
  Pectoralis major and minor
    C_5—T_1
  Serratus anterior C_5 – C_7
  Levator scapulae C_5
  Rhomboids $C_4 C_5$
  Supraspinatus C_5
  Infraspinatus C_5—C_6
  Teres minor C_5
  Biceps brachii C_5—6
  Brachialis C_5—6
  Deltoid

Sclerotomes

Bones:
  Area vertebra C_5—C_6
  Portions of humerus, scapula,
    proximal ulna
Joints:
  Acromioclavicular
  Glenohumeral
  Luschka
  Discs
  Elbow
  Zygapophyseal
  Sternoclavicular
Ligaments:
  Anterior longitudinal
  Posterior longitudinal
  Capsular
  Nuchal
  Ligamentum flavum
  Interspinous
(Pain perceived shoulder
  and arm, wider area than
  dermatome)

Table 2–3.   NEUROLOGIC ASSESSMENT: MOTOR FUNCTION, REFLEX, AND OTHER CLINICAL EXAMINATIONS FOR C_5

C5

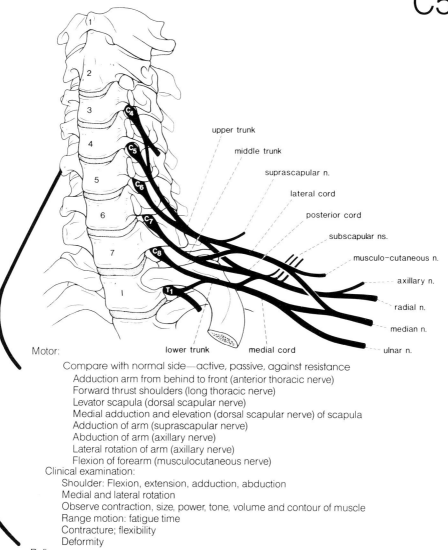

upper trunk
middle trunk
suprascapular n.
lateral cord
posterior cord
subscapular ns.
musculo-cutaneous n.
axillary n.
radial n.
median n.
ulnar n.
lower trunk   medial cord

Motor:
  Compare with normal side—active, passive, against resistance
    Adduction arm from behind to front (anterior thoracic nerve)
    Forward thrust shoulders (long thoracic nerve)
    Levator scapula (dorsal scapular nerve)
    Medial adduction and elevation (dorsal scapular nerve) of scapula
    Adduction of arm (suprascapular nerve)
    Abduction of arm (axillary nerve)
    Lateral rotation of arm (axillary nerve)
    Flexion of forearm (musculocutaneous nerve)
Clinical examination:
    Shoulder: Flexion, extension, adduction, abduction
    Medial and lateral rotation
    Observe contraction, size, power, tone, volume and contour of muscle
    Range motion: fatigue time
    Contracture; flexibility
    Deformity
Reflexes:
    Deltoid reflex: tap junction of upper and middle third lateral aspect humerus: contraction
      and abduction upper arm; C_5C_6 axillary nerve.
    Pectoralis reflex: arms midposition abduction and adduction; place index finger under
      pectoralis major tendon near crest greater tubercle humerus; tap finger: adductor and
      medial rotation arm of shoulder; C_5T_1 lateral and medial anterior thoracic nerve.
    Clavicle reflex: In hyper-reflexic state, tap lateral aspect clavicle causes extensive contrac-
      tion various muscle groups upper extremity; C_5T_1. Nonspecific: useful compare the two
      sides; indicates gross spread of reflex response.
    Biceps reflex: arm relaxed midposition; tap bicep tendon through examiner's thumb:
      biceps contraction and supination. C_5C_6 musculocutaneous nerve.
    Brachioradialis reflex(radial periosteal or supination reflex): tap styloid process radius
      with arm in semiflexion and semipronation: flexion of forearm and supination; sometimes
      flexion fingers associated, C_5C_6. Radial nerve: In pyramidal tract in midcervical cord
      lesion may see contraction of flexors of finger and hands without flexion and supination of
      the forearm(inversion radial reflex).
Sensory:
    Anterior aspect shoulder, arm, and forearm to wrist; lateral to ventral axial line; small area
      low posterior neck.

Table continued on following page

Table 2–3. DERMATOME, MYOTOME, SCLEROTOME DISTRIBUTION FOR C_6

C6

DERMATOMES

Ant.

Post.

MYOTOMES

Ant.

Post.

SCLEROTOMES

Ant.

Post.

Dermatomes

Anterior and posterior areas
of upper arm, forearm,
lateral to ventral axial line.
Anterior and posterior
areas of thumb.
Small area low posterior
neck and shoulder at this
level

Myotomes

Muscles:

Latissimus dorsi C_5—C_8
Coracobrachialis C_6—C_7
Pronator teres C_6—C_7
Flexor carpi radialis C_6—C_7
Flexor pollicis longus C_6—C_7
Abductor pollicis brevis
C_6—C_7
Flexor pollicis brevis
C_6—C_7
Opponens pollicis C_6—C_7
Extensor digitorum
communis

Sclerotomes

Bones:

C_6—C_7
Portions of radius, humerus,
first metacarpal bone, and
scapula
Area vertebrae and
periosteum

Joints:

Glenohumeral
Discs
Luschka
Elbow
Zygapophyseal

Ligaments:

Anterior longitudinal
Posterior longitudinal
Capsular
Nuchal
Ligamenta flava
Interspinous

Table 2–3. NEUROLOGIC ASSESSMENT: MOTOR FUNCTION, REFLEX, AND OTHER CLINICAL EXAMINATIONS FOR C_6

C6

Motor:

Wrist extension, C_{5-6} radial nerve
Medial rotation arm, C_{5-8} subscapular nerve
Adduction of arm front to back, C_{5-8} subscapular nerve
Adduction arm
Flexion forearm
C_6-C_7 musculocutaneus nerve
Pronation of forearm, C_{6-7} median nerve
Radial flexion hand, C_{6-7}
Flexion terminal phalanx thumb, C_6-C_7 median nerve
Abduction metacarpal thumb, C_{6-7} median nerve
Flexion proximal phalanx thumb, C_{6-7} median nerve

Clinical exam:

Carry out above anatomic movement, active passive, and against resistance
Observe for contour, weakness, range of motion, contraction, size, tone, volume of muscle

Reflexes:

Pronator reflex: tap styloid process, ulna, or postero-inferior surface of ulna with forearm semiflexed and wrist semipronated: forearm pronates and wrist adducts. Pronator teres and quadratus muscle C_6-T_1 reflex exaggerated in pyramidal tract lesion
Brachioradialis (radial periosteal or supinator reflex): tap styloid process radius: forearm flexion and supination, C_{5-6} radial nerve
Wrist extension reflex: Tap extensor tendon of the wrist with forearm pronated and wrist hanging down: contraction of extensor muscles and extension of the wrist, C_6-C_8 radial nerve.
Wrist flexion reflex: Tap flexor tendons of wrist on volar surface of forearm at or above transverse carpal ligament, hand supinated, fingers flexed: flexor muscles contract hand and finger; C_6-C_8 median, ulnar nerves.

Sensory:

Anterior and posterior areas of upper arm, forearm, lateral to ventral axial line. Anterior and posterior area of thumb. Small area posterior neck and shoulder at C_6 level

Table continued on following page

Table 2–3. DERMATOME, MYOTOME, SCLEROTOME DISTRIBUTION FOR C_7

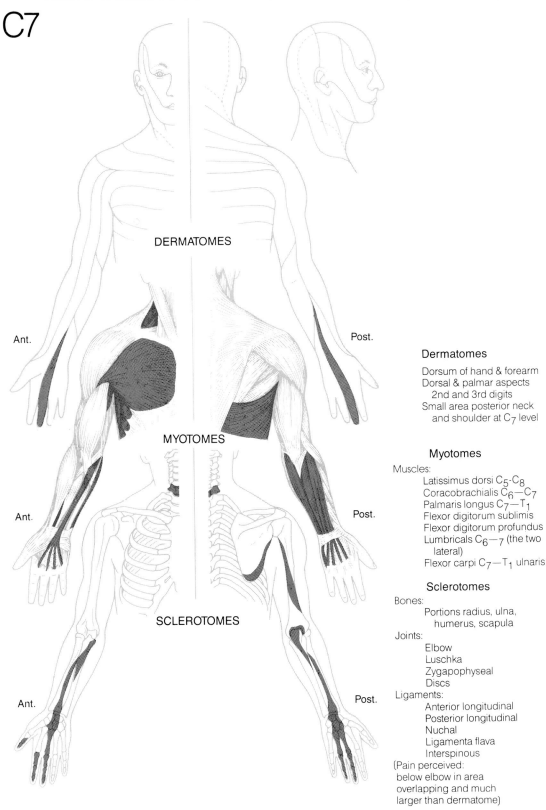

C7

DERMATOMES

Ant.   Post.

MYOTOMES

Ant.   Post.

SCLEROTOMES

Ant.   Post.

Dermatomes

Dorsum of hand & forearm
Dorsal & palmar aspects
  2nd and 3rd digits
Small area posterior neck
  and shoulder at C_7 level

Myotomes

Muscles:
  Latissimus dorsi C_5-C_8
  Coracobrachialis C_6—C_7
  Palmaris longus C_7—T_1
  Flexor digitorum sublimis
  Flexor digitorum profundus
  Lumbricals C_6—$_7$ (the two
    lateral)
  Flexor carpi C_7—T_1 ulnaris

Sclerotomes

Bones:
  Portions radius, ulna,
    humerus, scapula
Joints:
  Elbow
  Luschka
  Zygapophyseal
  Discs
Ligaments:
  Anterior longitudinal
  Posterior longitudinal
  Nuchal
  Ligamenta flava
  Interspinous
(Pain perceived:
 below elbow in area
 overlapping and much
 larger than dermatome)

Table 2–3. NEUROLOGIC ASSESSMENT: MOTOR FUNCTION, REFLEX, AND OTHER CLINICAL EXAMINATIONS FOR C_7

C7

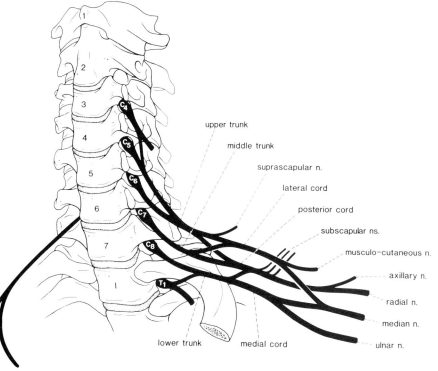

Motor:

Adduction arm, C_6-7 musculocutaneus nerve

Flexion forearm, C_6-7 musculocutaneus nerve

Flexion hand, C_7-T_1 median nerve

Flexion middle phalanx, index and middle fingers, C_7-T_1 median nerve

Flexion terminal phalanx index and middle fingers, C_7-T_1 median nerve

Flexion proximal phalanx and extension of 2 distal phalanges, index, middle, ring & little, C_6-C_7 median nerve

Ulnar flexion of hand, C_7-T_1 ulnar nerve

Clinical Examination

Carry out above anatomic movements, active, passive, and against resistance. Observe for size, power, volume, range of motion, contracture time, and volume of muscles.

Reflexes:

Triceps reflex: Tap triceps tendon just above insertion in olecranon process ulna, arm midway between flexion and extension: contraction triceps muscle, extension of forearm on the arm; C_6-8 radial nerve, center flexion of forearm indicates damage to area of triceps reflex, eg lesion C_7 C_8 cervical segment, flexion unopposed by biceps.

Thumb reflex: Tap tendons flexor pollicis longus: flexion distal phalanx thumb, C_6-T_1 median nerve.

Finger flexion reflex: Hand in partial supination, resting on table, fingers flexed; examiner places his middle and index fingers on volar surface phalanges patient's four fingers; taps his fingers lightly; response is flexion of patient's four fingers and distal phalanx, thumb—C_6-T_1 median and ulnar nerves.

Sensory:

Dorsum arm and forearm; dorsal and palmar aspects 2nd and 3rd digits; small area posterior neck and shoulder at this level.

Table continued on following page

Table 2–3. DERMATOME, MYOTOME, SCLEROTOME DISTRIBUTION FOR C_8

C8

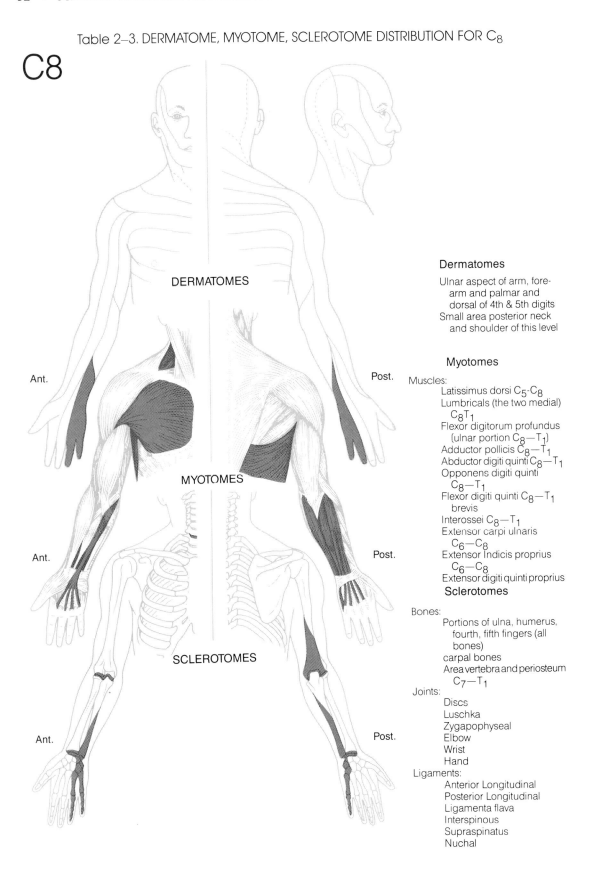

DERMATOMES

Ant.   Post.

MYOTOMES

Ant.   Post.

SCLEROTOMES

Ant.   Post.

Dermatomes

Ulnar aspect of arm, forearm and palmar and
  dorsal of 4th & 5th digits
Small area posterior neck
  and shoulder of this level

Myotomes

Muscles:
  Latissimus dorsi C_5-C_8
  Lumbricals (the two medial)
    C_8T_1
  Flexor digitorum profundus
    (ulnar portion C_8—T_1)
  Adductor pollicis C_8—T_1
  Abductor digiti quinti C_8—T_1
  Opponens digiti quinti
    C_8—T_1
  Flexor digiti quinti C_8—T_1
    brevis
  Interossei C_8—T_1
  Extensor carpi ulnaris
    C_6—C_8
  Extensor Indicis proprius
    C_6—C_8
  Extensor digiti quinti proprius

Sclerotomes

Bones:
  Portions of ulna, humerus,
    fourth, fifth fingers (all
    bones)
  carpal bones
  Area vertebra and periosteum
    C_7—T_1
Joints:
  Discs
  Luschka
  Zygapophyseal
  Elbow
  Wrist
  Hand
Ligaments:
  Anterior Longitudinal
  Posterior Longitudinal
  Ligamenta flava
  Interspinous
  Supraspinatus
  Nuchal

Table 2–3. NEUROLOGIC ASSESSMENT: MOTOR FUNCTION, REFLEX, AND OTHER CLINICAL EXAMINATIONS FOR C_8

C8

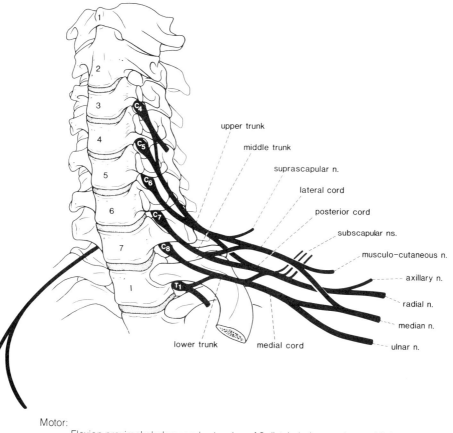

Motor:

Flexion proximal phalanx and extension of 2 distal phalanges ring and little fingers, C_8-T_1 ulnar nerve

Flexion terminal phalanx, ring and little fingers, C_8-T_1 ulnar nerve

Adduction metacarpal thumb, C_8-T_1 ulnar nerve

Abduction little finger

Opposition of little finger, C_8-T_1 ulnar nerve

Flexion of little finger, C_8-T_1 ulnar nerve

Flexion proximal phalanx, C_8-T_1 ulnar nerve, extension of two distal phalanges adduct and abduct fingers

Ulnar extension of hand, C_6-C_8 radial nerve

Extension index finger and hand

Extension phalanges little finger

Extension of hand, C_6-C_8 radial nerve

Clinical Examination:

Carry out above anatomic movements, active, passive, and against resistance; assess power, range of motion, size, volume, contactures, and tone.

Reflexes:

Pronation reflex-see above

Wrist extension reflex-see above

Wrist flexion reflex-see above

Finger flexion reflex-see above

Sensory:

Ulnar aspect arm, forearm, and palmar and dorsal aspect of 4th, 5th digits; small area posterior neck and shoulder at this level.

Table continued on following page

Table 2–3. DERMATOME, MYOTOME, SCLEROTOME DISTRIBUTION FOR T_1

T1

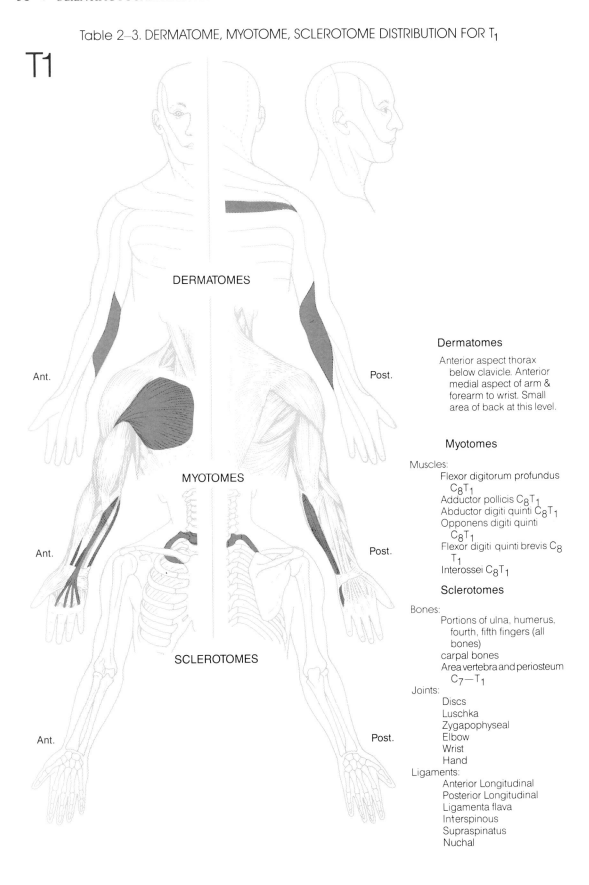

DERMATOMES

Ant.   Post.

MYOTOMES

Ant.   Post.

SCLEROTOMES

Ant.   Post.

Dermatomes

Anterior aspect thorax below clavicle. Anterior medial aspect of arm & forearm to wrist. Small area of back at this level.

Myotomes

Muscles:
Flexor digitorum profundus C_8T_1
Adductor pollicis C_8T_1
Abductor digiti quinti C_8T_1
Opponens digiti quinti C_8T_1
Flexor digiti quinti brevis $C_8 T_1$
Interossei C_8T_1

Sclerotomes

Bones:
Portions of ulna, humerus, fourth, fifth fingers (all bones)
carpal bones
Area vertebra and periosteum C_7-T_1
Joints:
Discs
Luschka
Zygapophyseal
Elbow
Wrist
Hand
Ligaments:
Anterior Longitudinal
Posterior Longitudinal
Ligamenta flava
Interspinous
Supraspinatus
Nuchal

Table 2–3. NEUROLOGIC ASSESSMENT: MOTOR FUNCTION, REFLEX, AND OTHER CLINICAL EXAMINATIONS FOR T_1

T1

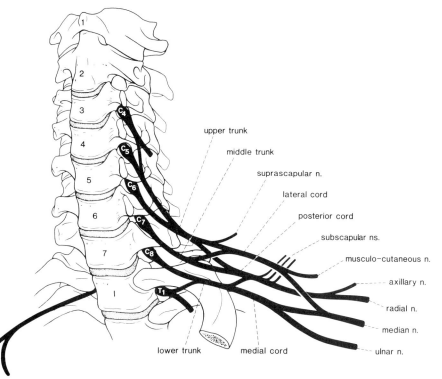

Motor:
   Flexion terminal phalanges ring and little fingers, C_8T_1 ulnar nerve
   Adduction metacarpal of thumb, C_8T_1 ulnar nerve
   Abduction little finger, C_8T_1 ulnar nerve
   Opposition little finger, C_8T_1 ulnar nerve
   Flexion of little finger, C_8T_1 ulnar nerve
   Flexion proximal phalanx
   Extension of two distal phalanges, adduction & abduction of finger, C_8T_1 ulnar nerve
Clinical Examination:
   Carry out the anatomic movements noted above; assess for power, range of motion, size, volume, contracture, and tone.
Reflexes:
   Wrist extension reflex. See above—C_6-C_8 radial nerve
   Wrist flexion reflex. See above—C_6-T_1 median & ulnar nerves
   Finger flexion reflex. See above—C_6-T_1 median & ulnar nerves
Sensory:
   Medial aspect arm slightly above and ⅔ below (above wrist) posterior elbow region and posterolateral area proximal and distal to the elbow.

In the 2nd year of life the condylar and squamous parts fuse, and by the 6th year the bone is in one piece, separated from the basisphenoid by a synchondrosis, which becomes ossified between the 18th and 25th years.

Before cartilage formation, the atlas is derived only from the bow of tissue seen in the upper cervical provertebrae. The perichordal portion contributing to the greater part of the body of a typical vertebra is fused to the body of the axis, thus forming the odontoid process.[4] The centers of ossification of the atlas differ widely; there are three centers: two (one for each of the two lateral masses) that appear about the 7th week of fetal life, and one (located in the anterior arch) that appears at the end of the 1st year of life. The one that appears later extends to and fuses with the anterior end of each articular facet during the 6th to the 8th year of life. The posterior arch is cartilaginous, ossifying from the lateral masses by two extensions that meet about the 4th year of life either directly or through an additional midline center of ossificiation.

The axis has five primary and two secondary centers of ossification. The true body (not the odontoid process) and each half of a neural arch ossify like the typical cervical vertebrae, each of which has one center. The centers for the arch appear about the 7th or 8th week of fetal life, and the body ossification center appears during the 4th or 5th month. The odontoid process (dens) or peg represents the caudally displaced ''old'' body of the atlas. The tip of the dens is formed by a bridge of cartilage. The true body of the axis and the caudal part of the odontoid process are joined together by circumferential bone but are separated centrally by cartilage until advanced age. Remnants of notochord are also found here, with occasional small fragments of bone reflecting ring epiphyses of the bodies of the atlas and the axis. Sometimes this secondary center of ossification appears on the tip of the odontoid process in the 2nd year of life.

The intervertebral discs are formed from the dense condensations of mesenchyme in the somites, getting contributions from both caudal and cranial halves of the adjacent sclerotomes. In earliest development the notochord and its definite sheath run through the whole vertebral column, but the tissue surrounding the notochord is a specialized cartilage and probably serves later as a potential source of growth of the nucleus pulposus. Ehrenhaft[3] thinks that this sheath forms the anterior and posterior longitudinal ligaments. While the cartilaginous vertebral bodies form and ossify, notochordal tissue degenerates, disappears, or is squeezed out of the discs to form the nucleus pulposus. Notochordal remnants and the cartilaginous cervical vertebrae in a 60-day human fetus show the specialized obliquely arranged fibers of the anulus fibrosus long before the vertebral column is subjected to any torque or compressive or external mechanical stresses. Vertebral bodies grow in girth greater anteriorly than posteriorly, resulting in the anterior position of the nucleus pulposus, the latter being avascular. The anulus itself has very little blood supply. The increase in size of the discs occurs at the expense of the hyaline cartilage end plates on the bodies of the vertebrae, and the increase in size of the nucleus pulposus is perhaps the result of mucoid degeneration of the persistent perichordal sheath substance.

The greatest embryonic instability in the axial skeleton occurs at the top and bottom, and it is here that congenital abnormalities occur in the greatest incidence. Congenital abnormalities of the occipital bone, cervical vertebrae, upper cervical spine, and the thoracic outlet are considered in Chapter 15, *Congenital Anomalies.*

SURFACE ANATOMY

Familiarity with surface anatomy is important to the clinician, since the main structures of the neck can be seen and felt easily in the thin patient; they are more difficult to see and feel in the obese, pyknic body type with a short neck. The sternocleidomastoid muscle runs from one corner to the other of a quadrilateral area formed by the anterior midline, the clavicle, and the leading edge of the trapezius; the mastoid-mandibular line divides the side of the neck into anterior and posterior triangles (Fig. 2–4A).

There is little to be seen in the posterior triangle, which is really a pyramid (Fig. 2–4B). The first rib is palpable at the base of the triangle, where it is crossed by the subclavian artery and the lower trunks of the brachial plexus. A cervical rib or its fibrous extension may be felt here. The spinal accessory nerve runs forward to the sternomastoid muscle, dividing the triangle into an upper ''safe''

Figure 2–4. *A,* Anterior right and left triangles are bounded by the anterior edge of the sternocleidomastoid muscle, the midline, and the lower border of the mandible. Some anatomists describe a large, upside-down triangle bounded by the two anterior borders of the sternocleidomastoid muscle and the two lower borders of the mandibles, with its apex at the sternal notch and its base at the mandibles. *B,* The posterior triangle bounded by the posterior border of the sternocleidomastoid muscle, the clavicle, and the leading edge of the trapezius muscle. *C,* Performing the valsalva maneuver, which raises intraspinal pressure. *D,* Platysma muscle in contraction. *E,* Palpation by a pincer technique involving the two stems of the hyoid bone. *F,* Lateral view of the four main landmarks to levels in the cervical spine: the hyoid bone (H, C3), the upper (C4–C5) and lower (C5–C6) margins of the thyroid cartilage (T), and the cricoid ring (C6), the first of the tracheal cartilage rings. The examiner's finger is at the lower margin of the thyroid cartilage. *G,* Pressing on the right carotid tubercle, the anterior tubercle of the transverse process of C6.

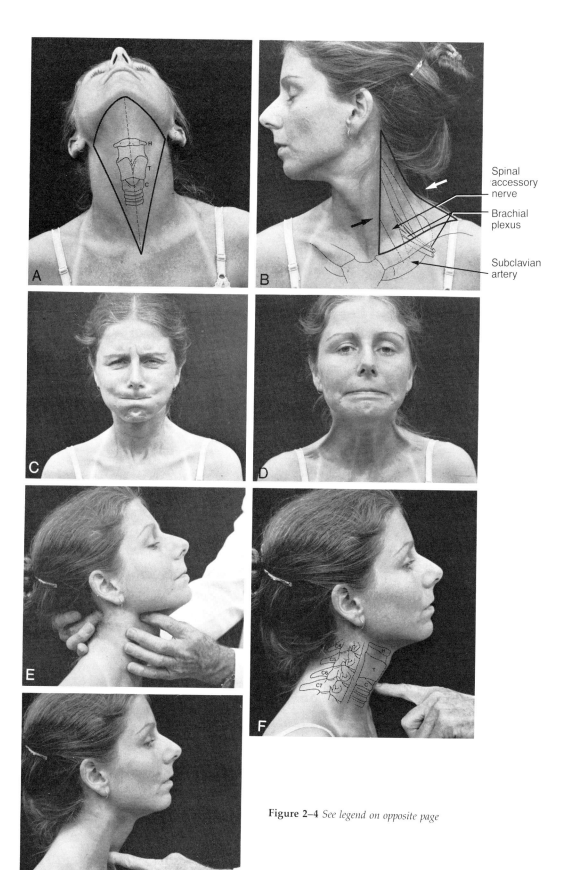

Spinal
accessory
nerve

Brachial
plexus

Subclavian
artery

Figure 2–4 *See legend on opposite page*

and lower "dangerous" area (see arrows). In the upper area the transverse processes of cervical vertebrae can be felt, though they are deep. The external jugular vein and the platysma muscle cross the sternomastoid muscle in the anterior triangle; both are prominent on breath holding (Fig. 2–4C, D). The pulsation of the carotid artery is easily seen.

The hyoid bone, a horseshoe-shaped structure, is felt at the level of C3 on a horizontal plane, above the thyroid cartilage. The anterior body of the bone and its two stems are readily felt by a pincer-like action of finger and thumb (Fig. 2–4E). With swallowing, the movement of the hyoid bone is easily palpable.

Moving down with the fingers, the upper edge of the thyroid cartilage is felt at the level of C4–C5. The lower border of the thyroid cartilage is at the level of C5–C6 (Fig. 2–4F). The thyroid cartilage also moves with swallowing and is, of course, the Adam's apple. The first bite of the forbidden apple was said to have stuck in Adam's throat—hence the name, Adam's apple.

Progressing downward, the first tracheal ring is felt immediately below the sharp lower border of the thyroid cartilage and at the level of the C6 vertebra. It is the only complete ring of the cricoid series and is an integral part of the trachea. The first ring is immediately above the site for emergency tracheostomy. Applying gentle pressure on palpation prevents initiating the gag reflex. With swallowing, the cricoid ring moves but does so less obviously than the thyroid cartilage. Moving laterally 1 inch from the first cricoid ring, we palpate the carotid tubercle, the anterior tubercle of the C6 transverse process. Although the carotid tubercle is small, located about 1 inch from the midline, and lies deep beneath overlying muscles, it is still clearly palpable! It is especially well detected by pressing posteriorly from the lateral position of the fingers (Fig. 2–4G). The carotid tubercles should be palpated separately, because simultaneous palpation of the carotid tubercles and other structures of the neck may occlude flow of both carotid arteries, resulting in the carotid reflex, a drop in blood pressure, and fainting. The carotid tubercle is the anatomic landmark for an anterior surgical approach to C5–C6 and the site for injection of the cervical stellate ganglion. The neurovascular bundle can be compressed against the carotid tubercle (level of C6 vertebra) (see Fig. 2–4F). At the apex of the triangle, the transverse process of the atlas can be felt as a small, hard lump just posterior to the internal carotid artery. It lies between the angle of the jaw and the mastoid process of the skull, just behind the ear. The examining finger tip rolls over the tip of the styloid process and the stylohyoid ligament.

The transverse processes of the atlas are the broadest in the cervical spine, readily palpable but of little clinical significance except that of being an easily identifiable anatomic point of orienta-

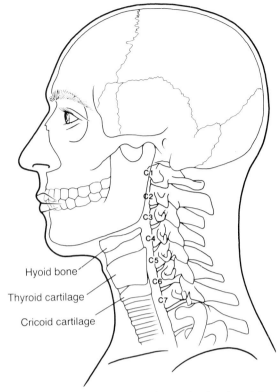

Figure 2–5. Drawing of lateral view landmarks of the cervical spine—hyoid bone, thyroid cartilage, carotid tubercle, and cricoid ring—in relationship to the whole cervical spine.

tion. The anterior arch of the hyoid bone, the notch of the thyroid cartilage, the cricoid, and the upper rings of the trachea are all readily felt in the anterior midline (Fig. 2–5).

The vertebra prominens, the spinous process of the seventh cervical and sometimes the first thoracic vertebrae, marks the lower end of the midline sulcus formed by the ligamentum nuchae, which extend from that spinous process to the occiput. The splenius capitis muscle forms a rounded ridge on either side of the sulcus; the trapezius muscle origin is tendinous, without muscle, and extends from the inion to the T12 spinous process. The dowager hump is the upper part of the vertebra prominens—always more obvious in obese people or in those with cervical osteoarthritis (Fig. 2–6).

The posterior landmarks of the cervical spine include the occiput, the inion, the superior nuchal line, and the mastoid process. The occiput is the posterior portion of the skull, including the floor. The inion ("bump of knowledge") is a dome-shaped bump in the midline of the occipital region and is the center of the nuchal line. The superior nuchal line is felt by moving laterally from the inion and is a small, transverse bony ridge extending out on both sides of the inion. Palpating laterally from the lateral edge of the superior

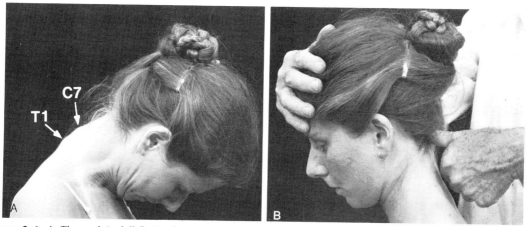

Figure 2–6. *A,* The neck in full flexion brings out the prominence of the spinous process of C7 and T1 vertebrae. *B,* The examiner's thumb is pressing on the spinous process of the axis, C2.

nuchal line, we find the rounded mastoid process of the skull (Fig. 2–7).

The spinous processes of the cervical vertebrae are in the posterior midline of the cervical spine. No muscle crosses the midline, so there is an indentation there. The lateral soft-tissue bulges outlining the indentation are made up of the deep paraspinal muscles and the superficial trapezius.

The C1 posterior arch of the atlas lies deep and has a small tubercle. The C2 spinous process, the axis, is large and easy to feel (see Fig. 2–5). The neck normally is in lordosis, but each spinous process can be felt. The cervical spinous processes are often bifid, having two small excrescences of bone (Fig. 2–8). The C7 and T1 spinous processes are larger than those above them. Normally the

Figure 2–7. Posterior aspect of head and neck with landmarks drawn in. The trapezius muscle originates from the inion, extends through all the thoracic vertebral spinous processes to T12, is inserted into the clavicle and scapula, and overlies all superficial structures in the posterior cervical spine.

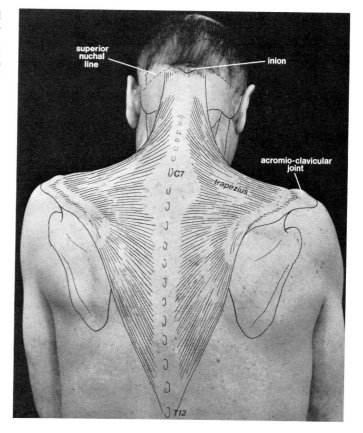

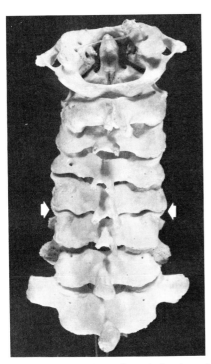

Figure 2–8. Posterior view of cervical spine. Arrows point to zygapophyseal joints clinically perceived as small domes lying deep to the trapezius muscle about 1 inch lateral to the respective spinous process. Note the bifid cervical spinous processes. The odontoid process is well shown, as are the atlantoaxial joints and the atlanto-occipital facets.

spinous processes are in line with each other. Misalignment can result from unilateral dislocation of a zygapophyseal joint or fracture of a spinous process due to trauma.

The zygapophyseal joints are palpable about 1 inch lateral to the respective spinous processes. They are often tender if abnormal, and they feel like little domes lying deep below the trapezius muscle. The patient should be completely relaxed for palpable perception of these facet joints. The vertebral level of any one of these posterior joints can be ascertained by lining up the joint level with the anterior structures of the neck—hyoid bone, thyroid cartilage, and first cricoid ring at C6.

The cervical spine is a superb example of the biologic principle of adaptation of structure to function. It supplies support for the head, a flexible and buffered tube for the transmission and protection of the upper spinal cord and the entry and exit of spinal nerves, and extremely serviceable mobility. Viewed from the front, it appears a truncated pyramid, widening from the axis downward; laterally, in neutral position, mild lordosis with the anterior convexity is present. Slight scoliosis to the left is normal at the cervicothoracic junction in 80% of people and to the right in 20% (Fig. 2–9).

MOBILITY

Erect posture, binocular vision, and cervical spine mobility allow human beings to look quickly behind themselves or over their shoulders or to gaze up at the stars or peer down a microscope far more efficiently than most animals. Many head and neck movements are social signals—nonverbal communication—indicative of mood, attitude of the moment, and emotion. We are not even aware of many of these signals. The cervical spine moves in flexion, extension, lateral flexion, and rotation. The latter two movements are always combined to some extent. Nodding occurs at the atlanto-occipital joints, with the atlantoaxial joint participating to some degree. Rotation mainly occurs at the atlantoaxial joints, principally the atlanto-odontoid rotation. The atlanto-occipital joints allow movement only in flexion and extension, not in rotation. Thus the atlas and skull move in rotation as a unit, and the position of the skull is a clear indication of the position of the atlas in rotation. The limiting factor in extension is the trapping of the posterior arch of the atlas between the occiput and the spinous process of the axis; lateral flexion is likewise so limited. Further extension is allowed by participation of the lower elements. About 25% of total extension occurs before the bony impingement limits further extension. Flexion is arrested when the posterior ligaments are taut and when the tip of the odontoid process (the atlas is tightly bound to it by the transverse ligament) abuts against the bony anterior lip of the foramen magnum. In these movements, the atlas does not move appreciably on the axis. With fusion of atlas and axis, flexion and extension are unchanged.

The atlantoaxial joints (all three) constitute the most complex joints in the body. Four distinct movements occur here: rotation, flexion, extension, and vertical approximation and lateral glide of the atlas on the axis (Fig. 2–10). Figure 2–11A shows an anteroposterior view (open mouth) of the atlas and axis joints. Figure 2–11B is a sagittal view of the atlas-axis-skull complex; the mastoid process is posterior and superior to the odontoid process.

The normal cervical spine can rotate as much as 160 degrees and, rarely, up to 180 degrees. Approximately 50% of the rotation occurs at the atlantoaxial articulation; the remainder occurs in joints below that level, with the joints rotating in decreasing magnitude. The atlas, like a wheel with an eccentrically placed axle, pivots around the laterally central but anteriorly eccentric odontoid process. The odontoid process is tightly bound to the occiput by the apical and the alar ligaments, which together with the capsule of the atlantoaxial zygapophyseal joints limit rotation each way to 45 degrees (see Fig. 2–10). Figure 2–12 is a view of the cervical spine from the top, looking down the "funnel" through the spinal canal of the atlas.

Thus, in rotation the wall of the spinal canal at

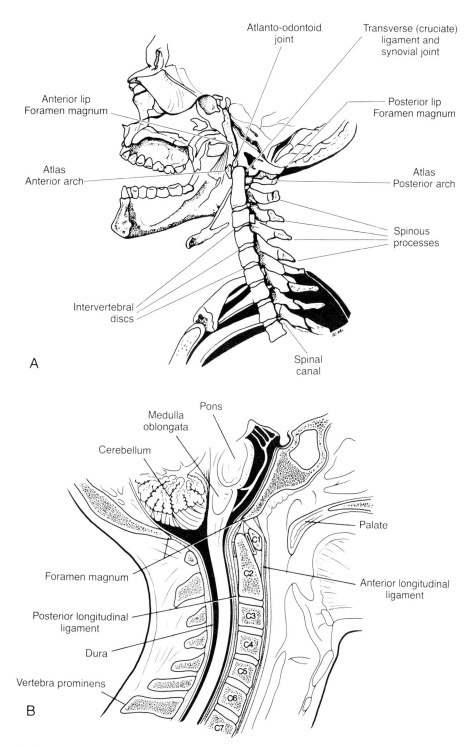

Figure 2–9. *A,* Sagittal view of the whole cervical spine showing relationship in that plane. (From Bland JH, Nakano KK: Neck pain. *In* Kelley, Harris, Ruddy, et al (eds): Textbook of Rheumatology. Philadelphia: W. B. Saunders Co, 1981.) *B,* Drawing of sagittal view of cervical spine showing the relationships of the brain stem, the medulla oblongata, the foramen magnum, and the spinal canal. The lower portion of the medulla is really outside and below the foramen. Thus, with subluxation of the atlas on the axis, compression of the brain stem can occur by pressure of the odontoid against the upper spinal cord and the lower medulla. Note that the anterior arch of the atlas is only millimeters from the pharynx.

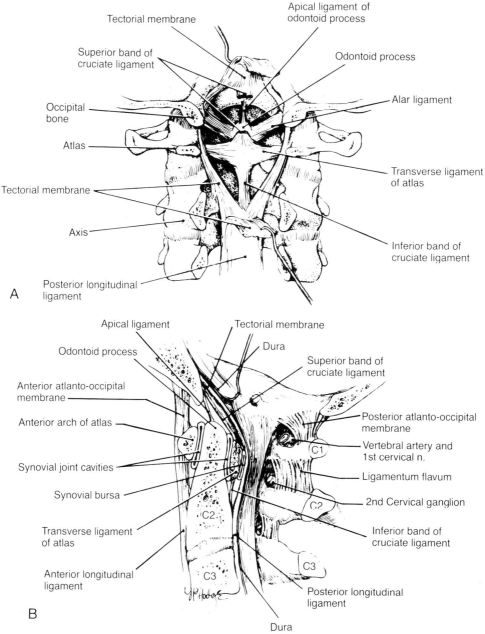

Figure 2–10. *A,* Coronal view of the upper cervical spine showing the critical transverse-cruciate ligaments, the apical and alar "check rein" ligaments of the odontoid. *B,* Sagittal view of the upper cervical spine showing the atlanto-odontoid joint with synovial joint cavities located anteriorly and posteriorly to the odontoid process. Note the vertebral artery rising out of the transverse foramen of the atlas in relationship to the first cervical nerve; the anterior arch of the atlas is only millimeters away from the pharynx. The cervical spinal canal is at its widest at the level of the foramen magnum. (Redrawn from Wilkinson M: Cervical Spondylosis. Philadelphia: W. B. Saunders Co, 1971.)

the atlas level swings laterally across the spinal canal of the axis level, narrowing the canal at this level by about one third (Fig. 2–13). Fortunately the canal is capacious here and accommodates such rotation. The diameter of the canal of C1 is equally occupied by the odontoid process, free space, and the cord. The free space allows for safe rotation. Ligamentous structures, remarkably

enough, are sufficiently lax to allow this wide range but are inelastic with high tensile strength and can limit further motion without impingement on vital structures. Lateral flexion of the head produces as much or more associated rotation of the axis than does simple rotation of the head. With head tilt, the spinous processes of the axis and of those vertebrae below rotate to the opposite

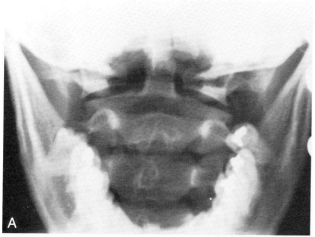

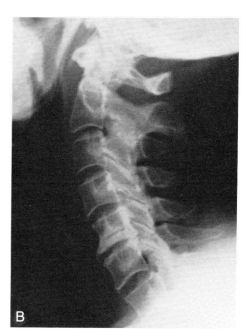

Figure 2–11. *A,* Note the atlantoaxial joints and the poorly seen atlanto-occipital joints. The spine is in slight lateral flexion, with lateral gliding of the atlas from the viewer's right to left. *B,* A sagittal view showing the atlanto-odontoid joint, the odontoid, the spinal canal, and the anterior and posterior arch of the atlas.

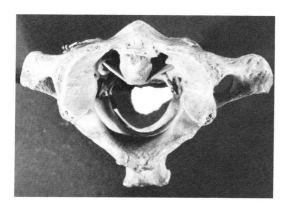

Figure 2–12. The cervical spine from the top. Note the foramina transversaria, the upper facets of atlas, the atlanto-axial (odontoid) joints. The spinal canal has a funnel-like shape, with the largest diameter at the top progressively narrowing from above downward. The rubber band posterior to the odontoid process represents the transverse ligament.

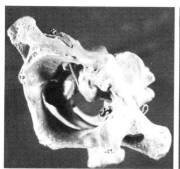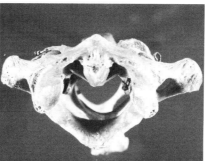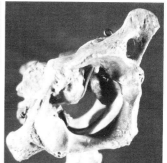

Figure 2–13. *Center,* Top view looking into the cervical spinal canal; note narrowing from above downward. *Right,* The atlas has rotated 45 degrees to the left on the odontoid peg, and the atlas wall of the spinal canal narrows it as it turns. *Left,* The rotation of atlas on odontoid process is the same, but turning is to the right, and narrowing of the cervical canal is at the atlantoaxial level.

side, to a greater degree in the upper than in the lower portions of the cervical spine.

Lateral glide occurs in normal people, with the atlas shifting to the side of the tilt. It is observable on radiographic film as a narrowing of the space between the odontoid process and the lateral mass of the atlas on the side of the tilt and a widening on the other side (see Fig. 2–11*A*). Flexion, extension, and vertical approximation depend on the shape of the lateral facets between the axis and the atlas. Axis facets are directed superiorly and laterally and are slightly convex; atlas facets are directed downward and medially and are not reciprocally concave but flat. These characteristics of the facets permit the atlas to rock backward and forward on the axis (flexion and extension). Telescoping, or vertical approximation of the atlas on the axis, occurs in rotation.

The vertebral artery enters the foramen of the transverse process of the sixth cervical vertebra and ascends through the foramina transversaria to enter the skull. It is protected in the foramen except between the axis and the atlas, where there is about 1.5 to 2.0 cm of artery lying outside the canal. In addition, the artery is clearly normally subject to the stress and stretch between atlas and axis, since it is situated at the periphery of the marked rotation. The artery is pulled forward and backward by the rotary action (Fig. 2–14). The

clinical consequences must be considered in any rotary dislocation, fracture, or malalignment of the atlas and axis.

Below the axis, rotation, flexion-extension, and lateral flexion occur in decreasing amount from the top down. The cervical spine normally is in slight lordosis, but a linear pattern is not necessarily abnormal. There is even reversal of the standard lordosis in a few normal people. During flexion, the cervical spine appears to lengthen; this seems to be attributable to straightening of the lordosis rather than to actual lengthening of the cervical spine.

Selective motion can occur between atlas and skull and between atlas and axis, without motion below the axis. Such is not the case with the vertebrae below the axis. One element cannot move without involving some or all of the others.

The cervical intervertebral discs are also involved in allowing motion. They are not mere cushions. Their physical properties of resilience permit motion and stop excessive motion, as ligaments and capsules are firmly attached to the vertebral bodies. In flexion and extension, associated normal disc formation and a sliding motion occur to a greater degree in the upper cervical region than in the lower. In lateral flexion and rotation the discs glide and deform and regain their resting states on completion of the motion.

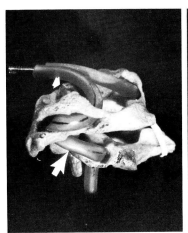 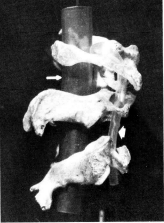 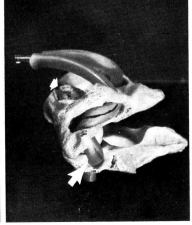

Figure 2–14. *Center,* Atlas, axis, and C3 are separated to show the course of the vertebral artery. The plastic tubing represents the spinal cord (narrow arrow). The clear tubing, representing the vertebral artery, is threaded through the foramina transversaria of C3, the axis (C2), and the atlas (C1). The artery must deviate out from C3 to C2 and sharply veer outward and upward through the transverse foramen of the atlas, where it must turn posteriorly around the lateral mass, making a complete U-turn to join its counterpart to form the basilar artery (thick arrow). Note the tortuous course, compression, kinking, and twisting the artery undergoes. This is all the normal circumstance. *Right,* The atlas and axis are shown with striped rubber tubing representing the vertebral artery (same caliber as the artery threaded through the foramina transversaria of the two vertebrae). The upper arrow points to the odontoid process and the atlanto-odontoid joint; the lower arrow points to the vertebral artery. Note the sharp deviation outward and upward that the artery must make from axis to atlas, followed by the complete U-turn about the posterior aspect of the lateral mass of the atlas before proceeding on to the clivus to join the other vertebral artery as the basilar artery. This is normal. Consider the situation with thick atherosclerotic plaques, narrow joint spaces, loss of intervertebral disc height, and extensive osteophytosis. *Left,* The atlas has been pulled down slightly and rotated to the right toward the viewer (short arrow). Note the "artery" segment between the axis and the atlas has been strikingly stretched and narrowed, thinning and almost obliterating the red stripe (large arrow). The U-turn portion is also narrowed and stretched.

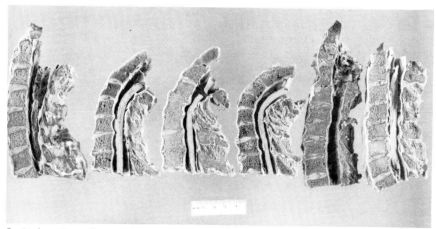

Figure 2–15. Sagittal sections of cervical spine from people increasingly older from left to right. The youngest, age 22 years, is on the far left, and the oldest, 91 years, is on the far right. Normal lordosis yields to increasing lordosis, then to straightening, and finally a reversed cervical lordosis (slight kyphosis) (far right). Note universal cervical intervertebral disc disease and osteoarthritis increasing from left to right.

Although range of motion between any two cervical vertebrae is not great below the axis, the summation of these movements permits the wide range of motion possible in the normal neck. Neck movement diminishes with increasing age, probably owing in great part to decreasing physical activity and relative immobilization rather than an intrinsic characteristic of chronologic age (Fig. 2–15). In childhood all motions are seemingly exaggerated, allowing considerable displacement of one vertebral body on another. The effect of neck movements on spinal cord nerve roots and blood vessels is considered later.

The overall extension range is greater than the flexion range; the ratio is 64 to 16 degrees. The full range in a healthy young adult, from maximal

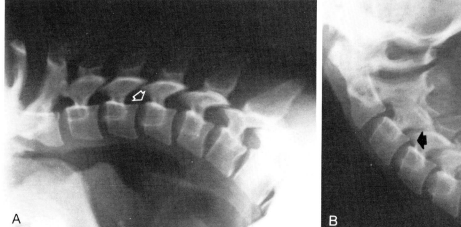
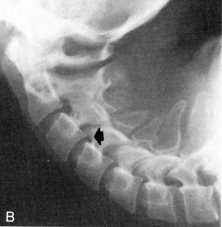

A

B

Figure 2–16. *A*, The neck in full flexion. The spine is concave forward, the anterior portion of the discs is compressed and narrow, and the posterior portion is widened and stretched. The superior articular facets slide forward in the inferior facets of the vertebrae below, and the vertebral bodies are subluxated forward in a mild stairstep–like arrangement. Arrow points to anterior subluxation. The zygapophyseal joints are spread open, and the capsules are stretched. The laminae and spinous processes are spread like a fan. The posterior longitudinal ligament is stretched, the anterior slack, the nucleus pulposus is displaced dorsally, and the elastic ligamenta flava are widely stretched. These characteristics are all normal and physiologic in a healthy young person. *B*, When the neck is in full extension, all changes noted in part *A* are reversed. Discs open anteriorly and compress posteriorly; vertebrae subluxate dorsally; the zygapophyseal joints close, and the capsules are slack. The laminae and spinous processes close. Note also the closed spaces between the occiput and the atlas. The space between the atlas and the axis closes in extension and spreads in flexion—all normal and physiologic. Arrow points to posterior subluxated vertebrae.

flexion to complete extension, is 90 degrees, with the greatest movement occurring at the C5–C6 level and the least at the C2–C3 and C7–T1 levels.

Clinically important in differential diagnosis are the following points: On full flexion the spine is concave and forward, and the anterior portions of the discs are compressed and narrowed, with the dorsal portions widened and stretched. The anterior longitudinal ligament is slack while the posterior is stretched; the nucleus is dorsally displaced; the paired superior articular facets of the vertebrae glide forward on the inferior facets of the vertebrae below, with slight forward displacement of the upper on the lower vertebral body. The laminae and spinous processes are open like a fan; the ligamenta flava and interspinous ligaments are stretched, and the posterior neck muscles, which are the most powerful limiting force, are under tension. The capsules of the zygapophyseal joints are stretched. Study Figure 2–16 carefully!

Extension of the neck reverses these events in the tissues. The limiting factors, however, are tension in the anterior longitudinal ligaments, the approximation and imbrication of spinous processes, and the locking of the lower border of the lower articular facets as the upper vertebrae glide downward and backward on the facets of the lower ones (see Fig. 2–16B). In left lateral flexion the upper facets glide upward and forward.

The size of the intervertebral foramina increases in flexion and decreases in extension by about one third. In lateral flexion or rotation, the ipsilateral foramen decreases in size, the contralateral increases (Figs. 2–17 and 2–18).

ZYGAPOPHYSEAL JOINTS

The zygapophyseal joints (also called the posterior joints, the joints of the vertebral arches, facet joints, and apophyseal joints) are paired, diarthrodial (freely movable) joints between the superior and inferior articular facets of adjacent vertebrae. The highest is located at the C2–C3 level, and the lowest at the C6–C7 level, though zygapophyseal joints at the C7–T1 level are indistinguishable from those at an upper level. Their surface area is about two thirds that of the intervertebral disc joints. There are fibrous capsules lax enough to permit fairly free movement. The joints are lined with synovial membrane and covered with hyaline cartilage and have a thin layer of subchondral bone at the chondro-osseous junction. We note in our study of 130 whole human cervical spines that virtually all diarthrodial joints, normal and abnormal, had a fibrofatty, fibrocartilaginous meniscus or disc that became proliferative as a pannus-like structure in osteoarthritis (Fig. 2–19).

The superior facets face forward and downward at an angle of about 45 degrees. The inferior surfaces face backward and upward also at an angle of 45 degrees. The curvatures of these facets do not fit each other perfectly, allowing the complex movements at these joints on lateral flexion and rotation of the neck. The zygapophyseal joints are not primarily weight-bearing, but they aid in stabilization of the motor segment—the intervertebral interface where movement occurs. Forward displacement of one vertebra on another is prevented by a "fail-safe" locking mechanism pro-

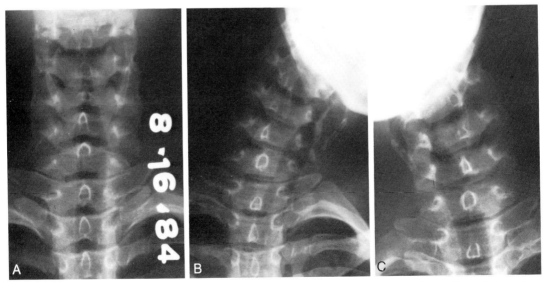

Figure 2–17. A, Anteroposterior view of the cervical spine in neutral position. Note the midline of the spinous processes, excellent lateral view of the joints of Luschka, faintly calcified thyroid cartilage, and zygapophyseal joints (far lateral). B, Right lateral flexion causes opening of the intervertebral foramina, the joints of Luschka, and the zygapophyseal joints on the left, compressing and narrowing the discs to the viewer's right and widening the discs to the viewer's left. C, Left lateral flexion reverses the events noted for right lateral flexion.

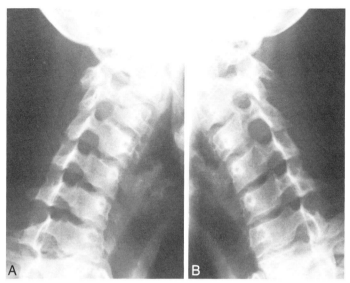

Figure 2–18. Right (*A*) and left (*B*) combination of lateral flexion and rotation in the oblique position opens the intervertebral foramina, the joints of Luschka, and the zygapophyseal joints to their maximum diameter (relieving nerve root compression if present, a useful clinical maneuver).

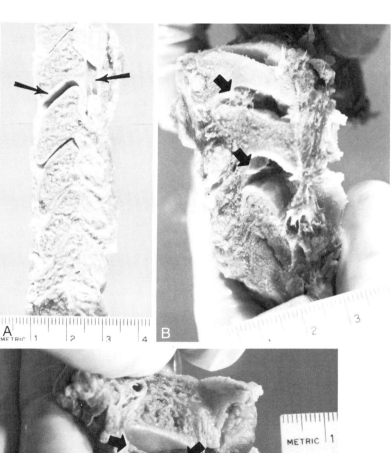

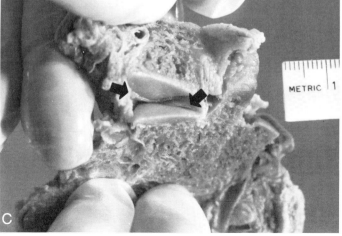

Figure 2–19. *A,* This sagittal section of whole cervical spine shows normal zygapophyseal joints slightly spread to reveal joint space, subchondral bone, and the layer of hyaline cartilage (arrow). A section of the vertebral artery is noted in the upper right; the nerve roots are in apposition to the zygapophyseal joints. *B,* Note the opened zygapophyseal joint with meniscus of fibrofatty, fibrocartilage tissue proliferating (upper arrow). A meniscus is noted in the joint below (lower arrow). *C,* The meniscus (arrows) is easy to see in this normal zygapophyseal joint.

vided by the abutment of the superior leading edge of the inferior facet into the angle of the joint above.

Joint capsules are richly innervated with proprioceptive and pain receptors much more than are the corresponding joints in the thoracic and lumbar segments of the spine. Striking awareness of head and neck movements is a function of the innervation. Though the zygapophyseal joint capsules and supporting ligaments of the neck are heavily innervated, the intervertebral discs are not.

LIGAMENTS OF THE CERVICAL SPINE

Occipitovertebral Ligaments. The transverse ligament of the odontoid process is diamond-shaped and holds the odontoid process tightly to the anterior arch of the atlas. There are two tough bands, one passing up to the occiput and the other down to the body of the axis, completing the cruciform ligament of the atlas. The vertical bands of the cross are relatively unimportant in containing the odontoid process, because the transverse ligament is the major ligament preventing subluxation. The apical ligament of the odontoid process, a vestigial remnant, attaches to the peak of the odontoid process and runs to the anterior lip of the foramen magnum. The alar ligaments run on either side from the tip of the

odontoid process to the margins of the foramen magnum. Both ligaments are enclosed in a sleeve of synovial membrane. These are very tough, robust cords that check atlantoaxial rotation (see Fig. 2–10).

The anterior atlanto-occipital membrane extends upward from the anterior longitudinal ligament to connect the anterior margin of the foramen magnum with the anterior arch of the atlas (see Fig. 2–10B).

The tectorial membrane is a fan-shaped continuation of the posterior longitudinal ligament to the basiocciput, and its fibers blend with the dura mater (see Fig. 2–10).

The posterior atlanto-occipital membrane arches over the vertebral artery and is much thinner than the ligamenta flava or the interspinous ligaments farther down the cervical spine.

The anterior longitudinal ligament is tightly adherent to the front of the vertebral bodies and loosely blends with each anulus as it crosses the disc spaces. The posterior ligament, to the contrary, is firmly bound to each disc but stands only loosely bound to the posterior concavity of the vertebral body. The space is occupied by retrocorporeal veins. By having only loose attachment to the vertebral body, the posterior longitudinal ligament allows the spinal canal to be a smooth-walled tube. Clinically any pathologic thickening or ossification of the ligament compromises the

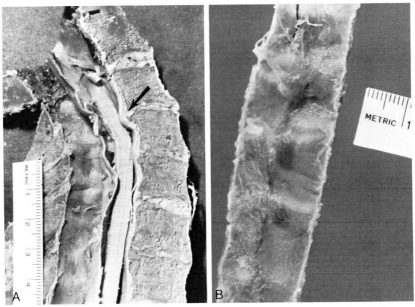

Figure 2–20. *A,* Sagittal section of a cervical spine with marked thickening and fibrosis of both dura and the posterior longitudinal ligament. The thickened and fibrotic ligament, coupled with osteophytes, has compressed the spinal cord. The arrow points to the dura and the ligament as separate entities. *B,* Coronal view of the anterior surface of the spinal canal shows thickened posterior longitudinal ligament. The filmy connective tissue is shown forming loose adherence between the dura and the spinal canal, mostly on the left.

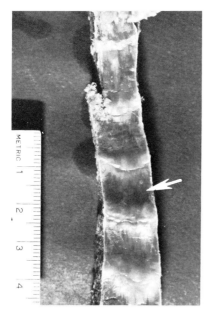

Figure 2–21. Laminae removed with ligamenta flava intact. The laminae are the light, banded areas, and the darker tissue is the very elastic ligamenta flava (arrow).

capacity of the canal even in the absence of osteophytosis or protrusion of the disc (Fig. 2–20).

The ligamenta flava are strong, very elastic ligaments spanning the space between the laminae in pairs, attached to the anteroinferior surface of the lamina above and the posterosuperior margin of the lamina below. They stretch laterally to the zygapophyseal joint and enter into the fibrous composition of the capsule. They lie at about the same level as the intervertebral discs. The ligamenta flava stretch under tension and retract and relax without undue bulging or folding in the normal state. Their function has been compared with that of the ligamentum nuchae in quad-

ripeds, supporting the neck in the erect position, aiding the muscles to extend the flexed neck, limiting motion of the zygapophyseal joints, and restraining abrupt movements between the vertebrae (Fig. 2–21; see Fig. 2–1 also).

CORD AND VERTEBRAL MOVEMENT

The length of the cervical canal increases as the head and neck move from full extension to full flexion. The anterior wall increases by 1.5 cm, and the posterior wall increases by 5 cm from T1 to the top of the atlas. The difference in length between extension and flexion of the vertebral canal is 2 to 3 cm. The cord is displaced upward in neck flexion; the dural sheath moves up, and increased tension is placed in the intrathecal nerve roots. The opposite occurs in neck extension (Fig. 2–22). Nerve roots may rub against the pedicle. These functional anatomic facts have clinical reflections and should be kept in mind by the clinician (Fig. 2–23).

VERTEBRAE

The atlas and axis have special architectural design (as have C1 and C2 in reptiles, birds, and mammals), whereas the lower five cervical vertebrae are constructed according to a common plan. This fact is very important in clinical considerations. The skull sits on the atlas. The atlas (Fig. 2–24) has no body and only an excuse for a spinous process. It is a solid ring of bone with two lateral pillars. The upper and lower surfaces of the atlas are articulating facets; the short anterior arch articulates in a vertical plane with the odontoid process of the axis (the old phylogenetic body of the atlas, complete with rudimentary disc); the longer posterior arch forms the posterior wall of the spinal canal. The upper facets, ellipsoid in shape, are cupped to articulate with the occipital condyles of the skull, and the lower ones are

Figure 2– 22. Schematic diagram showing the cervical spine in flexion and extension. Note the increase in length of cervical canal in flexion. The cord displaces upward in flexion, and tension is put on the nerve roots, which are slack in extension.

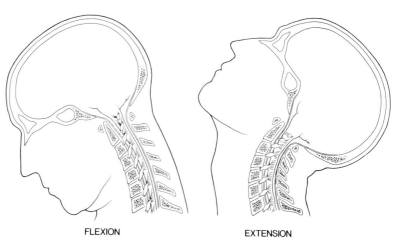

FLEXION   EXTENSION

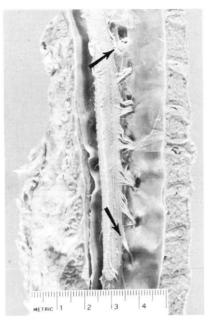

Figure 2–23. This anatomic specimen of a whole, opened cervical spine shows anterior spinal canal with osteoarthritic bars, fibrotic dura and dural root sleeves, hypertrophied ligamenta flava, anterior rootlets and roots (clearly seen) with traction and tension in the roots. Note that the higher nerve roots are deformed and directed upward (upper arrow), whereas the lower ones enter the root sleeves with increasing obliquity. The nerve roots above are lax; those below are stretched. Extension in this case predictably produced gross radiculopathies and myelopathic signs.

round, concave, face laterally and down, and articulate with the superior facets of the axis. The transverse processes of the atlas are wider than those of other vertebrae because of the muscle attachments and the leverage needed to rotate the head. Each has the transverse foramen for the vertebral artery, veins, and sympathetic nerve fibers. Just posterior to the facets are bony grooves around which the cervical spine veins and the vertebral arteries curve. The spinal canal at this level is spacious, and its sagittal diameter can be divided into three parts. The anterior one third is occupied by the odontoid peg and the anterior arch of the atlas; the cord occupies the middle third, and the subarachnoid space the posterior third. Cisternal puncture by the posterior or lateral approach is safe in experienced hands.

There is an oblique groove over the posterior arch of the atlas accommodating the vertebral artery after it has wound around the outside of the articular mass. The attachment of the posterior atlanto-occipital membrane arches over the artery at this point; this arch is sometimes outlined, completely or incompletely, by bone to form the arcuate foramen (see Fig. 2–24). The clinical significance of this bony arch is that it renders the atheromatous, tortuous vertebral artery more vulnerable to compression on rotation of the cervical spine.

The transverse width of the atlas is greater than that of any other cervical vertebra, subserving the function of providing leverage and mechanical advantage to the muscles inserted into the transverse process. The transverse process of the atlas

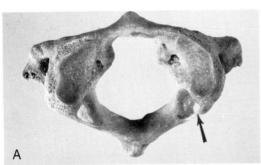

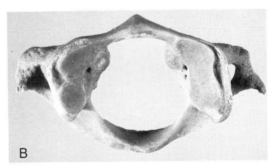

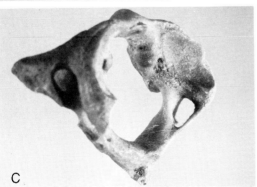

Figure 2–24. The atlas. No two atlases are exactly alike. Note the differences between part *A* and part *B*. The atlas shown in *B* has a larger spinal canal, differently oriented facets, and two hemifacets on the left. The lateral masses, anterior and posterior arches, and the transverse foramina are easily seen. In part *A*, a bony bridge is noted behind the posterior lateral mass, termed the arcuate foramen (arrow), through which the vertebral artery must wind. In *C* an atlas has been tipped up to show the arcuate foramen.

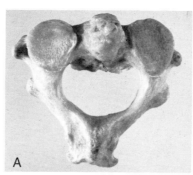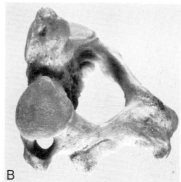

Figure 2–25. The axis. *A,* View from above shows the superior facets, the irregular and rough odontoid process (dens axis), and the spinous process. *B,* Posterolateral oblique view shows the transverse foramen and the anterior and posterior articular facets of the odontoid process.

is the only one in the cervical spine not grooved (intervertebral foramen), allowing exit and entrance of the nerve roots. The articular columns are broader and deeper than all the rest, for they shoulder the weight of the skull. The superior articular facets lie directly over the inferior, not behind them as do all the inferior facets of the subjacent zygapophyseal joints (see Fig. 2–24).

The obvious characteristic of the axis is the odontoid process, a peg rising perpendicularly from midbody, acting as an eccentric pivot about which the atlas rotates (Fig. 2–25). The anterior surface of the odontoid process has a facet articulating with the posterior surface of the anterior arch of the atlas. The posterior surface of the odontoid process also has a facet to accommodate the synovial bursa separating it from the transverse band of the critical cruciate ligament (see Fig. 2–10). On either side of the odontoid process are the inferior facets of the atlantoaxial joints. On the inferior side of the axis, it begins to take on characteristics of a typical cervical vertebra. Its laminae meet to form a bifid, often massive spinous process. The pedicles are thick, and their upper margins are continuous with the upper margin of the body. Unlike all other cervical vertebrae, the axis has no intervertebral foramen to accommodate the anterior and posterior nerve roots. The inferior facets lie below and behind the superior and subtend an angle of almost 90 degrees with the transverse process. The upper facets of C3 articulate with the lower facets of the axis (Fig. 2–26). The third through the sixth cervical vertebrae are so similar that it is difficult to identify any individualized bone. C7, the vertebra prominens, however, has a very large and prominent spinous process. In the articulated cervical column the vertebrae increase in size from the top down (Figs. 2–27 and 2–28). The bony margins are sharply defined about the superior rim; the posterolateral edge projects upward in a facet and articulates with a facet on the body of the vertebra above. This facet is known as the uncus or uncinate process, the ultimate joint of Luschka (Fig. 2–29).

The spinal canal is large to accommodate the

cervical cord enlargement. The laminae are slender, and in children each lamina overlaps the one below. The overlap increases remarkably with increasing age.

The zygapophyseal joints, uncinate processes, pedicles, and transverse processes are distinctive and peculiar to the cervical spine. Together they bound the intervertebral foramina and enclose the foramina transversaria (Fig. 2–30). Thus, there are no pedicles on the atlas and axis. The axis has very thick laminae (posterior arch) and a large, bifid, readily palpable spinous process. The transverse processes are remarkably small, with tubercles at their tips, and the transverse foramina to conduct the vertebral artery, veins, and nerves vertically. The artery must make a sharp upward and lateral bend between the transverse processes of the axis and atlas. This special design of C1–C2 precludes their having intervertebral foramina, and the first and second spinal nerve roots lie posterior to the articulating lateral masses. All lower roots lie anterior to the zygapophyseal joint facets and traverse their respective intervertebral foramina.

The lower five cervical vertebrae have characteristics in common—bodies, pedicles, laminae,

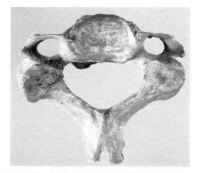

Figure 2–26. Typical cervical vertebra. The articulating facets are posterior (contrary to the atlas and axis) transverse processes and at an angle of 40 to 45 degrees. The spinous process is bifid; each typical vertebra has two (or paired) foramina transversaria, and the spinal canal is generally triangular.

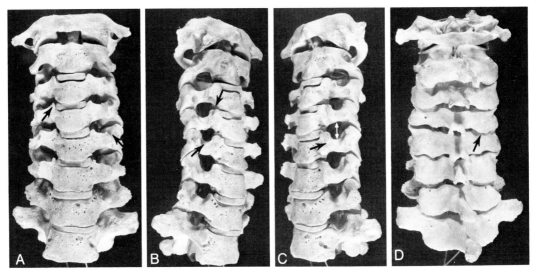

Figure 2–27. *A,* Anterior view shows the entire articulated cervical spine plus the first thoracic vertebra. Note the pyramid form, wide atlas, discs, zygapophyseal joints, and uncinate processes (Luschka joints [arrow on left] and the anterolateral intervertebral foramina [arrow on right] with their anterior and posterior tubercles). *B,* A right anterolateral aspect with a clear view of the intervertebral foramina bounded anteromedially by the joints of Luschka and posterolaterally by the zygapophyseal joints. The pedicles are easily seen. Upper arrow points to Luschka joint and lower arrow to intervertebral foramina. *C,* Left anterolateral aspect shows the tubercles (black arrow) to better advantage as well as the approximate 1-cm height (white arrow) of the foramen. *D,* A direct posterior view shows the bifid spinous processes, the zygapophyseal joints (arrow) with their approximate 30- to 45-degree increasing angularity from above down, and the overlapping laminae.

vertebral arches, and spinous processes (see Fig. 2–26). The vertebral arches arise from the posterolateral aspect of the bodies, giving rise to the pedicles, whose upper and lower surfaces are the articulating facets of the zygapophyseal joints. The arches face the bodies at an angle of 45 degrees, and the laminae arise from the pedicles and arch backward to meet in the midline, forming the bifid spinous processes, jutting down. In front of the facets the transverse processes arise laterally, projecting anteriorly and downward. Their upper surfaces are grooved and trough-like (like a gargoyle or rainspout from a roof), and they transmit

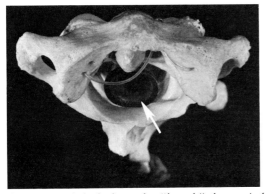

Figure 2–28. A look down the "funnel," the cervical spinal canal. Plastic tubing in the spinal canal represents the spinal cord (arrow).

the spinal nerves. Each transverse process except C7 has a foramen for the vertebral artery and its accompanying plexus of veins and sympathetic nerves. Anterior and posterior tubercles (homologous with thoracic ribs) on the transverse processes serve as attachments for the scalene muscles. Adjacent bodies are united by the intervertebral discs, and anterior and posterior longitudinal ligaments by the paired, posteriorly placed zygapophyseal joints, the ligamenta flava, the ligamentum nuchae, the intertransverse ligaments, and the interspinous ligaments (see Fig. 2–26).

The joints of Luschka (uncovertebral joints) are formed in the second decade of life, when the lateral margins of the superior surfaces of the lower five vertebrae are raised into lips (uncinate processes), and the corresponding margins of the vertebrae above become reciprocally beveled. Between lip and bevel is the Luschka joint, which only later develops articular cartilage and has capsular ligaments, synovium, and joint space. The joints of Luschka are of great significance in the cervical spine, since they act as barriers to the extrusion of disc material posterolaterally, preventing compression of nerve roots. Furthermore, the cervical nerve roots do not pass over the intervertebral discs and are protected from them; only posterior and posterolateral protrusions can occur. In the lumbar area the nerve roots lie directly over the posterolateral portions of the discs and are thus extremely vulnerable to disc protrusion. In the thoracic spine the nerve roots lie above the disc and are not as likely to suffer disc protrusion damage. In the cervical spine, discs cannot protrude into the intervertebral foramina—only posteriorly and into the cord—a fact not widely appreciated (Fig. 2–31).

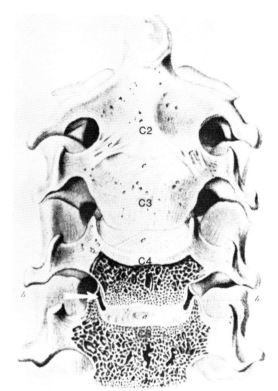

Figure 2–29. Hubert Luschka's original drawing of the joint bearing his name. The upper uncinate process C2–C3 is covered with ligament; the C3–C4 uncinate process is uncovered; the C4–C5 Luschka joint (arrow) shows the joint cavity, hyaline cartilage, and capsule. *Note:* Luschka's *a* indicates intervertebral disc at C4–C5; his *b* on both sides points to "his" joint.

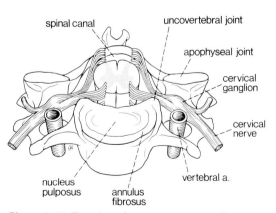

Figure 2–30. Drawing of transverse section shows relationship of Luschka and zygapophyseal joints, intervertebral foramen, nerve roots, transverse foramen, and the vertebral artery. Note the anterior nerve root is in apposition to the Luschka joint, and the posterior root to the zygapophyseal joint; the vertebral artery is anterior to the nerve root.

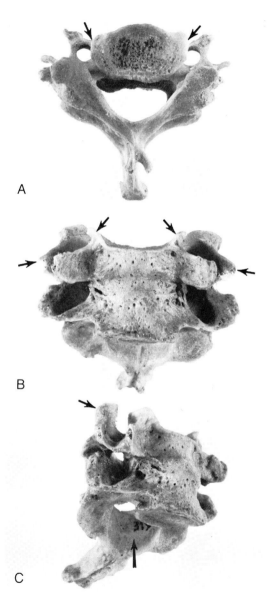

Figure 2–31. *A,* Anatomic specimen of a C4 vertebra with osteophytes projecting upward from the joint of Luschka, preventing disc protrusion into the intervertebral foramen (arrows). *B,* Coronal view of fused specimen with osteoarthritic Luschka joints projecting into the intervertebral foramen but occluding the disc protrusion (upper arrows). Note osteophytic tubercles on the intervertebral foramina (lower arrows). *C,* Inferoanterolateral view. Note spinal canal below (lower arrow). Also note two very osteophytic tubercles and a very large Luschka osteophyte at the top left of the foramen (upper arrow).

DISCS AND NUCLEUS PULPOSUS

There is no disc between the first and second vertebrae. The odontoid peg is separated from the body of the axis by a layer of cartilage, which ossifies before puberty. The cartilage is a notochordal remnant, not an epiphyseal plate.

In the second decade, clefts appear in the posterolateral area of the anulus just within the uncinate process. They are stress fissures—perhaps fatigue "fractures" of collagen produced by the major shearing forces involved. Like other diarthrodial joints, the clefts gradually develop synovial lining, true hyaline cartilage, and capsular and subchondral bone. They are the joints of Luschka (uncovertebral joints). Not so well known is that later—in the fourth, fifth, or sixth decade—other fissures regularly appear in the discs, and some may extend transversely across the entire disc (Fig. 2–32). These fissures are of varying size and extent, and some are synovial lined. In our study of 130 whole human cervical spines, this process of fissuring and clefting was universal in individuals 60 years of age and older. It surely is related to known dehydration of the nucleus pulposus and consequent loss of height. Such change in physical properties results in change in resistance to shearing forces, consequent cavity formation, and loss of height.

In radiographs of the cervical spine, one often sees the vacuum phenomenon, that is, gas, presumably nitrogen, in the disc. The known normal and physiologic subatmospheric pressures in diarthrodial joints probably apply to the intervertebral disc joints in the cervical spine. The intervertebral discs make up about one quarter of the length of the spinal column. They dehydrate (shrink) owing to weight-bearing during the day, and they rehydrate during rest at night, making us taller by one half to three fourths of an inch in the morning than at night. The discs are biconvex, conforming with the concavity of the vertebral bodies, but they are deeper anteriorly. This results in the normal cervical lordosis. Discs are relatively thick in the cervical spine (thickest at the C6–C7 level). The ratio of disc to vertebral body height ranges from 1:3 to 1:2. The thickness of discs in the cervical spine is a major factor in its extreme flexibility. Discs are thicker anteriorly than posteriorly; the sum of their anterior heights is 8 mm greater than of their posterior heights, again accounting for the cervical lordosis and anterior convexity. Discs are avascular (like hyaline cartilage) and are nourished by alternate compression, dehydration, and rehydration, and by diffusion of fluids from adjacent vertebral bodies as well as peripheral vessels of the anulus fibrosus[5, 6]

The disc is made up of anulus fibrosus and the

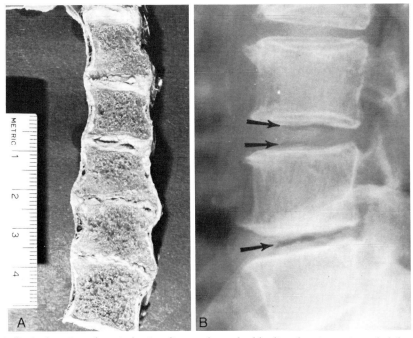

Figure 2–32. *A*, Sagittal section of cervical spine discs and vertebral bodies showing universal clefts across the discs anteroposteriorly. The same Luschka-to-Luschka clefts are seen in the coronal views. In life these usually show the vacuum effect—gas (nitrogen) in the disc—suggesting that there is subatmospheric pressure in the cervical disc, as there is normally in diarthrodial joints. *B*, Vacuum effect in L3–L4 and L4–L5 intervertebral discs. Arrows point to the gas pockets.

nucleus pulposus. The anulus is fibrocartilaginous, has some elasticity, and is made up of crisscrossing concentric lamellae between adjacent vertebrae, providing strength and stability but restricting excessive mobility. The anulus is reinforced in front and behind by fibers from the anterior and posterior longitudinal ligaments. Laterally, about the circumference of the vertebral body, the anulus blends with the periosteum but is bound down to the bone and can be separated only by incision. The nucleus is not in the center of the disc but lies a little anterior. It has a volume of 0.2 ml and is about 0.7 cm in diameter. It is a salt- and water-rich mixture of proteoglycan gel and a lattice of collagen fibers, with the remarkable property of absorbing and retaining water against physical and osmotic pressure. The nucleus becomes more and more fibrocartilaginous with increasing age, finally resembling the remainder of the disc; thus it loses its hydrophilic properties, an important clinical point.

The discs absorb stresses along the vertebral column. The viscoelastic nucleus changes its shape and distributes forces equally and uniformly in all directions, and it converts longitudinal to horizontal forces and transmits them radially to the circumferential anuli. The resilient anulus and the cartilage plate, capping the upper and lower surfaces of the vertebrae, absorb the shock energy.

INTERVERTEBRAL FORAMINA

The intervertebral foramina are short tunnels bounded ventromedially by the disc—with its covering posterior longitudinal ligament—and the uncovertebral joint (joint of Luschka) and dorsolaterally by the zygapophyseal joint and the superior articular process of the subjacent vertebra. The foramina open obliquely forward laterally and inferiorly from 10 to 15 degrees downward. Their shape is rather like a figure eight or the sole of a shoe with the heel positioned inferiorly (see Figs. 2–27 and 2–30). They are largest at the C2–C3 level, becoming progressively smaller down to the C6–C7 level. The average vertical diameter is 10 mm, the transverse 5 mm. The intervertebral foramina enclose and transmit the lateral termination of the anterior and posterior nerve roots—spinal radicular arteries, intervertebral veins and plexuses, and an extension of the epidural space with areolar and fatty tissue. Small arteries, veins, and lymphatics provide a protective cushion for the nerves. The roots occupy one quarter to one third of the foraminal space. The anterior root lies anterior and inferior to the posterior root and in close proximity to the uncovertebral joint; the posterior root is in close proximity to the zygapophyseal joint and especially to the superior articular process of the subjacent vertebra. The roots lie nearer the upper vertebral pedicle at the medial end of the foramen and nearer the lower vertebral pedicle at the lateral end.

VERTEBRAL CANAL

The vertebral canal is triangular in transverse section, with the posterior aspect of the vertebrae and the discs constituting the base or anterior wall of the triangle, which is covered by the posterior longitudinal ligament. The pedicles and the transverse foramina also contribute. The other two sides of the triangle laterally and dorsolaterally are the inner aspect of the zygapophyseal joints, the laminae and the ligamenta flava. The canal is funnel-like, widest at the atlantoaxial level and narrowing to the smallest sagittal diameter at the posteroinferior edge of the body of C5 and the lamina of C6 (Fig. 2–33).

The spinal cord is suspended and cushioned in the subarachnoid space by spinal fluid; the anterior and posterior spinal nerve roots traverse the subarachnoid space en route to their intervertebral foramina of exit. A capillary subdural space separates dura from arachnoid. The epidural space, with its areolar and fatty tissue, and the internal vertebral plexuses cushion the cord from moving laminae (see Fig. 2–33). The cervical canal is fairly roomy from the atlas to the level of C3, where the cervical enlargement of the cord begins, extending to T2. The cervical cord more nearly fills the canal here than at all other levels in the spine. A crucial factor in the pathogenesis of cervical myelopathy

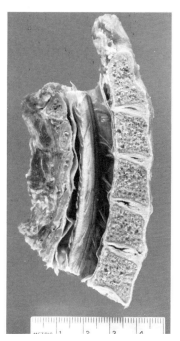

Figure 2–33. A sagittal section of a cervical spine showing the cut-away vertebral canal with the spinal cord laterally viewed, and posterior nerve roots penetrating the stiff, fibrotic, dural root sleeves on the right. The dura mater and the posterior longitudinal ligament can be seen as separate structures.

is the size of the vertebral canal relative to the cord, that is, how much space is available for the cord? The sagittal (critical) diameter of the vertebral canal and the size of the spinal cord differ significantly among individuals. Thus, the relative size of the vertebral canal and spinal cord is of great importance, and there are remarkable constitutional differences among individuals. The vertebral canal is narrower in women than in men (Fig. 2–34).

The sagittal diameter is readily measured on standard radiographs, the measurement being the shortest distance between the mid-dorsal surface of a given vertebral body and the ventral aspect of its spinous process in lateral radiographs. The sagittal diameter at the C4–C6 levels varies from 14.2 to 23 mm, with an average of 18.5 mm. An average accepted general figure for the sagittal diameter of C4 to C7 is 17 mm, whereas that for the transverse diameter is 30 mm (measured on AP radiographs as the interpedicular distance). Average sagittal diameter at the C1–C3 levels in adults is 21.4 mm, with a range of 16 to 30 mm. The variation in children differs only by 1 to 2.1 mm (see Chapter 6, *Radiologic Evaluation*).

The average sagittal diameter of the cervical spinal cord varies at different levels. It is 11 mm at C1, 10 mm at C2 and C6, and 9 mm to 7 mm distal to C6. The average transverse diameter of the cord between C4 and C6 is 14 mm, with a range of 10 to 17 mm (Fig. 2–34; see also Fig. 2–33).

In flexion and extension of the neck there is a sliding movement between vertebrae; in extension the posteroinferior margin of the upper vertebral body approximates the arch of the subjacent vertebra and protrudes into the cervical canal, narrowing the sagittal diameter by 1 to 2 mm. The posterior longitudinal ligament and the ligamenta flava are lax in extension, becoming stretched and thinner in flexion. The value for the intradural sagittal diameter is 2 to 3 mm lower in extension than it is in flexion. This, coupled with the fact that the cord is thicker in extension than in flexion, is an important clinical point in that the cord has less play in extension than in flexion (Fig. 2–35).

SPINAL CORD

The cervical enlargement of the spinal cord is thicker by far than the lumbar enlargement; its greatest circumference measures 48 mm at the C6 level. The cervical enlargement extends from C3 to T2; here all the long tracts for trunk and all limbs, ascending and descending, traverse the cord. During development the vertebrae and discs grow faster than the cord, which accounts for the discrepancy between spinal cord and vertebral levels. In the lower cervical spine a given spinous process overlies the cord segment located one below it numerically. For example, the C6 spinous process overlies the C7 cord segment. The usual

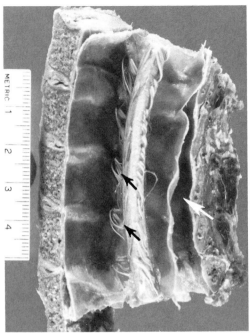

Figure 2–34. A cervical spine opened parasagittally shows the relative cord and canal size, the rootlets exiting the cord (black arrows), large osteoarthritic discal bars (left) and the dura mater, posterior longitudinal ligament, and the capillary subdural space separating the dura from the arachnoid. Also, the epidural space is seen on the right, with veins and areolar and fatty tissue. The internal venous plexuses cushion the cord from moving laminae (white arrow).

length of a cervical neuromere, the hypothetical cord segment, is 13 mm (Fig. 2–36). With increasing age the vertebra and discs lose height because the cord lengthens relative to the vertebral canal. In cervical osteoarthritis a cord segment and its emerging roots may be at the same level as the corresponding disc. The roots may thus have sharp angulations in their exit through the foramina (Fig. 2–37).

THE MENINGES

The dura, firmly attached only to the foramen magnum and the dorsal surfaces of the second and third vertebral bodies, is thrown into accordion-like transverse folds on extension of the neck, with bulging into the vertebral canal between the arches. In neck flexion the dura smooths out as the slack is taken up, and the dentate ligaments suspend the cord. The ligaments are thickenings of the pia mater between the anterior and posterior roots, and they attach firmly to the cord and laterally to the dural sheath itself by teethlike processes. The ligaments may be delicate tissue slips or tough and coarse fibrous structures. The physical properties of the liga-

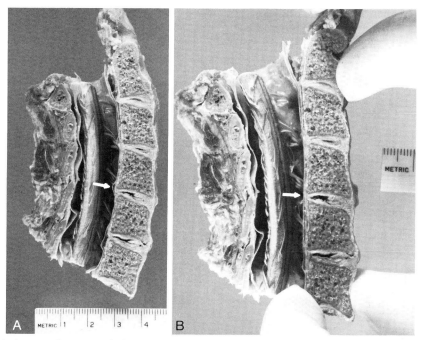

Figure 2–35. *A,* A cervical spine in slight extension. The lordosis shows the ligamenta flava posteriorly behind the cord and the dura mater buckling anteriorly into the vertebral canal (white arrow). *B,* With slight, forced flexion, the dura and posterior longitudinal ligament flattens (white arrow), and the ligamenta flava tend to extend, increasing the sagittal diameter.

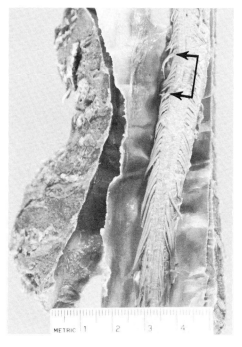

Figure 2–36. A cervical spinal cord with dura mater behind it. The average length of the neuromere and its rootlets (arrows) is 13 mm.

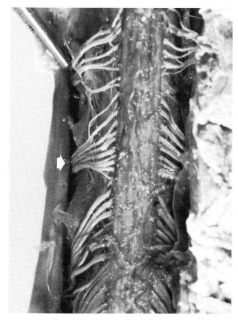

Figure 2–37. A cervical spinal cord, in situ, displays the posterior rootlets, which are fusing to form the root and are entering the spinal cord with increasing obliquity from above downward (arrow).

ments are factors in the pathogenesis of cervical myelopathy. The dentate ligaments, tense in flexion and slack in extension, allow extensive mobility of the cord. They seem to anchor the cord forward in its dural sheath, and the nerve roots themselves anchor the cord and the dural sheath to the vertebral canal (see Figs. 2–33 through 2–37).

THE NERVE ROOTS

The nerve roots are surprisingly short in their intrathecal course, the average length of C7 being 11.6 mm, with a range of 9 to 15 mm. The roots below the C1–C2 level course laterally downward with increasing obliquity the lower the level. As the cord lengthens relative to the spine in aging and in cervical osteoarthritis, the roots may even have to angle upward. Figure 2–34, an antero-oblique section of a cervical spine, shows the intervertebral foramina with the anterior and posterior roots.

The posterior root, comprised of a regular series of rootlets emerging from the dorsolateral sulcus of the cord, is three times thicker than the anterior root (except for C1 and C2) owing to the much greater amount of neural sensory traffic and the consequently greater number of fibers. The anterior root arises from the ventrolateral aspect of the cord by a less regular series of rootlets. The course and obliquity of the upper roots differ from those

of the lower ones—the upper roots often cross two discs, and the lower ones only one (Fig. 2–38).

The roots are invested in pia mater, and at their exit from the spinal canal they enter an outpouching of the dura, funnel-shaped "root pouch," allowing freedom of movement and a smooth transition from vertebral canal to intervertebral foramen (see Fig. 2–38A). At the bottom of the root pouch the posterior and anterior roots separately penetrate the dura and thus have pial and dural root sleeves. The dural sleeves are attached to the bony margin of the intervertebral foramen, with adherence becoming much firmer with age and in clinical osteoarthritis.

In cervical spine extension the root sleeves are slack and folded transversely, separating from the lower border of the pedicle. In flexion they are straightened and smooth and in contact with the inferior and medial margins of the pedicles. In lateral flexion the root sleeves are slack on the concave side and stretched on the convex side.

The root ganglia are quite variable in location, sometimes lying partly in the vertebral canal, or, particularly at the lower cervical levels, lying outside the intervertebral foramen in the gutter (gargoyle) of the transverse process, in close proximity to the vertebral artery. Beyond the ganglion, the two roots merge to form the composite spinal nerve with its anterior and posterior primary rami (divisions), each with contribution from both an-

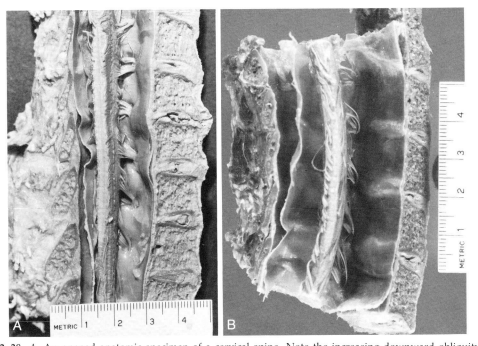

Figure 2–38. *A,* An opened anatomic specimen of a cervical spine. Note the increasing downward obliquity as the nerve roots enter the dural root sleeves. *B,* A lateral view of the opened spine with discal bar osteophytes, shortening of the spine, anterior and posterior rootlets leaving the cord, and the anterior and posterior roots entering fibrotic, stiffened dural root sleeves.

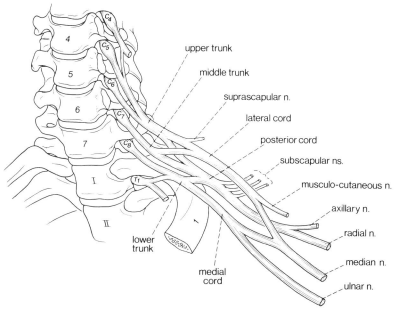

Figure 2–39. Drawing of the brachial plexus, which is made up of C4 through T1 nerve roots, shows trunks, cords, and peripheral nerves to the upper extremity. (From Bland JH, Nakano KK: Neck pain. *In* Kelley, Harris, Ruddy, et al (eds): Textbook of Rheumatology. Philadelphia: W. B. Saunders Co, 1981.)

terior and posterior roots. The posterior rami wind backward to supply skin, fascia, and muscle, C2 and C3 to the occipital nerve and the medial region of the back of the head, and the fourth and fifth vertebrae of the back of the neck. The anterior rami except for C1 and C2 are larger than the posterior and pass forward in close proximity to the vertebral artery. The upper four unite to form the cervical plexus; the lower four with the first thoracic vertebra form the brachial plexus (Fig. 2–39).

The cervical plexus supplies muscular branches to the sternocleidomastoid, the trapezius, and the levator scapulae and scalenus medius muscles; the sensory branches are supplied to the mastoid region, ear, lower cheek (great auricular nerve, C2 and C3), the anterolateral aspect of the neck, and skin above and below the clavicle. The dura in the posterior and lateral walls of the posterior fossa is supplied by C1 and C2. The brachial plexus supplies the upper limbs and most muscles of the shoulder girdle. Corresponding to each cord segment or neuromere is a territory of skin (dermatome), muscle (myotome), and skeleton (sclerotome). The territory is thus considerably larger than is usually clinically considered.

VERTEBRAL ARTERY

The vertebral arteries are inevitably linked with cervical spine syndromes because of their unusually tortuous course, close relationship to cervical nerves and cervical vertebrae, and their potential for causing bizarre and dramatic clinical reflections. The artery is the first branch from the subclavian trunk, proceeding to the transverse foramina of the sixth cervical vertebra. As it passes

through the transverse foramen from C6 to C2, it lies directly in front of the cervical nerves and medial to the intertransverse muscles (Fig. 2–40; see also Fig. 2–30). Accompanying the artery is the vertebral plexus of veins and the sympathetic fibers arising from the inferior (stellate) ganglion. They pass with the artery through the transverse foramen of the atlas, necessitating a sharp deflection outward, a tortuous course around the posterolateral aspect of the superior articular process of the atlas, and lying in the groove on the upper surface of the posterior arch of the atlas. The artery then runs upward through the foramen magnum into the cranial cavity, pierces the arachnoidea, and passes to the lower border of the pons, where it joins the opposite vertebral artery to form the basilar artery. The vertebral arteries give off spinal branches passing into the foramina to supply ligament, dura, and bone and to communicate with the posterior spinal arteries supplying the spinal cord, which are also branches of the vertebral arteries.

At the foramen magnum a branch comes off each vertebral artery to unite into the anterior spinal artery, descending on the anterior surface of the cord. These branches also give off branches (commonly through their posteroinferior cerebellar branches) to form the two posterior spinal arteries supplying the cord. These many vertebral branches supply the entire spinal cord to the level of T4. The vertebrobasilar system also supplies the inner ear, the cerebellum, most of the pons and brain stem, and the posterior portion of the cerebral hemispheres, especially the visual cortex. The vertebral arteries are vulnerable to disease and trauma throughout their course, often resulting in strange and unique clinical syndromes.

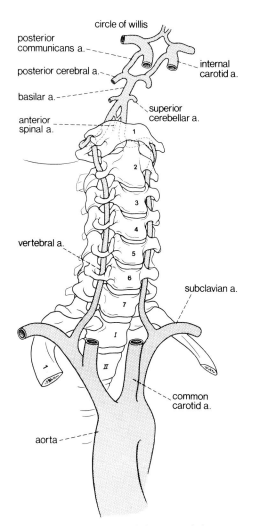

Figure 2–40. An anterolateral drawing of the course of the vertebral artery from C6 to C1 through the bony rings of the foramina transversaria. Note the double U-turn the artery makes from C2 to C1 and the posterior course around the lateral mass of the atlas. (From Bland JH, Nakano KK: Neck pain. *In* Kelley, Harris, Ruddy, et al (eds): Textbook of Rheumatology. Philadelphia: W. B. Saunders Co, 1981.)

Most vertebral arteries are markedly unequal in size; only 8% are equal. The diameter of one, usually the left, may be three times that of the right. One vessel may be congenitally absent (Fig. 2–41).

BLOOD SUPPLY OF CORD AND ROOTS

The blood supply to the cord and roots and its role in cervical myelopathy are controversial. The anterior spinal artery is very small; its direction of flow is usually caudad, and it has tiny penetrating branches entering the cord tissue itself. Circula-

tion may be precarious if continuity is interrupted by external pressure on the cord. Collaterals come into the vessel from the vertebral arteries. The most constant is a large feeder artery on one or both sides at the C6–C7 level, and it may give both ascending and descending branches to the cord. The proximal anterior spinal artery supplies only the upper half of the cord, and the lower half derives its supply from the main cervical radicular feeder. An interruption or reversal of flow is thought to explain cord signs cephalad to the apparent lesion in cervical osteoarthritis (Fig. 2–42).

The paired posterior spinal arteries descend in proximity to the emerging posterior nerve roots. This flow is thought to be caudad. In neck flexion, a disc protrusion may cause compression of the cord, with flattening, blanching, diminished pulsation, and obliteration of venous channels; neck extension or section of the dentate ligaments allows return of color and pulsation. The anterior spinal artery and its intramedullary branches may be thickened in cord changes of vascular insufficiency. Spinal artery thrombosis and myelomalacia have been reported. Cord ischemia may result from frictional damage by osteoarthritic ridges, compression of radicular branches in the intervertebral foramina, or atheromata, which are commonly found in these vessels. Vascular lesions may be transient or permanent, and the vulnerability is related to magnitude and location of osteoarthritic or traumatic lesions and anatomic peculiarities. Occlusion of the anterior spinal artery may produce ischemic change several segments below the level of vascular obstruction.

AUTONOMIC NERVOUS SYSTEM

The autonomic nervous system is connected to the central nervous system by afferent and efferent nerve fiber systems. It is concerned with regulation of all autonomic function, which involves the maintenance and regulation of the internal environment of the body and its stability. It is divided into two systems, sympathetic and parasympathetic. The parasympathetic system is connected with the central nervous system in the cervical area through the facial, glossopharyngeal, oculomotor, and vagus nerves.

The sympathetic nervous system arises in the mediolateral gray matter of the base of the anterior horns of the spinal cord from C4 through C8. The fibers of both parasympathetic and sympathetic systems run side by side in the same structures; a harmonious interaction of the fibers maintains a balance, though they are capable of antagonistic effects in pathologic states. Sympathetic fibers secrete epinephrine-like substances and are hence known as adrenergic fibers. Parasympathetic fibers secrete acetylcholine and are known as cholinergic fibers. The two systems respond differently to various drugs. The autonomic nervous

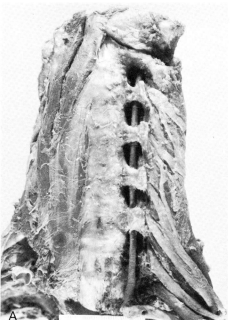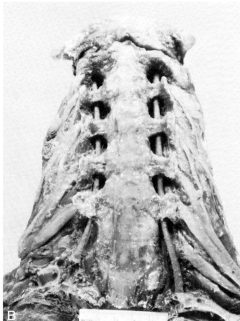

Figure 2–41. *A,* A close-up anterior view of dissection of the left vertebral artery. *B,* Note that the left vertebral artery (viewer's right) is clearly larger in caliber than the right artery (viewer's left).

system is not separate from but integral to the somatic and visceral peripheral nervous systems and the central nervous system.

The sympathetic nervous system is clearly involved in several cervical spine syndromes, notably the radiculopathies. The cervical nerves are connected with the sympathetic nervous system through the white rami communicantes of the upper two thoracic nerves, which join the sympathetic trunk through their anterior primary rami and proceed upward to the cervical ganglia. Postganglionic fibers, or gray rami communicantes, pass from the cervical ganglia to the anterior primary rami of the cervical nerve. The impulses are distributed with the divisions of the nerves. Other gray rami communications pass to most of the cranial nerves and peripheral branches to the pharynx, the heart, and the arteries of the head, neck, and arm.

Sympathetic cell bodies have been identified in the cervical portion of the spinal cord located in the mediolateral gray matter of the base of the anterior horns from C4 through C8. Preganglionic sympathetic fibers leave the spinal cord with somatic motor nerve fibers in the ventral roots of C5 through T1. Certain preganglionic neurons form a synaptic connection with postganglionic neurons in the small ganglia of the deep sympathetic chain. Other preganglionic neurons subverse the deep chain of small sympathetic ganglia in the foramina transversaria and join the sinuvertebral nerve by which they reach the cervicothoracic group. The deep chain is a seemingly tangled web

of sympathetic fibers, or macroscopically visible ganglia. It ascends along the posterior aspect of the vertebral artery from the C7 to the C4 level.

Classic sympathetic trunk in the cervical area comprises the superior, middle, and inferior ganglia connected by intervening cords. Motor branches supply the viscera of the neck and chest, and afferent branches form the vertebral nerve. The superior cervical ganglion has communicating rami with the ninth and twelfth cranial nerves. Gray rami communicantes join the anterior rami of the upper four cervical nerves. The internal carotid nerve passes upward with the artery to form the internal carotid plexus, and pharyngeal branches pass to the side of the pharynx communicating with the superior laryngeal nerve and join the pharyngeal plexus.

The fifth cervical spinal nerve root carries sympathetic fibers, joining the carotid plexus, and sympathetic innervation to the arteries of the head and neck. The sixth root carries sympathetic fibers to the subclavian artery and the brachial plexus. The seventh root has fibers reaching the cardioaortic plexus and subclavian and axillary arteries as well as the phrenic nerves.

Sympathetic fibers surrounding the internal carotid arteries give branches to the posterior orbit, orbital muscles, dilator muscles of the pupils, and smooth muscle of upper eyelid. Those surrounding the vertebral arteries and the basilar artery within the cranium reach the vestibular portion of the ear.

The right and left vertebral arteries and their

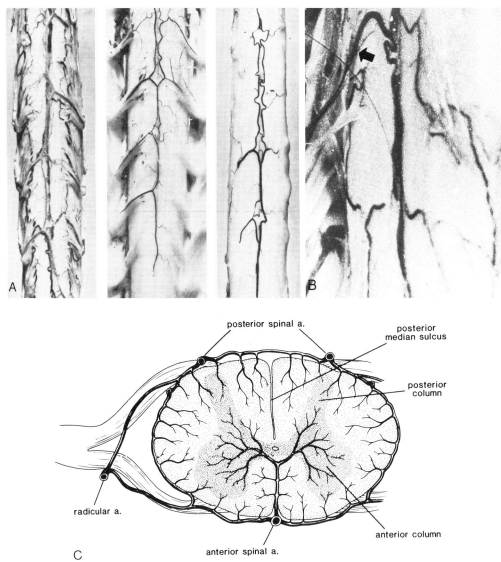

Figure 2–42. *A,* Anatomic specimen of the cervical spinal cord shows the anterior spinal artery, which is actually a longitudinal anastomotic chain formed by the division of the anterior radicular arteries near the midline into ascending and descending branches. These vessels arise from the vertebral, lumbar, and intercostal arteries, are variable in number, and enter the spinal canal through the intervertebral foramina. In the specimen on the left (dark vessels are veins) the arteries were injected, showing anterior radicular vessels at C4, C5, and C8 on the left and, on the right, at C6 and C7 only. A filter was used to make the photographs in the center and on the right so that veins would not be visible. Variability of the arterial pattern is apparent. (From: Payne EE, Spillane JD: The cervical spine: an anatomical-pathological study of 70 specimens [using a special technique] with particular reference to the problem of cervical spondylosis. Brain 80:571, 1957. Courtesy of Oxford University Press.) *B,* A close-up of an anterior spinal artery showing the radicular arterial "feeders" and the spinal nerve rootlets (arrow). *C,* A cross-sectional drawing of the cervical spinal cord illustrates its blood supply. On the left is a radicular "feeder" artery (from the vertebral artery), and the anterior and posterior spinal arteries are shown. Note that the arteries are end-arteries, without real anastomoses in the substance of the cord, enhancing the possibility of cord infarction. The anterior spinal artery and the illustrated anastomotic pial branching arteries supply about three fourths of the spinal cord tissue.

derivatives supply the cervical spine meninges, spinal cord, nerves, all plexuses, the contents of the posterior cranial fossa, and the visual cortex. The vertebral artery, supported in rigid, bony rings in the transverse processes, changes course from axis to atlas and then from atlas to the posterior cranial fossa, where the two vertebral arteries become the basilar artery. Inevitably the vertebral artery is moved with every movement of the spine and head. Shortening of the cervical spine caused by damage to discs and distortion of zygapophyseal joints leads to tortuosity and compression of the artery even in the absence of osteoarthritis surrounding it or atherosclerosis in its wall. There is a clear, "normal" reduction of the effective lumen of the vessel, particularly on rotation of the head. Cerebral circulation may be reduced to the point of syncope. The risk of reduction of supply of blood to cord and brain is increased not only because of the decreased lumen of the vertebral artery but also because of changes in bone and joint surrounding it, aggravating the distortion of the articular and radicular branches of the vertebral artery.

When the sympathetic nervous system in the cervical area is stimulated, clinical manifestations occur, including sudomotor, pilomotor, and vasomotor symptoms and signs, vertigo, blurred vision, tinnitus, deafness, pharyngeal and laryngeal paresthesias, paresthesia of shoulders, arms, hands, senses of heat and cold, tremor, tachycardia, and increase in rate and depth of respiration.

Thus many symptoms and clinical findings of cervical nerve root irritation are difficult to understand unless one evokes the autonomic nervous system mechanisms here described. The close association of the parasympathetic to the sympathetic nervous system makes it necessary that one understand the functions of both systems in the production of pain and the changes that occur as a result of nerve root compressions.

Pain-conducting afferent spinal nerve fibers from the blood vessels of the head, neck, and upper extremities traverse the sympathetic trunk. Postganglionic fibers communicate with recurrent spinal meningeal nerves before these nerves pass through the intervertebral foramina to supply the dura and ligamentous structures.

VENOUS DRAINAGE OF THE CERVICAL SPINE

Strangely, the venous drainage of the spinal cord does not mirror the arterial system except in the white matter, where drainage occurs circumferentially into the anterior spinal vein. The gray matter has a separate system, draining upward from the C1–C2 level. The two halves of the gray matter have discrete systems.

Veins of the cervical vertebral column have a continuous series of plexuses in the extradural space. The importance of this plexus in the spread of malignant disease has long been known through Batson's study of veins now named for him. The plexus communicates directly at every level with the vena cava and vena azygos systems. Most drainage of the cervical spine is to the confluence of sinuses at the basiocciput rather than to the segmental veins. Vertebral venography has been used in recent years as a diagnostic aid. It is safer in investigation of the cervical spine than arteriography.[7]

In recent years the importance of abnormalities of blood supply in disease of the cervical spine has been identified. Investigation is difficult because of the hazards of invasive radiologic study. Animals have been used extensively as experimental models.

MUSCLES

A high degree of finely coordinated muscle balance is required to support and move the head and neck. This is accomplished by paired lateral groups of muscles attached to the skull and the spinous and transverse processes. Converging deep cervical muscles ascend in front of the spine to be inserted in the midline to the vertebral bodies and to the anterior arch of the atlas. These muscles operating with the sternomastoids and the anterior neck muscles help resist any sudden or accidental backward movement of the skull. The spinous process of the second cervical vertebra is much larger than those immediately below that vertebra. From the axial spinous process and its neural arch, the various deep suboccipital muscles fan outward beneath the skull to be inserted in the occiput. These serve to balance the skull on the upper end of the spine. More superficially the semispinalis group arising from the spine and attached to the occiput constitutes the thick mass of muscle tissue at the back of the neck.

References

1. Brieg A: Biomechanics of the Central Nervous System. Chicago: Year Book Medical Publishers, 1960.
2. Brieg A, Turnbull IM, Hassler O: Effects of mechanical stresses in the spinal cord in cervical spondylosis. J Neurosurg 25:45, 1966.
3. Ehrenhaft JL: Development of the vertebral column as related to certain congenital and pathological changes. Surg Gynecol Obstet 76:282, 1943.
4. Ganguly DN, Roy KKS: A study on the craniovertebral joint in man. Anat Anz 114:433, 1964.
5. Levick JR: Joint pressure-volume studies; their importance, design and interpretation. J Rheumatol 10:353, 1983.
6. Levick JR: An investigation into the validity of subatmospheric pressure recordings from synovial fluid and their dependence on joint angle. J Physiol 289:55, 1979.
7. Batson OV: The vertebral vein system. AJR 78:195, 1957.

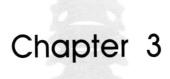

Chapter 3

Pathology

written in collaboration with
Professor Dallas Richard Boushey

The pathologic study of tissues in the cervical spine has not attracted the attention of investigators as much as the study of most other organs and tissues. Until recent years, the problem of obtaining whole specimens of human cervical spine precluded study in depth. In fact, morbid anatomy and gross and microscopic pathology in the field of rheumatology have all taken a back seat to immunology. With the rediscovery of rheumatoid factor in 1948 (Dr. Russell Cecil actually discovered it in 1927), modern rheumatology received an enormous impetus, and the greatest emphasis quickly became that of the immunologic implications in the relatively rare inflammatory arthritides. Rheumatology seemingly sprang fully formed into the modern world of molecular biology to the detriment of the more gradual development of clinical rheumatology, joint physiology, and gross and microscopic pathology. The essential process of scientific reductionism did not occur. Investigators catapulted from purely clinical researchers to supersophisticated molecular biologists, leaving basic joint and general connective tissue physiology—the study of the normal state—to the very few. Unfortunately, in rheumatology much of basic joint physiology is not applied in practical diagnosis and management, nor is the underlying pathology in the rheumatic diseases sufficiently appreciated and woven into modern research, practice, and education.

The cervical spine has been particularly neglected. The goal of this chapter is to present the morbid anatomy and gross and microscopic pathology of the cervical spine relative to three diseases—osteoarthritis, rheumatoid arthritis, and ankylosing spondylitis. Though there are many other diseases and disorders involving the cervical spine, the available pathology of these three diseases serves well as a background for the others. At the University of Vermont, the Rheumatology and Clinical Immunology Unit has long been involved in the study of the cervical spine, and the data here presented are based on anatomic, radiologic, pathologic, and clinical studies on 16 whole human cervical spines from patients with rheumatoid arthritis and 130 whole human cervical spines from patients with osteoarthritis of the cervical spine. The discussion is limited to pathologic characteristics in the cervical spine.

OSTEOARTHRITIS OF THE CERVICAL SPINE

Osteoarthritis is a common, almost universal disorder in vertebrate animals. It is a presumably slowly yet sometimes rapidly progressive disorder that occurs in mid- to late life and affects the movable joints, particularly weight-bearing joints. Clinical characteristics are pain, deformity, limitation of motion, and functional loss. Reversal or even arrest of the process is rarely considered. Histologic changes are focal, erosive lesions of the surface of hyaline cartilage; mitosis and formation of chondrocyte clones, with an increase in DNA–RNA turnover; increased synthesis of type II collagen and proteoglycan; and increased density of subchondral bone, with consequent microfractures and extensive remodeling of the entire ends of the bones, marginal osteophytes, and subarticular bone cysts. All intra-articular and periarticular connective tissues are ultimately involved.

Since Hippocrates' day it has been thought that articular cartilage that is injured or involved by disease has no capacity for repair. Interestingly, though, there was a period during the 18th and 19th centuries (when there was no cell biology or, indeed, little science) when thoughtful clinicians and investigators thought that joint healing could occur. William Hunter in 1743 discussed healing of articular cartilage,[1] as did Joseph Leidy in 1849;[2] in 1851 Peter Redfern's paper was titled, "On the Healing of Wounds in Articular Cartilage"[3]. James Paget in 1853 delivered a series of lectures on the healing of cartilage,[4] and Redfern[5] again wrote on the interrelationships of connective tissues in and about the joints in the healing process. Alexander Ogston, a surgeon, also presented evidence concerning healing of articular cartilage.[6] As recently as 1931 Shands[7] wrote extensively on the regeneration of hyaline cartilage in joints.

The evidence for healing of joints (in particular hyaline cartilage) presented by these giants of medicine was ignored until 1962, when a series of publications began to appear, again taking up the question of the regeneration and healing of these tissues.[8-14] Thus, the literature on reversibility of cartilage injury goes back more than 240 years. This literature is scarcely mentioned in the bibliographies of the most current writers and investigators on the subject. Could the potential for healing of joints, in particular hyaline cartilage, have been hiding in plain slight for all these years?

Theories of Initial Events in Osteoarthritis

Although there remains controversy as to whether articular cartilage can heal, there is uniform agreement that a first event, by whatever mechanism, at a molecular level is a decrease in the concentration of proteoglycan of hyaline cartilage. There is further general agreement that whatever the initial event is, two pathologic processes characterize osteoarthritis: (1) loss and ultimate ulceration of the bearing surface of the joint, and (2) proliferation and hypertrophy of new bone, cartilage, ligaments, tendons, and capsular tissues about the joint—most grossly, osteophytosis. Sokoloff[13] has described three separate general concepts of the sequential development of osteoarthritis: (1) A degeneration of articular cartilage occurs that leads to denudation of the joint surface. This is inconsistent with the fact that there is extensive bony remodeling; osteoarthritis occurs only rarely without remodeling, that is, it occurs only rarely with definite unrelated preceding inflammation or metabolic or genetic peculiarity in which mechanical abnormalities are primarily absent. (2) Fibrillation of the cartilage occurs, leading to secondary remodeling of the periarticular structures, particularly bony components. This view is the most widely accepted. There is little agreement as to which specific morphologic event precedes the others in sorting through the complicated changes observed in histologic sections. (3) Osteoarthritis begins because of changes in the stiffness of subchondral bone and is primarily due to increased stiffening of subchondral bone, with changes in cartilage occurring secondarily. The remodeling of the hyaline cartilage is not well explained by this formulation.

Fibrillation cannot be readily dissociated from remodeling of the bony tissues even in the earliest stages. Thus, the extensive remodeling of osteoarthritis (according to Wolff's law) results in alteration of both internal and external architecture of the tissues in and about the joint and implies that the removal of tissue is going on in tandem with the laying down of new tissue elsewhere. It seems that all tissues are in the process of remodeling but, more specifically, articular cartilage and bone; perhaps we should not make any intellectual effort to separate the various processes.

Morbid Anatomy of Osteoarthritis

The manifestation of osteoarthritis of the cervical spine differs slightly from that of osteoarthritis occurring elsewhere. First, some anatomic peculiarities of the cervical spine do make it somewhat different. In a study of 130 whole human cervical spines,[15] it was noted that virtually all of the joints of Luschka and the zygapophyseal joints in the cervical spine have meniscus-like structures, fibrofatty in nature, that have the capability of proliferation. The formation of pannus-like structures in these joints was also noted. Second, the grossly movable joints of the cervical spine have relatively little repetitive, impulsive loading in that their planes of articulation are at an angle of 35 to 45 degrees and their principal function is that of gliding and sliding on one another, permitting the extreme mobility of the cervical spine. Careful search disclosed no anatomic evidence of the ultimate occurrence of eburnation, as occurs elsewhere, in any of the joints of the cervical spine, particularly in the weight-bearing joints.

Figure 3–1 illustrates examples of the meniscus-like structures. Part *A* shows the normal anatomic structure, part *B* the proliferating meniscus over the surface, and part *C* the more gross pannus-like proliferation with loss of cartilage and joint space. Figure 3–2 illustrates the histologic features of the proliferating pannus. Both parts were taken from apophyseal joints of cervical spines in which prolonged immobilization by means of a cervical collar had been used therapeutically.

It is not possible to separate a single abnormality of the tissues of the joint in osteoarthritis of the cervical spine that is not associated with all of the manifestations described subsequently.

Changes in Cartilage. An initial, unidentified, widely variable event seems to trigger the cell and tissue changes in cartilage; these changes proceed simultaneously. The earliest identifiable morphologic change is a breaking up of the collagen net, especially at the surface of the joint. A velvet-like, shaggy, fissure-like change occurs, broadly known as fibrillation. Cartilage softening, or chondromalacia, occurs over the whole surface. Specific staining discloses a decrease in the concentration of proteoglycan in the hyaline cartilage of the zygapophyseal joint. These changes are securely

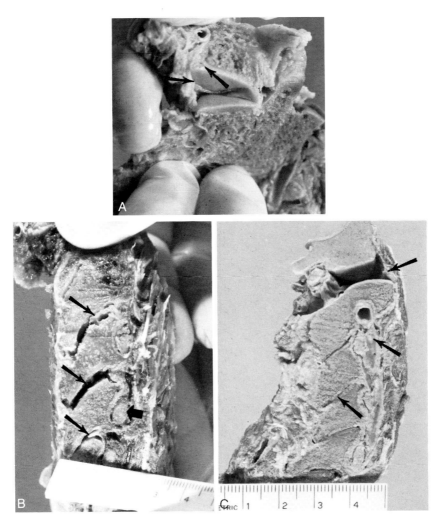

Figure 3–1. *A,* Zygapophyseal joint, atlantoaxial, showing fibrofatty meniscus-like structures (arrows). *B,* Three zygapophyseal joints. Upper joint shows proliferating meniscus of fibrofatty tissue, a pannus (upper arrow, left). Middle arrow (left) shows a zygapophyseal joint with erosions and loss of cartilage. Lowest arrow (left) points to fibrofatty meniscus. Thick, short arrow (right) points to the nerve root in the intervertebral foramen. *C,* Note loss of cartilage and obliteration of the joint space (lower arrow). The vertebral artery is shown in longitudinal section on the right (middle arrow), and the atlantoaxial joint is open above showing its fibrofatty meniscus (upper arrow).

secondary to a decrease in the amount of proteoglycan synthesized or are due to enzymatic depolymerization of the giant proteoglycan macromolecule or both. The first histologic change is a break in the very thin surface over the load-bearing hyaline cartilage, with resultant small ulcerations, erosions, flaking, and "pitting." These areas gradually enlarge, and the fissures at first tend to be tangential to the surface, later turning downward in a vertical direction, and ultimately penetrate to the subchondral bone. Chondrocytes, like central nervous system cells, and myocardial and skeletal muscle fibers do not display mitotic replication in the normal state. In osteoarthritis of the cervical spine these cells mitose, developing so-called brood capsules, which are clearly newly

proliferated clones. They are larely confined to areas of fibrillation or loosely textured matrix, and they tend to cluster around the margins of the clefts and fissures. Occasionally cell damage and focal cell necrosis is seen, but this is uncommon. A further interesting lesion in the cervical spine (as elsewhere) is the joint mouse, a tiny nidus of osteoarticular tissue that is detached from the joint surface into the synovial cavity. The bone loses viability, but the cartilage, not requiring a blood supply, gives rise to new cartilage arranged concentrically in synthetic layers about the nidus and within the synovial joint space.

The careful and astute pathologist will note evidence (as in inflammatory processes anywhere else) not only of inflammation but also of simul-

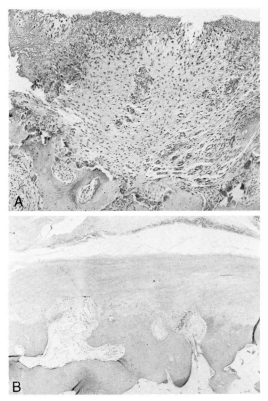

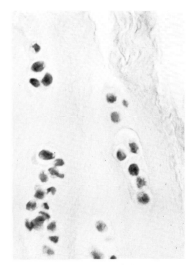

Figure 3–3. Note the clusters of chondrocytes in their lacunae. These chondrocyte clones represent mitosis from a single cell. There is increased DNA–RNA turnover and increased synthesis of proteoglycan and type II collagen. (From Sokoloff L: Pathology and pathogenesis of osteoarthritis. *In* Arthritis and Allied Conditions, 9th ed. Edited by DJ McCarty. Philadelphia: Lea & Febiger, 1979.)

Figure 3–2. *A,* Histologic section from zygapophyseal joint of patient with severe osteoarthritis. Note bony destruction below. Pannus has become very cellular and has active angiogenesis in process; note a more fibrous center area. *B,* Histologic sections from zygapophyseal joint in osteoarthritis. Pannus is more purely fibrotic but is proliferating over and destroying the cartilage surface.

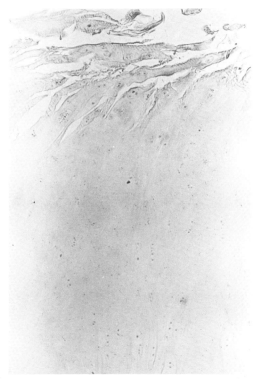

taneous healing or reparative processes, both in cells and matrix. The matrix shows a kind of disorderly reparative collagen appearing, synthesized by the chondrocytic clone. The macromolecules of reparative cartilage may come from the chondrocytes themselves, that is, intrinsic repair. Repair may also come from tissues outside the cartilage by metaplasia, synovial membrane, subchondral bone, or marrow cells that make their way through microfractures in the subchondral bone to reach the cartilage and proceed with synthesis of cartilaginous macromolecules. Both intrinsic and extrinsic reparative cartilage is usually seen. Grossly, this reparative cartilage appears as an irregular cobblestone layer of cartilage over the surface. Figure 3–3 depicts the chondrocyte clone as previously described. Figure 3–4 illustrates the early lesions on the surface of the cartilage—fissuring, small erosions progressing to larger erosions, and breaks in the continuity of the surface. The fissures soon tend to turn downward rather than remaining tangential to the surface. Figure 3–5, a gross specimen of a zyga-

Figure 3–4. The hyaline cartilage surface in osteoarthritis illustrates fibrillation, fissuring, cloning, and the turning of tangential fibrillation down to a vertical orientation, finally to penetrate to the subchondral bone. (From Sokoloff L: Pathology and pathogenesis of osteoarthritis. *In* Arthritis and Allied Conditions, 9th ed. Edited by DJ McCarty. Philadelphia: Lea & Febiger, 1979.)

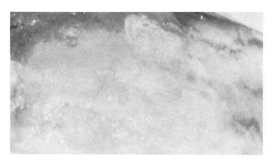

Figure 3–5. Cartilage surface of cervical zygapophyseal joint shows gross reparative cartilage surface, irregularities, and cobblestone appearance of the layering of new cartilage.

pophyseal joint surface, shows the cobblestone appearance of the layers of reparative cartilage.

Changes in Bone. As noted above, when any change occurs in and around the joint, all tissues are involved in the process, that is, osteoarthritis in the cervical spine, as elsewhere, is a disease not only of articular cartilage but also of bone, synovium, capsule, ligament, tendon, and even muscle.

While the hyaline cartilage is undergoing fibrillation and gradual diminution in thickness, the subchondral bone increases in density and proliferates, and microfractures occur resulting in and following callus formation. This bone undergoes focal pressure necrosis at its superficial layer as the microfractures occur. The increased density of subchondral bone is reflected in the radiographic changes. Figure 3–6 illustrates the increase in the density of subchondral bone in the intervertebral disc. Figure 3–7 shows increased density of subchondral bone in zygapophyseal and Luschka joints. New bone formations (osteophytes) also occur at the margins of the articular cartilage. These osteophytes really are a mixture of connective tissues, including a coating of fibrocartilage and islands of fibrocartilage and hyaline cartilage—even some tendon-like material may appear. Osteophytes show two patterns of growth: one is protrusion into the joint space, and the other is development just within capsular and ligamentous insertions into bone at the joint margin. The direction of osteophytic growth is a function of the lines of mechanical force exerted on the area of growth.

Osteophytic bone follows the contour of the joint surface from which the osteophyte springs. Bone of these osteophytes merges imperceptibly with other cortical and cancellous bone of the joint but is clearly not true bone alone. The layer of coating is both hyaline cartilage and fibrocartilage and is continuous with the adjacent synovial lining. Some authors believe the osteophytes are formed by metaplastic synovial cells. The rapid proliferation of subchondral bone will be most

evident in areas where the cartilaginous covering has been largely, if not entirely, removed.

Although it has been seen in cases of osteoarthritis in locations other than the cervical spine, the appearance of a glistening, very hard, ivory-like, polished surface—eburnation—was not seen anywhere in the cervical spine. Most of the osteoblasts in the eburnated surface elsewhere become necrotic and die, as noted by empty lacunae.

Cystic areas of rarefaction in the bone are common in osteoarthritis of most weight-bearing or very actively used joints but are rare in the cervical spine. These subchondral cysts represent diffusion of synovial fluid into the subchondral bone marrow, with a reactive response forming an "eggshell" of a cyst filled with debris. Rarely, cysts may appear in locations other than the cervical spine, and they are radiographically demonstrable before there is narrowing of the joint space or evidence of cartilage loss. In the rare instances in which we saw subchondral cysts, they were filled with debris, and trabeculae had undergone fibromyxoid degeneration. Fragments of dead bone, bits of cartilage, and amorphous debris are distributed within and around the cysts. Figure 3–8 illustrates the loss of cartilage, increased density of subchondral bone, and cyst formation in marrow space bone of a zygapophyseal joint in the cervical spine.

Changes in Synovial Membrane. As the cartilage and bone develop the changes described, the joint space collects increasing amounts of debris.

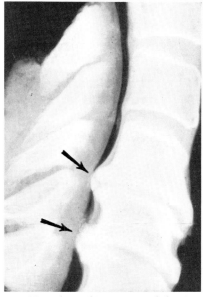

Figure 3–6. Note the striking increased density of subchondral bone in the lower two intervertebral disc spaces as compared with the density of subchondral bone in the two normal discs above. Note that there is spinal cord compression at the level of the large posterior osteophytes (arrows).

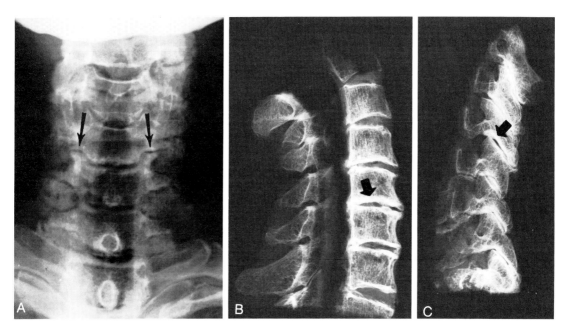

Figure 3–7. *A,* Note Luschka joints (arrows) showing gross involvement by osteoarthritis, marked increased density of subchondral bone, flattening, joint space narrowing, and joint destruction. Compare with the Luschka joints above those described. *B,* Anatomic specimen shows gross increased density of most vertebral end plates, especially as noted by arrows. *C,* Anatomic specimen shows sagittal view of zygapophyseal joints. Note the narrowing and irregularity of joint spaces and the striking increased density of the subchondral bone (arrow).

A polymorphonuclear response, that is, a phagocytic reaction of polymorphonuclear cells, follows, and the phagocytic synovial cells ingest the debris and digest it while the synovial membrane becomes very hypertrophic and hyperplastic. When the osteoarthritis is very active, a pannus-like lesion develops, reminiscent of rheumatoid ar-

thritis pannus but not having the same degree of intensity of cellular infiltration in the synovium (Fig. 3–9). Nevertheless, this osteoarthritic pannus can be quite aggressive, synthesizing and secret-

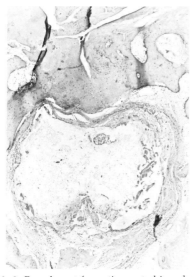

Figure 3–8. Pseudocyst formation noted in subchondral bone of zygapophyseal joint.

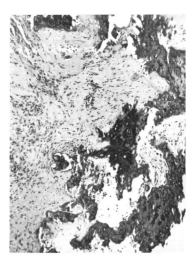

Figure 3–9. Synovial membrane proliferating pannus from osteoarthritic zygapophyseal joint, reminiscent of the pannus of rheumatoid arthritis. Bone destruction is in process. Note that pannus has been shown to produce large amounts of the enzyme collagenase in the course of osteoarthritis, thus destroying bone and other connective tissues.

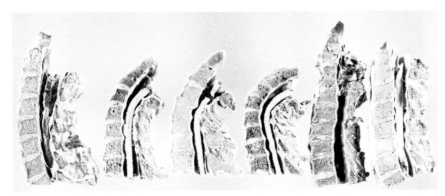

Figure 3–10. From left to right, a series of six sagittal sections of cervical spines illustrate gross changes that occur with increasing age and progressively greater intensity of the osteoarthritic process. Note the normal 24-year-old spine on the left. From left to right the increasing lordosis finally becomes straight, and on the far right (age 88) there is slight reverse lordosis. Note increasing osteophytosis, extensive remodeling, actual increasing bone volume in the vertebrae, spinal cord compression, narrowing and deformity of the disc spaces, large clefts in all the discs, and several fixed subluxations.

ing collagenase and prostaglandin. With increase in volume, hypertrophy, and hyperplasia of the synovial membrane, angiogenesis occurs, and capillary proliferation may be quite marked. When synovial tissue extends into the joint cavity like a pannus, it is traumatized between the surfaces, and micro- as well as macrobleeding occurs in the joint, with consequent hemosiderin staining of the synovial membrane and the appearance of an orange-brown color.

Normal synovial membrane carries out the proper nutrition for articular cartilage. The chronically inflamed, scarred synovial membrane of osteoarthritis loses this function, accelerating the chronicity of the osteoarthritic process.

Changes in the Joints as a Whole. The entire conformation of the cervical spine changes clinically, radiographically, anatomically, and histologically, as the overall process alters virtually all tissues of the spine. Figure 3–10 illustrates the changes that occur grossly with increasing cervical osteoarthritis and increasing age. With bony hypertrophy, hyperplasia, loss of cartilage surface, and increased density of subchondral bone, the base of the cervical spine and the lower vertebrae increase in volume; intervertebral disc spaces diminish; the joints of Luschka have osteophytic projections, as do the zygapophyseal joints. Synovial hyperplasia and the inflammatory component gradually increase. Figure 3–11 illustrates the gross cervical spine alterations. Figure 3–12 shows changes in the Luschka joints, including flattening, a marked increase in osteophytosis, subchondral bone density, and a limitation of gliding capability. Figure 3–13 illustrates the zygapophyseal joint changes with compromise of overall cervical spine mobility. So-called spondylotic bars occur on the posterior cervical spine surface owing to proliferation and hypertrophy of the posterior longitudinal ligament—the same type of osteo-

phyte occurs anteriorly. Hypertrophy of the ligamentum flavum posteriorly causes protrusions or "bars" into the spinal canal, often compressing the posterior spinal cord. Figure 3–14 illustrates

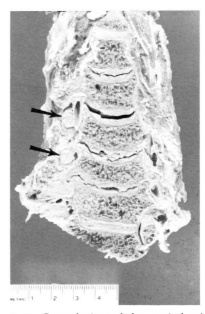

Figure 3–11. Coronal view of the cervical spine. All vertebrae have become extensively remodeled and widened from above down, and all intervertebral disc spaces have gross clefts extending from one Luschka joint to its counterpart on the opposite side (a universal finding). Disc spaces are narrow and deformed owing to the vacuum effect, which is usually seen by x-ray and suggests subatmospheric pressures on the clefts, and osteophytes are extensive. Subchondral bone is markedly increased in both thickness and density. Note the vertebral arteries on both sides (short area of coronal section of artery) and the nerve roots emerging lateral to the arteries (arrows).

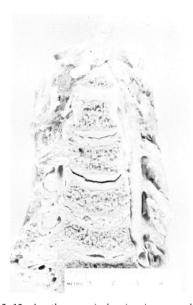

Figure 3–12. Another cervical spine in coronal section shows Luschka joint osteoarthritis almost throughout, with clefting connecting the two joints, and severe osteophytes and destruction of the joints. Note a dissection of the vertebral artery on the right, with extensive fibrous adhesions arising from both the Luschka and the zygapophyseal joints, which are normally in contact with the vertebral artery as it passes the intervertebral foramen.

posterior osteophytes and osteoarthritic bars along with anterior osteophytes. In this sagittal section, the vertebral artery is shown. Osteophytes from the zygapophyseal joints, those from the joints of Luschka, as well as vertebral osteophytes may compress the vertebral artery, interfering with brain stem and posterior fossa circulation. Figure 3–15 illustrates grossly hypertrophied ligamenta flava, with compression of the posterior spinal cord. Figure 3–16 illustrates a partial coronal section of an opened cervical spine, showing the posterior nerve roots as they exit through the dural root sleeves, and extremely severe osteoarthritic bars from the posterior spine leaving compressions on the anterior spinal cord. To the left of this illustration are seen four grossly hypertrophied ligamenta flava, which also compressed the posterior spinal cord.

An anatomic generality in osteoarthritis of the cervical spine is that there is clearly the greatest emphasis on intervertebral disc osteoarthritis in the lower three intervertebral disc spaces, C4–C5, C5–C6, and C6–C7. The joints of Luschka are maximally involved at the C2–C3 and C3–C4 levels, with overlaps at all three levels.[15] The basic process in the intervertebral disc is remarkably similar to that of any other joints, that is, the nucleus pulposus is fissured and deformed, the hyaline cartilage vertebral plates develop fibrillation, chondrocyte cloning occurs, and there is

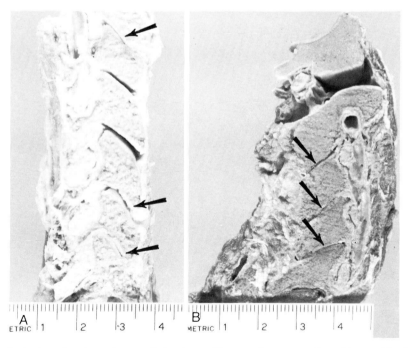

Figure 3–13. *A*, Sagittal section through a cervical spine to illustrate the zygapophyseal joints. The lower joints are grossly involved, as is the top joint in the specimen (arrows). *B*, A more involved group of zygapophyseal cervical joints (arrows).

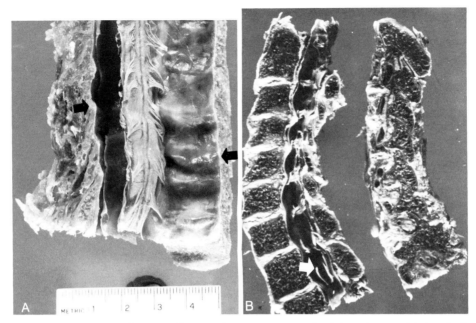

Figure 3–14. *A,* An opened cervical spine to illustrate the massive osteoarthritic bars (arrow, right) at the level of the intervertebral discs, with hypertrophy and hyperplasia of all tissue, nerve root compression as the nerve roots enter the dural root sleeves, and frequent anterior spinal artery compression (see center, spinal cord). On the left are markedly hypertrophied ligamenta flava bulging into the spinal canal, compressing the posterior spinal cord (arrow, left). *B,* Sagittal section of a whole cervical spine with the spinal cord removed. Note at all levels the posterior protruding bars and uniformly narrow, degenerated discs (there were visible spinal cord compressions at all levels). The anterior and posterior spinal nerve roots, cut from the cord, are also visible (arrow).

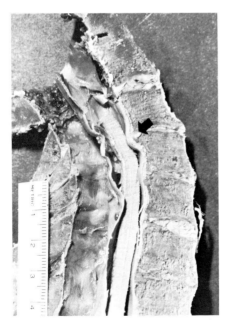

Figure 3–15. Sagittal section of opened cervical spine shows massive ligamentum flavum hypertrophy with posterior cord compression (left). A localized posterior osteophyte, osteoarthritic discal bar, compresses the anterior cord (see arrow, right). Note all discs are severely involved, and some are completely destroyed.

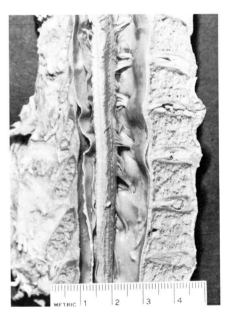

Figure 3–16. Partial coronal section shows the nerve roots as they enter the dural root sleeves. Note the upper roots are entering at an angle above the horizontal plane, whereas the lower roots enter with increasing obliquity from above down, a consequence of the loss of cervical spine height due to extensive disc destruction. Note vertebral remodeling, clefts and narrow disc spaces, and osteoarthritic bars.

increased density of subchondral bone, with fewer formations of pseudocysts than elsewhere. Sclerosis of the subchondral plate also develops. These processes are readily identifiable in the zygapophyseal and Luschka joints.

Osteoarthritis in the cervical spine does not characteristically proceed to ankylosis. Nevertheless, a related condition, diffuse idiopathic skeletal hyperostosis, or the ankylosing vertebral hyperostosis of Forestier and Rotés-Querol, though having few characteristics of osteoarthritis, is thought by some authors to be related in some obscure way. This condition manifests itself in the cervical spine, though more often in the thoracic portion and less so in the lumbar spine. Another related disorder of the cervical spine has been titled physiologic vertebral ligamentous ossification of the cervical region.[16] Ankylosis does occur in humans, as it commonly does in other species.[17] Thus ankylosis may complicate very severe cervical osteoarthritis. The disc space becomes strikingly narrowed, destructive changes occur in the bony cortex, and new bone formation extends into the anterior longitudinal ligament. Radiologically this suggests avulsion of the ligament from the osteophyte, followed by repair and remodeling. This lesion has been confused with ankylosing spondylitis. Osteoarthritis of the cervical spine, when the rare event ankylosis occurs, may be related to the relatively limited mobility of the intervertebral disc and the strikingly extensive mobility of the cervical spine as a whole via the zygapophyseal and Luschka joints. Baastrup's syndrome is an osteoarthritis-like alteration in the distal portions of "kissing" dorsal spinous processes. Its occurrence is associated with the most severe cervical osteoarthritis—a rarity in roentgenologic investigation.

In the spine as a whole, sites of osteoarthritis are most common in the areas of maximal lordosis or kyphosis, specifically C5, T8, and L3–L4. These sites are farthest from the body's center of gravity and thus are areas of maximal spinal motion. It is interesting that although osteoarthritis occurs in the thoracic spine, it is almost always asymptomatic. Perhaps the reason for this is that this area is minimally mobile.

Acute cervical intervertebral disc protrusion is more common in younger people and is an uncommon cause of cervical radiculopathy. Narrowed intervertebral discs caused by ostearthritis are commonly responsible for neck pain, radiculopathy, spinal cord compression, and vertebral artery compressive syndromes. Intervertebral disc syndromes may occur because of nuclear herniation without actual neural structure compression, anular protrusion, or dehydration or fissuring of disc material. Disc space narrowing occurs, and osteophyte formation proceeds both anteriorly and posteriorly. As fragmentation increases, the nucleus pulposus bulges outward through tears in the anulus fibrosus. This continues as the

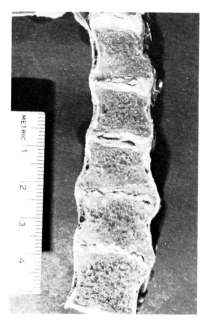

Figure 3–17. Anatomic specimen in sagittal section illustrates the grossest type of intervertebral disc osteoarthritis. The lower discs are practically completely obliterated; all discs are cleft through and through; vertebral bodies are extensively remodeled; ligaments are hypertrophied and thickened.

nucleus pulposus is held by the longitudinal ligament. Intradiscal pressure decreases, and the anulus bulges. Vertebral end plates can approximate. Figure 3–17 illustrates the gross type of intervertebral disc osteoarthritis.

An anatomic consideration is that the cervical spine is made up of two functional segments. The upper one is the atlanto-occipital (skull and C1) and the atlantoaxial (C1–C2) joint. The first two cervical vertebrae, C1 (atlas) and C2 (axis) have no posterior articulations, and there are no intervertebral foramina traversed by cervical nerves (as there are in the lower cervical spine). Most of the movement of the cervical spine occurs between C1 and C2 as the atlas rotates around the odontoid process (50% of total neck rotation occurs between C1 and C2 before any rotation occurs in the remainder of the cervical spine).

The second segment (C_3 to T_1) is of similar functional subunits, but the anterior aspect (intervertebral discs and vertebrae) serve a weight-bearing, shock-absorbing function, whereas the posterior aspect has a guiding, gliding function.

RHEUMATOID ARTHRITIS OF THE CERVICAL SPINE

The second most common area of involvement of rheumatoid arthritis is in the cervical spine, with particular emphasis on the upper cervical spine.[20] A reasonable generality about rheumatoid arthritis is that where there is the most motion there will be the most granulomatous, destructive disease. The upper cervical spine is the most mobile portion of the body. Current evidence strongly favors the issue that changes in the diarthrodial joints start in the synovial tissue, and this is as true in the cervical spine as it is elsewhere. The morbid anatomy of rheumatoid arthritis of the cervical spine is quite variable depending upon duration and intensity of disease—high titer rheumatoid factor and rheumatoid subcutaneous nodules as well as nodules in other areas (tendons, ligaments). Those patients with involvement of the cervical spine that be-

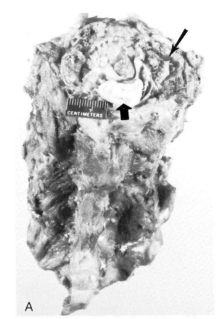

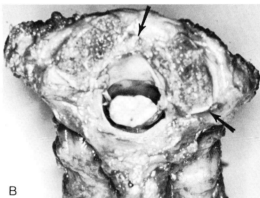

B

Figure 3–19. *A*, A whole rheumatoid spine viewed from above and posteriorly. The occipital condyles and the atlanto-occipital joints are included (thin arrow). These joints were nearly destroyed by the granulomatous process. All tissues in and about the foramen magnum were grossly invaded. The odontoid process compressed the spinal cord (thick arrow) and had a collar of thick, invasive rheumatoid granuloma about it. An atlantoaxial subluxation of 12 mm (by radiographic measurement) was noted, and it was found that the odontoid process and atlantoaxial complex had subluxated vertically into the foramen magnum. *B*, Looking into the spinal canal from a superior position. The odontoid process is grossly eroded (top arrow), and pannus covers the surfaces of both the atlanto-occipital (lower right arrow) and the atlantoaxial joints. An 11-mm subluxation of the atlantoaxial-odontoid joint was noted, and a thick collar of synovial rheumatoid granuloma surrounded the odontoid process.

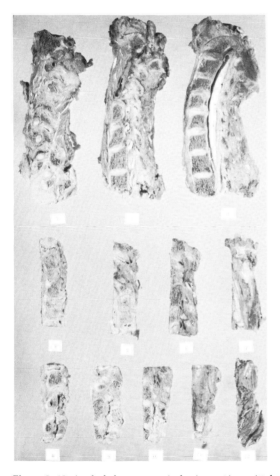

Figure 3–18. A whole human cervical spine cut in sagittal slabs, from one side to the other, in order to study lesions, gross and microscopic, caused by rheumatoid arthritis. By using serial sections one can build up a three-dimensional view of any tissue desired: joints of Luschka, zygapophyseal joints, discs, ligamenta flava, intervertebral foramina, ligaments, and their contained nerve roots, vertebrae, or spinal cord. (This specimen was prepared by Dr. Leon Sokoloff.) (From Bland JH: Rheumatoid arthritis of the cervical spine. J Rheumatol 1:319, 1974.)

comes grossly symptomatic usually have the most severe synovial inflammation—destruction of bone, ligament, tendon, and capsule—and cervical spine rheumatoid arthritis generally consti-

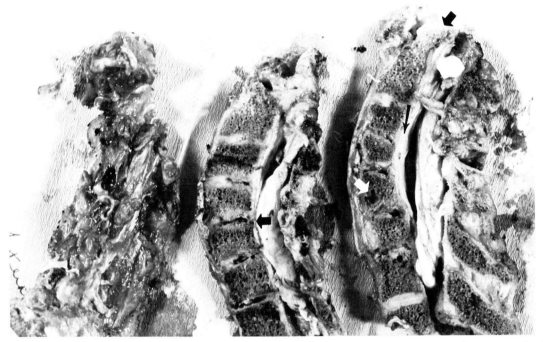

Figure 3–20. A sagittally cut rheumatoid cervical spine showing the middle slabs. There is virtually no uninvolved tissue. All discs are involved, and each is filled with the granuloma (black arrow, center). All vertebrae were infiltrated (white arrow). A rheumatoid pachymeningitis is visible grossly (thin arrow), and all zygapophyseal and Luschka joints have been destroyed. The odontoid process has practically eroded away (top arrow), and the anterior arch of the atlas is exceedingly thin. Spinal cord compression due to atlantoaxial and subaxial subluxation was noted in several areas.

tutes a poorer prognosis for those patients than for patients without symptomatic cervical spine disease. Figure 3–18 is a whole human cervical spine in sagittal, sectional slabs. Figure 3–19 illustrates the posterior aspect of a whole human cervical spine viewed from above. Figure 3–20 depicts three sagittal slabs in a rheumatoid arthritic cervical spine. Note the gross destruction of bone as well as cartilage. The upper spine on the right shows an almost destroyed odontoid process and extremely proliferative synovium all about the odontoid process, anteriorly and posteriorly. The anterior arch of the atlas is grossly damaged. Histologically, rheumatoid pachymeningitis was noted. Figure 3–21 shows a rheumatoid cervical spine from directly above.

Figure 3–21. A view directly above a rheumatoid cervical spine in which there was grossly more rheumatoid granuloma than other recognizable tissue. The odontoid process (top arrow) and the spinal cord (bottom arrow) are shown.

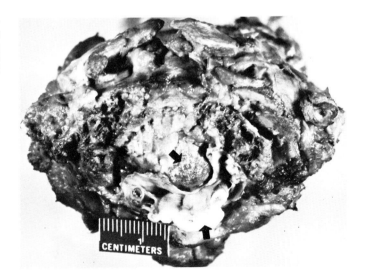

The principal clinical reflections of the involvement of bone, ligament, tendon, capsule, and joint are atlantoaxial subluxations, the most common of which are anterior dislocations. Upward dislocation may occur, bringing the odontoid process into the foramen magnum, making compression of the brain stem or upper spinal cord more likely. Posterior dislocation is much less common.

Collapse of the lateral mass of the atlas due to bony destruction also occurs. The neurologic consequences are legion, but the actual frequency of occurrence of this clinical syndrome in a whole population of patients with rheumatoid arthritis is quite uncommon. Sudden death, though one would suspect it would occur commonly, is actually rare. In our study we showed that the joints of Luschka were very commonly involved and that the granuloma would move into the intervertebral disc, destroying it and resulting in very narrow discs, particularly in the upper cervical spine without osteophytosis—a pathognomonic sign of rheumatoid arthritis.[18, 19]

Thus in the cervical spine there are vertebral lesions. Rheumatoid nodules have been reported in all tissues, tendons, ligaments, striated muscles, peripheral nerves, and arteries—from post-

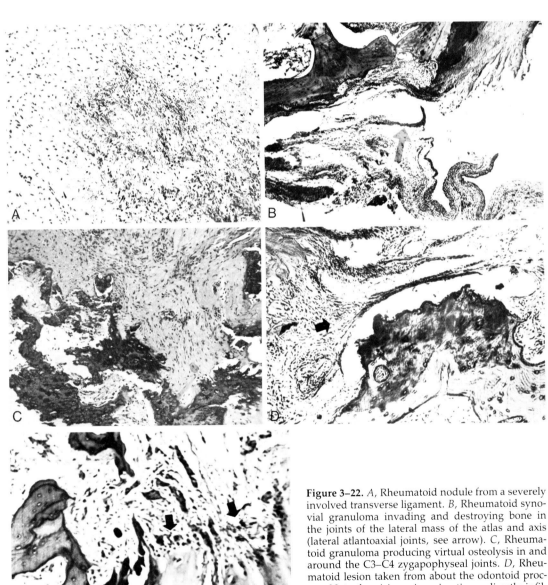

Figure 3–22. *A,* Rheumatoid nodule from a severely involved transverse ligament. *B,* Rheumatoid synovial granuloma invading and destroying bone in the joints of the lateral mass of the atlas and axis (lateral atlantoaxial joints, see arrow). *C,* Rheumatoid granuloma producing virtual osteolysis in and around the C3–C4 zygapophyseal joints. *D,* Rheumatoid lesion taken from about the odontoid process. Note the vicious, invasive tissue directly infiltrating and digesting cartilage and bone (arrow). *E,* Rheumatoid granuloma overlying and destroying bone, the anterior arch of the atlas (arrows).

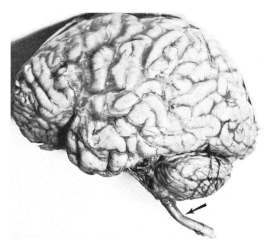

Figure 3–23. Brain and spinal cord from a rheumatoid patient in which the cord was chronically and finally acutely compressed just below the brain stem. Note the compressed area in the cord (arrow).

capillary venules to the large vessels traversing the cervical spine.

The histologic lesion is the same as occurs elsewhere—the characteristic rheumatoid granuloma, with synovial cell transformation to collagenase- and prostaglandin-secreting cells causing enzymatic digestion of the tissues of the cervical spine. Figure 3–22 illustrates the destructive process histologically—the granuloma in the process of destroying bone in and around the odontoid process, the atlas, axis, atlanto-occipital joint, vertebrae, and zygapophyseal and Luschka joints—all histologic sections of tissue in rheumatoid arthritis of the cervical spine illustrating the destructive process. This includes sections of ligament flavum, synovitis of zygapophyseal and Luschka joints, spinal cord involvement, and the pachymeningitis. Figure 3–23 illustrates a case in which the spinal cord and brain stem were compressed, resulting in sudden death. Note the compression of the spinal cord just below the brain stem.

PATHOLOGY OF ANKYLOSING SPONDYLITIS

The primary lesion of ankylosing spondylitis is an enthesopathy—an inflammatory process at the site of junction of tendon, ligament, and capsule into bone, the area of Sharpey's fibers. Specifically this is an inflammation, an osteitis, and ultimately an ossification of tendonous, ligamentous, and capsular insertions into bone throughout the spine, or even about peripheral joints, or at some distance from the joints. About 25% of patients with well-documented ankylosing spondylitis do have peripheral arthritis in the diarthrodial joints. The pathologic changes that occur in the diarthro-

dial joints of the spine (zygapophyseal joints), the sacroiliac joints, and the peripheal joints are very much like those that occur in peripheral rheumatoid arthritis, except the former are not as severe as the latter. Bony ankylosis is very rare in rheumatoid arthritis but is the rule in ankylosing spondylitis. The degree of ankylosis is highly variable, with the exception of severe disabling ankylosis. Osteolytic resorption occurs at the margins of the vertebral bodies where the anulus fibrosus inserts, an enthesopathy. This inflammatory infiltrate in bone or disc tissue has been observed only rarely early in the course of the disease. A metaplastic ossification (not a calcification) of the anulus fibrosus occurs, penetrating the margin of the vertebral bodies into the atlas. The spinal ligaments are not involved nearly to the extent that the anulus fibrosus is. Such is anatomically apparent on inspection of the bony bridges in the anteroposterior radiologic projections and on the lateral aspects of the vertebral body. Remember that the longitudinal spinal ligaments are anterolateral and posterior, not lateral. This ossification of soft tissues is remodeled, ultimately forming a continuous bony structure. Similar pathologic events occur in juvenile polyarthritis, psoriatic arthritis, and Reiter's disease in the cervical spine. Clinically in rheumatoid arthritis, subcutaneous nodules and vascular lesions occur. These are very rare in ankylosing spondylitis of the cervical spine.

A major risk that patients with ankylosing spondylitis have with cervical spine ankylosis is frac-

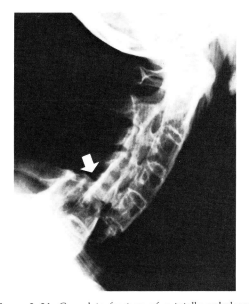

Figure 3–24. Complete fracture of a totally ankylosed cervical spine in a patient with ankylosing spondylitis (arrow). Note that the cervical spine was one whole bony unit; even the atlas was ankylosed to the skull. This is an exception in the population of people with ankylosing spondylitis.

ture. They tend to fall as gross unit, with little in the way of reflex regulation of absorbing the shock of a fall. Through-and-through fracture, fairly common in the patient with a completely anky-losed cervical spine, poses a major threat. Figure 3–24 illustrates a through-and-through fracture of the cervical spine in a patient with ankylosing spondylitis. The fracture resulted in instant death.

References

1. Hunter W: On the structure and diseases of articu-lating cartilage. Philosophical Trans Roy Soc London 9:267, 1743.
2. Leidy J: On the intimate structure and history of the articular cartilage. Am J Med Sci 17:277, 1849.
3. Redfern P: On the healing of wounds in articular cartilage. Month J Med Sci 13:201, 1851.
4. Paget J: Healing of cartilage: lectures in surgical pathology. Proceedings of the Royal College of Sur-geons 1:263, 1853.
5. Redfern P: Observations on the development and nutrition of bone and cartilage and on the relations to each other in health and disease. J Anat Physiol 32:96, 1897–1908.
6. Ogston A: On articular cartilage. J Anat Physiol 10:49, 1875–1876.
7. Shands AR: The regeneration of hyaline cartilage in joints, an experimental study. Arch Surg 22:137, 1931.
8. Calandruccio RA, Gilmer WS: Proliferation, regen-eration and repair of articular cartilage of immature animals. J Bone Joint Surg 44A:137, 1962.
9. Cruess L: Cartilage repair. J Bone Joint Surg 53B:365, 1971.
10. Radin EL, Burr DB: Hypothesis: Joints can heal. Semin Arthritis Rheum 13:293, 1984.
11. Bland JH: The reversibility of osteoarthritis. Am J Med 74:16, 1983.
12. Bland JH, Cooper SM: Osteoarthritis: A review of the cell biology involved and evidence for reversi-bility. Management rationally related to known gen-esis and pathophysiology. Semin Arthritis Rheum 14:106, 1984.
13. Sokoloff L: The remodeling of articular cartilage. *In* Schattesskirchner M (ed): Rheumatology. Basel: S. Karger, 1982, vol. 7, p. 11.
14. Sandy JD, Adams ME, Billingham MEJ: In vivo and in vitro stimulation of chondrocyte metabolic activity in early experimental osteoarthritis. Arthritis Rheum 27:388, 1984.
15. Bland JH, Boushey DR: An anatomical, clinical, radiologic and histologic study of 130 whole human cervical spines. Semin Arthritis Rheum 1987 (in press).
16. Smith CF, Pugh DG, Polley HF: Physiologic verte-brae ligamentous calcification: An aging process. AJR 74:1049, 1955.
17. Sokoloff L, Snell KC, Stewart HL: Spinal ankylosis in old rhesus monkeys. Clin Orthop 61:185, 1968.
18. Bland JH, Davis PH, London MG, et al: Rheumatoid arthritis of the cervical spine. Arch Intern Med 112:892, 1963.
19. Bland JH, VanBuskirk FW, Tampas JP: A study of roentgenologic criteria for rheumatoid arthritis of the cervical spine. AJR 95:949, 1965.
20. Bland JH: Rheumatoid arthritis of the cervical spine. J Rheumatol 1:319, 1974.

Chapter 4

Clinical Methods

For anatomic and clinical reasons, the cervical spine is the most complex component of the entire locomotor system. The neck is seldom in the same position for any length of time, waking or sleeping. It is a dense, concentrated conglomerate of skeletal, muscular, articular, ligamentous, nervous, and vascular structures situated in a relatively small area. Precise diagnosis in a pathologic process requires that the source or cause of the abnormality as well as the involved structures be clearly identified—not an easy task in the cervical spine, where so many tissues are crowded together. Nevertheless, all pain has a source that is clinically identifiable. The great variety of pathologic and physiologic changes that may affect the cervical spine adds to diagnostic difficulty. Because of the intimate relationship of the bones, joints, muscles, blood vessels, spinal cord, and nerve roots, a lesion of the cervical region may produce local as well as widely referred symptoms. Hence, examination of the neck must include neurologic examination of the head, neck, upper extremities, and even elsewhere as indicated.

The most frequent causes of cervical clinical syndromes are the rheumatic disorders and trauma; however, congenital anomalies, inflammatory disease, neoplasms (primary and metastatic), infection, metabolic bone disorders, Paget's disease, and primary neurologic syndromes all may be in the differential diagnosis—or there may be quite asymptomatic, radiologically gross cervical osteoarthritis with a few trivial neurologic signs! Also, a cervical syndrome may arise in structures adjacent to or even far distant from the neck, albeit perceived in the neck!

All successful treatment must start with accurate diagnosis. The obvious diagnosis is not always the correct one. We should not focus on the initial assumption but give attention and thought to all possible diagnoses. Incorrect diagnosis and consequent improper treatment follow hurried and careless evaluation. To reach accurate diagnosis, it is necessary to deal with musculoskeletal disorders in an orderly manner and employ a logical sequence of thoughts. Performing a careful evaluation requires (1) knowledge of the regional anatomy (this is no substitute for thorough knowledge of general anatomy in assessing musculoskeletal disorders); (2) a precisely recorded history; (3) a thorough physical examination; (4) appropriate laboratory studies, tests to verify clinical findings, and radiographic studies; (5) knowledge of the complete differential diagnosis. When these data are assembled, the doctor can synthesize and analyze them, make an accurate diagnosis, and initiate proper management.

Clinical examination is the most reliable means of reaching secure diagnosis. It so happens that the cervical spine lends itself satisfyingly to simple and hence sophisticated clinical analysis. Historical elicitation and physical examination are the major means of data gathering in the diagnosis and management of cervical syndrome pain and the least likely to be done well.[1] Laboratory studies are not important generally. Radiographic examination may be quite important but usually is performed to confirm the clinical formulation. In concept, the examiner should have in mind the enormously broad range of clinical possibilities in cervical spine disease and injury, that is, local cervical syndromes, cervicocephalic syndromes, cervical brachialgic syndromes, syndromes of bony, muscular, articular, or neurogenic origin, nerve root syndromes, myelopathic clinical reflections, shoulder and upper thoracic spine and scapular syndromes, vertebral and vertebrobasilar arterial insufficiency with headache, esophageal symptoms and signs, vertigo, auditory and visual disturbances, drop attacks, psychologic and psychiatric disorders, Raynaud's syndrome, and the various thoracic outlet abnormalities with cervical spine reflections.

The goal of this chapter is to present a systematic and logical approach to clinical historical data collection and physical examination plus a series of special examinations useful in diagnosis and formulation of pathophysiology of the cervical spine and its disorders.

HISTORY

During the first visit, the doctor must instill confidence in the patient. Proper rapport between doctor and patient is a necessity to optimum results. Because of previous failure of treatment, many patients with cervical spine disorders are discouraged and pessimistic. Many feel the doctor regards them as psychoneurotic, that "nothing can be done," that "it's all in my head." The patient's faith in the physician is the sine qua non of a treatment or management measure. The doctor must convey an attitude of calm consideration and confidence that all that can be done to solve the problem will be done and done well. Patients need to see that their unique individuality is recognized and that their pain is significant to someone other than themselves—that the doctor, office assistants, and colleagues are empathic and sympathetic. The doctor should express full confidence in the method of management by explaining why and how it will work. In general, 1 hour should be reserved for the first visit of a patient who has a cervical spine disorder.

The detailed history is surely the most important aspect of clinical data gathering. With skillful interpretation and careful analysis of historical data, a highly probable diagnosis is forthcoming prior to physical examination. The doctor has accumulated very definitive information regarding the emotional and psychologic background of the patient. During the period of historical elicitation, the best possible rapport can be established, as the doctor interacts with the patient in a friendly, courteous, empathic, and sympathetic manner and appears well informed, scientifically sound, and deeply interested in and totally focused on solving the patient's problem. The systems review, medical history, family history, and social history are sought just as they would be for any other medical problem. It is important to take the time to obtain this information.

Much of the physical examination can be done during history taking. The patient should be undressed. We learn much more in physical examination from observing than from listening, thumping, or feeling. Thus, the expert clinician is very alert to making all clinical observations possible during the interview. When we touch the patient we tend to stop looking! Table 4–1 summarizes relevant historical data that can be elicited during the initial interview.

Age and Occupation. Knowing the age and occupation of the patient is of major importance. Cervical osteoarthritis with its myriad syndromes is a disease of later life. Trauma and "crick"

Table 4–1. SUMMARY OF HISTORICAL DATA RELEVANT TO CERVICAL SPINE

Age and sex	Congenital defects
Race	Posture (head, neck)
Occupation	Bifocal glasses worn
Body type	Have radiographs been
Medications used and	taken?
results	History of head or neck
Emotional resources	trauma
Pain (detailed	Neurologic loss
description)	Headache, occipital
Radiation of pain	neuralgia
(referred)	Pseudoangina
Local or diffuse pain	Dysphagia
Weakness	Eye, ear, throat symptoms
Paresthesia	Vertigo
Gait	Fainting
Swelling	Respiration
Tenderness at pain sites	Stiffness (morning,
Degree and course of	duration, generalized,
pain	localized)
Effect of weather, rest,	Crepitus, "cracking"
exercise, drugs, mood,	Drop attack
heat, cold, sleep	Flaccidity, spasticity
Sleep position	Atrophy of muscles,
Pillow (type, how long	especially intrinsic
used)	hand muscles
Weight loss (infection or	
malignant disease)	
Deformity (neck, limbs,	
back, leg length, limp,	
gait, atrophy, irregular	
pant or dress length)	

(spasmodic torticollis) occur in younger people. An occupation requiring continued or intermittent hyperflexion, hyperextension, or over-rotation of the cervical spine may cause production and prolongation of symptoms. The patient's job may necessitate chronic cervical spine flexion (most commonly), but extension and lateral flexion postures on the job are also not rare.

Previous Injury. Details of previous injury are of primary importance. These include the "when" and "how" of an accident; the position of the patient in an automobile; whether it was a collision from the back, front, or side; the patient's recollection of the detailed events before and after the injury, such as sudden pulls or thrusts of arms, a turn or a jerk of the head, somersaults, or a fall of any kind. Symptoms may appear gradually, immediately, or hours to days after a given event. An event in the distant past may be relevant, such as a head injury sustained during childhood or adolescence, concussion, unconsciousness, a fall from a bicycle, or sports injuries. Permanent but trivial upper motor neuron signs from a previous injury may be misleading.

When interpreted properly, a history of past or present chiropractic or osteopathic manipulation of the spine may provide meaningful information. One needs to know the specific movements to which the patient has been subjected.

If the patient's symptoms are absolutely un-varying—nothing makes them better or worse, they are uninfluenced by rest or exercise, and they are the same day and night—the problem is surely not of mechanical origin. This scenario suggests malignant disease, occult infection, hysteria, malingering, and other psychologic mechanisms producing pain syndromes.

If your assessment on early interview is that the problem is very severe, the patient is inordinately irritable, and the nature of the disorder suggests a serious disease, it is sound to proceed to a neurologic examination. If this produces negative (normal) results, proceed to a systematic historical survey and objective physical examination, with gross and objective neurologic physical signs. An emergency may exist, such as acute myelopathy, spinal cord infarction, or rapidly progressing neurologic dysfunction.

Bifocal Glasses. Use of bifocal glasses may be pertinent, because it may require extension at the occiput-atlas-axis complex and flexion in the lower cervical spine. A syndrome of posturally induced neck pain and occipital and retro-orbital headache may be thus explained, especially with recent change of glasses to bifocals.

Pillow. Inquiring about the type of pillow the patient uses, if any, frequently brings out useful information. The physician should find out how long the patient has used the pillow, and the patient's sleep position should be characterized. Is the cervical spine in extension or lateral flexion while the patient sleeps? Is the arm hyperabducted or placed under the pillow? Does the patient sleep in the fetal position? Ask the patient to bring the pillow to the office to demonstrate how he or she sleeps. A simple change of pillow solves many cervical spine problems (see the section entitled *Pillows* in Chapter 12).

Physical Characteristics. Observe such physical characteristics as a very long or short neck, a receding mandible, a high, arched palate, crooked teeth and asymmetry of facial bones and muscles (sternocleidomastoid), and general poor development of the head and neck. These findings constitute strong evidence of congenital deformities of the cervical spine, especially at the occiput-atlas-axis complex, in explanation of the clinical syndrome presented.

Temporomandibular Joint. Inquiring regarding the temporomandibular joint function is important and rewarding. Painful bite, limited jaw opening, or swelling of the temporomandibular joint area, past or present, may lead to proper diagnosis. Temporomandibular joint malfunction may mimic cervical spine syndromes or independently accompany them.

Pain Characteristics. Three phases or periods of the patient's pain history should be covered during the interview: onset, course, and present status. Obtain detailed information regarding date, hour, and minute of onset and all the circumstances contributing to the possible cause. Ascertain the location, size, distribution, quality, intensity, severity, and duration of the first pain. Sharp, dull, aching, burning, throbbing, cramping—such characteristics aid in differentiating the site of origin, the pain-sensitive structure. Bone pain is generally described as dull, deep, nagging; fracture pain is sharp, severe, intolerable; muscle pain is cramping, sometimes gradually increasing in intensity; descriptions of joint pain vary because of the variety of tissues involved. Is the pain worse at night (Paget's disease, osteomyelitis, and osteoid osteoma)? Inquiry about any associated sensation is important, including sensory, motor, or autonomic disturbances apparent at first onset of pain. Figure 4–1 illustrates patterns of reflexly referred pain from visceral and somatic structures.

Learning about the course of the pain involves determining whether the pain has disappeared, remained constant, intermittently reappeared, or changed in any way. Has there been any change in location of pain? Has it become better or worse with passage of time? Has quality, severity, and relation of pain to time of day or night changed? Have associated sensations—sensory, motor, or autonomic—changed? What is the relationship to motion, weight-bearing, use? Most musculoskeletal pain is relieved by rest. Pain that is not relieved by rest suggests another, usually more serious source.

In assessing the present status of the pain, ask the patient to describe the characteristics of the pain at the time of examination. The following questions could be asked: "What do you think caused your pain?" "What has increased or relieved the pain?" "Can you make it stop by changing your position or moving?" "Does it prevent sleep?" Determine how weather, drugs, cold, heat, exercise, cough, sneeze or straining affect the pain. The effect of deep breathing on severity, quality, and distribution of pain should also be considered. Pain accentuation by cough, sneeze, or jolt suggests an intracranial component, whereas accentuation by movement in certain directions indicates a musculoskeletal cause. Ask the patient what has been done to alleviate the pain, and with what degree of success or failure. Inquire as to the time of day the pain is felt least, and when it is felt most. Active osteomyelitis under pressure becomes increasingly painful and is not relieved by rest. Did an injury or illness, such as streptococcal sore throat, migratory polyarthralgia, or arthritis, precede the symptoms? A lesion at the level of C7–C8–T1 with neurologic signs, decreased or absent sensation, absent reflexes, and atrophy of the intrinsic hand muscles is usually ominous, suggesting a more serious diagnosis, such as cervical spine metastatic malignancy or osteomyelitis. Table 4–2 lists common disorders of the cervical spine resulting in neck and shoulder pain.

Stiffness with consequent limitation of motion

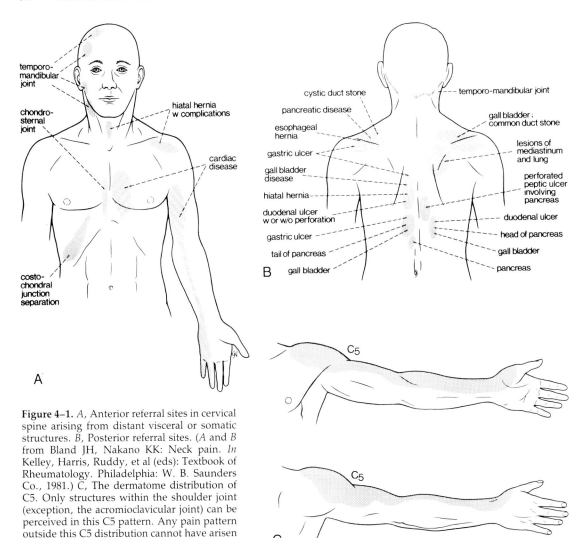

Figure 4–1. *A*, Anterior referral sites in cervical spine arising from distant visceral or somatic structures. *B*, Posterior referral sites. (*A* and *B* from Bland JH, Nakano KK: Neck pain. *In* Kelley, Harris, Ruddy, et al (eds): Textbook of Rheumatology. Philadelphia: W. B. Saunders Co., 1981.) *C*, The dermatome distribution of C5. Only structures within the shoulder joint (exception, the acromioclavicular joint) can be perceived in this C5 pattern. Any pain pattern outside this C5 distribution cannot have arisen from structures within the shoulder.

of neck, shoulder, elbow, wrist, and even fingers may occur. Such stiffness can be due to previous injury response, actual articular involvement, nerve root irritation, or reflex sympathetic dystrophy. It is very informative to determine whether the limitation of motion is caused by pain or stiffness or by actual tissue change in and around the joints.

Strangely, tenosynovitis, tendonitis, tennis elbow, and carpal tunnel syndrome frequently accompany syndromes of the cervical spine. They may involve tendon members of the rotator cuff or tendons about the wrist or hand, where stenosis or fibrosis of tendon sheaths and palmar fascia occurs. A causal connection with the cervical spine disorder is presumed, such as vasospasm or atypical reflex sympathetic dystrophy or other circulatory changes due to immobilization secondary to pain. Swelling of the fingers is common

and contributes to the sense of stiffness of the hands.

Cervical nerve root irritation causes a well-localized area of pain, whereas severe but poorly defined areas of pain arise from deep connective tissue structures—muscle, ligament, bone, joint, or disc. The patient's ability to describe the pain may provide an important clue.

The patient who "hurts all over" and cannot clearly describe the sensation is suspect as emotionally unstable. Head pain, bilateral or unilateral, retro-orbital, temporal, and occipital, is common, reflecting the referral pattern of atlas, axis, and C3, and their surrounding structures. Pain may occur in any part of the neck—the back portion, the sides, or the front segment—and may radiate to the upper thoracic spine, shoulders, scapular areas, and into one or both arms, extending to the finger tips. It may be produced, re-

Table 4–2. COMMON DISORDERS OF THE
CERVICAL SPINE CAUSING NECK AND
SHOULDER PAIN

Spasmodic torticollis
Intervertebral disc protrusion
Cervical osteoarthritis
Fibrinolytic syndrome
Trauma, cervical spine fracture
Injuries caused by hyperflexion or
    hyperextension (whiplash)
Rheumatoid arthritis of cervical spine
Ankylosing spondylitis of cervical spine
Infection of cervical spine
Thoracic outlet syndromes
Metastatic malignant disease of cervical
    spine
Carotid and vertebral artery atherosclerosis

lieved, or exaggerated by various normal movements of the cervical spine. Pain may be persistent or intermittent, sharp or dull, aching or burning. The patient may relate how it can be relieved or aggravated by various postural maneuvers, drugs, heat, or cold—important information in identifying the pain-sensitive structure. The designated areas of pain may be tender—for example, the transverse process, spinous process, apophyseal joints, anterior vertebral bodies, and all muscles innervated by the cervical or brachial plexus. All of these areas can be palpated directly or indirectly. Proximal pain of the leg and arm may occur secondary to cervical myelopathy or as an isolated phenomenon unrelated to cervical syndromes. Pain is the most common presenting symptom of cervical syndromes, although it varies in duration, degree, character, and location.

Paresthesia. Numbness and tingling occur in the segmental distribution of the nerve roots, often with no demonstrable objective sensory change. The symptoms may be present on one or both sides and upon awakening. They are often relieved by changing position of the neck and arms. Paresthesia may be intermittent or constant and may occur at any time. Paresthesia of the face, head, or tongue indicates involvement of the upper three nerve roots of the cervical plexus; numbness of the neck, shoulder, arm, forearms, and fingers indicates involvement of the C5–T1 roots or may be due to circulatory compromise.

Weakness. Weakness is not common but requires inquiry. Patients may have trouble balancing their heads because of muscle weakness. Weakness of an arm, inability to work with arms over the head, grip weakness, dropping things from one or both hands, breaking dishes, or difficulty eating or writing are all important symptoms. Weakness can be assessed in 6 grades: grade 5—normal—complete range of motion against gravity with full resistance; grade 4—good—complete range of motion against gravity with some resistance; grade 3—fair—complete range of mo-

tion against gravity only; grade 2—poor—complete range of motion with gravity eliminated; grade 1—trace only—evidence of slight contractility but with no joint motion; grade 0—no evidence of any contractility.

The signs of anterior radiculopathy are those of a lower motor neuron lesion, weakness, hypotonia, and fasciculation (during active degeneration). Muscles are almost always innervated by more than one root; hence, when all or several roots are involved, muscle atrophy may be extreme. Some weakness may be functional in that it is due to pain and guarding; a motor lesion may cause sensory symptoms, such as a feeling of heaviness of the limbs. The common symptoms of stiffness and clumsiness are difficult to trace to their precise cause, whether it is motor, sensory, or even autonomic in origin. (See the discussion under *Embryologic Development of the Cervical Spine* in Chapter 2. See also Tables 2–1, 2–2, and 2–3 on the dermatome, myotome, and sclerotome distribution patterns.)

Headache and Occipital Neuralgia. Head pain is common in and characteristic of cervical syndromes. It has been attributed to root compression, vertebral artery pressure, compression of sympathetic nerves, autonomic imbalance, posterior occipital and nuchal muscle spasm, and the osteoarthritic lesion of the zygapophyseal joints of the upper three cervical vertebrae.[1]

The headache is invariably occipital and occurs in the age groups in which osteoarthritis is common. It is often associated with pain in the neck and upper limbs and occipital or cervical paresthesias. It may spread to the eye region on one or both sides. The ache is dull and nagging, not pulsating, and it is aggravated by strain, sneeze, and cough as well as by movements of the head and neck. The headache often starts on rising, and it may wake the patient at night. It may worsen or pass as the day goes on. Headaches sparing the occipital region are not likely to be due to cervical syndromes.

Pseudoangina. A lesion at the level of C6–C7 may cause neurologic or myalgic pain and real muscular tenderness in the precordial or scapular region, raising the question of angina pectoris. The pain may be compressive, increased by exercise, referred down the arm in the ulnar distribution, aggravated by neck movement, or associated with torticollis or neck muscle spasm. Heart disease is ruled out by the presence of other evidence of radiculopathy, the absence of shock and fever and leucocytosis, and a normal electrocardiogram. Both angina and pseudoangina may be present in the same patient.

Eye Symptoms. Eye symptoms and signs are common in cervical syndromes. Blurring of vision with frequent change of glasses without improvement, intermittent visual blurring relieved by changing neck position, increased tearing, pain in one or both eyes, retro-orbital pain, strange descriptions of eyes being pulled backward or pushed forward are all common symptoms. They are probably due to irritation of the cervical sympathetic nerve supply to eye structures via the plexuses surrounding the vertebral and internal carotid arteries and their branches. The extraocular muscles may develop spasm and venous congestion with consequent peculiar eye sensations.

Ear Symptoms. Changes in equilibrium occur from irritation of sympathetic plexuses surrounding the vertebral arteries or result from vascular insufficiency. Difficulty with gait or balance is common, with veering off to the side of involvement, bumping into door jambs, or actual falls. Frequently these symptoms are misdiagnosed as Meniere's disease, prompting repeated unnecessary consultations with otolaryngologists. Tinnitus and deafness, constant or transitory, result from vascular insufficiency due to vasospasm or vertebral or basilar arterial obstruction.

Throat Symptoms. Dysphagia is not unusual in cervical syndromes and can be due to muscle spasm, anterior osteophyte compression of pharynx and esophagus, or abnormalities of the cervical cranial nerve connections and sympathetic communications (Fig. 4–2).

Miscellaneous Symptoms. A large group of bizarre symptoms, which seem unrelated, are explicable in terms of multivariate pathogenetic mechanisms. These symptoms and mechanisms include the following: a cervical syndrome of dyspnea ("can't get a deep breath") due to C3–C4–C5 lesions whose roots innervate the dia-

phragm and other respiratory muscles; cardiac palpitation and tachycardia on assumption of unusual positions or hyperextension of the neck caused by irritation of the C4 root supplying the diaphragm and pericardium or by irritation of the cardiac sympathetic nerve supply; nausea and vomiting; ill-defined pain and paresthesia due to cord compression; drop attacks caused by abrupt loss of proprioception; and collapse without loss of consciousness, often with the ability to rise and continue with the previous activity.[1]

Differential diagnosis between psychoneurosis and cervical syndromes is a common problem, usually reflecting the examiner's inexperience with the enormous and complex variety of symptoms and signs explicable as nerve root compression, sympathetic nervous system involvement, cervical cord compression, vascular insufficiency, and diseases and trauma of cervical bone, muscle, and joint. An extensive knowledge is required of the basic anatomy, kinesiology, physiology, and pathophysiology of the extensive intricacies of structure and function of the cervical spine to assess and interpret the clinical data.

CLINICAL EXAMINATION

There are two parts to physical examination of the musculoskeletal system: (1) the examination of the patient as a whole—the same as the internist's complete clinical study—with emphasis on thoroughness and systematic, traditional inspection, palpation, percussion, and auscultation (look, feel, percuss, and listen!); and (2) the musculoskeletal examination proper, with focus on a particular region, such as the cervical spine. The patient should be undressed and in a good light. With a unilateral syndrome, always compare the involved with the uninvolved side.

The examination includes head, neck, upper thoracic spine, shoulders, arm, forearm, wrist, and hand. The patient must be undressed at least to the waist. The principles of examination that apply elsewhere in the musculoskeletal system apply here as well. From the historical data, the examiner gets some indication of the tissue site and origin of symptoms. When the site is identified, all tissues there are tested, one after the other, until the pain-sensitive or paresthesia producing structure is precisely recognized.

We tend to divide the examination of the spine into regions: cervical, thoracic, and lumbar spine clinical studies. This is a mistake. The three units are closely interrelated structurally and functionally—a whole person with a whole spine. The cervical spine may be symptomatic because of a thoracic or lumbar spine abnormality, and vice versa! Sometimes treating the lumbar spine will relieve a cervical spine syndrome, or proper management of cervical spine will relieve low backache. If the patient slouches in a chair during the examination and loses his or her normal lumbar

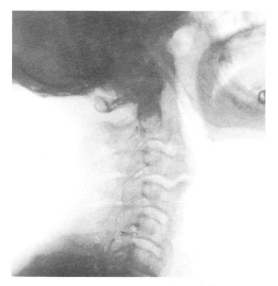

Figure 4–2. Diffuse idiopathic skeletal hyperostosis. Note the laminar bone at the C3–C4 level has pushed the esophagus forward, stretching the tissues and causing dysphagia. The disc spaces are preserved contrary to pathologic events in osteoarthritis.

lordosis (flat lumbar spine), cervical spine range of motion is clearly diminished (normally). During examination of the cervical spine, the patient should sit or stand, maintaining the best posture possible.

The patient's posture, movements, facial expression, gait, and sitting, standing, and supine positions provide important data. Observe the patient as he or she walks, undresses, sits, and moves from chair to examining table. Look for sacral base-level fullness, symmetry of supraclavicular fossae, pelvic tilt, equality of height of iliac crests and of scapulae, forward head carriage, lordosis, kyphosis, kyphoscoliosis, and long-leg or short, detailed postural analysis. The patient, slumped in the chair, bobbing the head about while talking, or gesturing with head and neck, has little or no pain from cervical spine structures. As the patient walks in, observe how the head is held and how naturally and rhythmically the head and neck move with body movement. The head and neck are normally perpendicular to the floor, not held stiffly to one side or the other. Nor is the neck normally either flexed or extended much beyond the neutral position. The normal cervical lordosis is checked.

The neck is inspected for normal landmarks, hyoid bone, thyroid cartilage, thyroid gland, first cricoid ring, scars, or pigmentation (Fig. 4–3). Examine the skin for color, scars, old incisions, ecchymoses, marks. The osteoporotic patient has very thin skin; patients with neurofibromatosis have light brown pigmentation over the body (café au lait). Palpate any area that seems suspicious, swollen, tender, deformed, or warm, but palpate with a kind, gentle, warm hand, avoiding unnecessary roughness. You will be able to feel more in relaxed patients than in tense ones, whether they are children or adults! Assess skin temperature, bones, muscles, and any localized tenderness. Increased skin temperature denotes increased vascularity, usually inflammation. Hyperemia occurs in a rapidly growing neoplasm. Assess bulk and tone of muscle, that is, spasm. Decide whether a swollen joint is due to increased synovial fluid or increased synovial membrane and capsular proliferation or both. When feeling bony structures, evaluate general contour, abnormal prominence, local landmarks, and tenderness. Mark sites of tenderness with a "magic marker" pencil. Try to correlate these sites with a local structure. Compare with the opposite side; it is your "control" structure!

Deformity is easy to detect, but do look for it! If pain is present, abnormal gait is characteristic. The patient walks gingerly to avoid any jar or jolt to the neck. The chin may be supported by the hand. Wry neck (torticollis) is the most common deformity, and pain is increased with any movement. Wry neck of young people lasts days to weeks and disappears. If it has been present for several years, asymmetry of the face appears.

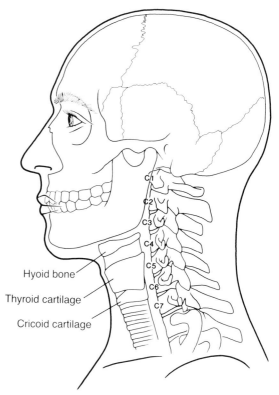

Figure 4–3. Drawing in lateral view of landmarks in the cervical spine. Note the hyoid bone is at the level of the C3 vertebra, the upper and lower margins of the thyroid cartilage are at C4 and C5 respectively, and the cricoid ring cartilage is at the C6 level. Each level allows clinical assessment of localization.

Patients who can touch each shoulder with the chin and then the ear, have very serviceable cervical spine movement.

The neck may be held in an asymmetric posture. Observe whether the deformity is a pure lateral list or whether rotation is also present. If pain is present, the deviation can be either toward or away from the painful side. Careful observation may disclose a compensating thoracic curve. If so, the etiology of the asymmetry may be adolescent scoliosis, Klippel-Feil deformity, previous thoracoplasty, or unilateral cervical rib.

Observing the posterior chest, note the level at which the scapulae lie. Downward and lateral displacement occurs in trapezius muscle weakness for a variety of reasons, including accidental section of the eleventh cranial (spinal accessory) nerve during an operation for "glands" in the neck. One shoulder higher than the other in the absence of scoliosis suggests a leg-length disparity. Prominence of the vertebral border of one scapula (winged scapula) suggests long thoracic nerve neuritis with paralysis of one serratus anterior muscle (Fig. 4–4). Winging of both scapulae

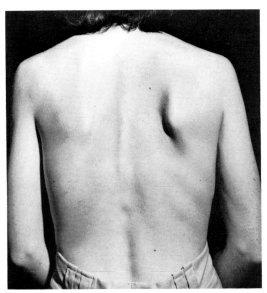

Figure 4–4. A case of unilateral, long thoracic nerve neuritis with winging of the right scapula. This lesion reflects the C5–C6 cervical level.

with weak serratus anterior function occurs in myopathic lesions of the muscle. Thoracic kyphosis in children and in asthenic, thin adults results in prominent low angles of the scapula, the bone thus standing out. Atrophy of the infraspinatus muscle is readily observed and felt. Etiologies include rupture, myopathic lesions, trauma, suprascapular neuritis, or severe arthritis of the shoulder, such as rheumatoid arthritis (Fig. 4–5). Sprengel's deformity, congenital elevation of the scapula, is readily identified by fixation of one

scapula at a higher level than the other. The levator muscle of the scapula is replaced by abnormal bone, termed the suprascapular bone. Clavicle enlargement as a manifestation of Paget's disease, and dislocation or inflammatory involvement of the sternoclavicular joint are all readily diagnosed. Cleidocranial dysostosis, congenital absence of the clavicle (always bilateral), results in such extensive mobility of the scapulae that the shoulders may meet in front of the sternum (see Chapter 12, *General Management Methods*).

There is no lesion that can possibly cause abrupt total inability to move the head in an otherwise healthy patient. This clinical finding is a characteristic of hysteria, when active movement may suddenly become impossible in all directions. Careful examination displays the gross exaggeration, and the effort to examine passive movement is met with striking resistance. Examination may gradually be allowed, and a full range of passive movement may be disclosed, with no pain experienced at the extremes.

Examination of Bony Structures

Palpation of bony structures is best done with the patient supine to relax overlying muscles. The bony contour is explored. In the root of the neck, accessory ribs may be felt or even seen (Fig. 4–6). Focal tenderness, skin temperature, and the cervical lymph nodes are assessed, with the neck slightly flexed for better assessment of the cervical lymph nodes. In palpating the anterior part of the neck, stand at the patient's side and support the neck from behind with one hand, palpating with the other, relaxing the spine as much as possible. The horseshoe-shaped hyoid bone is above the thyroid cartilage (Adam's apple) and is at the level

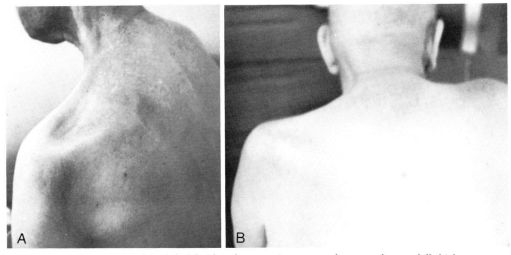

Figure 4–5. *A*, Marked atrophy of the left deltoid and supraspinatus muscles secondary to full-thickness tear of the rotator cuff. *B*, Atrophy of the left supraspinatus muscle caused by granulomatous destruction of the rotator cuff in rheumatoid arthritis. Deltoid muscle atrophy is also apparent.

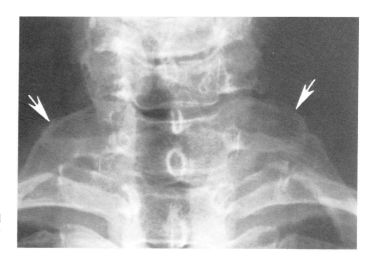

Figure 4–6. Cervical ribs. The C7 cervical ribs (arrows) are readily palpable clinically in the posterior triangle.

of the C3 vertebra. Figure 4–3 shows cervical spine landmarks. Feel with index finger and thumb in a pincer-like position to palpate the stem of the horseshoe. When the patient swallows, the hyoid bone moves up and then down. The thyroid cartilage has a superior notch and a flaring upper portion, the top of which is the Adam's apple. The upper border of the cartilage is at the C4 level, and the lower border is at C5. Just below the lower border of the thyroid cartilage and opposite the C6 vertebra, the first cricoid ring is palpable; this is the upper border of the trachea and is just superior to the site of emergency tracheostomy. The cricoid ring also moves with swallowing. About 2 to 3 cm lateral to the first cricoid ring, the carotid tubercle can be felt. It is the anterior tubercle of the transverse process of C6 (Fig. 4–7, see also Fig. 4–3). Though deep, it is clearly palpable. The carotid arteries are adjacent to the tubercle, and the pulse is palpated. If both carotid tubercles are palpated simultaneously, the carotid arterial flow may be restricted,

resulting in the carotid reflex, an unpleasant and surprising experience. The tubercle is used as a landmark when the stellate sympathetic ganglion is injected. It also is a landmark for anterior surgical approach to C5–C6. The hard bump of the transverse process of C1 is palpable between the angle of the jaw and the styloid process of the skull. Because it is the broadest transverse process of the cervical spine, it is easily palpated; indirect evidence of normality of the atlanto-occipital and the atlantoaxial joints and bony structures can be obtained by performing a lateral sliding movement, holding the atlas between the thumb and index finger by the transverse processes.

The posterior landmarks of the cervical spine are the occiput, the inion, the superior nuchal line, the mastoid process, the spinous process of each vertebra, and the zygapophyseal joints (Fig. 4–8). The occiput is palpated first, and the inion, the dome-shaped "bump of knowledge," marks the center point of the superior nuchal line; the line is felt as a transverse ridge extending out on both sides of the inion. The round mastoid process is at the lateral edge of the superior nuchal line. The spinous process of the axis (C2) is easy to feel just below the indented area immediately under the occiput. The posterior arch of the atlas is usually not palpable, but spinous processes from C2 to T1 are readily felt. The bifid spinous processes of C3–C6 can sometimes be perceived; the spinous processes of C7 (the vertebra prominens) and T1 are larger than the others. The spinous process alignment is noted. The zygapophyseal joints are palpated as small, rounded domes deep into the trapezius muscle and about 1 inch lateral to the spinous processes. The patient must be quite relaxed and without muscle spasm and tension for effective palpation of these joints. The joint involved can be identified by lining up the hyoid bone with C3, the thyroid cartilage with C4 and C5, and the first cricoid ring with C6. These joints are often tender with osteoarthritis, espe-

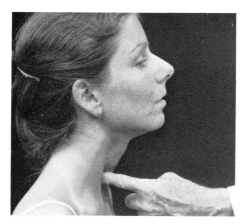

Figure 4–7. Examiner's finger points to the right carotid tubercle on the sixth cervical vertebra.

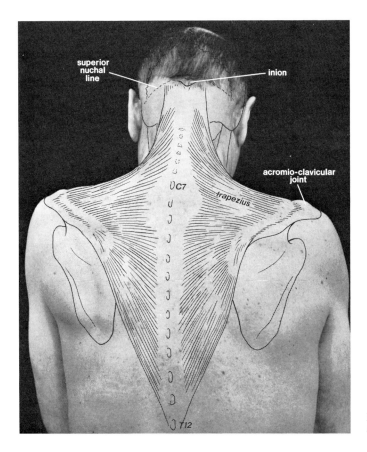

Figure 4–8. Landmarks of the posterior aspect of the cervical spine.

cially in the upper cervical spine. At the C5–C6 and C6–C7 levels, however, osteoarthritis in the intervertebral discs is more often the case (Fig. 4–9).

Examination of Soft Tissues

Systematic examination of soft tissues in the neck is divided into two anatomic areas, anterior and posterior. The anterior area is bordered laterally by the two sternocleidomastoid muscles, superiorly by the mandible, and inferiorly by the suprasternal notch—roughly an upside-down triangle. The posterior aspect includes the whole area posterior to the lateral border of the sternocleidomastoid muscle (Fig. 4–10).

The patient is best examined in the supine position. Anteriorly the sternocleidomastoid muscle is noted by asking the patient to turn the head to the opposite side, the muscle then stands out sharply and is palpable from origin to insertion. The opposite muscle is compared for any discrepancies in size, bulges, or power. The muscle is often overstretched in hyperextension injuries, with resultant hemorrhage into the tissue. Localized swelling may be due to hematomas. The muscle is always involved and clinically evident in serious torticollis.

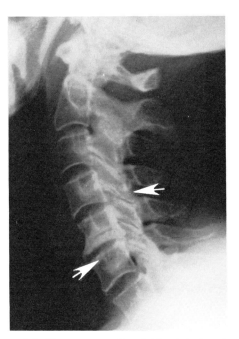

Figure 4–9. The arrow on the right points to osteoarthritic involvement of a zygapophyseal joint in the upper cervical spine. The arrow on the left points to intervertebral disc osteoarthritis at the C5–C6 level of the lower cervical spine.

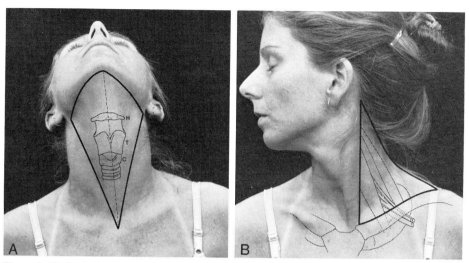

Figure 4–10. Surface anatomy. Anterior (*A*) and posterior (*B*) cervical triangles and their contents.

The lymph node chain along the medial border of the sternocleidomastoid muscle is usually not palpable, but small, definitive nodes, often tender, can be felt if enlarged. This suggests tumor, metastases, or throat or ear infection. Also, node enlargement may cause torticollis.

The thyroid gland lies below the thyroid cartilage in an "H" pattern; the bar is the isthmus, with the two lobes situated laterally. The gland is normally smooth and commonly palpable without enlargement; one may note diffuse enlargement, cysts, nodules, or tenderness.

The two carotid artery pulses, best felt near the carotid tubercle on C6, should be examined separately because the carotid reflex may be tripped off if both vessels are felt simultaneously. The pulses are usually equal in volume—a point always to be assessed. Listen with stethoscope for bruits on both sides. Remember that the vagus nerve and the internal jugular vein are there too.

The parotid gland overlies part of the sharp angle of the mandible and is usually indistinct to palpation; but if the parotid gland is enlarged, the usually sharp and bony angle of the mandible feels soft and boggy owing to overlying glandular tissue, as in mumps, Sjögren's syndrome, or other exocrinopathies.

The supraclavicular fossa, which is above the clavicle, is examined for nodes, unusual excursion with respiration, swelling, fat accumulation, and asymmetry relative to the opposite side. The platysma muscle crosses the fossa but is too thin to alter its contour. Observation during voluntary platysma contracture may reveal lumps or asymmetry (Fig. 4–11). The apex and dome of the lung extend up into the fossa; cervical ribs are sometimes palpable (see Fig. 4–6). Behind the sternocleidomastoid muscle are the anterior scalene muscles, with the medial and posterior scalenes

behind them. The brachial plexus passes through them. Deep palpation at the base of the posterior triangle (supraclavicular) reveals the subclavian artery, and the small mass of tissue felt comprises the cords of the brachial plexus. Application of severe pressure to this point brings people to their knees with pain. Thus one must palpate gently. Deep palpation enables one to feel the transverse processes of the atlas and axis as well as other cervical vertebrae. The atlas can be slid gently laterally on the facets of the axis. The spinal nerves can be pressed against the transverse process if pressed very gently.

The apical portion of the lung is located above the clavicle, and a Pancoast's tumor may grow into that space and produce swelling, asymmetry, and pain—symptoms of one of the thoracic outlet syndromes. The pain is related to breathing; it increases or appears upon inhalation. Pseudoarthrosis of an old clavicular fracture may be felt.

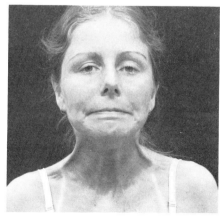

Figure 4–11. Contracting the platysma muscle.

An exostosis on the first rib is also palpable. Hypertrophy of a pectoralis minor muscle can compress the brachial plexus or the subclavian artery or vein, resulting in neurologic and vascular clinical symptoms and signs.

The posterior aspects, examined with the patient sitting, presents the trapezius muscle, the lymph nodes, the greater occipital nerves, and the superior nuchal ligament. The trapezius origin extends from the inion to the spinous process of T12 and inserts laterally in a continuous arc into the clavicle, the acromion, and the spine of the scapula (see Fig. 4–8). The muscle should be felt systematically from origin to insertion, beginning high on the neck. Flexion injuries may traumatize the trapezius, and it is often the site of focal points of pain and tenderness in fibrositis syndrome; hematoma in the muscle is common. The two trapezius muscles are best palpated bilaterally and simultaneously. The clinician looks for tenderness, lumps, swelling, and asymmetry of the two muscles and examines along the entire insertional sites—clavicle, acromion, and spine of the scapula. Embryologically the trapezius and sternocleidomastoid muscles form as one muscle, later splitting, but they retain a common attachment along the base of the skull to the mastoid process; their nerve supply is the same, the eleventh cranial (spinal accessory) nerve.

The significant lymph node chain, located at the anterolateral border of the trapezius muscle, is not normally palpable but may enlarge and be tender. The greater occipital nerves are lateral to the inion, extending well up in the scalp and are easily palpable and very tender if inflamed. A neuritis here is a fairly common cause of headache; flexion-extension injuries of the cervical spine result in traumatic inflammation and swelling of these nerves.

The superior nuchal ligament arises from the inion and extends to the C7 and T1 spinous processes. It is just under the examining finger when the spinous processes are palpated, and it may be tender, irregular, or lumpy if overstretched or injured.

Individual Muscle Actions in Range of Motion

The relatively large range of motion of the cervical spine provides a wide scope of vision, subserves the senses of sight, hearing, and smell, and is essential to the necessary acute sense of balance. The basic movements of the neck include flexion, extension, lateral flexion (right and left), and rotation (right and left). These movements and the many combinations of them give the head and neck extremely diversified motion. About one half of the total flexion and extension occurs at the occiput and C1–C2 level; the other half is equally distributed among the other six cervical vertebrae, with a slight increase at the C5–C6 level. About one half of rotation occurs at the

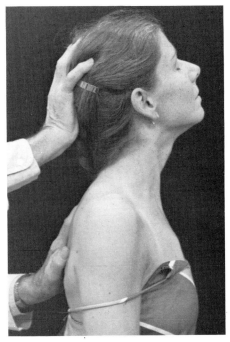

Figure 4–12. Method of testing cervical spine extension against resistance. Patient gradually increases extensor power.

atlantoaxial joint (odontoid process), and the other half is equally distributed among the other five vertebrae. All vertebrae share in lateral flexion. A decrease in a specific motion may be due to blocking at a joint, pain, fibrous contractures, bony ankylosis, muscle spasm, mechanical alteration in joint and skeletal structures, or a tense and uncooperative patient. Other causes of spasm are injury to muscles, involuntary splinting over painful joints or skeletal structures, and irritation or compression of cervical nerve roots of the spinal cord.

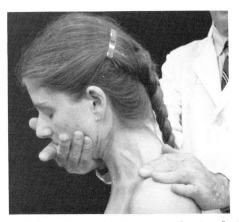

Figure 4–13. Method of testing cervical spine flexion against resistance.

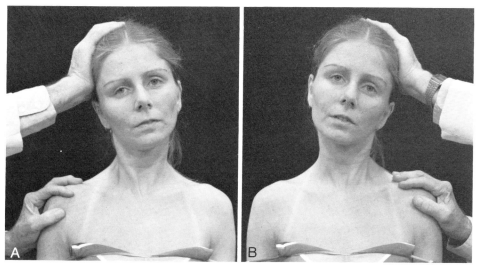

Figure 4–14. *A*, Method of testing right lateral flexion against resistance. *B*, Method of testing left lateral flexion against resistance.

The examiner assesses the primary extensors (paravertebral extensor mass, splenius capitis, semispinalis capitis, trapezius, eleventh cranial nerve) and secondary extensors (small intrinsic neck muscles) by placing the left hand over the upper posterior chest and scapular area, with the right palm cupped over the occiput; the patient then gradually increases neck extension to a maximum force. The trapezius is noted to contract and strain, and its tone and power can be assessed (Fig. 4–12).

Primary flexors of the neck are the anterior group, sternohyoid, sternothyroid, and the thyrohyoid. Forced flexion against resistance identifies any weakness and confirms function (Fig. 4–13).

Lateral flexors (the three scalenes, anterior primary division of cervical nerves C2–C3 and C3–C4, and the small intrinsic neck muscles) are examined by placing the left hand on the patient's shoulder (to stabilize him or her) with the right palm (fingers extended) against the side of the patient's head; the patient then flexes laterally against resistance to maximum power. Both directions are examined and compared (Fig. 4–14).

In testing the rotators (sternocleidomastoid and intrinsic neck muscles) for left lateral rotation, the examiner places the stabilizing left hand on the patient's left shoulder and the right hand along the right side of the mandible, and the patient rotates with maximum power (Fig. 4–15*A*). Figure

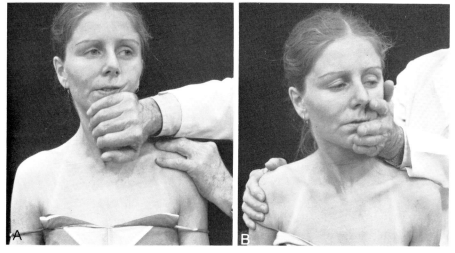

Figure 4–15. *A*, Method of testing left rotation against resistance. *B*, A second method of testing left rotation against resistance. Right rotation against resistance is tested on the right side of cheek and chin.

4–15B depicts a second method to test left rotation. The reverse procedure is used to test right rotation. One sternocleidomastoid functioning alone provides the main pull to the side being tested. The two sides are compared, and degree of power is assessed as well as evidence of pain, paresthesia, stiffness, or appearance of other symptoms and signs. The sternocleidomastoid muscle is supplied by the spinal accessory nerve, which is the eleventh cranial nerve.

Movement: Active, Passive, and Against Resistance[2]

In the clinical study of moving parts, one causes pain—or any other symptoms—by applying selective tension to the suspected part. The diagnosis may rest on the demonstration of which movements cause pain and which do not. Selective stretching, or tension, is applied to each tissue or structure, one by one, and the patient describes the effect of each movement on his or her symptoms. The pain-sensitive structure thus emerges, and the reproducibility is confirmed by a few repetitions. Examination for tenderness should be deferred until the tissue at fault is identified.

Various movements are noted as normal and others as painful or producing "pins and needles" or weak or limited motion. Negative findings can be just as important as positive findings; that is, if certain movements elicit familiar pain and implicate a particular tissue or structure, the lack of pain in all other movements relating to other tissues and structures can help confirm the diagnosis. Thus positive findings in conjunction with negative findings often help one arrive at an accurate conclusion.

If all ranges of motion are grossly decreased, one is dealing with either a severe physical problem or hysteria. Virtually always in cervical spine disorders at least one or two motions, if performed slowly enough, are pain-free, full range, and normal. Generally flexion and lateral flexion are preserved, and extension with the combination of rotation and lateral flexion is most likely to result in pain in the affected side because this set of movements puts the zygapophyseal joints in close-pack positions and narrows the intervertebral foramina the most. The patient's eyes should be open and observed by the examiner, because nystagmus, a vertebral artery syndrome, may occur during cervical spine movements and be easily overlooked.

Cervical Spine Movements

The neck movements assessed during examination include active motion, passive motion, and motion against resistance. This assessment is best accomplished while the patient stands or sits, maintaining his or her best posture. If the patient is slumped in a chair and normal lumbar lordosis is absent, optimal cervical spine range of motion is normally diminished. There are classically six movements of the cervical spine: flexion, extension, right lateral flexion, left lateral flexion, right rotation, and left rotation (Fig. 4–16). During active motion, examination of the range is noted, including observations regarding pain or stiffness and inquiries regarding a painful arc (pain at the mid-area of motion). The painful arc may be noted at the mid-range of one or two active movements of the cervical spine, but rarely, if ever, is it noted at more than two movements.

When observing active motion, the examiner studies mobile contractile structures (muscle and tendon). In fact, strongly resisted contraction of a muscle with the joint held immobile still puts tension only on the muscle and tendon. Stretching in the opposite way may hurt. When observing passive motion (patient relaxing all muscles), the examiner studies noncontractile structures (ligaments, capsules, bursae, nerve roots and trunks, and the meninges—dura mater mainly). Pain originating in nonmobile structures usually hurts only on stretching.

Active movements yield three types of clinical data: range of motion, motor power, and the status of the patient's voluntary control or "willingness" to do as much as he or she can. Some psychologic disorder is probable if there is a gross discrepancy between active and passive ranges of motion or muscular power.

If active range of motion fails to elicit the pain pattern or paresthesia, two further techniques are useful in bringing them out. One is overpressure. For example, have the patient maximally, serially, and systematically flex, extend, laterally flex, and rotate the cervical spine, holding it at the extreme of each motion for 10 to 30 seconds. If no symptoms occur, the examiner should put increased pressure on the maximally achieved motion, stretching muscles, ligaments, and capsules (see Figs. 4–12 through 4–15). The other maneuver is to increase the rate, rhythm, and velocity of the movement through, for example, rapid nodding, rotation, extension, and lateral flexion. This may elicit the familiar pain or paresthesia.

It is best to start with extension because it causes close-pack position as the inferior facet of the zygapophyseal joints glide posteriorly on the superior facet of the vertebra below, narrowing the foramen and tending to compress the nerve root. Lateral flexion and combined rotation may cause pain, numbness, or paresthesia in the shoulder, arm, or hand. By beginning with extension, one avoids undue pain and paresthesia and allows a prompt diagnosis.

Extension movement tests patency of the intervertebral foramen. The position of combined extension, lateral flexion, and rotation is the "quadrant position." The foraminal diameters are altered by head positioning. The patient's eyes should be open and observed should there be nystagmus due to vertebral artery compression

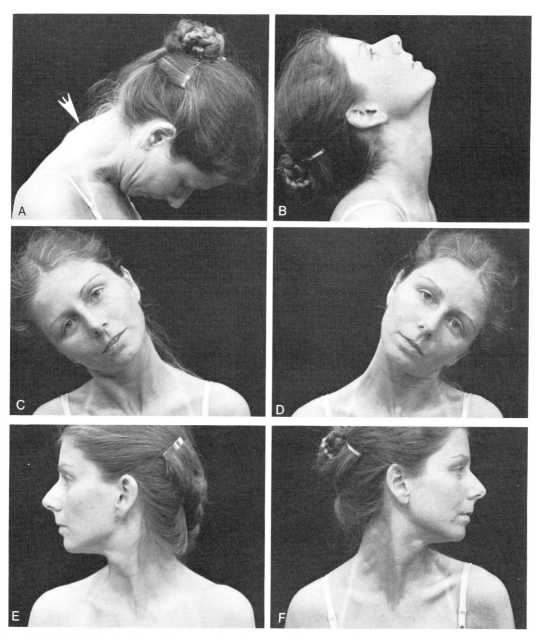

Figure 4–16. *A,* Full flexion. The chin approaches the upper chest. Normally, the examiner's index finger can be compressed between the chin and the sternal manubrium. Note that C7, the vertebra prominens (arrow), and the T1 spinous process are easily visible. The patient's mouth must be closed completely for accurate assessment. *B,* Full extension. The examiner's finger normally can be compressed between the inion and the C7 spinous process. Note that the upper and lower borders of the thyroid cartilage are easily visible. *C,* Right lateral flexion. Patient attempts to touch right ear to shoulder (can be done only rarely). Note the prominent contracted sternocleidomastoid muscle, right more than left. The edge of the trapezius is easily seen, and the anterior and posterior triangles can be readily inspected. *D,* Left lateral flexion. Note that the right lateral flexion is greater than the left, a usual clinical observation. *E,* Right rotation. Note very prominent sternocleidomastoid muscle contraction, supra- and infraclavicular fossae, jugular vein, edge of the trapezius, and upper border of the thyroid cartilage. The posterior triangle is especially well seen for clinical observation and palpation. *F,* Left rotation.

and local loss of blood supply to the brain stem and cerebellum.

Passive movements with maximal muscle relaxation illustrate whether full range of motion at the cervical joints exists, and they provide clinical correlation with the data on active movement. The patient should be standing or sitting when examined, since a greater range of motion exists in the supine position. The postural tone of muscles in the erect position limits motion slightly.

Passive movement allows the assessment of function of nonmobile (noncontractile) structures and excludes the effects of muscle power and willingness. Certain patterns emerge: (1) A capsular pattern is characterized by pain on passive movement of the involved joint and definite limitation of range of motion. This reflects a contracted, usually inflamed and fibrotic capsule, as seen in arthritis. This pattern varies from joint to joint but is very reproducible at any one joint or set of joints. (2) A noncapsular pattern is noted when range of passive motion is fully or marginally restricted; ligaments or tendons and their sheaths about the joint (extra-articular) may be sites of inflammation, fibrosis, and adhesion. Movements that stretch the ligaments hurt and limit motion, compromising full range of motion; such movements are normally pain-free. (3) Abnormalities of menisci or intra-articular flakes of cartilage may block a joint's motion; such loose bodies may move about with consequent pain, abrupt and severe, quite unlike the capsular pattern. Virtually all the joints in the cervical spine have menisci and fibrofatty structures intra-articularly, though presently we know little of their clinical effects. Intra-articular, loose bodies usually cause pain on one side of the joint. If the full capsular pattern (pain and equal limitation of all movements except flexion, which is hardly restricted at all) emerges in examination of the cervical spine, the presence of an internal derangement is very unlikely.

Cyriax[2] provides useful and diagnostic descriptions of the sensations perceived by the examiner as the end of passive motion is reached. The "end feel" of bone on bone (example is full passive extension of the elbow) is a hard stop, and further forcing produces no more movement. "Elastic stretch" is a sensation of continuing stretching that one can push farther (normal in shoulder, hip, or elbow in passive rotation—a rubbery, elastic sensation). When nonarticular tissues are approximated about a joint, the movement is stopped. For example, forearm muscles press against the biceps muscle on full elbow flexion, and little definitive resistance is felt. This "empty feel" is evident before the normal extreme range of motion is reached. The patient's refusal of further movement generally indicates more serious disease, such as bursitis, sepsis, or metastatic malignancy. Passive motion can be abruptly and unexpectedly stopped by acute muscle spasm, as seen in cases of fracture or acute synovitis. A "springy block" is suggestive of a free piece of meniscus or an intra-articular fragment of bone or cartilage.

Movements against resistance are tested for all muscle groups. The patient contracts the muscle with all his strength while the examiner provides enough resistance to prevent any joint movement. Each muscle and its origin and insertion are examined. If there is a full, passive range of motion and one resisted movement hurts, the diagnosis is a muscle lesion. If a few contradictory resisted movements cause pain, the muscle is not the pain-sensitive structure. A weak muscle without increase in pain suggests a neurologic lesion or a complete rupture of a tendon. A primary tendonitis or tenosynovitis does not limit passive movement.

Search for tenderness should follow identification of the pain-sensitive structure. The term painful arc describes appearance of pain in the wide range of joint movement, notably in the shoulder at about 60 degrees of abduction, indicating a supraspinatus tendonitis. The lesion then lies between two bony surfaces and is pinched at that point—the arc of movement (Fig. 4–17).

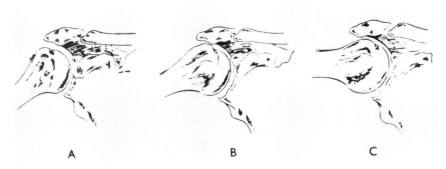

A   B   C

Figure 4–17. Painful arc in the shoulder. *A* shows abduction to about 45 degrees. *B* illustrates abduction to 60 degrees, and the greater tuberosity of the humerus is sliding under the acromion, the site of compression of the inflamed supraspinatus tendon. *C*, the greater tuberosity is now beneath the acromion, and the painful arc is relieved. (From Codman EA: The Shoulder. Boston: Thomas Todd Co Printers, 1934.)

There may be extra-articular reasons for limitation of movement. For instance, straight-leg raising, which involves hip flexion, may be limited by failure of neck flexion. When the leg reaches a certain point, posterior thigh pain appears. Further neck flexion increases the pain, and the structure whose mobility is impaired is the dura mater and its extension, the sciatic nerve sheath.

Clinical experience shows that resisted movement seldom causes pain; the exceptions are fracture of a first rib, lymphadenopathy in the cervical spine, and acute adult torticollis. The interpretation here is that cervical spine joint lesions predominate and muscle lesions are uncommon. The clinical data on muscle performance against resistance, collected during examination, are often useful in identifying hysteria, psychogenic disorders, malingering, or "compensationitis."

Pathophysiologic Interpretation of Cervical Spine Movements

Flexion of the neck stretches both cervical and thoracic dura mater. Such movement elicits pain in cases of cervical as well as thoracic disc lesions. Either central or unilateral pain at any scapular level can occur. Precise interpretation is determined by whether cervical or thoracic movements are painful. Pain on scapular approximation almost always means that the thoracic spine is the site of a lesion, because this movement pulls up the thoracic but not the cervical dura mater. The capsular pattern at cervical spine joints is as follows: (1) no limitation of flexion, (2) equal limitation of lateral flexion and rotation, and (3) marked limitation of extension. Painless limitation of motion in an elderly person means osteoarthritis, a painless stiffness. Pain produced by any passive movement except flexion, particularly if unilateral, is interpreted as a disc lesion in the symptom-free osteoarthritis joint.

Gradual onset of marked limitation of passive movement in a young person is characteristic of ankylosing spondylitis. When this limitation of movement is present, the thoracic and lumbar portions of the spine are usually already ankylosed, and the perception of bone-to-bone end feel is apparent at the extremes of passive rotation and side flexion of the neck (Fig. 4–18).

Rapid onset (within weeks or a few months) of gross limitation of movement in the capsular pattern that is associated with pain and increases in severity is strong evidence of metastatic malignant disease. Involvement at C4 to C7 is readily detected by neurologic signs in the upper extremities even though no pain has appeared in the arm. At the C1–C3 level, muscle weakness is rare and detection difficult. In metastatic malignancy, the presence of metastases in muscles, bones, and joints causes marked pain on rotation against resistance. The pain is often too severe for the patient to cooperate by hard pressing. Gentle passive movements with the patient supine may cause the perception of abrupt onset of muscle spasm in the presence of metastases, muscle spasm end feel.

Multiple myeloma involving the cervical spine has a much more gradual onset with subtle compromise of movement. Later involvement of a nerve root, with radiation of pain and paresthesia in the upper limb, often extreme and bilateral, or lasting too long, provides the lead to diagnosis.

Differential diagnosis of decreased cervical spine movements in the capsular pattern at the cervical joints includes rheumatoid arthritis, osteoarthritis, recent fracture, ankylosing spondylitis, postconcussion adhesions, and metabolic bone disease.

Osteoarthritis at the occipito-atlanto-axial level results in ligamentous scarring, adhesion, and contracture, with resultant pain in the occipital area and the forehead. The pain is worse in the morning and often occurs upon nodding the head. Inability to turn the head prohibits the patient from the routine activity of backing up the car. Osteoarthritis at the lower level of the cervical spine usually causes no symptoms but does cause painless stiffness.

The great majority of patients with ankylosing spondylitis do not suffer great disability. Those who do, however, experience increasing fixation and ultimate ankylosis in flexion. Stiffness in the joints precedes by many years the radiographic evidence of ankylosis. There is clinical evidence that stretching exercises carried out daily can prevent ankylosis.[3, 4] When the disorder has progressed painlessly in the lumbar and thoracic portions of the spine, the diagnosis may be obscured during the period of cervical spine stiffness, with very gradual compromise of motion but with normal radiograms. The radiographic appearance of the sacroiliac joint enables the physician to make the proper diagnosis.

Fracture of a cervical vertebral body, untreated, is symptom-free in a few weeks. Years later osteoarthritis may appear, but osteophyte formations at the joints of the cervical spine are quite compatible with painless function. However, in some elderly patients with ligamentous capsular contracture causing limitation of all cervical movement, the radiogram may not show osteophytes. Osteophytes in the cervical spine tend to remodel themselves away or do not form in the first place in the markedly restricted or immobilized neck.

In rheumatoid arthritis, destruction of the intervertebral disc occurs as pannus invades the disc tissue from the joints of Luschka. The presence of osteophytes in this situation is unusual. The joints are lax and loose and have the characteristic empty end-feeling on passive movement; that is, the movement ends without any bony or heavy ligamentous contact—in fact, movement ends short of how far the joint can actually go structurally.

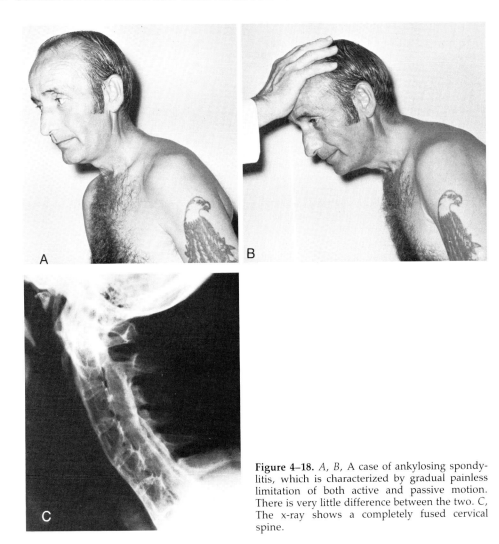

Figure 4–18. *A, B,* A case of ankylosing spondylitis, which is characterized by gradual painless limitation of both active and passive motion. There is very little difference between the two. *C,* The x-ray shows a completely fused cervical spine.

Forced immobilization results in bizarre cervical spine syndromes. For example, in postconcussional syndrome in which the patient is immobilized in bed for months for fracture of the skull, with no possibility of physical exercise, extreme atrophy of muscles, tendons, and ligaments occurs. The upper cervical joints and their muscular attachments are often sites of pain. The cause of pain is falsely attributed to psychoneurosis. Physical therapy, gentle stretching, and massage to muscle origins together with cervical spine exercises and gentle manipulation have been found useful in prevention of pain and in the return to a normal state, which requires at least a year.

A very unusual condition, subacute arthritis of the atlantoaxial joint, has been noted. It usually occurs in men between 25 and 40 years of age. Several weeks of increasing stiffness and pain in the upper cervical spine are characteristic when there is no previous history of neck disorder.

Patients demonstrate a full range of flexion, extension, and lateral flexion, but gross limitation of rotation, restricted to 10 to 15 degrees in both directions, may occur. It is a very unusual finding. There are no systemic symptoms or signs, and there is no local tenderness. The end feel of passive rotation is a soft stop, unlike the hard end-feel of ankylosing spondylitis or the end feel of osteoarthritis, intervertebral disc lesion, or muscle spasm.[2] It seems likely that this cervical spine syndrome is a consequence of atypical and self-limited rheumatoid arthritis involving the upper cervical spine. The clinician needs to know that cervical spine syndrome can be mimicked by disease in distant visceral and somatic structures. Parts *A* and *B* of Figure 4–1 illustrate sites of diseases and conditions that may be perceived in the neck. Part *C* shows the C5 dermatome. Since many clinical problems in the shoulder overlap cervical spine syndromes, it is useful to know that if the pain is perceived outside the C5 dermatome, myotome, and sclerotome, the pain-sensitive structure cannot be in the shoulder. All shoulder structures except the acromioclavicular joint derive from the original C5 somite, dermatome, myotome, and sclerotome (see Chapter 2, *Anatomy and Biomechanics*).

Scapular Movements and Clinical Impressions[2]

Appreciation of normal scapular movements is required in this area of assessment (Fig. 4–19). The clinician asks the patient to move his or her shoulders and determines whether the scapulae have normal mobility in relation to the thorax. Crepitation may be perceived. Scapular mobility can be compromised by pulmonary malignancy, arthritis of the sternoclavicular joint, metastatic malignant disease in the scapulae proper, contracture of the costocoracoid fascia and, in ankylosing spondylitis, ankylosis of the acromioclavicular joint. In the latter instance the arm cannot be elevated over the horizontal level. Paresthesia in the hands with the scapulae elevated for 60 seconds in strong evidence for one of the thoracic outlet syndromes. Hyperabducting the arm maximally and bringing the scapulae sharply backwards may eliminate the radial pulse if the space between the clavicle and the first rib is abnormally small. This does occur in normal persons with no symptoms but also suggests thoracic outlet syndrome (see Adson test, p. 105).

The following resisted scapular movements are tested (Fig. 4–20): upward movement seen in the full shrug (trapezius and levator scapulae muscles); forward movement of the scapulae (pectoralis major and minor and serratus anterior muscles); backward movement (rhomboids and lower trapezius muscles); upward and lateral movements (arms over the head, palms facing each other, maximal scapular migration); forward movement (patient presses against a wall [serratus anterior muscles]; winging of the scapulae [see Fig. 4–4]). Note that active scapular movements influence joints at either end of the clavicle (acromioclavicular and sternoclavicular joints). Approximation of the scapulae stretches the dura mater through traction in the upper thoracic nerve roots, sometimes causing pain in the chest suggesting a thoracic disc lesion at any level.

Pathophysiologic Interpretation of Scapular Pain[2]

In the following section, eight cases are described, and the pathophysiologic interpretation of scapular pain is given for each case.

1. Active and passive movement of and elevation of the scapulae are painful; forward and backward movements are not painful, and resisted movements are painless. Passive scapular movements are performed by the examiner lifting and rotating the arm and shoulder, with the patient as relaxed as possible. The differential diagnosis is (a) arthritis of the sternoclavicular joint—pain may be perceived at the posterior unilateral side of the neck if the posterior ligaments of the joint are involved; (b) stretching of the costocoracoid fascia—complete elevation of the arm is painful in the pectoral scapular area; and (c) dense scarring in the apex of the lung, limiting the mobility of costocoracoid fascia.

2. Resisted movements are not painful, but all active and passive scapular movements hurt. These symptoms are characteristic of a first or second thoracic root lesion. Occasionally radiation occurs to the ulnar border of the forearm and the palm (T1 level) or to the medial aspect of the arm on the inner side of the elbow (T2 level).

3. Active and passive elevation of scapulae is painful and limited, but resisted movements are painless. If the patient has a history of trauma and no skeletal damage, a hematoma in contact with a costocoracoid fascia will explain the syndrome. If the patient has no history of trauma, an apical pulmonary malignancy is suspected—carefully examine the pupil of the eye and the small muscles of the hand. Plain radiographs or laminograms may confirm the diagnosis.

4. Passive movement of the scapulae up and down is uncomfortable and crepitant, though rarely audible to others. This indicates scapulothoracic syndrome.

5. Active and passive approximation of the scapulae is painful, and resisted movements are painless. An upper thoracic intraspinal lesion with dura mater compression is suspected. This is usually a thoracic disc protrusion and may be associated with a positive Lhermitte's sign.[5]

6. Unilateral pain at the root of the neck is induced by flexion and lateral flexion toward the painless side, active and passive scapular elevation, and complete elevation of the arm. A lesion at the joint between the first rib and the transverse process of the first thoracic vertebra is suspected.

7. Active and passive elevation of the scapulae is painful in the pectoral area, with pain occurring also on resisted depression of the scapulae. These symptoms indicate that the subclavius muscle is abnormal.[2]

8. Pain in the scapular area is uninfluenced by neck or scapular thoracic movements, and radiographic findings of lungs and ribs are normal. Pleuritis, herpes zoster, or peripheral neuritis is indicated. The "shingles" vesicles often appear in 3 or 4 days, and the neuritic pain lasts 3 to 4 weeks. Neuralgic amyotrophic brachial pain reaches a crescendo in a few days and subsides; thus pain that continues for more than a month with spreading suggests visceral disease, such as atypical angina pectoris.

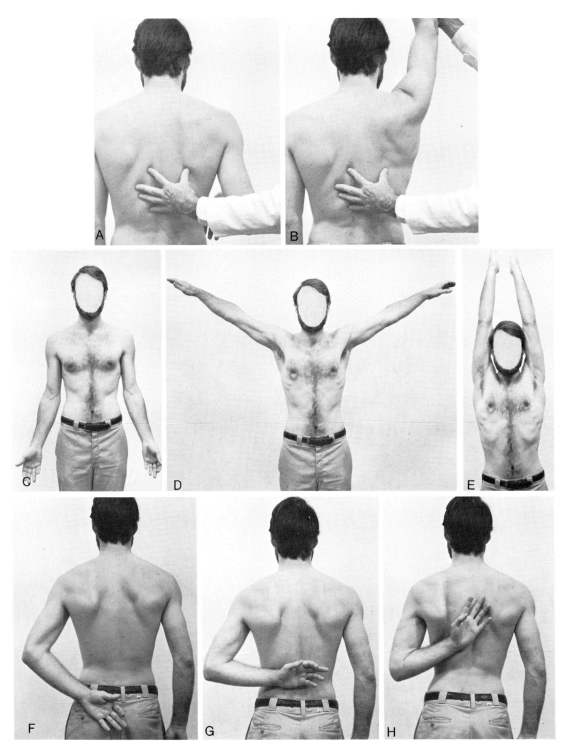

Figure 4–19. *See legend on opposite page*

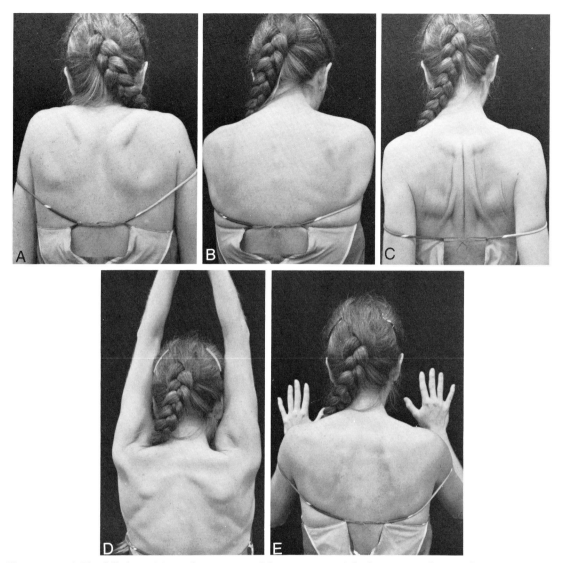

Figure 4–20. *A*, The full shrug. Maximal contraction of the trapezius and the levator scapulae muscles. Note scapular elevation and contracted muscle masses. *B*, Forward movement of both scapulae on maximal contraction of the pectoralis major and minor and the serratus anterior muscles. *C*, Scapulae almost approximate each other (medial migration) on contraction of the rhomboid muscle and the lower trapezius muscles. *D*, Upward and lateral motion of the arms over the head (palms meet) shows maximal scapular migration. Virtually all scapular muscles are in contraction. *E*, Pressing forward against a wall (serratus anterior muscle) causes scapular fixation. If there is long thoracic nerve neuritis or a primary myopathy, winging of the affected side occurs (see Figure 4–4).

Figure 4–19. Scapular movements. In ruling out shoulder disorders and examining the scapular movements in cervical spine disorders, one needs to know and interpret normal scapular movements. *A*, Examiner's thumb is at the inferior angle of the scapula. The bone is somewhat prominent and slightly shrugged with the elbow flexed. *B*, On passive abduction followed by hyperabduction and medial humeral rotation, the scapula glides anteriorly, upward, and laterally over the upper lateral chest wall. *C*, Active movement. Normal anatomic position. *D*, Arms abducted to just above 90 degrees until humeri are medially rotated, palms facing down. Moving the arms the next 60 degrees requires further humeral and scapular rotation. *E*, Palms facing each other, scapulae have rotated, allowing 60 degrees more hyperabduction and elevation. Moving the arms the last 30 degrees to touch the head is achieved by abduction of the humerus across the front of the scapula, the coracoid process, and the acromion. *F*, Limited shoulder motion detected by finding that the patient can medially rotate the shoulder only enough to have hand on upper buttock. *G*, With increased range of motion, the patient can reach the flank. *H*, The normal range of motion allows the hand to reach the interscapular area. Note the increased winging of the scapula.

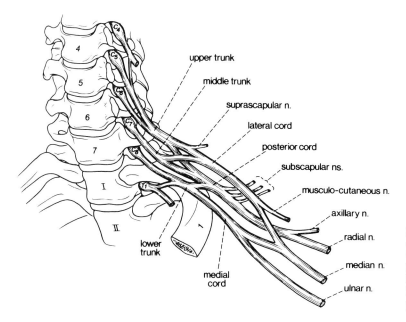

Figure 4–21. The brachial plexus consists of nerves emerging from C4 through T1. (From Bland JH, Nakano KK: Neck pain. *In* Kelley, Harris, Ruddy, et al (eds): Textbook of Rheumatology. Philadelphia: W. B. Saunders Co, 1981.)

TESTS TO ASSESS LEVEL OF INVOLVEMENT (C5–T1)

Many abnormalities in the cervical spine are perceived clinically as neurologic symptoms and signs in the upper extremity. This is understandable, since the C4 through T1 nerves provide innervation for the entire upper extremity. The clinical tests, discussed subsequently, determine whether pathologic changes in the neck account for upper extremity neurologic symptoms and signs. The tests examine motor power, reflexes and sensation by neurologic level C4 to T2.

There are eight paired spinal nerves in the cervical spine but only seven vertebrae. The first through the seventh exit above the vertebra of corresponding number; for example, the first exits above the atlas, and the seventh exits above the seventh vertebra. The eighth cervical nerve, however, exits below the seventh vertebra and above the first thoracic vertebrae, and the first thoracic nerve exits below the first thoracic vertebra. The brachial plexus is composed of nerves emerging from C4, C5, C6, C7, C8, and T1 (Fig. 4–21). The nerves exit, pass between the scalene muscles (anterior and medial), and C5 and C6 immediately join to form the upper trunk. C8 and T1 join to form the lower trunk, and C7 independently constitutes the middle trunk. All trunks pass beneath the clavicle and then divide to form cords. The upper trunk (C5 and C6) and the lower trunk (C8 and T1) contribute to the middle trunk to form the posterior cord. The middle trunk sends fibers to connect with C5 and C6 to form the lateral cord, and the remainder of C8 and T1 forms the medial cord. Branches—musculocutaneous, median, ulnar, radial, and axillary nerves—emerge

from the cords. Sensation of all sorts is supplied according to the dermatome, myotome, and sclerotome distribution patterns. (*Note:* Refer to Tables 2–1, 2–2, and 2–3 for further clarification of the following discussion.)

C5 Level. Muscles reflecting C5 nerves are the deltoid and biceps brachii—the deltoid entirely by C5, and the biceps brachii by C5 and C6 (musculocutaneous nerve). The deltoid is a three-part muscle flexing in its anterior portion, abducting in the middle, and extending the shoulder in its posterior portion. Thus, the examiner resists shoulder flexion, abduction, and extension. The biceps brachii flexes the shoulder and elbow and supinates the forearm. It is tested by offering resistance to flexion and supination. The brachioradialis muscle, the other main flexor of the elbow, is also of musculocutaneous innervation, and flexion in resistance will identify C5 integrity via this test. The reflex of the biceps brachii reflects the integrity of both C5 and C6, and even a slightly decreased reflex is significant. The skin of the lateral arm is the area of C5 sensation, which is supplied by the axillary nerve (Fig. 4–22*A–D*).

C6 Level. The C6 muscles are the biceps brachii (in part) and the wrist extensors—extensor carpi radialis longus, extensor carpi radialis brevis, and extensor carpi ulnaris. The wrist extensors have C7 contribution; thus, the muscle tests are not pure. Power of wrist extension against resistance is assessed as well as shoulder flexion, and any difference in the two sides are noted. The brachioradialis reflex is tested where the muscle becomes tendinous before inserting into the radius near the wrist. The biceps reflex is also elicited. Sensation supplied by C6 via the musculocutaneous nerve is in the lateral forearm, the thumb, index finger, and one half of the middle finger (Fig. 4–22*D*–*G*).

C7 Level. The C7 muscles are the triceps and the wrist flexor group. The triceps muscle, supplied by C7 via the radial nerve, extends the elbow and is tested by extension against resistance. The wrist flexor group, flexor carpi radialis (median nerve) and flexor carpi ulnaris (ulnar nerve), is tested by the patient's making a fist and flexing against resistance. The finger extensors—extensor digitorum communis, extensor digiti indicis, and extensor digiti minimi—are also supplied by C7. Finger extension is tested by pressing on the patient's extended fingers, noting the power present (see Fig. 4–22*I*). The triceps tendon reflex is elicited by tapping the tendon where it crosses the olecranon fossa at the elbow. Sensation of the middle finger is largely a C7 function (Fig. 4–22*G*–*I*).

C8 Level. C8 has no reproducible reflex. The C8 muscles are finger flexors, flexor digitorum superficialis (proximal interphalangeal joints) and flexor digitorum profundus (distal interphalangeal joints), from the median and ulnar nerves. To examine finger flexion, curl and lock your fingers into the patient's flexed fingers and try to pull them out of flexion. C8 supplies sensation to the ring fingers, the little fingers, and the distal half of the ulnar side of the forearm (Fig. 4–22*J*).

T1 Level. T1 has no identifiable reflex. The muscles of T1 are the finger abductors, the dorsal interossei, and the adductor digiti quinti. Muscle testing is done by squeezing the abducted fingers together; adduction by having the patient try to hold a dollar bill between the adducted fingers. T1 supplies sensation to the medial side of the upper half of the forearm and to the lower half of the arm via the medial brachial cutaneous nerve (Fig. 4–22*K*–*O*).

All clinical examination methods used in studying C5 to T1 are presented in Figure 4–22.

SPECIAL TESTS, OBSERVATIONS, AND SYNDROMES IN CLINICAL DIAGNOSIS

Head Compression Test (Spurling Test).[6] Brought about by narrowing of the intervertebral foramina, pressure and shearing forces on the zygapophyseal joint surfaces, intervertebral disc compression, and pressure on stiff ligamentous and muscular structures all may cause pain or increased pain on compression of the head with force transmission to the cervical spine. A pain pattern may be perfectly reproduced, allowing location of the neurologic level. If radicular pain or paresthesia with referral to the upper extremity occurs, nerve root irritation is assured; if the pain is confined to the neck, soft connective tissues or joints are more likely the pain-sensitive structures.

The test is done with the patient sitting. Place one hand across the other on the top of the patient's head and gradually increase downward pressure, with the patient noting pain or paresthesia and its distribution. Pressure may also be applied with head tilted to either side, backward, or forward (Fig. 4–23).

Distraction Test. This test provides some prediction of the effect of cervical spine traction in relieving pain or paresthesia. Nerve root compression may be relieved, with disappearance of the symptoms and signs, if the intervertebral foramina are opened or the disc spaces extended. Pressure on joint capsules of apophyseal joints is also decreased by distraction. Muscle spasms of any cause may be relieved (Fig. 4–24).

The test is done with the patient sitting. Place the open palm of one hand under the patient's chin and the other under the occiput and gradually increase the force of lifting, removing the weight of the skull and distracting the foramina, discs, and joints. Continue for 30 to 60 seconds.

Valsalva's Maneuver. This test, holding the breath against a closed glottis, raises intrathecal pressure and may result in pain secondary to an intraspinal tumor or a herniated disc, or the pain may radiate to a dermatome distribution of a nerve root. Voluntary hard cough or sneeze likewise may elicit cervical spine pain (Fig. 4–25).

Supraclavicular lymph nodes may sometimes be demonstrated during Valsalva's maneuver.[7] The maneuver increases intrathoracic pressure, with bulging of the apical pleura and consequent elevation of deeply situated lymph nodes, which puts them within reach of the examiner's hands. This maneuver is especially useful in the physiologically thin or cachectic patient because, in those patients, there is less subcutaneous tissue between the lymph nodes and the examining fingers.

Dysphagia Test. Ask patient to swallow food, preferably solid food. Pain or some restriction to swallowing may be due to soft tissue swelling, hematoma, vertebral subluxation, or osteophytic projection into the esophagus or the pharynx.

Examination of Eyes and Ears. Pupillary signs may differ from one side to the other or vary from one time to another, indicating irritability of the sympathetic nerve supply, which is located in the neck and controls the pupillary muscles. This is not Horner's syndrome, which follows complete interruption or paralysis of sympathetic fibers, with constriction of the pupil on the immobilized side, vasomotor changes, and a drooping of the upper eyelid. These pupillary changes come and go; a change of glasses is useless.

Ear symptoms accompanying cervical spine disorders are difficult to relate precisely to the pathology. Treatment of the cervical spine problem often relieves ear symptoms, and a proper therapeutic trial of cervical spine traction is often useful diagnostically.

Vertigo is not common in cervical spine disease, but its presence rules out other causes of upper cervical spine and brain stem dysfunction. Table 4–3 lists causes of vertigo.

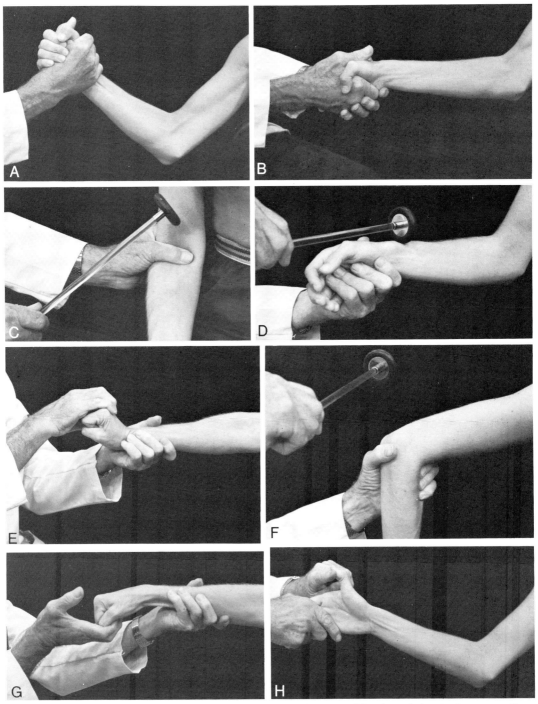

Figure 4–22. *A*, Examiner offering resistance to flexion of the biceps and brachioradialis. *B*, Examiner offering resistance to supination on testing the power of the biceps muscle. *C*, Eliciting the biceps muscle reflex, C5–C6. *D*, Eliciting the brachioradialis muscle reflex. *E*, Examining wrist extension for power against resistance. *F*, Eliciting the triceps reflex, C6–C7. *G*, Examiner testing wrist flexion against resistance. *H*, Testing the power of the adductor pollicis, C8–T1.

Illustration continued on opposite page

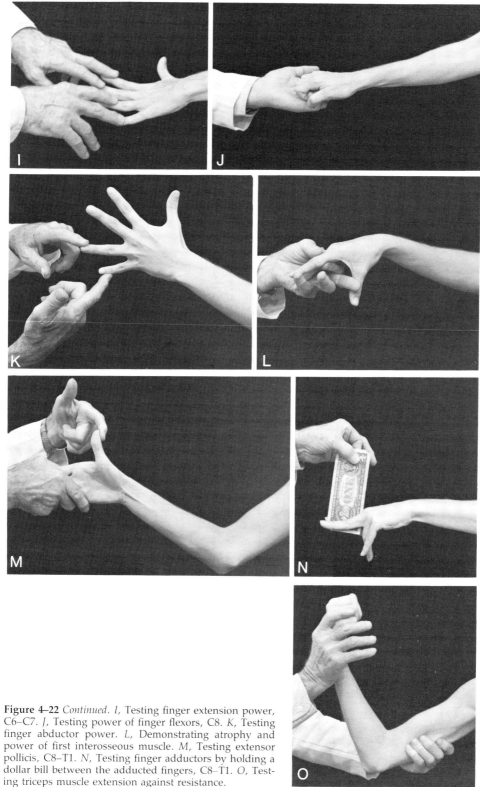

Figure 4–22 *Continued. I,* Testing finger extension power, C6–C7. *J,* Testing power of finger flexors, C8. *K,* Testing finger abductor power. *L,* Demonstrating atrophy and power of first interosseous muscle. *M,* Testing extensor pollicis, C8–T1. *N,* Testing finger adductors by holding a dollar bill between the adducted fingers, C8–T1. *O,* Testing triceps muscle extension against resistance.

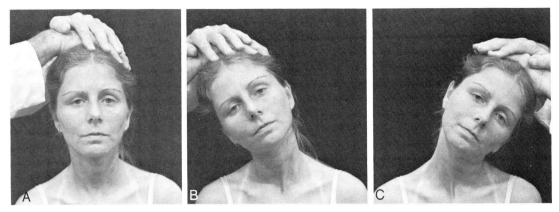

Figure 4–23. Spurling test, compression of the cervical spine. Examiner applies pressure first directly downward (*A*) with gradual increase and maintenance of constant pressure for 30 to 60 sec. The same procedure is repeated in right (*B*) and left (*C*) lateral flexion, since this tends to close the intervertebral foramina on the side of the flexion, reproducing the familiar pain or paresthesia.

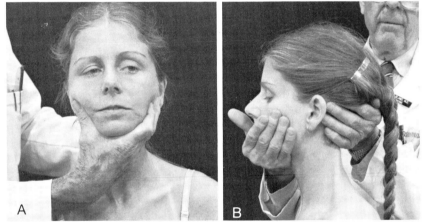

Figure 4–24. *A*, Distraction of the cervical spine, with upward traction by hand, patient seated. Traction force is gradually increased and held for 30 to 60 sec. *B*, Note that in lateral view the cervical spine can be clearly lengthened by manual traction. Note the edge of the trapezius muscle.

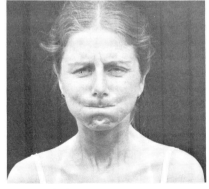

Figure 4–25. Valsalva's maneuver, exhalation against a closed glottis, raises intraspinal and peripheral venous pressure. This maneuver may elicit a familiar pain by creating pressure on intraspinal structures.

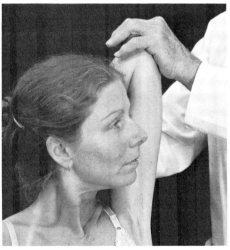

Figure 4–26. Adson test.

Table 4–3. CAUSES OF VERTIGO

Otologic	**Cardiac**
Acute serous otitis media	Arrhythmia
Acute labyrinthitis	Myxoma embolization
Vestibular neuronitis	Aortic stenosis
Cholesteatoma	Bradycardia
Purulent otitis media	Poor pump efficiency
Petrositis	Hypertension
Poststapedectomy	Orthostatic hypotension
syndrome	
Perilymph fistula	**Metabolic and**
Meniere's disease	**Hematologic**
Benign positional vertigo	Glucose intolerance
Acoustic neuroma	(diabetes mellitus)
(intracanal)	Hypoglycemia
Ototoxic drugs	Hypoadrenalism
	Syphilis
Central Nervous System	Hyperthyroidism
Stroke	Hypothyroidism
Transient ischemic	Salt-losing syndrome
attacks	Anemia
Multiple sclerosis	Polycythemia
Trauma	Leukemia
Metastatic tumor	
Primary tumor	**Drugs**
Neurosyphilis	Streptomycin
Meningitis	Kanamycin
Encephalitis	Diazepam
Fainting	Sedatives
Posterior fossa tumor	Opiates
Vertebrobasilar artery	Alcohol
insufficiency	Neuroleptics
Temporal lobe epilepsy	Aspirin
Drug	Nicotine
Migraine and migraine	Caffeine
equivalents	Prochlorperazine
Vertiginous epilepsy	
	Infections
Neck	Influenza
Trauma	Herpes zoster oticus
Osteoarthritis	Measles
Subclavian steal	Mumps
syndrome	
Vertebral artery disease	**Other**
Acromegaly	Temporomandibular joint
	syndrome
	Heatstroke

Adson Test. The Adson test is performed to examine the subclavian artery when it may be compressed by a cervical rib, the scalene muscles, or another thoracic outlet abnormality. The patient's radial pulse is continually felt as the examiner abducts, extends, and externally rotates the arm; the patient then takes a deep breath and rotates the head maximally toward the side being tested. With compression of the subclavian artery there is a marked decrease in volume or an absence of the radial pulse. The maneuver may elicit a tingling sensation, paresthesia, pain, or sensations of heat and cold if portions of the brachial plexus are compressed (Fig. 4–26). Both decrease in pulse volume and even absent pulse may occur normally.

The Adson test may be performed according to Adson's original description, in which the patient, with breath held, hyperextends the neck and turns the head toward the affected side. In addition to a decrease in pulse amplitude or an absent pulse, the patient may experience tingling sensations in the hand and arm and a sense of coldness. The vascular or neural compression may occur between the first rib and the clavicle or under the pectoralis minor muscle. The hand on the affected side is usually somewhat swollen, recognized by careful clinical comparison with the normal side in a good light. Grip strength is commonly reduced on the affected side, perhaps related to the swelling. Carpal tunnel edema may cause carpal tunnel syndrome in the various thoracic outlet syndromes.

An added important technique is to auscultate with the stethoscope over the subclavian artery. In this case, auscultation should be performed both supra- and infraclavicularly as well as both primarily and during the hyperabduction maneuver. One may hear a bruit that changes its character and intensity during the maneuver as the arterial lumen is narrowed. Exercises of shoulder, arm, and hand may reduce swelling. Such patients tend not to move and use the hand, arm, and shoulder, exaggerating swelling. Holding the hand above the head periodically may reduce swelling and improve symptoms.

Electromyographic study of C7–T1 nerves and muscles can be confirmatory if not diagnostic. A simple, exaggerated military posture with some shrug and with arms back in extension and abduction closes the space between the first rib and the clavicle. Hyperabduction stretches the pectoralis major, resulting in decreased pulse volume, coldness, tingling, and pain in the arm and hand.

Blood Pressure. Blood pressure often varies in the two arms in cervical spine disorders, presumably owing to irritating cervical sympathetic nerve supply and vasoconstriction of arteries supplied by sympathetic fibers. Muscle spasm secondary to nerve root irritation may contribute. Spasm of scalene muscles secondary to C2–C3 and C3–C4 nerve root irritation may compress the subclavian artery, with a consequent difference in blood pressure. Radial pulses may be obliterated for the same reason.

Atherosclerotic stenosis also may result in variable blood pressures. A reduction of blood pressure in one arm and a bruit heard over one or both subclavian arteries strongly suggests the diagnosis of subclavian steal syndrome,[8] a condition often presaging a stroke. Such varied symptom combinations of paresis, numbness, dysphasia, vertigo, diplopia, and dysarthria may occur. Atherosclerotic stenosis or occlusion of one subclavian artery proximal to the origin of the vertebral artery results in a reduction of pressure distally, causing that blood, instead of flowing upward in the corresponding vertebral artery and supplying the basilar region of the brain, actually to flow downward (in reverse), draining blood away from the basilar system and into the subclavian artery.

Shoulder Depression Test. This test determines indirectly whether there is irritation or compression of nerve roots, dural root sleeve fibrosis or adhesions, foraminal encroachment, or adjacent joint capsule thickening and adhesions. The examiner, standing beside the patient who tilts the head to one side, places one hand on the shoulder and the other on the side of the patient's head, and exerts downward pressure on the shoulder and lateral flexion pressure on the head in the opposite direction. The test places a tug on nerve roots, and with root sleeve fibrosis, foraminal osteophytes, or adhesions, radicular pain or paresthesia often results (Fig. 4–27).

Muscle Weakness and Atrophy. Weakness of muscles may be difficult to assess because shoulder girdle and muscles of the arm, forearm, and hand are innervated by two or more roots. Weakness may vary day to day or week to week depending on the magnitude of nerve root irritation and the rate of loss of function. Dynamometer readings of the gripping muscles, serially taken, may be useful in early detection of denervation atrophy. Circumference measurements of the forearm and midportion of the arm, recorded at each visit, may warn of rapid progression to clinical loss of function. Denervation atrophy can occur in 3 to 4 weeks. Atrophy may follow, owing to lack of use or to pain. Atrophy of the interossei muscles in the hands is often striking in cervical spine disease.

Examination of Related Areas. Shoulder lesions may closely mimic cervical spine disease, and a complete shoulder examination is necessary to rule them out as a contributor.[9] The shoulder syndromes usually have little or no neurologic component. Rotator cuff tendonitis, calcareous deposits in tendons, and capsulitis are often associated with cervical spine disease; reflex sympathetic dystrophy may occur, with the triggering pain mechanism arising in the cervical spine. The coexistence of shoulder syndromes and cervical spine disease is common. The same changes may occur at the elbow, wrist, and fingers. Finger motion may be limited owing to swelling secondary to circulatory reflex ischemic changes caused by sympathetic nerve irritation. Fibrous nodules and contracture of palmar fascia occur following cervical spine disease or injury.

Examination of Temporomandibular Joint, Teeth, Lower Jaw, and Scalp (Referred Pain). Infection of the temporomandibular joint, teeth, lower jaw, or scalp may refer pain to the temporomandibular joint area and to the neck. These structures should be examined (Figure 4–28). The interincisor distance allows three fingers (about 6 cm). The temporomandibular joint is examined by inspection during opening and closing of the mouth and by direct palpation during which the examining finger falls into a depression on opening and is pushed out on closing. The posterior aspect of the joint can be easily felt with the fifth finger pressing forward in the external auditory canal.

Tendon Reflexes. The tendon reflexes in the upper extremities depend on the balance between the upper and lower motor neuron lesions. When the lower motor nerves (anterior horn cells) are involved in a myelopathy, the tendon reflexes tend to decrease, finally to disappear. But when the corticospinal tract (upper motor neurons) is involved in the myelopathic process, the deep tendon reflexes are exaggerated. If a nucleus pulposus herniation occurs and compression is just above the cervical enlargement, all reflexes in the upper extremities are exaggerated. More commonly, the cervical enlargement itself is involved, and the scattered combination of decrease in some reflexes and exaggeration of others is seen. The biceps reflex is most commonly decreased or lost because the C5–C6 level is most commonly involved.

A common finding in upper extremity reflexes is the inverted radial reflex. If a lesion of the fifth cervical segment involves the corticospinal tract (through which pass the nerve pathways mediating the radial reflex), the tendon reflexes mediated by lower segments of the cervical cord, especially the flexor finger jerk, become exaggerated. So, in tapping the lower radius, the normal brachioradialis reflex is diminished or absent, but the stimulus by irradiation causes reflex flexion of the fingers, the inverted radial reflex. Increased flexor finger jerks can be elicited by tapping the flexor surfaces of the finger directly or by Hoffmann's reflex. In this situation the triceps reflex is often exaggerated, with upper motor neuron signs in the lower extremities. These signs may occur in any cord lesion that involves the fifth cervical segment.

Superficial abdominal reflexes are commonly diminished but rarely absent. The absence of

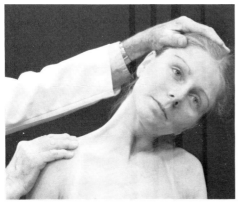

Figure 4–27. Shoulder depression test.

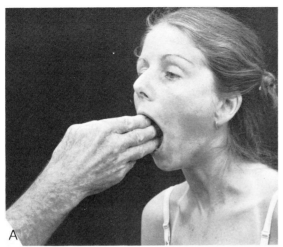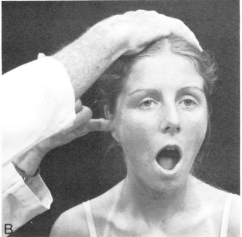

Figure 4–28. *A,* Mouth is opened to an estimated 6 cm. *B,* Examiner's fifth finger tip, placed in the external auditory canal, presses forward on the temporomandibular joint. Also an index finger placed just anterior to the ear, with applied pressure, may elicit tenderness and pain. The joint may be visibly swollen. In the patient with a normal temporomandibular joint, the examiner's finger tip causes no pain as the patient opens and closes the mouth.

abdominal reflexes is a common sign early in the course of disseminated sclerosis. Clonus, usually abortive, not sustained, and exaggerated patellar and ankle jerks occur, and reflexes in the lower limb show spasticity and extensor plantar responses. Sphincter control is rarely if ever lost in cervical spine lesions as it is in lumbar cord lesions.

Upper motor neuron signs (spinal cord signs) that identify incipient or established myelopathy include hyperactive, often asymmetric, patellar and Achilles reflexes and clonus that is intermittent early and then later constant; positive Babinski's and Hoffmann's signs; positive palmomental reflex; odd sensation of gait; awkward walking; variable hyper-reactive biceps, triceps, and brachioradialis reflexes; senses of heat or cold in the lower extremities; diminished vibratory sensation; hypesthesia, hyperesthesia, paresthesia; and anesthetic spots on the skin—more on the lower than on the upper extremity. Frequently lower motor neuron signs occur in the upper extremities and upper motor neuron signs occur in the lower extremities.

Jaw Jerk. The jaw reflex, mediated by the fifth cranial nerve and involving the masseter and temporalis muscle, is stimulated by placing the index and middle fingers on the mental area of the chin, with the patient's mouth in rest position (slightly open); the fingers are tapped with the reflex hammer, and the jaw reflexly closes (Fig. 4–29*A*). Another method is to place a wooden tongue depressor on the lower molars with the patient's mouth open and tap the tongue depressor (Fig. 4–29*B*). An absent or decreased reflex suggests abnormality in the course of the trige-

minal nerve, and a brisk reflex suggests an upper motor neuron lesion. The reflex is useful in separating cervical spine disease from primary trigeminal nerve disease. A normal jaw jerk plus exaggerated, deep tendon reflexes in the upper extremities strongly suggests a lesion below the foramen magnum; however, an exaggerated or absent jaw jerk indicates a lesion at or above the level of the pons, an upper motor neuron lesion.

Lidocaine (Xylocaine) Test. Irritation or compression of cervical nerve roots with radiation of pain is accompanied by diffuse, deep tenderness at the site of pain, the myotome and dermatome areas. Segmental areas of deep tenderness may not be painful until palpated. Injection of a local anesthetic (1% lidocaine) into myalgic areas momentarily reproduces the radicular pattern of pain, often resulting in dramatic relief for days, weeks, and months. Injection of a local anesthetic into a painful area in which there is no associated tenderness causes only fleeting relief of pain and no reproduction of the radicular pain. In that case one should consider other lesions as responsible for this pain, notably a lesion of a visceral or somatic structure having the same segmental nerve supply. This test also readily identifies malingerers, who deny any relief at all.

Atlantoaxial Subluxation Clinical Test. Subluxation of the atlas on the axis, even of minor proportions, produces a bulge in the posterior pharynx that can be easily seen by lifting the soft palate with a tongue depressor. Normally the anterior arch of the atlas is only a few millimeters from the pharyngeal wall; a 5-mm subluxation can be seen. By the same token, a bulge of the spinous process of the axis appears in the upper posterior

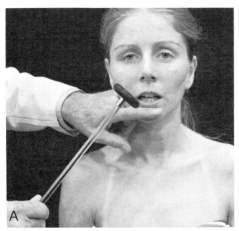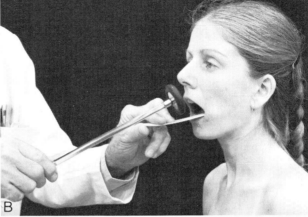

Figure 4–29. *A,* The jaw reflex, mediated by the fifth cranial nerve, involves the masseter and temporalis muscles. The examiner places the index finger in the chin, with the jaw relaxed, and taps the finger. Reflex closure occurs. *B,* The tongue blade method is a more sensitive technique that is more often clinically useful. The examiner places the tongue blade along the lower molar teeth and strikes the tongue blade. Absent, normal, and hyperactive reflexes are all clinically useful and significant.

neck as the head and the atlas slide forward in subluxation and the posterior arch is displaced in a forward direction (Fig. 4–30).

Sharp-Purser Test. The palm of one hand is placed on the patient's forehead, and the thumb of the other is placed on the tip of the spinous process of the axis. As the patient gently flexes the neck, the examiner presses backward with the palm. A sense of the head and atlas sliding backward on the axis is perceived, often with a sound—a clunk—as the subluxation is reduced. The subluxation may be clearly perceived[10, 11] (Fig. 4–31).

Short Neck. Short neck is seen in marked up-

ward subluxation of the odontoid process in rheumatoid arthritis, much the same as that seen in congenital platybasia. Flattening of the usual cervical lordosis also occurs. Here, the process is best termed basilar invagination.

Crepitus. Crepitus can be heard and felt, especially during cervical spine flexion. It can be readily heard normally by placing the stethoscope over the upper posterior cervical spine.

Absence of Signs. Fifteen per cent of patients with rheumatoid arthritis and atlantoaxial subluxation and those with severe osteoarthritis of the cervical spine may have no cervical signs.[10, 12]

Vibratory Sense. If a patient senses vibration

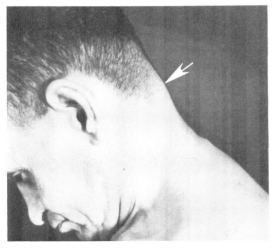

Figure 4–30. Note the bulge in the posterior neck caused by the atlas subluxation forward, bringing the spinous process of the axis into prominence beneath the skin (arrow). (Courtesy of Harold S. Robinson, MD, Vancouver, British Columbia.)

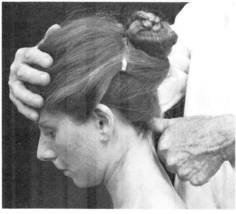

Figure 4–31. The Sharp-Purser test. The examiner's right hand is cupped over the forehead, and the left thumb is placed firmly over the spinous process of the axis. The head is gently pushed posteriorly. A sense of gliding movement or a sound or clunk is heard as the atlas and skull subluxate forward and backward.

on one side of the skull and not on the other, it should be noted. In cases of so-called whiplash there are often major problems in identification of the mechanism of symptom production. Is the syndrome due to hysteria, psychoneurosis, or "compensationitis"? Is it due to cervical spine trauma and disability? To perceive vibration on one side of the skull and not on the other can occur only through hysterical mechanisms. Thus, the test of skull vibratory sense is occasionally very useful.

Lhermitte's Sign. Actually a symptom, this "sign" is a sudden, severe, electric shock–like sensation arising in the cervical or thoracic spine and spreading down the body on flexion of the head or trunk. It was first described by Lhermitte, Bollak, and Nicholas[13] in 1924 in a patient with multiple sclerosis. The symptom is not indicative of multiple sclerosis; it does indicate a spinal cord lesion of many possible causes: trauma, neoplasm, osteoarthritis, arachnoiditis, radiation, myelopathy, syringomyelia, Pott's disease and subacute combined degeneration.[14] The "electric" sensation is elicited by anterior neck flexion. Uncommonly, the symptom occurs in trunk flexion, not cervical spine flexion, and reflects a lesion of the thoracic spinal cord.[15]

Signs of Trigeminal Nerve Impairment. Decreased or absent corneal reflex, usually unilateral, may be seen in atlantoaxial subluxation, both horizontal and vertical (upward translocation of the odontoid process into the foramen magnum). Trigeminal nerve involvement, usually in the territory of the first division, may occur, causing decreased or absent light touch and pain sensation in the face.[16]

The corneal reflex change indicates a lesion above the foramen magnum, as does trigeminal nerve involvement. The corneal reflex has occasionally been useful as an early sign of brain stem involvement in atlantoaxial subluxation in rheumatoid arthritis.[17]

Signs of Vertebral Artery Syndrome. Extension or lateral flexion or rotation is most likely to result in partial or complete vertebral artery occlusion, causing dizziness, nystagmus, vestibular signs, and a host of potential symptoms induced by ischemia to the cerebellum, visual cortex, vestibular apparatus, and the brain stem. The simplest and safest test is to have the patient lie supine on the examining table with the head over the end of the table and supported by the examiner's hands. The patient keeps both eyes open while the head and neck are gently extended. The examiner carefully looks for nystagmus. The patient reports any symptoms. If symptoms appear and there is no nystagmus, the neck, completely but comfortably extended, is rotated and laterally flexed. Each maneuver may be held for 10 to 30 seconds to determine whether symptoms or signs appear. If symptoms, signs, or nystagmus appears, the maneuver is stopped. One should never

proceed in an effort to learn, for instance, whether it is a right or left vertebral artery occlusion. This is purely academic. Do not get academic with the vertebral artery!

Breathing Pattern and Beevor's Sign. Breathing pattern is observed to note whether the intercostal muscles are functioning or whether the movements are entirely abdominal. If the C3, C4, C5 nerve roots (diaphragm) are intact and a spinal cord lesion is present (caused by trauma or tumor) and the intercostal muscles are paralyzed, respiratory movements will be entirely abdominal. If abdominal musculature is paralyzed on one side only, the umbilicus tends to be pulled to the normal side on inspiration. On coughing, the paralyzed side bulges farther than the unaffected side. When the patient flexes his head and neck toward the trunk, the equal tension of the entire abdominal musculature keeps the umbilicus in a central position. With a spinal cord lesion causing paralysis of the lower abdominal muscles and not the upper, the umbilicus rises. This is Beevor's sign.

Tumor Signs and Symptoms. *Tumors High in the Cervical Spine (C1, C2, C3, C4).* These tumors characteristically cause pain in the neck and the postauricular region, usually causing the patient to hold his or her head in an abnormally cocked position (cock-robin position). When a tumor is at C4, the pain is felt on the superior aspect of the shoulder. Deep and superficial cervical muscles are usually atrophied, and the dermatomes of these nerves may show hypo- or hyperesthesia. Sensory and motor loss below the level of the lesion is not unusual, but extensive atrophy of the muscles of the upper limbs sometimes occurs, even though these muscles are supplied by anterior nerve roots and motor cells of segments below the area of tumor compression. This may be due to anterior spinal artery occlusion. Such atrophy is commonly preceded by perception of a sense of coldness, stiffness, or pain in the arms. The sternocleidomastoid muscle may be in spasm and later atrophy, as may the levator scapulae and the trapezius. A sensation of constriction around the neck and a feeling of suffocation is frequently reported and may be assessed by an uninformed examiner as psychoneurotic manifestation or hysteria. With a tumor at C4, diaphragmatic muscle paralysis may occur, as may paralysis of the serratus anterior and the supra- and infraspinous muscles. Light touch is usually little disturbed even by extramedullary tumors at this level.

Tumors Low in the Cervical Spine (C5, C6, C7, C8, T1). These tumors are clinically characterized by radicular and segmental disturbances in the upper extremities. Reflex changes occur early before atrophy or paralysis. Decrease or absence of the biceps reflex with weakness of the biceps muscle (C5), the pronator reflex (C6), the triceps reflex with weakness of that muscle (C7), or the finger flexor reflex with weakness of that movement (C8). Inversion of the reflexes of the upper extremity occurs with tumors in the lower cervical region. A tumor at the level of C7 causes the triceps reflex to disappear, but the biceps reflex, whose center lies above the tumor, may be preserved. Percussing the triceps muscle near the point of attachment will not cause extension of the elbow but may, for an instant, increase the angle at the elbow, mechanically stretching the bicipital tendon, resulting in a reflex contraction of the biceps muscle and arm flexion.

Low cervical tumors cause pain early in their development, first in one arm, depending on the level of the tumor, and then in both arms. With tumors at C5 and C6, the pain is in the shoulder or on the radial surface of the forearm and thumb. Tumors at C7 and C8 cause pain on the inner side of the arm and in the fingers. Sensory loss with these tumors extends upward to involve the inner aspect of the arm. Muscular weakness due to tumors at C5 and C6 principally involve the shoulder girdle and proximal arm, but all muscles of the upper extremity are affected to some degree. Extension to C4 results in atrophy of the pectoralis major, the pectoralis minor, and the scapular muscles, while extension downward to C7 causes atrophy and paralysis of the triceps muscle; involvement of C8 and T1 adds intense atrophy to the smaller muscles of the hand and flexors of the finger. Loss of power in the lower extremities occurs first in the ipsilateral lower limb, next in the contralateral lower limb, and then in the contralateral upper limb.

Tumors High in the Thoracic Spine. Tumors at T1 and T2 result in very little paralysis or atrophy in the upper limbs. The intrinsic muscles of the fourth and fifth fingers may be involved, and sensory loss from a tumor at T1 may extend to the inner aspect of the upper arm. The sympathetic innervation of both the eye and the face is usually involved, with enopthalmos of the ipsilateral eye, decrease in the size of the pupil on that side, and narrowing of the palpebral fissure (Horner's syndrome). Vasomotor changes and alteration in sweat secretion on the face are common. Sympathetic symptoms and signs in the head and neck result from an intraspinal tumor at any level of the cervical cord affecting the descending supranuclear sympathetic fibers. The presence of these symptoms and the absence of paralysis or atrophy of the upper extremities characterize high thoracic tumors. Beevor's sign is positive when a patient with a tumor of the middle thoracic area attempts to raise his head from a recumbent position; the umbilicus moves upward, and the upper superficial abdominal reflexes may be present, whereas the lower are lost.

Naffziger's Test. Radiating pain and paresthesias are commonly produced in gross herniations of the intervertebral discs or in intraspinal obstruction secondary to tumor. These conditions raise intracranial and intraspinal fluid pressure. Coughing, sneezing, straining to move the bowels, twisting the back by stooping, lifting hard, and just being on the feet for a long period of time may cause such pain and paresthesia. The pain reflects an increase in intraspinal fluid pressure and can also be produced by compressing the jugular veins in the neck, thus increasing the intracranial and intraspinal pressure by distending intraspinal veins.

Clinical Reflections of Spinal Cord Trauma. Radiographic study usually determines the site of traumatic lesions such as fracture and dislocation. The neurologic symptoms and signs also localize the lesion. Crushing lesions of the spinal cord destroy the long pathways as well as anterior horn cells at the level of the crush and usually destroy or grossly irritate the anterior and posterior roots, resulting in pain, hyperalgesia, segmental sensory losses, and segmental atrophies. Such cord lesions result in hemiplegia, monoplegia, and hematomyelia. Injuries involving the level of C1–C2 usually either kill the patient promptly or result in complete quadriplegia. Upper cervical spine stiffness and pain are severe, with radiation through the distribution of the upper cervical nerves and the greater and lesser occipital nerves to the posterior scalp. Severe hyperpnea, hyperpyrexia, and striking vasomotor disturbances occur below the lesion, and priapism may last until death. Death often occurs by slight movements during handling of such a patient.

With trauma involving C3 and C4, the origin of the phrenic nerve, respiratory symptoms are prominent, and may, if survival occurs, result in pneumonia due to deficient pulmonary ventilation. Quadriplegia and a fairly sharp sensory level localize the lesion. Sensory defects are of three types: (1) absence of all forms of sensation below the lesion; (2) segmental loss of sensation at the level of the lesion due to tearing of the posterior horn or root; (3) hyperalgesia in the adjacent upper dermatome caused by irritation of the next higher intact posterior root. Atrophy is segmental and corresponds to segmental anesthesia of the posterior horn or root origin. Trauma at the C5–C6 level results in the characteristic posture, with adductors of the upper arm and extensors of the forearms and hands paralyzed; consequently upper arms are abducted and externally rotated, with flexed forearms and flexed wrists (Thorburn's position). The biceps reflex is absent and, if the C6–C7 cord level is involved, upper arms are abducted and forearms flexed secondary to paralysis of the deltoid and triceps muscles. Flexors of the fingers are paralyzed. The triceps reflex is absent and may be inverted to give a flexor response. Biceps reflex is usually hyperactive, and the muscle is strong. At the C8–T1 level, the expected sensory loss occurs over the entire inner or ulnar side of the upper arm, forearm, and hand. The more extensive the lesion, and the deeper it is in the cervical cord, the more the musculature of the upper extremity is spared. At T1 and T2, the oculopupillary fibers are caught, resulting in Horner's syndrome, miosis, enophthalmos, and ptosis. Localization at the remaining thoracic segments is accomplished by eliciting appropriate truncal sensory levels. If the lesion is below the eighth thoracic segment and above the eleventh, Beevor's sign is positive; that is, on raising the head, the umbilicus moves upward, since the upper part of the rectus abdominalis is still innervated, and the lower part is paralyzed.

Brown-Séquard's Syndrome. Brown-Séquard's syndrome may be due to cervical spine disease or trauma involving the spinal cord. It is a partial or incomplete unilateral lesion of the cord often caused by knife wounds but may be due to meningeal or vertebral disease or extramedullary cord tumors; the syndrome may be also caused by osteoarthritis or infectious diseases, with incidental unilateral destruction of the spinal cord.

On the side of the lesion, destruction of the lateral tracts causes paralysis of voluntary motion, striking increase in muscle tone, exaggeration of deep tendon reflexes, clonus, and positive Hoffmann's and Babinski's sign (upper motor neuron signs). These occur on the ipsilateral side because the motor fibers have already decussated in the medulla. At the level of the lesion, severance of the anterior horn cells or roots and the posterior roots results in ipsilateral segment atrophy and sensory loss. On the contralateral side, analgesia and thermoaesthesia develop a few segments below the lesion, since the spinothalamic fibers contain crossed fibers from below. The difference in lesion levels and the loss of pain correspond to the distance the pain and temperature fibers ascend on the same side of the cord before decussating. This distance may be 2 to 4 segments. Tactile sensibility is usually, but not always, intact because of the many crossed as well as uncrossed fibers. Proprioception, muscle and joint sensibility, is compromised on the ipsilateral side. By nature of the lesions causing Brown-Séquard's syndrome, lesion sections are rarely exact. Thus, pressure from meningeal and bony vertebral disease, extramedullary cord tumors, knife wounds, trauma, and degenerative or infectious disease by accidental unilateral destruction of the cord may all result in Brown-Séquard's syndrome.

Spinal Stroke (Hematomyelia). Hemorrhage into the substance of the spinal cord is common in cord injuries, particularly crushing injuries. It occurs usually in circumstances in which the trauma is massive and multiple, rendering the hematomyelia of relatively little clinical significance. Spinal stroke results in the clinical picture of a sudden stroke-like seizure: the patient sinks to the ground, with paraplegia. Complete paralysis is the rule, with loss of sphincter control and

striking vasomotor changes below the level of the lesion. These symptoms continue for a few days, increase in severity, and then level off. Extremities have no muscle tone for some days to weeks, though an extensor plantar response is usually elicited. The presence of deep tendon reflexes is a function of the extent of the spinal shock.

Direct injuries to the spinal cord occur, even though no bony vertebral injury has been suffered; contrecoup, fractures, and dislocations of vertebrae may occur but do not crush the cord. Sudden, sharp head-bending, stooping, or diving may produce hematomyelia. It may result from falling with great force onto the buttocks. Occasionally, relatively slight exertion or strain in lifting results in spinal stroke, perhaps owing to some abnormal blood vessel fragility. Blood dyscrasias, hemophilia, or any hemorrhagic diathesis may cause spinal stroke. Heavy explosions and severe vibration during war with heavy artillery fire have also caused the lesion. Alcoholism seems to predispose one to it.

Special tests and physical signs used in clinical diagnosis of abnormalities of the cervical spine are listed in Table 4–4.

Table 4–4. SPECIAL TESTS AND PHYSICAL SIGNS IN CLINICAL DIAGNOSIS

Posture	Scapular movement
Gait	Active
Facial expression	Passive
Decreased range of motion	Against resistance
	Hyoid bone
Deformity	Thyroid gland and cartilage
Anterior landmark changes	First cricoid ring
Posterior landmark changes	Parotid gland
	Corneal reflexes and trigeminal nerve impairment
Crepitus	
Lymph nodes	
Carotid pulses	Vibratory sense, skull
C1, C2, C3, C4 cervical plexus	Short neck
	Distraction test
Reflex changes	Valsalva's maneuver
Motor changes	Dysphagia
Sensory changes	Eye and Ear signs and symptoms
C5, 6, 7, 8 brachial plexus	
Deep tendon reflexes	Adson test
Reflex changes	Blood pressure
Motor changes	Shoulder depression test
Sensory changes	Muscle weakness and atrophy
Lhermitte's sign	
Spurling test (head compression test)	Shoulder and temporomandibular joints
Sharp-Purser test	Jaw reflexes
Cervical spine range of motion	Lidocaine (Xylocaine) test
Active	Radiologic study
Passive	Electromyographic study
Against resistance	

References

1. Brain WR: Some unsolved problems in cervical spondylosis. Br Med J 1:771, 1963.
2. Cyriax J: Textbook of Orthopedic Medicine, 5th ed. London: Tindall and Cassell, 1964.
3. Sharp J: Personal communication. Unpublished data.
4. Swaim LT: The orthopedic treatment of Strumpell-Marie arthritis. J Bone Joint Surg 21:983, 1939.
5. Lhermitte J: Étude de la commotion de la moelle. Rev Neurol (Paris) 1:210, 1932.
6. Spurling RG, Scoville WB: Lateral rupture of the cervical intervertebral discs. Syn Gyn Obst 78:350, 1944.
7. Keuper DH, Papp JP: Supraclavicular adenopathy demonstrated by the Valsalva maneuver. N Engl J Med 280:1007, 1969.
8. A neurovascular syndrome—the subclavian steal (editorial). N Engl J Med 264:912–913, 1961.
9. Bland JH, Boushey DR, Merritt JA: The painful shoulder. Semin Arthritis Rheum 7:21, 1977.
10. Sharp J, Purser DW: Spontaneous atlanto-axial dislocation in ankylosing spondylitis and rheumatoid arthritis. Ann Rheum Dis 20-47, 1961.
11. Stevens JC, Cartledge NEF, Saunders M, et al: Atlantoaxial subluxation and cervical myelopathy in rheumatoid arthritis. Q J Med 40:391, 1971.
12. Serre M, Simon L, Jonicil JY, et al: Les affections rheumatismales de la charnière cervico-occipital. Rev Rhum 30:518, 1963.
13. Lhermitte J, Bollak P, Nicholas M: Les douleurs à type de décharge électrique dans la sclérose en plaques. Un cas de forme sensitive de la sclérose multiple. Rev Neurol (Paris) 2:56, 1924.
14. Brody IA, Wilkins RH: Lhermitte's sign. Arch Neurol 21:338, 1969.
15. Leveson JA, Zimmer AE: A localizing symptom in thoracic myelopathy. Ann Intern Med 76:769, 1972.
16. Rana NA, Hancock DO, Taylor AR, et al: Atlanto-axial subluxation in rheumatoid arhritis. J Bone Joint Surg 55B:458, 1973.
17. Rana NA, Hancock DO, Taylor AR, et al: Upward translocation of the dens in rheumatoid arthritis. J Bone Joint Surg 55B:471, 1973.

Chapter 5

Rheumatologic Neurology

The challenges in clinical diagnosis and management of diseases, disorders, and injuries of the cervical spine are to determine the type of pathologic changes present (inflammatory, metabolic and endocrine, congenital, mechanical, neoplastic, infectious, degenerative (osteoarthritic), or traumatic); to identify the neurologic level, location, and extent of the process; to assess the probable course of future clinical events (prognosis); and to design a therapeutic and management program geared to influence the pathophysiologic characteristics favorably. This is done mainly by elicitation of detailed historical data and physical examination and, in particular, neurologic examination. Essentially this involves noting the following information: identification of the pain-sensitive structures (all pain sensation is neurally transmitted and traceable to some tissue); presence or lack of motor power; atrophy or hypertrophy of muscle, ligament, tendon, bone (other connective tissue structures); presence or absence of position and vibratory sense; pain, temperature, and touch perception; presence of numbness, paresthesia, hyperesthesia, hypesthesia, dysesthesia, or anesthesia; proprioceptive function; cervical range of motion; analysis of reflexes; presence or absence of normal gait.

The classic clinical neurologic approach takes into account only the dermatome distribution. I regard scrutiny of the dermatome distribution pattern as 33% of what can and should be done on rheumatologic neurologic clinical analysis which should include an assessment of dermatome, myotome, and sclerotome distribution. Please refer to Table 2–3. This extensive table illustrates the dermatome, myotome, and sclerotome distribution and referral patterns at each cervical spine level (C1–T1) as the patient may perceive them clinically. Specific structures and areas are listed, that is, skin (dermatomes), specific nerves and muscles (myotomes), and liga-

ments, bones, and joints (sclerotomes). Generally only dermatome distribution is considered in clinical practice. However, knowledge of and clinical application and use of myotome and sclerotome distributions allow perception and understanding of many cervical spine syndromes. Accompanying each listing is the anatomic drawing of the dermatome, myotome, and sclerotome distribution patterns for each cervical vertebra (C1–T1). In addition, the clinical examination methods for each level are listed, including motor and sensory function tests, pertinent reflexes, and other corresponding observations to be made for accurate and complete neurologic and rheumatologic assessment of the cervical spine. The dermatomes (with considerable neighboring dermatomal overlap) are the areas of skin supplied by a single efferent nerve fiber from a single dorsal root. This is also the case with the myotomes and sclerotomes, which do not necessarily follow the distribution patterns of the dermatomes. Muscle, ligament, tendon, bone, capsule, and fascia all have their individual segmental motor and sensory nerve supply, and their tissues are as involved in disease and trauma as the dermatomes (if not more so). Thus, all areas should be included in clinical assessment (see Chapter 2, *Anatomy and Biomechanics* and Chapter 4, *Clinical Methods*).

The goals of this chapter are to review pertinent neuroanatomy briefly and to present a systematic clinical method and approach to examination by neurologic level. The effect of pathologic events in the cervical spine is manifested in the head, neck, upper trunk, shoulder, and the upper extremity. Such is true of pathologic involvement of all structures in the cervical spine, spinal cord, nerve roots, and peripheral nerves, bone, muscle, tendon, ligament, joint, and cartilage. Clinical characteristics of each level of the spinal nerves, from C1 through T1, are presented systematically.

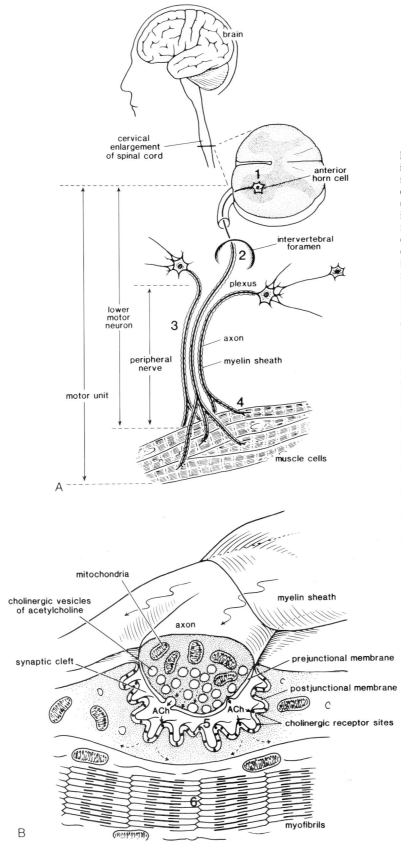

Figure 5–1. *A,* Diagram illustrating upper and lower motor neuron. The upper motor neuron originates in the cerebral cortex (Betz's cell) and terminates with its synapse in an internuncial neuron or in the anterior horn cell itself. Injury or functional compromise at any point results in symptoms and signs of upper motor neuron lesions. The lower motor neuron begins in the anterior horn cell and terminates in muscle, ligament, skin, or other connective tissue. Interruption or functional compromise at any point results in symptoms and signs of lower motor neuron lesions. Arabic numbers 1 through 6 in *A* and *B* indicate sites at which disorders and disease may interfere with lower motor neuron function. *Key:* 1: anterior horn cell; 2: anterior and posterior nerve roots in the intervertebral foramina; 3: peripheral nerve; 4: myoneural junction (or other peripheral termination); 5: synaptic cleft; 6: the peripheral muscle cell (or other cells) itself. *B,* Diagram illustrating the termination of the peripheral nerve in a muscle cell. The nerve is depicted as branching axons, one of which has entered its myoneural junction in muscle. The impulse initiates the secretion of acetylcholine across the prejunctional membrane into the synaptic cleft, where it binds to cholinergic receptor sites in the postjunctional membrane, finally initiating and converting chemical energy into mechanical energy by triggering the contractile proteins to shorten and proceed with normal muscle metabolism.

A BRIEF REVIEW OF NEUROANATOMY

When a person has a "thought," that person voluntarily initiates nerve impulses arising from the cerebral cortex (motor cortex). The impulses travel through long descending nerve fibers extending in the pyramidal system, cross to the opposite side of the body in the medulla (left to right and right to left), and synapse, first to cells of voluntary motor nuclei of the cranial nerves and then descending through the medulla to the spinal cord, synapsing with the anterior horn cells (motor cells) in the cord. Without the motor cortex (Betz's cells), voluntary motion is impossible and paralysis occurs. There are internuncial neurons connecting the pyramidal fibers with the anterior motor horn cells. Because the fibers cross over (decussate), the right cerebral cortex has voluntary control of the left side of the body, and the left cerebral cortex controls the right side of the body. Conventionally there are two parts of the pathway from Betz's cell in the motor cortex to the muscle fiber itself: the upper motor neuron (corticospinal tract or pyramidal fibers) and the lower motor neuron (anterior horn cell and peripheral nerve fibers). The term motor unit is used to describe the anterior horn cell, the peripheral nerve, the neuromuscular junction, and the contractile proteins of the muscle cells themselves. The term lower motor neuron describes the anterior horn cell and peripheral nerve to the neuromuscular junction (Fig. 5–1).

Upper motor neuron fibers are classified into three groups: (1) corticospinal tract (pyramidal tract), (2) corticobulbar tract, (3) corticomesencephalic tract. The latter two have no special pertinence to the cervical spine, but the corticospinal tract and its system of descending fibers require clinical understanding and application (Fig. 5–2). The corticospinal tract (pyramidal), originating in the Betz's cells of the cerebral cortex, descends from the white matter of the brain to the internal capsule (a large aggregation of all the nerve fibers) upper motor neuron to the cerebral peduncle, pons, and pyramid, and finally crosses to the opposite side (decussates) in the medulla, further traveling down the lateral corticospinal tracts to their synapse with an internuncial neuron or directly to the anterior horn cell. Some few fibers do not cross over, descending in the anterior funiculi of the cord as uncrossed anterior pyramidal tract. This tract ends in the cervical enlargement of the cord, for it does finally cross over, synapsing with the lower motor neuron in the cervical cord.

Of course, the number of fibers decreases as they travel more distally in the cord because fibers are continually reaching their termination. Fibers controlling the arm are in the most medial part of the lateral corticospinal tract, and those controlling the legs, bowel, and bladder are in the most lateral part. Knowledge of the location of these fibers

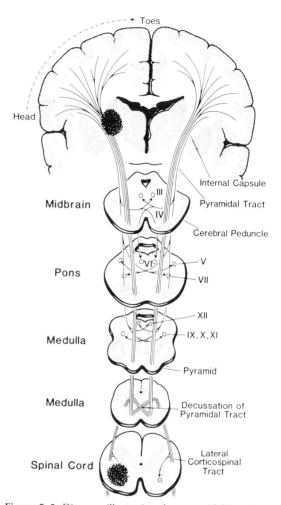

Figure 5–2. Diagram illustrating the pyramidal (corticospinal) system of descending fibers described in text. Note the black, oval lesion in the internal capsule area (upper left), designating an upper motor neuron lesion. Note also the round, black lesion at the spinal cord level, designating a lower motor neuron lesion involving the anterior horn. Note the 12 cranial nerve nuclei. The 9 cranial nerves that exert voluntary control over certain skeletal muscles are designated by Roman numerals (III, IV, V, VI, VII, IX, X, XI, XII). They essentially follow the same pattern and may be affected by both upper and lower motor neuron lesions. This fact is often especially important in the accurate diagnosis of cervical spine disorders. Phylogenetically these nuclei and their peripheral nerves may be regarded as "higher cervical nerves," since they were such in more ancient animals.

allows diagnosis of certain clinical syndromes, such as central versus lateral cord compression.

Rootlets enter the spinal cord posteriorly in the lateral sulcus, and the bundles of fibers from the anterior horn cells (lower motor neurons) exit anteriorly. The posterior and anterior roots join to form the common spinal nerve. Besides synapsing

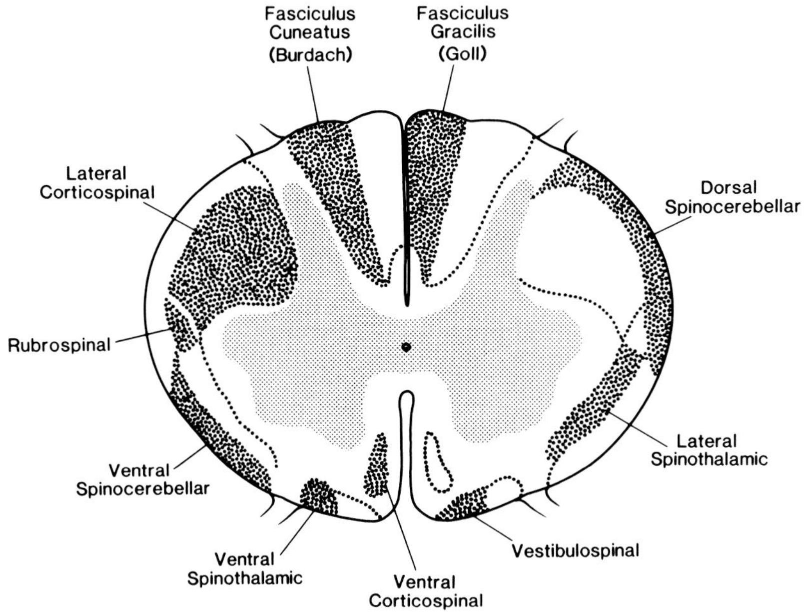

Figure 5–3. Diagram of a cross-section of the cervical spinal cord at the level of the enlargement illustrates the clinically important motor and sensory tracts. Note that the illustration is designed such that part of each tract is dotted black, while the opposite and corresponding part of each tract remains white. It is necessary to know the anatomic location of the tracts to relate the historical data and physical signs in identifying and localizing a lesion according to the functional compromise, both subjective and objective. The functions of the major motor and sensory tracts are listed in Table 5–1.

with the pyramidal tract, the anterior horn cells also synapse with extrapyramidal motor fibers and sympathetic, parasympathetic and association fibers. Other less well understood synapses also take place. These synapses all contribute to connecting reflex circuits, resulting in rhythmic, coordinated, mechanically efficient motion (see Fig. 5–2). Figure 5–3 is a drawing of a cross-section of a spinal cord, showing the major motor and sensory tracts and their geographic locations in the spinal cord. Table 5–1 lists the functions of these important tracts. Tables 5–2 and 5–3 list the location of upper motor neurons and lower motor neurons, the general and specific clinical symp-

toms associated with dysfunction of each, and specific diseases and disorders of both.

All connective tissue structures in the shoulder joint derive mainly from the C5 dermatome, myotome, and sclerotome. Thus, nearly all symptoms and signs originating in anatomic structures in the shoulder are perceived in the C5 distribution. Since cervical syndromes and diseases originate in structures derived from the C4–C5 through T1 somites, clinical problems of the shoulder and arm are always in the differential diagnosis of cervical spine clinical disorders. Figure 5–4 illustrates the C5 distribution; this knowledge permits diagnosis of shoulder lesions, either separate from or related

Table 5–1. FUNCTIONS OF THE MAJOR MOTOR AND SENSORY TRACTS

	Tract	*Function*
Sensory	Fasciculus gracilis (Goll)	Lower half of body: motion, position, vibratory sense
	Fasciculus cuneatus (Burdach)	Upper half of body: sensation, deep pain
	Dorsal and ventral spinocerebellar	Involuntary regulation of muscle coordination, balance, and proprioception
	Lateral spinothalamic	Pain and temperature (superficial sensations)
	Ventral spinothalamic	Light touch (superficial sensations)
Motor	Lateral corticospinal (pyramidal)	All voluntary muscular movement, mainly extremities
	Ventral corticospinal (pyramidal)	Voluntary muscular movement of trunk
	Vestibulospinal	Equilibrium and position sense
	Rubrospinal	Function not clear in human beings

Table 5–2. UPPER MOTOR NEURONS

Anatomic Location
Brain
Brain stem
Cerebellum
White matter
Lateral and posterior horns of gray matter of the
spinal cord
General Clinical Signs of Lesions
Spastic paralysis or paresis
Absent atrophy (only atrophy of immobilization)
Absent fasciculations
Absent trophic changes
Hyperactive deep tendon reflexes
Diminished to absent superficial reflexes
Clonus—ankle, patella, wrist
Specific Clinical Signs of Lesions
Babinski's reflex (posterior), Hoffmann's reflex
(posterior)
Exaggerated finger flexor reflexes (Wartenberg's
sign)
Unilateral or conspicuous palmomental reflex
Diminished to absent superficial abdominal,
cremasteric, palmar grasping, gluteal reflexes
Vigorous, voluntary flexion of fingers against
resistance results in adduction and flexion of
thumb
Active extension of arms causes abduction and
hyperextension of the fingers (Souques's finger
sign)

Specific Clinical Signs of Lesions *Continued*
Failure of pronation of hand on being loosely
shaken
Positive head retraction reflex test. Procedure:
patient is in supine position and raises head from
examining table; examiner places finger over
patient's upper lip, strikes briskly with reflex
hammer. Positive test: quick, backward jerk of
head (indicates bilateral, supracervical, direct,
and interrupted corticospinal tract (disease). False
positive results are not usual
Absent automatic accessory movements, such as
pendular swinging of the arm on walking and
extension of the wrist in flexing fingers
Mass flexion movements of the upper extremity on
painful stimulation by scratch, pinch, or prick to
palms, inner surface of forearm, axilla, or upper
chest
Toe dorsiflexion positive in variations of Babinski's
sign (Gordon's, Schaefer's, Chaddock's,
Throckmorton's, Gonda's, and Allen's signs)
Specific Diseases and Disorders
Neoplastic disease
Stroke
Cerebral palsy
Multiple sclerosis
Transverse myelitis
Trauma

Table 5–3. LOWER MOTOR NEURONS

Anatomic Location
Final common pathway
Anterior horn cell
Spinal cord axons of anterior horn cells (of brain
stem, spinal cord, and peripheral nerves)
Myoneural junction of muscles concerned
General Clinical Signs of Lesions
Flaccid paralysis
Atrophy, marked and rapid development
Fasciculations (especially if onset is extremely slow)
Trophic changes (reaction of degeneration 10 to 14
days past onset)
Diminished to absent deep tendon (stretch) reflexes
Specific Clinical Signs of Lesions
Loss of muscle tone, volume, and contour
Weakness of muscles
Abnormalities reflecting mixed function of
peripheral nerves and loss or perversion of
function of motor, sensory, and autonomic
functions
Hypotonic, flaccid muscles
Peripheral nerves may change size, consistency,
and contour; tenderness and pain (both increase
in passive stretching); irritability of nerve,
neuromas, and neurofibromas; infiltration of
nerves

Specific Clinical Signs of Lesions *Continued*
Loss of electric reaction
Spasm and overactivity of antagonistic muscles
may cause joint contractures
Anesthesia with absent pain on pressure
Both deep and superficial reflexes absent distal to
the lesion
With partial interruption, complete clinical loss of
function for a period of time, followed by
resumption of normal conduction by the intact
fibers
In regeneration, autonomic fibers are restored first,
noted by improvement in color and texture of
skin
Specific Diseases and Disorders
Poliomyelitis
Progressive spinal muscular atrophy
Myasthenia gravis
Muscular dystrophy
Guillain-Barré syndrome
Herpes zoster

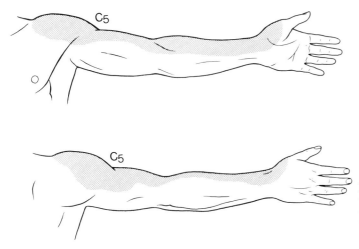

Figure 5–4. C5 dermatome distribution pattern. Any lesion producing symptoms and signs outside this pattern cannot be located in structures within the shoulder—with the exception of the acromioclavicular joint.

to cervical spine disorders. Figure 5–5 illustrates the dermatome distribution pattern of voluntary cranial nerves and C1 through T5. Figure 5–6 is a diagrammatic sketch of the brachial plexus; knowledge of the brachial plexus is also necessary for precise diagnosis in cervical spine syndromes.

Spastic Muscle Paralysis

If the pyramidal tracts are destroyed anywhere between the origin in Betz's cell and the synapse at the anterior horn cell, voluntary motor impulses do not arrive at the anterior horn cell below the level of the lesion (see Fig. 5–1A). Thus muscle

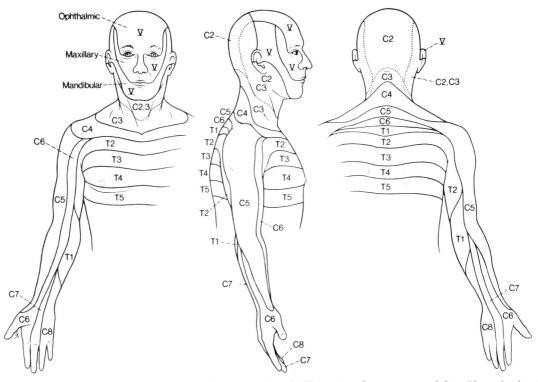

Figure 5–5. Dermatome distribution pattern for the C1 through T5 somites. Roman numeral five (*V*) on forehead and face refers to the fifth cranial nerve distribution (trigeminal nerve). Three divisions are designated with *V*: frontal, maxillary, and mandibular. (From Bland JH, Nakano KK: Neck pain. *In* Kelley, Harris, Ruddy, et al (eds): Textbook of Rheumatology. Philadelphia: W. B. Saunders Co, 1981.)

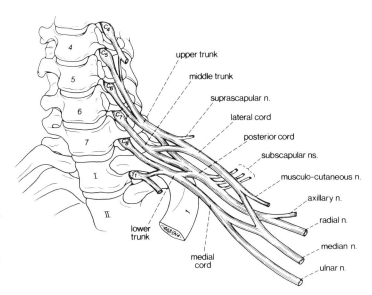

Figure 5–6. Drawing of the brachial plexus, showing roots, trunks, cords, and peripheral nerves. (From Bland JH, Nakano KK: Neck pain. *In* Kelley, Harris, Ruddy, et al (eds): Textbook of Rheumatology. Philadelphia: W. B. Saunders Co, 1981.)

paralysis occurs in muscles whose upper motor neuron is supplied by these cells. Abrupt destruction results in complete absence of motor function below the level of injury; stretch reflex and deep tendon response are absent. In days to weeks, stretch reflex gradually reappears, and after a variable interval the reflex is more active than it was normally—that is, hypertonicity occurs as illustrated by firmness and stiffness of the muscles themselves or as perceived in the clinical attempt to move, particularly in the leg. Passive motion of the joints is stiff owing to muscle resistance. Gradual application of passive motion results in sudden release of the resistance. Deep tendon reflexes are overactive and clonus is present. Positive Babinski's reflex, absent abdominal and cremasteric reflexes, Hoffmann's response, and often a positive palmomental reflex are all characteristic.

Flaccid Muscle Paralysis

If the anterior horn cells, ventral nerve roots, or motor fibers of peripheral nerves are destroyed, all voluntary and reflex responses are absent. Muscles are flaccid to floppy and without tone, and reflexes are totally absent. Atrophy of the muscles occurs within a few weeks; it occurs in greater magnitude than it would if the muscles were simply immobilized. Muscle requires the continual "instruction" by peripheral nerves in order to maintain its metabolic activity. Shortly after the disappearance of muscle tone and voluntary and reflex responses, muscles show fibrillations and fasciculations; the latter are simply coarser spontaneous twitchings of the muscle (see Fig. 5–1). As noted by the arabic numerals on the drawings, there are potentially six sites, beginning with the anterior horn cell, at which a lesion resulting in flaccid paralysis may occur.

Afferent Paths

The dorsolateral fasciculus, the lateral spinothalamic tract, and the spinotectal tract carry the perceptions of pain and temperature (see Fig. 5–3). These axons pass through the ganglion (dorsal root), enter the spinal cord running to the tip of the dorsal horn, and divide into ascending and descending branches for just one or two segments. Individual fibers go to only two to three segments, but in the aggregate they form a tract that extends the entire length of the spinal cord, mediating pain and temperature. These fibers then decussate ventromedially in the ventral white commissure and ascend as the lateral spinothalamic tract in the lateral funiculus. The fibers carrying pain and temperature sensations in the cervical area are the most medial and the most ventral in the spinothalamic tract; sacral area fibers are the most dorsal, and thoracic area fibers are a little more medial. The spinotectal tracts are similar to those of the lateral spinothalamic tracts, and after reaching the opposite ventrolateral white matter, the fibers ascend along the medial border of the lateral spinothalamic tract (see Fig. 5–3). The spinotectal tract carries the sensation of pain and probably carries some other sensations that are not completely sorted out. The lateral spinothalamic tract may be sectioned to relieve intractable pain. Generally, bilateral section must be done to block intractable visceral pain completely.

Position Sense and Proprioception

Fibers representing proprioceptive pathways enter the spinal cord and run by three different routes: (1) directly to lower motor neurons in the anterior horn cell, (2) to spinocerebellar pathways, and (3) straight upward in the posterior funiculus.

The direct fibers to lower motor neurons are afferent fibers of the two neurons that make up the stretch reflex arc. They arise in a muscle spindle and end in a synapse of motor cells within one or two spinal segments at the level entering the cord. Those fibers entering the spinocerebellar tract proceed to the cerebellum, reporting the instantaneous activity of muscle groups to the cerebellum, which then modifies the actions of muscle groups so that movements are accurately, rhythmically, and smoothly performed. Other proprioceptive impulses arising from receptor end organs in neuromuscular connective tissue, neurotendinous spindles, and pacinian corpuscles ascend in the posterior funiculus, cross to the opposite side, enter the medial lemniscus, and proceed to the thalamus—ultimately to the cerebral cortex in the so-called somesthetic area (see Fig. 5–2). The conscious recognition of body and limb posture requires cortical involvement. Other fibers having to do with sense of touch traverse posterior funiculi, medial lemniscus, and thalamus to the postcentral gyrus, where stereognosis, the tactile discrimination of form, is located.

Touch Perception

Touch perception is divided into two forms, simple light touch and tactile discrimination; the latter includes sense of deep pressure, spatial localization, and appreciation of size and shape of objects. The afferent nerve begins in tactile corpuscles in the dermis and in certain networks of nerve terminals about hair follicles, oil glands, and sweat glands. The impulse enters the dorsal root, synapsing with cells in the inner portion of the posterior gray columns, the nucleus proprius. Some synapse in adjacent segments, but some extend longitudinally 10 to 12 segments upward before synapsing. These fibers decussate in the anterior white commissure and go up into the anterior spinothalamic tract of the opposite side (see Figs. 5–2 and 5–3). The fibers terminate in the thalamus, synapse, and, via thalamocortical fibers, transmit sensory impulses to the cerebral cortex. Light touch is the least likely to be abnormal in spinal cord lesions affecting only one side of the cord.

Deep-Structure Pain

The innervation of skeletal, articular, and muscular structure is segmental, but deep-structure pain differs a great deal from superficial-structure pain. The pain is never perceived at the site of the structure unless the structure is in the body image. The area of pain is quite large relative to the size of the lesion in the tissue from which the pain arises. Deep-structure pain is the most severe type of pain known, and there is no real difference between the perceptive experiences of pain in visceral deep structures and that of pain in somatic deep structures. The pain is delayed in onset and is not affected by anesthetizing the area of pain perception (not the site of the pain-sensitive structure). Deep pain radiates both proximally and distally from the site of perception, and the radiation varies with the severity of pain. Such pain is most severe at the site of insertion of tendon, ligament, and capsule into bone. Muscles in the surrounding area become tender, and bony points, sites of insertion of ligamentous structures, are the most tender. Clinical manifestations of deep-structure pain include sweating, blanching, nausea, and sudomotor, pilomotor, and vasomotor responses—even collapse. This radiation of pain follows neither the distribution patterns of major nerve trunks nor those expected in dermatomes. The fact that myotome and sclerotome distributions represent the embryonic migration of these deep structures, which carry with them their nerve supply in early embryonic life, provides explanation for these peculiar pain behaviors.[1]

HISTORICAL DATA IN CERVICAL SPINE DISEASE AND TRAUMA

The usual complete historical elicitation is required unless there is an emergent situation such as spinal cord injury, cervical vertebral fracture or dislocation, or brain stem lesion. Information regarding the time and characteristics of an injury, evidence of laceration or abrasion about the head and face, and type of force and mechanism of injury—such as cervical hyperextension from a forehead blow—all are needed. Inspection and palpation about the neck may show local tenderness, torticollis, deformity, gibbus, or strikingly tender cervical spinous processes at the site of injury. Observation of the breathing pattern is often very informative and requires 1 to 3 minutes of observation. Pain perception should be examined early; pin prick is the best single stimulus. The examiner begins in the foot and progresses upward, noting a decrease or an absence of sensation and a sensory level of cord involvement.

Immediately after injury, a transverse myelitis is characterized by absent deep tendon responses below the level of the lesion. This absence of response is replaced by hyper-reflexia over a period of weeks. Early demonstration of Babinski's response indicates a favorable prognosis. Stretch reflex is absent in hyporeflexia.

There are three very serious cervical spine syndromes other than complete transverse myelitis. (1) The Brown-Séquard syndrome is produced by injury to one half of the spinal cord, resulting in paralysis and loss of sensation, both incomplete. The pyramidal and extrapyramidal system damage causes paralysis on the same side as the lesion, and as in transverse myelitis, the muscles are flaccid at first and spastic later. Loss of the lateral spinothalamic tract results in loss of pain and temperature on the opposite side; with reticulospinal and ligamentospinal systems gone, Horner's syndrome appears. (2) Acute anterior spinal cord syndrome is that of complete paralysis below the level of the lesion, with preservation of touch, proprioception, and often vibratory sense. This syndrome may be caused by an intervertebral disc protrusion or bone fragment, the so-called "tear drop" fracture.[2] (3) Acute central cervical syndrome involves hyperesthesia, hypalgesia to the level of the lesion, partial loss of touch and vibration sensation, and preservation of motion and position sense. Bladder and bowel dysfunction are usual. This syndrome is probably common, with the most likely etiologies being a hyperextension injury and secondary anterior spinal artery obstruction. Clinical improvement may be early and dramatic, with return of bladder function. The sensory changes first return to normal in the lower extremities, followed by the trunk and arms, in that order. *Since the neuropathologic change suggests damage to the central portion of the cord, laminectomy could only accelerate the clinical condition.*

Lesions of the lower cranial nerves and dysfunction in the medulla can be produced by pathologic processes at the junction of the medulla and the cervical cord. The symptoms of pain, paresthesia, numbness, and dysesthesia are very important. Pain may arise from vertebral, joint, or other connective tissue sources as well as from the cord or nerve roots. In the case of nerve roots, the pain is well localized, usually described as sharp or lancinating, and precipitated or aggravated by minor postural changes of the head and neck. Physical activity and increased intraspinal pressure, cough, sneeze, and straining may exaggerate the pain. *If the pain arises from the cervical cord itself, it is far more diffuse and poorly defined.* Furthermore, the pain is usually perceived in areas several segments below the level of the lesion. Bony destructive lesions result in a localized, deep, nagging ache or pain that can precede radiographic changes by months. Paresthesias along specific dermatomes are common owing to radicular stretch or inflammation. They are usually not associated with objective sensory changes.

I regard numbness as a vague, poorly described, and poorly understood, very common, and quite significant symptom. In speaking of pain, the patient may mean such diverse sensory changes as pain, paresthesia, hypesthesia, dysesthesia, hypoalgesia, or even anesthesia. If the source is intramedullary in the cord, the symptoms are likely to be more diffuse and disassociated, not following an expected radicular pattern.

Determining the level of a cervical spine lesion requires knowledge of cross-sectional anatomy, especially with details of the longitudinal axis. The higher the lesion in the cervical spinal canal, the more extensive the loss of motor, sensory, and autonomic function, that is, a high cord or low medullary transection of the cervical cord results in complete quadriplegia with respiratory impairment—almost always immediately fatal. Lesions involving multiple segments of the cervical cord are incomplete and may be manifested by the simultaneous occurrence of upper and lower motor neuron signs and variably long sensory tract and autonomic symptoms and signs. Patients with acute quadriplegia due to injury are very likely to have other injuries (life-threatening injuries to the head, abdomen, or chest), particularly about the head, and may perhaps require more direct and immediate attention. A ruptured spleen is readily overlooked. Bradycardia is common with spinal shock.

In medical cervical spine problems, examination of the back of the neck and occiput may sometimes require removal of hair. Cutaneous angiomas and telangiectases may point to spinal cord arteriovenous fistulae, café au lait spots, intracutaneous nodules, or tumors of the peripheral nerve suggesting neurofibromatosis. Both medical and surgical problems of the cervical spine require knowledge of complete and incomplete lesions. Each patient is a new challenge and requires individual clinical assessment. Table 5–4 lists general clinical neurologic symptoms and signs arising in disorders of the cervical spine.

Table 5–4. SYMPTOMS AND SIGNS ARISING FROM TISSUES IN THE CERVICAL SPINE

Symptoms	Signs
Pain	Falling
Headache	Tender scalp
Dizziness	Tender bones
Vertigo	Anesthesia
Paresthesia	Hyperesthesia
Fatigue	Dysesthesia
insomnia	Atrophy
Restless arms and legs	Weakness (upper extremity)
Cough	
Sneeze	Asymmetry
Nausea	Sweating (or lack of)
Diarrhea	Nystagmus
Threatened faint	Tender muscles
Visual disturbance	Fasciculation
Auditory disturbance	Pathologic gait
Drop attack	Transient loss of hearing, consciousness, sight
Arm and leg pain and ache	Drop attack
Stiff neck	Ataxia
Torticollis	Spastic gait
Gait disturbance	Reflex changes
Balance poor	
Speech disturbance	
Muscle twitch	
Mood depressed	
Tinnitus	
Diplopia	

CRANIAL NERVES IN CERVICAL SPINE DISORDERS

The examination of cranial nerves is a most important aspect of rheumatologic neurology and requires careful and detailed clinical study. Ten of the 12 cranial nerves have voluntary fiber tracts that connect to Betz's cells in the cerebral cortex, as in any other upper and lower motor neuron system. These nerves can be properly regarded as simply "high" cervical nerves with brain and cord representation, anterior and posterior rootlets and roots, peripheral nerves, and both motor and sensory function (see *Phylogenetic Implications* in Chapter 1). Reptiles that have no extremities have four more upper cervical vertebrae and cervical nerves than animals with extremities. The evolutionary development of extremities, occipital bone, and cerebral cortex has included the paired cervical nerves. The last two behave in structure and function like the paired spinal nerves and react in the same way to disease processes. The first two cranial nerves, olfactory (I) and optic (II), and to some extent the third auditory (III), react more as does the brain proper.

The cranial nerves are best examined individually and in consecutive order. One must understand their anatomic relationships and functions to comprehend and interpret the significance of symptoms and signs secondary to their dysfunction.

Disease and disorder of cranial nerves are conveniently divided into those that involve the peripheral nerve fibers or trunks (infranuclear lesions), those that affect the nuclear center (nuclear lesions), and those that involve central connections (supranuclear lesions). There are cerebral cortical areas governing function of the motor cranial nerves, and there are sites of termination of the sensory impulses for recognition and interpretation. The peripheral nerves run from their nuclei to the ultimate distribution of their fibers; part of their course often lies in the brain tissue.

Even though a peripheral cranial nerve may be involved independently of its nucleus, if the nucleus is damaged, there follows inevitable degeneration of the nerve, as occurs with loss of the primary neural cell body anywhere else. Because of the close proximity of many of the cranial nerve nuclei, particularly in the brain stem, and their proximity to other structures, only rarely will a single nucleus be involved without involvement of other nuclei and other neural structures.

Clinical assessment and interpretation of the status of individual cranial nerves allow clinical localization of the disease process in the central nervous system and also permit diagnosis of systemic disease. Identifying cranial nerve dysfunction leads to diagnosis of cervical spine, cord, and intracranial lesions; reflects rising intracranial pressure; suggests such diffuse processes as meningitis, vasculitis, generalized infection, sarcoidosis, and diabetes mellitus; or may even reflect a primary pathologic process at some distant site.

Clinical Examination of Cranial Nerves

Olfactory Nerve (I). Smell is tested by the use of nonirritating volatile oils or liquids, such as oil of wintergreen, tar, oil of roses, oil of clove, oil of turpentine, and vanilla. Many substances (chloroform, menthol, camphor, ammonia) are unsatisfactory because they stimulate gustatory (taste) end organs or the peripheral endings of trigeminal nerves in the nasal mucosa. Olfactory nerves themselves are rarely the seat of disease but may be involved in association of disease or injury of surrounding structures.

Optic Nerve (II). Optic nerve is essentially a sensory nerve carrying impulses having to do with the special sense of vision. Light rays pass through cornea, lens, and vitreous and penetrate the retina to reach the outer surfaces of the rods and cones. By nerve fibers, impulses are carried to consciousness for recognition of light, form, and color in the visual cortex. Another function is mediation of afferent impulses for light and visual reflexes. Clinical tests are those of vision (acuity), fields of vision, and special components (color vision and day and night blindness). The optic nerve is the only cranial nerve that can be examined directly (ophthalmoscopy). One looks for local ocular changes, cataract, conjunctival irritation, corneal scarring or opacity, iritis, uveitis, glaucoma, anulus or arcus senilis, Kayser-Fleischer rings (Wilson's disease), the optic disc, retinal venule pulsation, light reflections, arteriole and venular characteristics, evidence of blurring of the disc margins or nerve head edema, and the macula.

Oculomotor Nerve (III). This nerve supplies the superior, medial, and inferior rectus muscles and the inferior oblique extraocular muscles. It also supplies the levator palpebrae superioris, which elevates the musculature of the eyelid. Some innervation is supplied by the orbicularis oculi (with which fibers of the levator are closely intermingled), the pupillary sphincter (pupil constriction), and the ciliary muscle.

Complete paralysis of the third nerve results in ptosis, paralysis of gaze (medial and upper), paresis of downward gaze, and dilation of the pupil. The patient is unable to raise the eyelid and unable to turn the eyeball medially, downward, laterally, or upward. The eyeball deviates laterally and somewhat downward. Third nerve paralysis may not be complete.

Trochlear Nerve (IV). The trochlear is the smallest of the cranial nerves. It supplies the superior oblique muscle, which depresses the eye (especially if it is in abduction), abducts the eyeball, and rotates the abducted globe so that the upper end of the vertical axis is inward. In a nuclear lesion of the fourth nerve, the contralateral superior oblique muscle is paralyzed, but in a lesion along the course of the nerve (peripheral) after its decussation, the ipsilateral nerve is involved.

Abducens Nerve (VI). The sixth cranial nerve supplies a single muscle, the lateral or external rectus, which abducts the eyeball or deviates it laterally. In paralysis of the sixth nerve, the eyeball is turned medially and cannot be moved laterally. *Because of its long intracranial course, this nerve is more frequently involved in disease processes than are the other cranial nerves.* An increase in intracranial pressure or exudate from inflammatory processes or hemorrhage may produce compression between the pons and the clivus and interrupt its continuity. In such circumstances there may also be bilateral involvement of the sixth nerve.

The third, fourth, and sixth cranial nerves are considered together because they are the ocular motor nerves.

Trigeminal Nerve (V). The fifth cranial nerve is a mixed nerve with both motor and sensory fibers, and it is the largest of the cranial nerves because of its connections with the third, fourth, sixth, seventh, ninth, and tenth cranial nerves and with the sympathetic nervous sytem in one of the most complex interconnections. Nuclei of the trigeminal nerve are located in the midportion of the pons. The trigeminal nerve is divided into three branches, the ophthalmic, the maxillary, and the mandibular divisions.

Motor Functions. Motor functions of the trigeminal nerve include supplying motor power to the muscles of mastication involving weakness or loss of power in raising, depressing, protruding, retracting, or deviating the mandible. In unilateral paresis, the jaw is deflected toward the side of the involved nerve, and the patient is unable to deviate it toward the nonparalyzed side. In bilateral paresis, the jaw droops, owing to the pull of gravity, and all muscle power is lost.

In examination, the patient clenches the jaw while the examiner feels contraction of the masseter and temporal muscles on each side. The patient opens the mouth (pterygoid muscle function internal and external); the patient moves the jaw from side to side against resistance. In unilateral paralysis of the fifth nerve, the patient is able to move the jaw to the paralyzed but not to the nonparalyzed side. The examiner asks the patient to protrude and retract the jaw and notes any tendency toward deviation. The patient bites on a tongue depressor with the molar teeth, and the examiner compares the depth of the teeth marks in the wood on both sides. If the examiner can pull out the tongue blade while the patient is biting on it, there is weakness of the muscles of mastication. The jaw reflex is tested (discussed subsequently). Tone, volume, and contour of the muscles of mastication are noted.

The other muscles supplied by the fifth cranial nerve cannot be adequately examined; nevertheless, if there is paralysis of the mylohyoid muscle and the anterior belly of the digastric muscle, one may note on palpation some flabbiness or flaccidity of the floor of the mouth. If there is paralysis of the tensor muscle of the velum palatini, the uvula may be slightly tilted to the affected side, and the palatal arch on that side may appear broader and lower than normal. Paralysis of the tensor muscle of the tympanic membrane is not apparent objectively, but the patient may complain of difficulty hearing high notes or of dysacusis for high tones.

Sensory Function. Perceptions of superficial pain, heat, cold, and light touch are examined individually in the same manner as elsewhere in the body. Corneas, conjunctivae, nostrils, gums, tongue, and insides of the cheeks are also examined. One should try to differentiate between sensory changes of peripheral origin (one or more of the primary divisions of the nerve) and changes in the segmental distribution resulting from lesions in the cerebrospinal axis. In differentiating physical from hysterical anesthesias of the face, it is important to remember that there is less crossing at the midline on the face than there is elsewhere on the body and that the skin over the angle of the jaw is not supplied by the fifth nerve but by the second and third cervical nerves through the great auricular nerve. In trigeminal neuralgia and other neuritides there is increased sensitivity at the emergence of the various sensory branches through their individual fascial sheaths and foramina—"trigger" or pain producing zones that may on pressure precipitate severe attacks of pain.

Reflexes of the Trigeminal Nerve. Jaw, masseter, or mandibular reflex. Examiner places index finger over the middle of the patient's chin, holding the mouth slightly open and relaxed; examiner taps the finger with a reflex hammer; the response is a contraction of the masseter and temporal muscles, causing a sudden closing of the mouth. An alternative to the procedure just outlined involves placing a tongue blade over the lower molar teeth and tapping the tongue blade outside the mouth. Both procedures elicit a bilateral response. A unilateral increase in, decrease in, or absence of reflex is sometimes elicited by tapping the angle of the jaw or by placing the tongue blade over the lower molar teeth. *Zygomatic reflex (modification of the jaw reflex).* Percussion over the zygoma causes ipsilateral deviation of the mandible. *Head retraction reflex.* With the head slightly bent forward, the upper lip is sharply tapped just below the nose. Positive response is a quick, involuntary, backward jerk of the head. This reflex usually is not elicited in normal persons but is obtained if there is exaggeration of deep reflexes. *Head retraction reflex is present in bilateral supracervical lesions of the pyramidal tract;* the reflex centers are in the upper cervical portion of the spinal cord.

Corneal reflex. The examiner touches the cornea lightly with a wisp of cotton, a piece of string, or a strand of hair. The cotton should be moistened to avoid irritation. The patient turns the eye in one direction, and the examiner approaches from the opposite side to eliminate the blink (visual palpebral reflex). Both the lower and upper portions of the cornea should be tested. A positive response is blinking or closing the ipsilateral eye (the direct corneal reflex) and also closing the opposite eye (the consensual corneal reflex). In a unilateral trigeminal lesion with consequent corneal anesthesia, stimulation fails to produce either the direct response on the involved side or the consensual response on the opposite side. Stimulation on the opposite (uninvolved) side elicits both responses. With a seventh nerve lesion and paralysis of the orbicular muscle of the eye, the direct response is absent on the involved side, but the contralateral consensual reflex is maintained. When the opposite cornea is stimulated, the direct response appears, but the consensual reflex is absent. *Conjunctival reflex.* This may be absent in normal individuals who have a high threshold of pain and it is also often absent in individuals suffering from hysteria. The conjunctival reflex is much less significant clinically than the corneal reflex. *Nasal, sneeze, or sternutatory reflex.* Stimulation of the nasal mucous membrane by tickling with a hair or a cotton wisp is followed by contraction of the nasopharyngeal and thoracic muscles resulting in a sneeze, violent expulsion of air from the nose and mouth. The afferent portion of the reflex arc is carried from nasal mucous membrane through the trigeminal nerve, and the efferent impulses are carried through trigeminal, facial, glossopharyngeal, and vagus nerves and through the motor nerves of the cervical and thoracic portions of the spinal cord—a widespread reflex response.

Facial Nerve (VII). The seventh cranial nerve is predominantly a motor nerve that innervates the muscles of facial expression. It does carry parasympathetic secretory fibers to the salivary and lacrimal glands and to the mucous membranes of the oral and nasal cavities. It conveys several types of sensation from the region of the eardrum, taste sensation in the anterior two thirds of the tongue, general visceral sensation from salivary glands and mucosa of the nose and pharynx, and proprioceptive sensation from the muscles it supplies. The motor nucleus of the seventh nerve is deep in the reticular formation of the lower part of the pons, medial to the nucleus of the descending root of the fifth nerve, anterior and lateral to the nucleus of the sixth nerve, and posterior to the superior olivary nucleus. Examination consists of assessment of the action of the muscles of facial expression. The examiner inspects the patient's face, noting mobility of facial expression, asymmetry or abnormality of muscles, "one-sided appearance" while talking or smiling, inequality of palpebral fissures, infrequent and asymmetric blinking, and smoothness of the face (absence of normal wrinkling or increased wrinkling). Each of these areas may provide clues to facial nerve involvement.

Specifically, the patient is asked to contract the various muscles individually and in unison. The examiner asks the patient to frown, wrinkle the forehead, raise the eyebrows and corrugate the brow, and close the eyes singly and bilaterally—first lightly, then tightly, and then against resistance. The patient is asked to draw back the angles of the mouth, show the teeth, grimace, blow out the cheeks, purse the mouth, whistle, and retract the chin muscles. Platysma function is tested by having the patient try to open the mouth against the resistance of firmly clenching the teeth. Tone of muscles and facial expression are noted, and atrophy and fasciculations are sought. Weakness of stapedius muscle is not apparent objectively, but the patient may complain of hyperacusis, especially for low tones.

Reflexes of the Facial Nerve. Sucking reflex and palmomental reflex. Orbicular oculi reflex is the reflex closing of the eyes in response to a loud noise, a sudden fright, or tapping the root of the facial nerve. *Orbicular oris reflex*: percussion of the upper lip or side of the nose causes a contraction of the ipsilateral quadratus labii superioris and caninus—elevation of the upper lip and angle of the mouth occurs. Chvostek's sign—spasm or tetanic contraction of the ipsilateral facial muscles—is elicted by tapping over the exit of the facial nerve anterior to the ear.

Sensory Function. Sensory function of the seventh nerve is not easily tested. Gustatory sense, or taste, is closely associated with smell. Also, taste is carried through the glossopharyngeal nerve and probably through the vagus nerve, thus making it difficult to separate sensory function.

Secretory Function. Secretory function of the facial nerve can be assessed by noting increased or decreased lacrimation (historically) and by noting the amount of tear secretion produced by hanging a strip of litmus paper or filter paper in each lower lid (Schirmer's test). The lacrimal reflex (secretion of tears), usually bilateral, can be produced by stimulating the cornea or by mechanically or chemically stimulating the nasal mucosa.

Acoustic (Auditory) Nerve (VIII). This nerve is composed of two fiber systems blended into a single nerve trunk, the cochlear nerve and the vestibular nerve. The cochlear nerve end receptors (end organs) are hair cells (auditory cells) in the organ of Corti within the cochlea of the internal ear. Impulses are carried to the bipolar cells of spinal ganglia of the cochlea from which central fibers pass to the cochlear nerve. Hearing is tested by using voice, whispering, rubbing thumb and index finger together close to the ear, studying high and low pitches, and using the more sophisticated audiograms. Other tests include the watch tick test, Rinne's test, and Weber's test.

Disturbances in cochlear nerve function are

manifested by loss of hearing (with or without tinnitus) and rarely by auditory hallucinations or auditory aphasia.

The most characteristic symptom in disease of the vestibular system including the nerve is dizziness, or vertigo—sensation of movement often accompanied by feelings of unsteadiness and loss of balance. True or vestibular vertigo is usually rotatory in type and is said to be objective if external objects seem to be rotating around the individual and subjective if the individual seems to be rotating. Nystagmus is due to vestibular stimulation. Noting postural deviation and performing the rotation test while observing for nystagmus are some of the simple clinical identifying studies.

Glossopharyngeal Nerve (IX). The glossopharyngeal and the vagus nerves are intimately related and similar in function, as both have motor and autonomic branches with nuclei of origin in the medulla. Both conduct exteroceptive and general and special visceral sensations to similar or identical fiber tracts in the brain stem. The two nerves leave the skull together and course through the neck in a similar manner, and in many instances both supply the same structure. They are frequently affected in the same disease process. Thus, it is sound to consider them together.

As its name indicates, the glossopharyngeal nerve is distributed mainly to the tongue and pharynx. Motor fibers originate in the cells of the nucleus ambiguus in the reticular formation of the lateral portion of the medulla. The functions of the ninth nerve are difficult to test because the areas of distribution are supplied by other nerves, some of which are more important, and because many of the structures it supplies are inaccessible. The motor supply of the ninth nerve probably goes only to the stylopharyngeal muscle. Autonomic function of the glossopharyngeal nerve can be evaluated by noting the function of the parotid gland, that is, the copious flow of saliva from Stensen's duct on eating highly seasoned food. The nerve supplies taste perception to the posterior third of the tongue. Examination of pharyngeal and palatal reflexes is an important part of the examination of the glossopharyngeal nerve. The pharyngeal or gag reflex is elicited by placing a tongue blade or an applicator on the posterior pharyngeal wall; the reflex center is in the medulla. The palatal or uvula reflex is elicited by stimulating the lateral and inferior surfaces of the uvula or soft palate with a tongue blade or cotton applicator. A positive result is simultaneous elevation of the soft palate and retraction of the uvula. Carotid sinus reflex, which affects control of respiration, blood pressure, and heart rate, has an afferent supply from the glossopharyngeal nerve. Lesions of the glossopharyngeal nerve are not common. The nerve is small and well protected.

Vagus Nerve (X). The vagus nerve is the longest and most widely distributed of all cranial nerves. Nuclei of origin are similar to and in many respects identical to those of the glossopharyngeal nerve. In spite of its great size, its multiple functions, and its importance in the regulation of essential visceral processes, clinical testing of the vagus nerve is difficult and techniques for examination inadequate. Motor branches supply the soft palate, pharynx, and larynx and are more accessible for clinical testing than most other branches of the nerve. Asymmetries of the soft palate may be seen. Weakness of the soft palate or deviation of the uvula to one side or the other may provide a clue. A nasal quality of speech, dysphagia more marked for liquids than solids, and regurgitation of fluids into the nose when swallowing are symptoms. In bilateral vagal paralysis, the palate cannot be elevated on phonation, although it may droop markedly, owing to the action of normally functioning tensors of the palate. Palatal reflex is absent bilaterally. The nasal cavity is not separated from the oral cavity, and, on speaking, air escapes from the nasal into the oral cavity, causing difficulty with palatal and guttural sounds such as K, Q, and CH. The sound B becomes N, the sound E becomes M, D becomes N, and K becomes NG—similar to a patient with cleft palate. Pharyngeal functions are tested by noting contraction of the pharyngeal muscles on phonation and by observing elevation of the larynx on swallowing. Dysarthria occurs in pharyngeal paresis. Coughing or loss of the cough reflex may be seen. In examination of the larynx, the character and quality of the voice, abnormalities of articulation, difficulty with respiration, and cough impairment are noted. Mirror examination of the larynx or direct laryngoscopic examination should be carried out if there is hoarseness not explained by other mechanisms.

The vagus is the most important parasympathetic nerve in the body, but its autonomic functions are not readily tested clinically. The pulse rate may become slower in the event of medullary or upper cervical spine compression or increased intracranial pressure, so monitoring the pulse rate is useful in following intracranial disease. Tachycardia occurs when the vagus is paralyzed, whereas stimulation of the vagus causes bradycardia. Obviously cardiac rate changes are due to many causes. Vagal paralysis may also cause depression, acceleration or irregularities or respiratory rate, and alterations of gastrointestinal function.

Reflexes to be studied are the vomiting reflex, gag reflex, swallowing reflex, cough reflex, nasal or sneeze reflex, sucking reflex, and hiccups (singultus). Yawning is occasionally a clue. The carotid sinus reflex is also regulated by the vagal nerve. Total paralysis of one vagal nerve is accompanied by sensory and autonomic changes and paresis of the soft palate, pharynx, and larynx on the involved side.

Spinal Accessory Nerve (XI). This nerve has two distinct portions, the cranial part and the spinal part (the major portion). The fibers of this nerve arise from motor cells of accessory nuclei in the ventral horn of the spinal cord from the lower end of the medulla to the fifth or even the sixth cervical segment. Rootlets from these nuclei pass through the lateral funiculus to the cord and unite from a single trunk, which ascends within the dura between the dentate ligament and the posterior roots of the spinal nerve. This trunk enters the skull from the foramen magnum and is directed toward the jugular foramen, where it joins the cranial portion of the nerve for a short distance. The eleventh nerve is entirely motor in function. Functions of the cranial portion of the eleventh nerve are so closely related to those of the vagus that they cannot be distinguished from them clinically or examined separately.

The sternocleidomastoid and trapezius muscle are supplied by the eleventh cranial nerve. Function of the sternocleidomastoid is assessed by inspection and palpation as the patient rotates the head against resistance. The muscle stands out well. Its contours are distinct even at rest, and its contractions are readily seen. In a unilateral paresis, one may see little change in the position of the head in the resting state, and rotation and flexion can be carried out fairly well by other cervical muscles. However, a weakness of rotation can be seen readily by having the patient counteract the resistance of the examiner's hand, which is placed against one side of the patient's chin. The trapezius muscle is tested by having the patient shrug and retract the shoulders against resistance. Such movements are observed, and contraction can be seen and palpated. Muscle power should be compared on the two sides. In unilateral paralysis of the trapezius, the shoulder cannot be elevated and retracted, the head cannot be tilted toward that side, and the arm cannot be elevated beyond the horizontal. There is dropping of the arm on the affected side, and the finger tips touch the thigh at a lower level than on the normal side. If the palms are placed together with the arms extended anteriorly and slightly below the horizontal, fingers on the affected side extend beyond those of the normal side. The upper portion of the scapula tends to fall laterally, with its inferior angle drawn inward—even some "winging" of the scapula occurs.

Hyperkinetic manifestations with tonic or clonic spasm of the muscles supplied by the eleventh cranial nerve are fairly common. Torticollis (wryneck), due to muscular contractions that cause a turning or deviation of the head and neck, is the most common single manifestation.

Hypoglossal Nerve (XII). The motor nerve to the tongue has origin in the cells of the hypoglossal nucleus. The nucleus extends almost the length of the medulla; its upper portion is beneath the floor of the fourth ventricle, close to the midline, and its lower portion is located in the gray matter in the ventrolateral aspect of the central canal. The hypoglossal nerve leaves the medulla in 10 to 15 rootlets (very similar to the anterior and posterior rootlets of the conventional cervical spine).

Examination of the hypoglossal nerve consists of assessment of the motor functions of the tongue. Motor power is tested by noting the position of the tongue on protrusion and at rest as well as the strength and rapidity of movement in all directions. Weakness, paralysis, atrophy, and abnormal movements are observed. Position of the tongue at rest in the mouth is observed first. The patient is asked to protrude it, move it in and out, side to side, upward, downward, both slowly and rapidly, and to press it against the cheek while the strength of the pressure is noted by the examiner, whose finger is placed outside of the patient's cheek. The patient should be asked to curl the tongue upward and downward over the lips and to elevate the lateral margin.

If there is unilateral paralysis or paresis of tongue muscles, the tongue deviates toward the involved side on protrusion, owing to the muscle action of the normal genioglossus muscle, which is stronger than other tongue muscles. Peripheral or central lesions of the hypoglossal nerve cause paresis or paralysis of the tongue. A unilateral paralysis may be grossly asymptomatic, with speech and swallowing little affected. However, in bilateral paralysis the tongue cannot be extended or moved laterally, impairing the first step in deglutition and causing speech difficulty, particularly in producing lingual sounds. Tongue paralysis, or glossoplegia, may be due to a supranuclear, nuclear, or infranuclear lesion.

Surgical and Medical Lesions at the Level of the Upper Cervical Spine and Foramen Magnum

Lesions of all sorts, particularly acute and complete, are invariably fatal without immediate respiratory support. Lower cranial nerves and their nuclei may be involved with incomplete lesions, as may the pyramidal decussation, sensory and motor tracts and their nuclei, respiratory and autonomic centers and their tracts as well as the anterior and posterior nerve roots of C1, C2, and C3. The posterior fossa may be invaded by large lesions, resulting in either neurologic reflections of cerebellar and brain stem compression or hydrocephalus. Vertebral artery or anterior spinal artery syndromes are particularly likely to result in ischemia or gross infarction, suggesting to the examiner damage of the upper cervical cord and brain. Upper cervical spinal cord lesions may produce a strange pattern of sensory loss over the face, described as the "onion peel" pattern. This results from functional compromise of the descending tract of the fifth cranial nerve, extending as far as the level of C4.[3] The distal portion of this tract conducts impulses from the periphery of the face, whereas the central areas are conducted by impulses from a higher level. Pain and temperature perception are altered in a centripetal manner from the outermost portion of the face as the lesion in the fifth nerve tract extends upward—thus this pattern of sensory loss is termed "onion peel." The dorsal root of C2 supplies the posterior scalp; C1 has no dorsal root. However, pain arising from ligaments, joints, bones, such as transverse ligaments, interspinous ligaments, atlanto-occipital joints, and atlantoaxial joints, is perceived in the retro-orbital and temporal areas. For example, in rheumatoid arthritis a subluxation of atlas on axis is perceived in this area.

Suboccipital headache is almost universal in patients with lesions in the area of the upper cervical spine and foramen magnum. Peculiar head and neck postures ("cock robin" posture) may be due to the pain. Because the fibers conducting dorsal column sensation from lower and upper limbs are medial and lateral in the posterior column, there may be selective impairment, depending on the portion of the posterior columns involved. The sternocleidomastoid and trapezius muscles are innervated by the spinal accessory nerve, which arises from the rostral cervical cord segment, and their function may be compromised.

With involvement of the pyramidal decussation, odd and various patterns of weakness and spasticity are seen, ranging from ipsilateral monoparesis to quadriplegia. Most corticospinal fibers cross over in the first cervical segment, or at the junction with the medulla. This anatomic characteristic explains a variety of motor changes in lesions at the foramen magnum level. Mass lesions in the upper cervical spinal cord or in structures about the cord may appear first as a spastic monoparesis of the ipsilateral arm, followed by the ipsilateral leg, and later, the contralateral leg and the opposite arm.[4] Paralysis of both upper limbs, with sparing of the legs, can occur if disease involving the midline and upper part of the pyramidal crossover occurs, for example, fractures and mass lesions of the odontoid process, hyperextension cervical spine injuries, or basilar impression.

Respiratory disturbances are very common and are consequent to phrenic nerve compression or irritation. Hiccups, dyspnea, and cough follow destruction of this nerve and paralysis of the diaphragm. Bradycardia is not common, but when it occurs, it is due to involvement of fibers ascending to the cardiovascular center in the medulla. Vertebral artery occlusion and anterior spinal artery thrombosis with high cervical cord infarction are followed by quadriplegia, impairment of many sensory modalities, bladder and bowel dysfunction, and the respiratory, cardio-

vascular, and vasomotor changes. The level of the C1–C2 spinal cord segments is very vulnerable to injury. A direct blow on the vertex of the skull may have its impact transmitted to the C2 segment of the cord, identified clinically and experimentally as a definite syndrome.[5, 6] The atlantoaxial joints can be disrupted by abrupt, severe force from above, and acute torsion of the cervical spine can damage vertebral arteries as they wind around the lateral masses of the atlas and enter the skull. Such an event is far more likely to occur in patients with cervical osteoarthritis and atherosclerosis involving the artery. Finally, the upper three cervical segments have relatively few radicular vessels to supply the anterior spinal artery, rendering that vessel more likely to produce ischemic and infarcted cervical cord.[7]

Cautionary Clinical Notes

Lesions high in the cervical spine, foramen magnum, and at C1–C2 may result in objective clinical signs of weakness in the interosseous and lumbrical muscles in the hand closely mimicking a C7–T1 lesion. This is understandable as it results in an ischemic lesion in the lower cervical segments by interruption of blood flow in the anterior spinal artery.

The direction of blood flow in the anterior and posterior spinal arteries is not well comprehended. The venous outflow is thought to be up, and it has been suggested that high cervical venous obstruction may have a pathologic effect on the lowest and most dependent cervical areas.[8]

The clinical separation of true intracranial lesions from cervical cord disease and trauma is difficult, and each may mimic the other. Hemiparesis occurring with supratentorial tumors may be difficult to diagnose early on if facial sparing occurs. Computed tomography resolves such problems nowadays, precluding the necessity for myelogram. Also, false localization may occur with lesions at the junction of the medulla and cervical cord, and contralateral weakness is seen because of corticospinal tract involvement above the decussation.

Spinal Shock

Spinal shock is a term used to describe the areflexia and flaccidity immediately following severe injury or transection of the spinal cord. There is marked hypotonia and complete areflexia, *except for the anal reflex*. This clinical characteristic demonstrates that, in primates at least, cord function is very dependent on influences from above the site of the lesion. Function of the spinal cord is much more independent in lower animals.

Spasticity appears after the period of spinal shock, which usually lasts a few weeks. The mechanism is an interruption of descending inhibitory fibers in the corticobulboreticular and caudatospinal and cerebelloreticular and reticulospinal pathways. Muscle hypertonicity, hyper-reflexia, and clonus are seen—a result of repeated stretch reflexes conducted through simple mono-synaptic pathways. Reflex activity (except for the deep tendon reflex responses) precedes the ap-pearance of spasticity. These reflexes are of two kinds: (1) the sacral parasympathetic response with reappearance and strengthening of both the anal and bulbocavernous reflexes, (2) a primitive withdrawal response, which is variable but seen as flexion of the knee and flexion and adduction of the hips, often associated with Babinski's re-sponse (extension of the great toe and fanning of the lateral toes). These reflexes can be elicited by stimulation from many areas on the lower extrem-ity. A mass reflex may occur, later characterized by violent bilateral flexion and abduction of the legs and striking abdominal contraction, with bladder and bowel emptying. Reflex sweating also occurs. This is interpreted as a broad spectrum of activity in much of the isolated cord. Flexor spasm is a third characteristic; the spasms are frequently violent, initiated by seemingly minor stimulation of skin. Reflex sweating occurs in reflex contrac-tion of the detrusor muscle of the bladder.

Complete absence of sensory perception is pres-ent with complete lesions, often associated with a zone of hyperesthesia at the level of injury. Though the phrenic nerves are primarily motor, their small sensory component may transmit sen-sation. They enter the cord at the C3–C4–C5 levels and thus may be partly above the cervical lesion in any individual. Neural impulses may also move along autonomic nervous system pathways; an-other mechanism associated with autonomic hy-per-reflexia is reflex vasoconstriction in the para-lyzed area, resulting in hypertensive crisis, with severe headache, stuffiness of the nose, tachycar-dia, and flushing. Phantom sensations are also reported, sometimes involving localized areas, such as the genitals.

A vascular type of shock occurs in the acute period following cervical injury and is caused by sudden loss of sympathetic control in the ventro-lateral white matter. Blood pressures are low for 1 to 2 days, and postural hypotension is present, sometimes persisting for weeks after the injury. This can be identified by tilt-table examination and is caused by slow return of vasomotor tone. Bladder involvement is usual.[9] There is no active or reflex contraction of the bladder's detrusor muscle, and the bladder thus distends behind the passive obstruction at the bladder neck. This re-sults in overdistension and eventual overflow in-continence. The period of bladder shock is about the same as that of spinal shock (1 to 6 weeks). Reflex detrusor contractions finally appear. These contractions may occur before the reappearance of the deep tendon reflexes through the mecha-nism of afferent and efferent reflex arcs at S2, S3, and S4, paralleling the monosynaptic reflex for

skeletal muscle. A full, automatic bladder seems to follow in about 25% of men with paraplegia. This is not true in women.

Sexual dysfunction is likewise a consequence of compromise of the control of the autonomic ner-vous system. In the male, priapism and passive engorgement are common in the acute phase. Reflex erections return later, at about the same time as reflex detrusor action does. Bors[10] reports an overall figure of 86.6% for reflex return at all spinal sites. This frequency is clearly higher for cervical lesions than for lower lumbar lesions with lower motor neuron involvement. Ejaculations are not usually possible with complete cervical cord lesions, since such requires more complicated in-tegrated reflex activity in the lumbar sympathetic system. Orgastic sensations are absent with com-plete lesions, but alternate site or similar feelings may occur above the level of transection.

Gastrointestinal function is likewise impaired. Bowel distension and fecal retention are expected. An automatic emptying of the rectum (as with the bladder) usually develops. Absence of sweating is a significant problem, since 80% of heat produced must be lost through the skin. Of course, such patients are not physically active, nonetheless, very minor physical activity may overcome their heat dissipation capacity. The higher the lesion—a lesion of the cervical spine, for example—the more common the problem and the more difficult it is to control heat regulation. Late adaptation occurs only partially.

References

1. Lewis T: Pain. New York: Macmillan Publishing Co, 1942.
2. Schneider RC: The syndrome of acute anterior cer-vical spinal cord injury. J Neurosurg 12:95, 1955.
3. Humphrey T: The central relations of the trigeminal nerve. In Kahn E, Crosby E, Schneider R, et al (eds): Correlative Neurosurgery, 2nd ed. Springfield, Il: Charles C Thomas, Publisher, 1969.
4. Davis L, Davis RA: Principles of Neurologic Surgery. Philadelphia: W. B. Saunders Co, 1963.
5. Gosch HH, Gooding E, Schneider RA: Mechanism and pathophysiology of experimentally induced cer-vical cord injuries in adult rhesus monkeys. Surg Forum 21:455, 1970.
6. Schneider RC, Crosby EC, Russo RH, et al: Trau-matic spinal cord syndromes and their management. Clin Neurosurg 20:424, 1972.
7. Turnbull IM, Brieg A, Hassler O: Blood supply of the cervical spinal cord in man: A microangiographic cadaver study. J Neurosurg 24:951, 1966.
8. Taylor AR, Byrnes DP: Foramen magnum and high cervical cord compression. Brain 97:472, 1974.
9. Nathan P, Smith M: The centrifugal pathways for micturition with the spinal cord. J Neurol Neurosurg Phychiatry 21:177, 1958.
10. Bors F: Sexual function in patients with spinal cord injuries. Proceeding of symposium on Spinal inju-ries. Edinburgh: Royal College of Surgeons, 1963, p 62.

Chapter 6

Radiologic Evaluation

With development and refinement of diagnostic methods such as computed tomography (CT) and nuclear magnetic resonance (NMR) there have developed a complacency and a lack of interest in the older and deeply established technologies of plain film radiography and standard tomography. Bone and joint radiologists are relatively few. Those of us interested in musculoskeletal disease should become as highly skilled as possible in plain film radiology through experience and continuing education. This chapter, indeed this book, emphasizes maximum application of clinical skills to the cervical spine and the integration of radiology into all aspects of clinical practice, research, and education. Radiology is a tool to be used along with all of our other methods. Always read your patients' films yourself!

Radiologic study of the cervical spine contributes to diagnosis of disorders and to the ongoing assessment of disease progress in healing. It also furthers our understanding of cervical biomechanics and pathology. Study of films other than those of the cervical spine often allows more precise interpretation of those of the cervical spine.

It is wise to remember always that the diagnosis of cervical osteoarthritis is essentially a radiologic one, that is, it is based on radiologic signs shown on a radiograph. On films of middle-aged and elderly people, these signs are the rule, not the exception. They are perhaps a more reliable sign of middle age than gray hair. Eighty per cent of normal (control) subjects have cervical spondylosis (cervical osteoarthritis of the discs). It seems logical for etiologic purposes to study the unusual 20% of men over age 50 who do not have it!

Clearly the great majority of patients with cervical osteoarthritis are asymptomatic. A significant number do have intermittent stiff neck; a sizable proportion have asymptomatic but trivial neurologic signs indicating minor lesions of nerve roots or long tracts of the spinal cord; bothersome but clinically unimportant paresthesias and hypesthesia may occur in hands and feet; a very few patients develop more or less disabling syndromes referable to nerve root or cord damage. Arrest and even reversal of symptoms are well documented and occur either spontaneously or with conservative management. An irremediable, inexorable, downhill course is not at all likely. The ubiquitousness of the radiographic changes of cervical osteoarthritis calls for special caution in attributing etiologic and pathogenetic significance to radiologic signs. Surgeons who plan an anterior spinal fusion for cervical radiculopathy should place their own films next to those of the patient. They may see little or no difference!

RADIOLOGIC ANATOMY
Normal Standard Films of the Cervical Spine

Standard films for clinical study of the cervical spine include (1) frontal or anteroposterior view (AP); (2) AP view of the upper cervical spine taken through the open mouth (odontoid view); (3) lateral views—neutral, full flexion, and extension—to include the whole cervical spine; (4) 45-degree oblique views (right and left). One must know which side is which. In the left oblique view, the left zygapophyseal and uncovertebral (Luschka) joints and the left intervertebral foramina are outlined. "Left" in this context means that the patient is rotated 45 degrees to the right, and his or her left side is nearer the tube (Fig. 6–1).

The anteroposterior views show the uncovertebral joints best (see Fig. 6–1A); the zygapophyseal joints are visible in the AP view but better seen in detail in the lateral views. The measured distance between the zygapophyseal joints in the

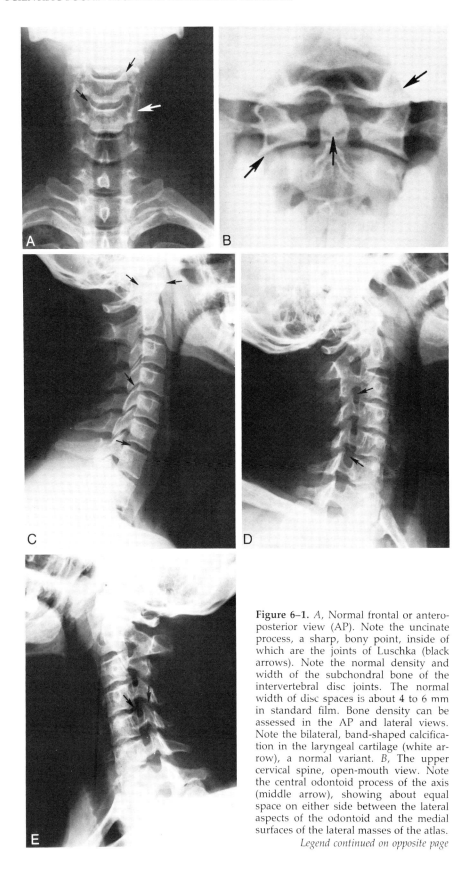

Figure 6–1. *A*, Normal frontal or antero-posterior view (AP). Note the uncinate process, a sharp, bony point, inside of which are the joints of Luschka (black arrows). Note the normal density and width of the subchondral bone of the intervertebral disc joints. The normal width of disc spaces is about 4 to 6 mm in standard film. Bone density can be assessed in the AP and lateral views. Note the bilateral, band-shaped calcification in the laryngeal cartilage (white arrow), a normal variant. *B*, The upper cervical spine, open-mouth view. Note the central odontoid process of the axis (middle arrow), showing about equal space on either side between the lateral aspects of the odontoid and the medial surfaces of the lateral masses of the atlas.

Legend continued on opposite page

AP view provides a rough idea of the minimal coronal diameter of the spinal canal, an average of 30 mm. If there is vertebral subluxation, the coronal diameter will be obscured. The AP view of the upper cervical spine taken with the mandible moving shows the skull-atlas-axis complex, especially the odontoid process, the lateral masses of the atlas, and the atlantoaxial joint (see Fig. 6–1B). The shadow of the central incisor teeth is occasionally misread as a bifid odontoid process.

The lateral view (see Fig. 6–1C, lower arrow) should include the whole spine and best shows the intervertebral disc joints, the zygapophyseal joints (middle arrow), and the skull-atlas-axis complex (upper arrows). The uncus shadow (lower uncovertebral joint) is seen. Vertebral subluxations are best seen in the lateral view. The normal cervical curve is that of lordosis with posterior concavity. Change in the lordosis to straight or flattened cervical spine, even reversed lordosis, may be clinically significant, reflecting muscle spasm, injury to the neck, or early cervical osteoarthritis. Figure 6–1D shows the oblique view demonstrating the intervertebral foramina, the joints of Luschka, and less well, the intervertebral disc and zygapophyseal joints. Figure 6–1E is the opposite oblique view. These films all showed normal findings. There is a range of normal postural lordosis, and a straight cervical spine may be within normal limits (Fig. 6–2). A localized lesion may be suspected by alteration in the shape of the curve in a symptomatic patient.

The sagittal diameter of spinal canal is roughly one half the coronal diameter. The sagittal diameter can be measured in millimeters between the posterior edge of the vertebral body and the site of junction of the laminae (spinolaminar line) from C1 (odontoid process) to the middle of the posterior arch of the atlas and from C2 through C7. The spinal canal is like a funnel, with the sagittal diameter diminishing from the top down. The average sagittal diameter at C1 is 21.6 mm, whereas that in the lower cervical spine is 17.0 mm. Spinal cord compression is likely to occur if the sagittal diameter is less than 10 mm. Figure 6–3, a cervical vertebra, illustrates well where the sagittal and transverse diameters are measured.

If there is an interruption of the normal funnel shape as noted by the measurements from the top down, an expanding intraspinal mass is suspected. A decrease in the sagittal diameter of the vertebral body and flattening of the normal convexity of the spinolaminar line also indicate an expanding intraspinal lesion. This can be drawn on a good quality lateral film[1] (Fig. 6–4).

The cervical spine has an enormous range of motion, though the range of movement between any two vertebrae is not great. The summation of these intersegmental movements allows a wide range of motion in the normal neck. The atlanto-occipital joints between the atlas and skull permit only flexion and extension. Motion between the atlas and axis allows flexion and extension, rotation, vertical approximation, and some lateral gliding. Separation or widening between the anterior arch of the atlas and the odontoid process normally is less than 3 mm in the adult and less than 5 mm in the child. Displacement beyond this limit without bony change suggests laxity or other derangement of the transverse ligament. The odontoid process serves as a pivot, like an eccentrically located axle in the ring of the atlas, permitting rotation of 45 degrees to the left or the right. (Fig. 6–5). With lateral gliding, the odontoid process appears asymmetrically placed between the lateral masses of the atlas because the articular surfaces are offset 2 to 4 mm. This asymmetry is a normal finding, not a subluxation (Fig. 6–6).

The application of cervical traction of 20 pounds for 20 minutes to the normal adult neck results in radiologic straightening of or loss of the normal cervical lordotic curve, widening of the normal intervertebral discs and the intervertebral foramina, and separation of facets of the zygapophyseal joints. There is little effect on the atlanto-occipital or the atlantoaxial joints. The changes occur from C2 to T1. These are physiologic events.[2]

Cervical spine movement decreases with in-

Figure 6–1 *Continued.* The atlantoaxial joint is easily seen (left arrow), and the atlanto-occipital joint is poorly seen (right). The transverse process of the atlas is readily seen. Note the spurring on the atlas, laterally at the atlantoaxial joint, a common normal variant. Note the bifid spinous process of the axis and C2, also normal (midline). C, The lateral view shows the atlanto-odontoid joint. The right arrow points to the anterior arch of the atlas, and the posterior arrow (top) to the odontoid process. Note the anterior arch of the atlas is only a few millimeters from the superior pharynx. Even slight subluxation of the atlas on the odontoid process produces a bulge on the pharyngeal wall, easily visible on elevation of the soft palate with a tongue blade. The discs are normal (lower arrows), and a good view of all zygapophyseal and intervertebral disc joints is noted. Normal cervical lordosis is present, with the concavity posterior. D, a 45-degree oblique view shows the intervertebral foramina (arrows), the joints of Luschka, and the zygapophyseal joints. The pedicles overlie the vertebral bodies as dense, bony rings. A good view of the styloid process of the temporal bone is present. The atlanto-odontoid joint is seen in its oblique view. Note that the joints of Luschka and the zygapophyseal joints appear on either side of the intervertebral foramen where the nerve roots exit. E, The opposite oblique view illustrates more clearly the intervertebral foramina and, on either side, the joints of Luschka (left arrow) and the zygapophyseal joints (right arrow). (From Bland JH, Nakano KK: Neck pain. *In* Kelley, Harris, Ruddy, et al (eds): Textbook of Rheumatology. Philadelphia: W. B. Saunders Co, 1981.)

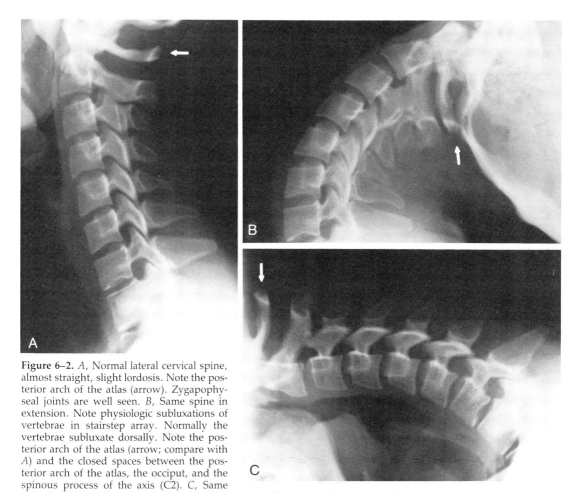

Figure 6–2. *A*, Normal lateral cervical spine, almost straight, slight lordosis. Note the posterior arch of the atlas (arrow). Zygapophyseal joints are well seen. *B*, Same spine in extension. Note physiologic subluxations of vertebrae in stairstep array. Normally the vertebrae subluxate dorsally. Note the posterior arch of the atlas (arrow; compare with *A*) and the closed spaces between the posterior arch of the atlas, the occiput, and the spinous process of the axis (C2). *C*, Same spine in flexion. Note the physiologic subluxation of C3 through C7 in strained but painless flexion. The vertebrae subluxate in stairstep fashion, each upper one being more ventral than the one below it. The atlanto-occipital and atlantoaxial spaces open in flexion.

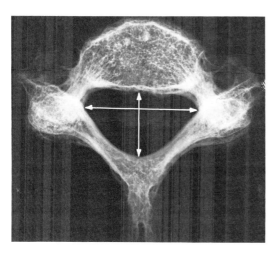

Figure 6–3. The fourth cervical vertebra (C4). Note the transverse process with foramen transversarium, a bifid spinous process, pedicles, and laminae. The spinal cord is faintly visible, as are the meninges. The horizontal arrows illustrate where the transverse diameter is measured, and the vertical arrows show where the sagittal diameter is measured.

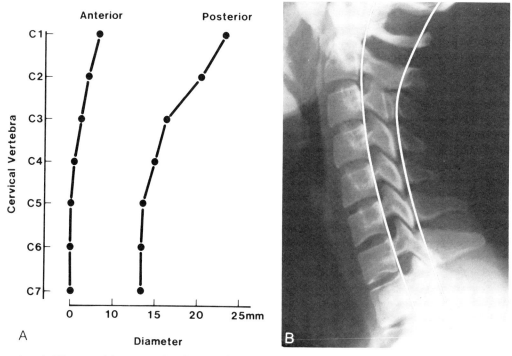

Figure 6–4. *A,* Diagram of the maximal and minimal sagittal diameters taken from *B,* a lateral film of a cervical spine.

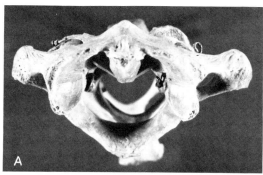

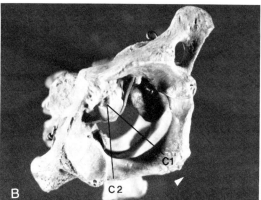

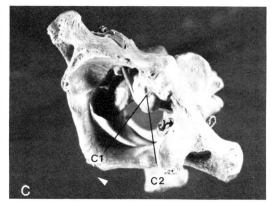

Figure 6–5. *A,* The atlas is set squarely on the axis and viewed from above; note the open spinal canal. *B,* The atlas is rotated to the left, and the spinal canal is encroached upon; the atlas rotates about 45 degrees on the odontoid process. The posterior arch of the atlas (C1) moves in an arc, with the odontoid process (C2) as the pivot point. *C,* The atlas is rotated to the right, again reducing the size of the spinal canal.

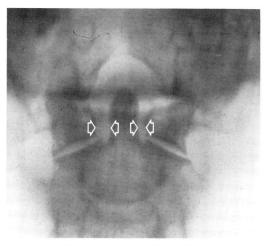

Figure 6–6. Atlanto-odontoid joints with the odontoid process in the center and the foramen magnum in the background. Note that the space between the odontoid process and the lateral masses of the atlas is wider on the observer's left than on the right (see arrows)—a normal variant that is dependent on posture and general flexibility.

creasing chronologic age, though it is unclear whether this is because of increasing immobilization, the universal occurrence of cervical osteoarthritis, or loss of hydration of intervertebral discs and hence loss of height. There is good physiologic evidence that continuing motion, stretching exercises, and use of the cervical spine will, in considerable degree, prevent this loss of motion. Osteophytes about surgically fused vertebrae remodel themselves, eventually disappearing altogether—a predictable phenomenon. People who have undergone surgical fusion of the cervical spine show increased mobility above and below the site of fusion, though the fusion site itself is rigid. These changes are entirely consistent with Wolff's law, which states that any bone will remodel itself according to the lines of stress applied to it. The stability of the cervical spine depends on bony structures only to a minor degree; stability depends to a major degree on the ligamentous structures.

Radiologic Criteria for Diagnosis of Osteoarthritis

There are four events occurring at varying rates in osteoarthritis at the cell and tissue level that have radiologic reflection.[3] These four steps in the pathophysiology of osteoarthritis are

1. Microenvironment of chondrocytes changes; chondrocytes mitose, produce clones that increase rates of all export products, proteoglycans, collagen, enzymes.

2. Subchondral bone osteoblasts increase rates

of synthesis; density of subchondral bone increases; stiffness increases; microfactures follow.

3. Osteophytes form at periphery of joint (metaplastic synovial cells); active inflammatory process (synovitis) occurs.

4. Pseudocysts form in trabecular bone below subchondral bone; volume and density of all articular and periarticular structures, capsules, tendons, ligaments, and bones increase.

With the great increase in synthesis of macromolecular components of bone, cartilage, ligament, tendon, capsule, and synovium in osteoarthritis, radiographic changes occur. The application of the following four radiologic criteria to plain films will assure precise diagnosis of osteoarthritis. The diagnosis is not always easy. The radiologic criteria for osteoarthritis are

1. Irregular or asymmetric narrowing of the joint space;

2. Increase in density of subchondral bone;

3. Osteophyte formation;

4. Pseudocysts in marrow cavity.

Figures 6–7, 6–8, and 6–9 illustrate the underlying anatomic and radiologic features of osteoarthritis. Ideally all four characteristics should be present to make an accurate diagnosis. Pseudocysts, however, are much less common in the cervical spine than in other joints with osteoarthritis.

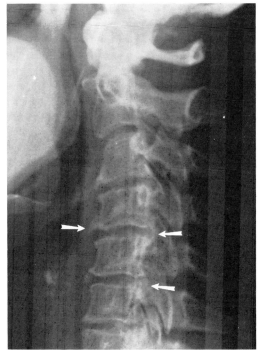

Figure 6–7. Radiograph of the cervical spine, with irregular narrowing of the intervertebral disc joint spaces and the anterior and posterior osteophytes (arrows).

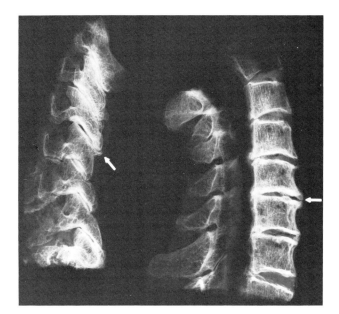

Figure 6–8. Film of an anatomic specimen. *Left*, note the marked increase in density of the subchondral bone, irregular disc space narrowing, and anterior and posterior osteophytes (white arrow). The spinal cord is faintly visible. *Right*, the zygapophyseal joints show the same findings (white arrow). In the second and third joints from the bottom, subchondral pseudocysts are present.

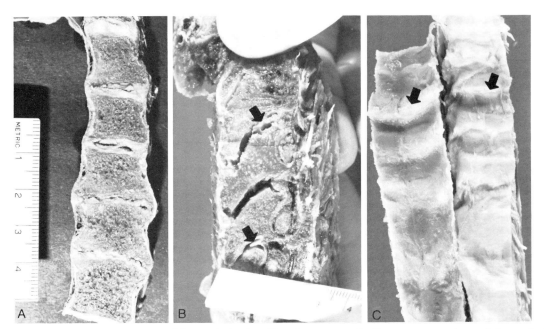

Figure 6–9. *A*, Anatomic specimen of the cervical spine. Note the asymmetric disc space narrowing and the marked remodeling and enlargement of the lower three vertebrae, with anterior and posterior osteophytosis. Marked thickening of the anterior and posterior longitudinal ligaments has occurred. *B*, Anatomic specimen. Zygapophyseal joints with irregular loss of cartilage, synovial proliferation, asymmetric joint space narrowing, and fibrofatty meniscal proliferation in a pannus-like lesion (seen in most of our cervical spine studies) (upper arrow). Note in lower joint a relatively normal meniscus compared with the upper joint (lower arrow). *C*, Two anatomic specimens of the posterior vertebral surface, anterior spinal canal. Note the large osteoarthritic bars and nodular lesions at the level of the intervertebral discs (arrows). Histologically, these are osteophytes with a mixture of cartilage and bone. The lesions compressed the anterior spinal cord in this case.

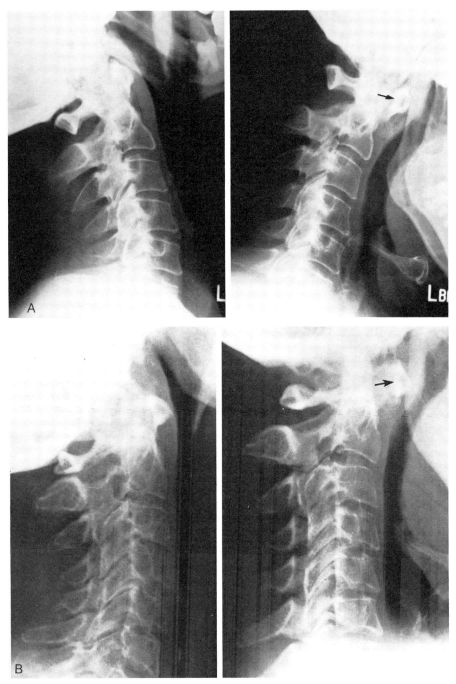

Figure 6–10. *A,* Example of atlantoaxial subluxation on flexion of the neck (extension on the left and flexion on the right). The arrow shows the gross 10-mm subluxation and change in the orientation of the atlas. The disc spaces between C3–C4 and C4–C5 are narrow without osteophytes, a characteristic of rheumatoid arthritis. *B,* Another example of the atlantoaxial subluxation on even slight neck flexion (arrow, right). Note that the atlantoaxial relationship is normal in slight extension (left), with a 9-mm subluxation in slight flexion (right). The atlas is seen to slide as well as tip forward. There are vertebral body end-plate erosions, C3 zygapophyseal erosions, and narrow disc spaces without osteophytes.

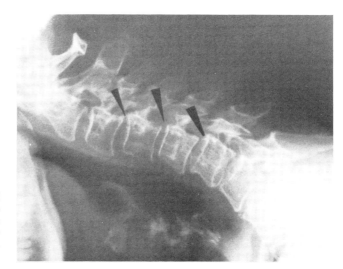

Figure 6–11. Illustration of multiple vertebral body subluxations (arrowheads), stairstep subluxation. There are also atlantoaxial subluxations, vertebral end-plate erosions, narrow disc spaces without osteophytes, and zygapophyseal joint erosions.

Radiologic Criteria for Diagnosis of Rheumatoid Arthritis of the Cervical Spine

Bland et al[4, 5] studied ten criteria for the diagnosis of rheumatoid arthritis involving the cervical spine, concluding that if five or more criteria are present, the diagnosis of rheumatoid arthritis is secure. The radiologic criteria for diagnosis of rheumatoid arthritis of the cervical spine are as follows:

1. Atlantoaxial subluxation of 2.5 mm or more.

2. Multiple subluxations of C2–C3, C3–C4, C4–C5, and C5–C6.
3. Narrow disc spaces with little or no osteophytosis.
   a. Pathognomonic at C2–C3 and C3–C4.
   b. Probable at C4–C5 and C5–C6.
4. Erosion of vertebrae, especially vertebral plates.
5. Odontoid process: small, pointed, eroded, loss of cortex.
6. Basilar impression ("platybasia-like").
7. Zygapophyseal joint erosion; blurred facets.

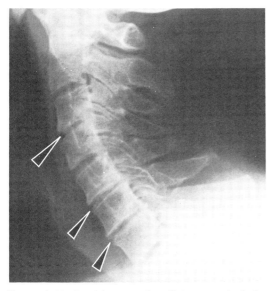

Figure 6–12. In this example, all intervertebral disc spaces are narrow without osteophytosis (arrowheads)—a pathognomonic sign of rheumatoid arthritis. Also seen are one vertebral body subluxation, C4 on C3, and many vertebral erosions and zygapophyseal joint erosions.

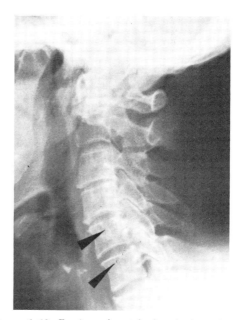

Figure 6–13. Erosion of vertebral end plates (arrowheads). Narrow disc spaces, erosions of the odontoid process, and a settling of the atlas downward over the odontoid process are also apparent.

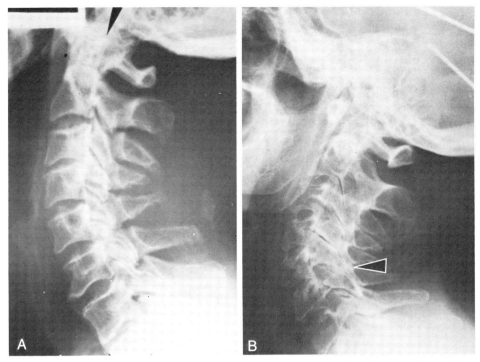

Figure 6–14. *A,* Odontoid process erosions. The odontoid process is small with swiss cheese–like erosions (arrowhead); virtually all ten radiologic signs of rheumatoid arthritis are present here. Note that in extension the atlantoaxial subluxation is reduced. *B,* Note the sharply pointed odontoid process and the presence of virtually all other characteristics of radiologic lesions. The arrowhead points to zygapophyseal joint erosions.

8. Osteoporosis: generalized, cervical spine.
9. Wide space (5 mm or more) between posterior arch of atlas and spinous process of axis (flexion to extension).

10. Osteosclerosis: secondary, atlanto-axial-occipital complex.

Figures 6–10 through 6–19 are examples of all the criteria.

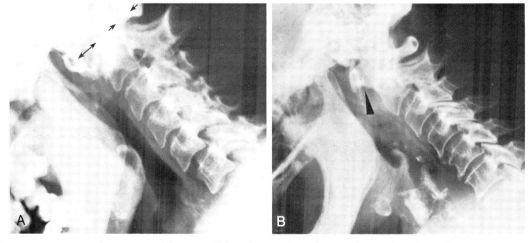

Figure 6–15. *A,* Note the vertical subluxation of the atlanto-odontoid joint, placing the odontoid process directly in the foramen magnum. Gross anterior subluxation is present, and most other signs of rheumatoid arthritis are noted. Strangely, this patient had no neurologic signs. Arrows indicate space behind and in front of the odontoid process. The posterior space is occupied by the spinal cord and is extremely narrow. *B,* Anterior (arrowhead) and vertical subluxation, with the odontoid process occupying the foramen magnum. Most of the odontoid process is above McGregor's line. Note narrow disc spaces and vertebral erosions.

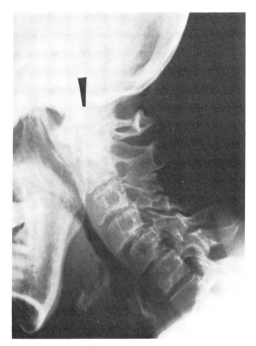

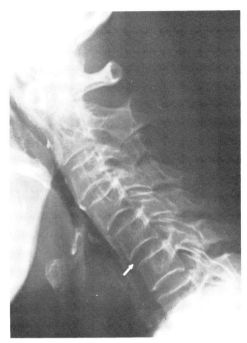

Figure 6–16. Zygapophyseal joint erosions, vertical sub-luxation (arrowhead), atlantoaxial subluxation, vertebral erosions, narrow disc spaces without osteophytes, and dislocated lower vertebrae.

Figure 6–17. Gross osteoporosis, giving the vertebrae an appearance of little boxes. Vertebral subluxation, ballooning of the discs without osteophytes (arrow), and vertebral plate and zygapophyseal joint erosions noted.

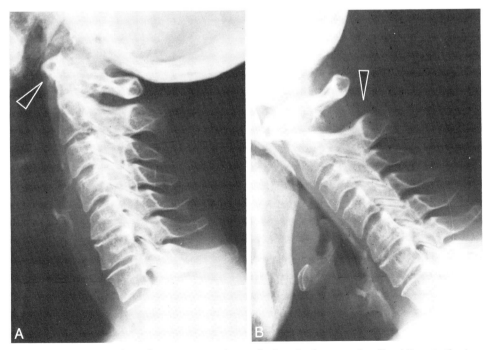

Figure 6–18. Tipping the atlas from flexion to extension to flexion. In the extension film (*A*), note the 1-mm space between the posterior arch of the atlas and the spinous process of the axis. In the flexion film (*B*), this space increases to 10 mm (arrow). If the difference in measurement from flexion to extension is greater than 7 mm, it indicates ligamentous laxity and the tipping atlas.

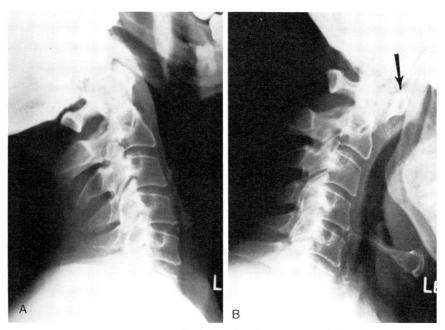

Figure 6–19. Osteosclerosis about the anterior arch of the atlas, the occiput, and the odontoid process (arrow). We noted this in rheumatoid arthritis and interpret it as indicating secondary osteoarthritis. Note that antlantoaxial subluxation occurs in flexion even with extensive osteosclerosis.

RADIOLOGIC METHODS FOR CERVICAL SPINE STUDY

Plain, routine radiographs are considered to serve well for evaluation of most skeletal and soft-tissue structures. Coned-down views, specialized projections, tomograms, and fluoroscopy may supplement and complement plain films.

Conventional Tomography. Tomographic evaluation still has an important place in cervical spine study. It is particularly useful in the study of the atlanto-occipital, atlantoaxial, and uncovertebral joints and in the assessment of anterior, posterior, vertical (into the foramen magnum), or lateral subluxation of the atlas on the odontoid process of the axis. The intervertebral disc joints and the cervical vertebrae themselves are well visualized for the study of erosions, subluxations, compression fractures, osteoporosis, and osteomalacia. Tomograms in an oblique projection may best show uncovertebral and zygapophyseal joints, whereas frontal and lateral projections are preferable for the vertebrae and atlanto-occipital and atlantoaxial joints. Tomograms are very useful in the assessment of cervical spine osteomyelitis because they precisely identify areas of cortical disruption and sequestra, that is, foci of active disease. Refer to Figure 6–20. Part *A* is a tomogram showing severe atlantoaxial subluxation with spinal cord compression. Part *B* shows a lateral subluxation of the atlas to the left. Parts *C* and *D* show an anatomic specimen with the odontoid

process in vertical subluxation in the foramen magnum, a case of rheumatoid arthritis.

Computed Tomography (CT). The CAT scan is the greatest advance in radiology since Roentgen discovered the x-ray in 1896. In less than 10 years, it has had a meteoric rise in use, revolutionizing diagnosis in most medical disciplines, particularly neurology, neurosurgery, orthopedics, and rheumatology. Essential components of a CT system are a scanning gantry frame with a patient table, an x-ray generator, and a data processing system.

CT is always preceded by study of standard films or views produced by other conventional imaging procedures, such as tomography or xeroradiography. CT examination is indicated only in the following situations: (1) when correct diagnosis cannot be made otherwise, (2) to demonstrate the extent of the disease process, or (3) for specific and necessary planning of surgical medical management. It should not be used to confirm information determined by other radiologic methods.

In the cervical spine, CT provides accurate data on (1) intraspinal masses, (2) the coronal and sagittal diameters of the cervical canal, (3) encroachment by soft or hard tissue on the spinal cord, and (4) marginal fractures and subluxations. Spinal stenosis and other congenital or acquired disorders compromising spinal cord or nerve root function are readily identified by CT. The cross-sectional display allows precise visualization of the spinal canal diameter as well as narrowing of

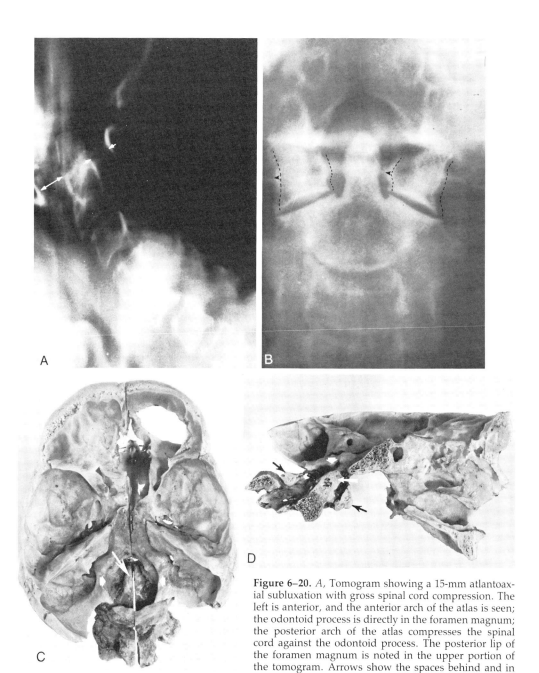

Figure 6–20. *A,* Tomogram showing a 15-mm atlantoax-ial subluxation with gross spinal cord compression. The left is anterior, and the anterior arch of the atlas is seen; the odontoid process is directly in the foramen magnum; the posterior arch of the atlas compresses the spinal cord against the odontoid process. The posterior lip of the foramen magnum is noted in the upper portion of the tomogram. Arrows show the spaces behind and in front of the odontoid process. *B,* A lateral subluxation of the atlas, to the observer's left. The atlanto-occipital joints are grossly eroded, right more than left. The arrows point in the direction of lateral (left) subluxation, and the dotted lines outline lateral masses of the atlas. *C, D,* Anatomic specimen of a skull with the odontoid process situated on the foramen magnum. *C,* A view from above with the calvarium removed. The short arrows point to the foramen magnum, and the longer arrow shows the odontoid process (sawed down the middle) occupying the foramen magnum. *D,* The sagittal view shows the foramen magnum with its anterior and posterior lips (short white arrow) and the odontoid process in the foramen (long white arrow). The anterior and posterior arches are shown with black arrows.

the neural foramina and lateral recesses. CT may someday replace myelography. CT also allows needle biopsy localization of relatively inaccessible sites and is a diagnostic aid in primary or metastatic malignancy in the cervical spine. Many soft-tissue masses are about the same density as muscle, the CT scan can differentiate them clearly and show soft-tissue masses in sharp contrast to subcutaneous fat. Fatty neoplasms are well demonstrated by CT. The potential for bone mineral analysis is developing because CT clearly defines a specific volume and precisely measures the density of that volume. It has the capability of measuring cancellous bone of the axial skeleton, including the cervical spine, which is incidentally a skeletal area very sensitive to metabolic and endocrine regulation and stimuli. Hence CT can diagnose osteoporosis and osteomalacia as well as assess bone mineralization serially in the metabolic and endocrine bone diseases (Fig. 6–21).

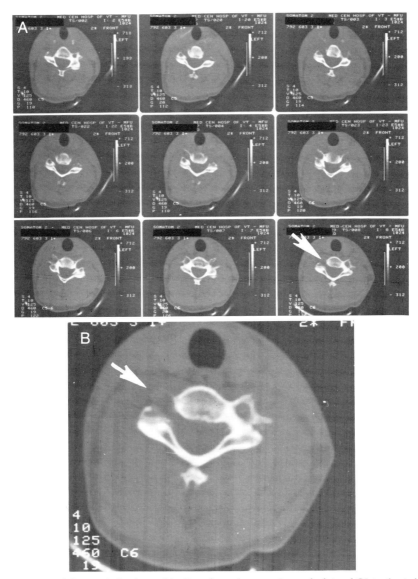

Figure 6–21. *A,* CT scan of the cervical spine, with slices from the superior end plate of C5 to the inferior end plate of T1. The sections are read from left to right. The intervertebral foramina, the vertebral artery, the foramina transversaria, and the zygapophyseal joints are well visualized. Mass lesions and bone destruction are not identified. The facet and the Luschka joints are normal. *B,* Enlargement of the lowest right section of *A,* showing a tangential cut through the intervertebral foramen on the left and the foramen transversarium on the right. The nerve is swollen in the C6 area (arrow).

Illustration continued on opposite page

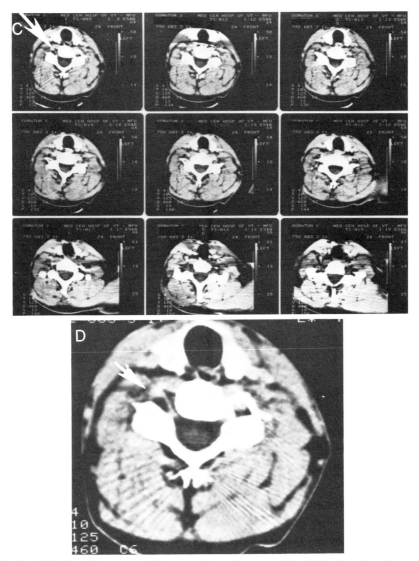

Figure 6–21 *Continued C,* The C6 nerve root is unusually well seen and is diffusely enlarged, suggesting a very swollen C6 nerve root (arrow), etiology unknown. Clinically the patient had a severe proximal C6 radiculopathy, and an electromyogram revealed denervation of the right C6 myotome. *D,* Enlargement of a C6 section showing the swollen nerve.

Myelography. Development of radiologic study for intraspinal pathology dates back to the 1920s in the United States and Europe. Contrast media have been of three types. Air or oxygen (gas) injection into the spinal canal came first, a negative contrast medium appearing radiolucent in the film. Positive contrast media were developed later, appearing radiodense on the film because of absorption by the x-ray beam. The two media currently in use are (1) iophendylate (Pantopaque), an oily 30.5% iodine in an oily ester, and (2) metrizamid (Amipaque), a water-soluble, nonionic substance. Other imaging modalities for intraspinal disorders include spinal arteriography (carotid and vertebral arteries in the cervical spine),

venography, discography, and epidurography. Cervical extradural compression of the spinal cord and nerve roots is relatively common, mostly at the C5–C6 and C6–C7 levels. Men are affected more commonly than women, and older patients are affected more commonly than younger patients.

Plain films show both anterior and posterior vertebral osteophytes, disc space narrowing, zygapophyseal and uncovertebral joint sclerosis, and hypertrophy with protrusion of osteophytes into the intervertebral foramina. The myelogram shows extradural compression of the spinal cord and nerve roots caused by the combination of vertebral osteophytosis, herniated nucleus pul-

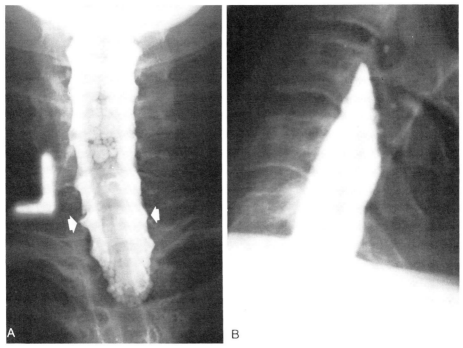

Figure 6–22. *A,* Myelogram showing an anteroposterior view of a cervical spine. Visualization of the spinal cord and subarachnoid space is excellent. There is no evidence of a herniated disc or other intra- or extradural lesions. Arrows point to the root pouches. *B,* Myelogram showing a lateral view of the same cervical spine. Again, findings were normal.

posus, joint sclerosis, and osteophytosis and hypertrophy of the posterior longitudinal ligament and the ligamenta flava. Multilevel changes may be seen, necessitating precise clinical correlation. Main findings are amputation of the nerve root sleeves, spinal cord compression, thinning of contrast column, "spondylotic bars," and displacement of the subarachnoid space (Fig. 6–22). Thus, myelography is useful and indicated in detecting effects of pathologic events on the subarachnoid space and its contents. Its limitation is that although it can detect the extraspinal extent of the pathologic process, it cannot detect associated disease in other organ systems. *When a myelogram is performed, the strong implication is that surgical, radiation, or chemotherapy treatment is being considered seriously. In most cases of osteoarthritis of the cervical spine, myelography discloses little or nothing that is not already known, that is, the procedure is rarely required.*

Cineradiography. Cineradiography means radiographic movies. Of the many techniques used to analyze cervical spine motion, cineradiography is the most valuable. An image intensifier is used, and the image is recorded on electromagnetic tape. The basic components of cineradiography are an x-ray source, a fluoroscopic screen, an image intensifier, a television or motion picture camera, and film. Image intensification means an increase in image brilliance without a corresponding increase in radia-

tion dosage. The electron optical image intensifier has made the science of cineradiography practical and universally accepted. The image can be intensified over 1000 times with today's equipment.[2]

Clearly cineradiography is the best method for the study of biomechanics and dynamics of motion in the cervical spine. Relying on memory or visual acuity of the observer is unnecessary because the films are permanent records. The films have great educational value, can be used repeatedly, and are helpful for diagnostic and prognostic purposes when compared with a patient's previous films or with films showing a disorder at a more advanced stage.

The determination of normal motion, sites of greatest and least motion, contribution by joints, discs, ligaments, tendons, and muscles to motion (and their limitations), and the biomechanics of normal motion of the occiput-atlas-axis complex all have been studied very successfully through cineradiography. Clinical application of full knowledge of the normal allows recognition of the abnormal.

Magnification Radiography. Magnification techniques have expanded in clinical practice and research. The quality of the radiographic image is important in precise and detailed assessment of subtle skeletal abnormalities. High-resolution radiographic techniques can maximize diagnostic information gathering. Magnification techniques

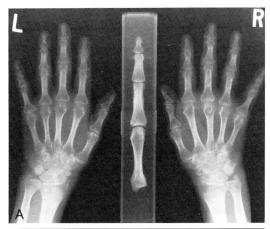

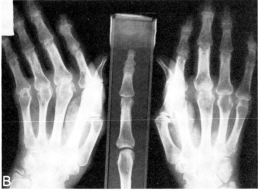

Figure 6–23. Normal and enlarged radiographic images of hands. *A* shows normal-size films, and *B* illustrates films enlarged by optical magnification. The hands in *B* completely took up the space of a 14- by 17-inch film (size of chest radiograph). The enlargement clearly allows diagnosis of lesions not perceived by the usual technique.

in skeletal radiology have been widely developed and used.

Two techniques allow high-resolution magnification. The first is simple optical magnification of fine-grain films, and the second is direct radiographic magnification. Optical magnification is done by contact exposures using conventional radiographic equipment and fine-grain industrial films, such as Kodak type M. The image is viewed with optical enlargement (Fig. 6–23). Direct radiographic magnification is used less often. It requires the newly developed x-ray tubes that have small focal spots (100 to 150 mm) and enough output for clinical examination. Initial results are encouraging, and uses for both thick and thin body parts are being established.[6] Magnification methods are used in the diagnosis of cervical spine disorders.

Ultrasonography. Diagnostic ultrasonography plays a central role in the assessment of many clinical problems in obstetrics, medicine, and surgery; its application in bone, joint, and soft-tissue

diagnosis is limited. The mechanism of ultrasonographic imaging is the transducer, which converts electric energy to sound energy and back again. A crystalline material (barium titanate) is physically deformed by an electric current, with consequent production of sound waves. The sound waves return from the body and deform the transducer crystal in a similar way, producing an electric current. This property of certain crystals is termed the piezoelectric effect and is the means for clinical application of ultrasonography.

The descriptive terminology in ultrasonography is straightforward, characterizing lesions or normal structures as either cystic, solid, or complex—for example, pancreatic cyst, popliteal cyst (Baker's cyst), distended urinary bladder, or arterial aneurysm. Detection of tumors or abscesses of bone and soft tissue is well done by ultrasonography and thus may have occasional application in the cervical spine.

Xeroradiography. This technique involves an electrostatic imaging system that utilizes selenium as a photoconductor. The method is derived from the xerographic process used in photocopying, hence the name. The xerographic process was discovered by Carlson in 1937. The image is produced by first charging a metal plate to a high positive potential, then placing the plate in a cassette, where it becomes an image receptor (like the conventional screen-film system); when the x-

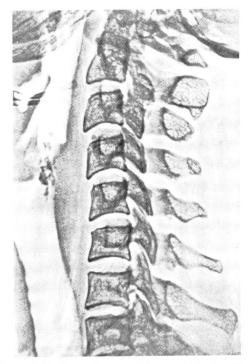

Figure 6–24. Xeroradiogram of the cervical spine. Note the marked and sharp delineation of both hard and soft tissue boundaries.

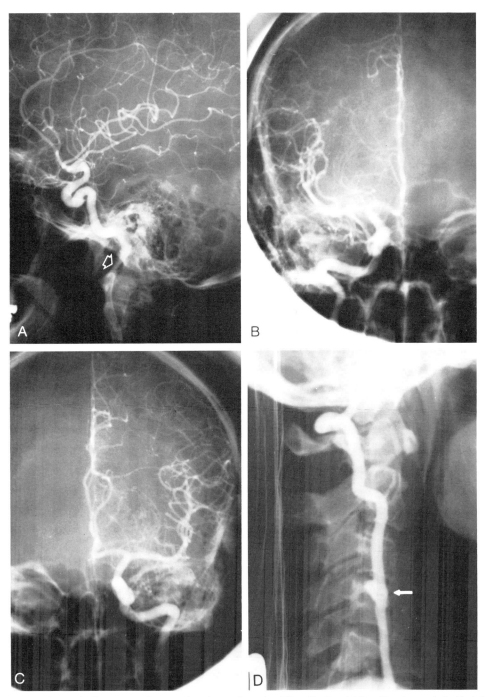

Figure 6–25. *A,* A vertebral artery angiogram showing a stenosis at the atlantoaxial junction (arrow). *B, C,* A bilateral carotid artery angiogram with normal findings (*B,* left; *C,* right). The pericollosal arteries and the internal cerebral veins are in the midline, and neither aneurysm nor arteriovenous malformations are identified. Vascular spasm and vasculitis are absent, and the lateral ventricles as defined by the thalamostriate veins are not enlarged. *D,* A vertebral artery angiogram showing a trauma-induced aneurysm at the level of C4 (arrow).

rays strike the selenium plate, photoconduction occurs, resulting in a latent charge image of the object. The latent image is then made visible by the use of charged developer particles—so-called toner particles that are brought in close proximity to the plate. The powder image is transferred to paper and thermally fused, resulting in a permanent opaque image (Fig. 6–24). A unique feature of the xeroradiogram is the edge enhancement, strikingly delineated at osseous as well as soft-tissue edges or boundaries.[7]

Xeroradiography provides very high-quality images of the cervical spine and ribs, recording many tissues of differing density and thickness—bone, fat, muscle, air, and joint—all of which are well shown on a single image. This method can provide as much information on a single print as a number of tomograms, without exposing the patient to as much radiation. It is useful in soft-tissue injuries of the neck.[8]

Bone Scanning With Radionuclides. Skeletal bone scanning with radio isotopes is as effective in diagnosing bone disease in the cervical spine as it is anywhere else in the skeleton. Technetium-99m that is labeled methylene diphosphate or ethylene hydroxydiphosphonate is the best isotope because it has low toxicity and is safe for repeated studies. Radionuclide scans measure bone turnover, and increased metabolic activity in bone shows up as areas of increased density in the print. The image resolution in the cervical vertebrae is not as good as it is in the rest of the spine. Bone scanning is useful in the diagnosis of bone and joint inflammation, infection, and metastatic and primary bone tumors of the cervical spine.

Arthrography, Tenography, and Bursography. Contrast opacification of joint cavities (arthrography), tendon sheaths (tenography), and bursae (bursography) is widely used in diagnosis and assessment of these structures in rheumatologic and orthopedic practice. There is very little requirement for these procedures in disorders of the cervical spine. Discograms may occasionally be used.

Vertebral Angiography. Obstructive lesions of the cervical vertebrobasilar arterial system are increasingly identified. Unhappily, the risks entailed in vertebral angiography are too often greater than the risks of the arterial lesion investigated. Surgically treatable lesions at the upper cervical level may be revealed by vertebral angiography and are only just worth the risk; vertebral angiography is a necessary procedure in investigation of disease of the posterior fossa. Myelography (and even high-quality plain oblique films) may locate the site of maximum vertebral artery obstruction. It is probably safer for the neurosurgeon to decompress the artery surgically during anterior fusion for cervical myelopathy than to carry out vertebral angiography in patients over 60 years of age. In general, the procedure is not justified in the treatment of cervical myelopathy secondary to cervical osteoarthritis (Fig. 6–25).

Vertebral Venography. The cervical venous system is well described.[9] Venograms do not predictably show normal flow pattern. Filling defects can represent some abnormal structure, such as a prolapsed disc. The interpretation of findings in relation to plain films, clinical data myelography, and angiography has not been satisfactorily worked out for predictable clinical use.[9]

Normal Anatomic Variants Simulating Disease in the Cervical Spine

There are many normal variants often mistaken for disease in day to day bone and joint radiology. So few radiologists have had the rare opportunity to see "population" films of people from different age groups who are not seeing doctors. Thus the normal never becomes established in their diagnostic considerations. To determine what is normal and what is not is the radiologist's primary function. To recognize the abnormal, full knowledge of the normal is the primary requirement. There are many "look alikes" in radiology, normal variation in curvature, density of tissue, defects in projection, overlap of structures, trabecular patterns in bone—in a word, pseudolesions.[10, 11]

In the cervical spine, the zygapophyseal joints at the C2–C3 level are poorly seen, giving the impression of fusion. This is due to overlapping shadows and occurs in most plain films (Fig. 6–26).

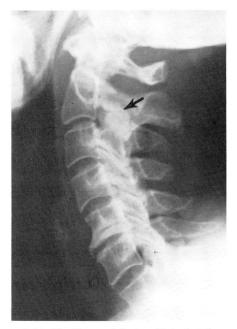

Figure 6–26. C2–C3 pseudofusion. Note that the zygapophyseal joint between C2 (axis) and C3 (arrow) appears abnormal, as though fused. This and similar appearances occur in most lateral cervical spine films.

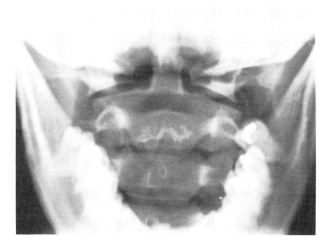

Figure 6–27. Physiologic subluxation of the atlas on the axis. Lateral flexion to the observer's left results in lateral glide, and the space on the left between the lateral mass of the atlas and the odontoid process is wider than that on the right. Obviously this requires no treatment.

The odontoid process normally has variable shape—a pointed configuration, often with small osteophytes. The superior aspect of the anterior arch of the atlas often has some new bone formation. Both may suggest erosion (see Figs. 6–10, 6–14, 6–15 and 6–19).

In extreme lateral flexion, the atlas slides laterally to the side of flexion by 1 to 3 mm, varying with the intrinsic flexibility of the person. This normal variant is much more marked and apparent in children than in adults. A child who has had a head or neck injury is at risk of being put in skull tongs and traction for the "subluxation," which is a normal variant and may be 5 to 6 mm (Fig. 6–27). The fully flexed spine also shows anterior subluxation for C2–C7 of 1 to 2 mm in the person with normal, lax, and flexible connective tissue. The same is true in full extension (see Fig. 6–2).

The zygapophyseal joints in the midcervical spine may give the impression of fusion, subluxation, or even erosive disease because of positioning of the spine or overlying shadows in the direction of the x-ray beam. Oblique projection usually resolves this by showing well-defined joint surfaces in the normal subject.

Faulty positioning and slight rotation of the spine at the time the film is taken may create the illusion of factitial calcification of the posterior longitudinal ligament. Actually two posterior aspects of the vertebral bodies are seen. Repeated study with correct positioning resolves this problem also.

The superior zygapophyseal joint surfaces of C5, C6, and C7 in some normal people have a groove or a depression, which should not be mistaken for bone or joint trauma or an erosive process.

The normal cervical lordosis may be "normally" less lordotic, straight spine, or even reverse lordosis, that is, even slight kyphosis, and still be within physiologic and normal limits (see Fig. 6–1).

The foramen transversarium of the atlas may occasionally be seen as a ring or an area of decreased density in the lateral aspect of the lateral mass of the atlas at the AP open-mouth view. It can be confused with an erosive process. Figure 6–28 shows the arcuate foramen—a variable anatomic feature of the atlas—formed by an arc of bone over the groove on the posterior aspect of the lateral mass, enclosing the vertebral artery in its tortuous course around the lateral mass and up to the clivus to join its opposite vertebral artery to become the basilar artery.

Sialoliths are the most important calcific shadows observed in the soft tissues of the neck. They are salivary calculi projected into the region below the mandible (the shadow of the mandible). They are characterized by their density and a certain homogeneity.

Earrings of semiopaque material may cause

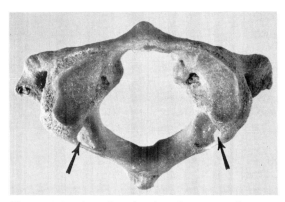

Figure 6–28. An atlas showing the arcuate foramen (arrows), a ring of bone over the groove on the posterior aspect of the lateral mass of the atlas.

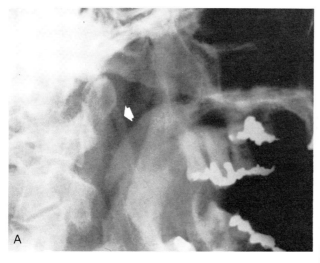

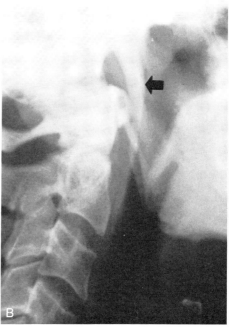

Figure 6–29. Arrow (*A* and *B*) points to a long styloid process that is really an ossified stylohyoid ligament. It was symptomatic in this case, necessitating removal.

shadows leading to misinterpretation when the head is in an oblique position during the filming. Streaks of calcium are often seen in the scar tissue of keloids in the soft tissue of the neck. Calcification of lymph nodes is the most frequent of all calcific deposits. The calcium has a definite granular appearance.

The styloid process of the temporal bone develops to varying lengths in different individuals. Its tip may just reach the anterior border of the atlas, or it may override this arch and appear as a small, protruding tip of bone, giving the impression of an exostosis on the anterior arch of the atlas. Sometimes it is very long, 10 cm or more, and is

then an ossified stylohyoid ligament (Fig. 6–29). It has been confused with a swallowed fish bone and has led to attempts at surgical removal of the "foreign body." The styloid process and the stylohyoid ligament may cause symptoms of dysphagia or of strange aches and pain in the throat unrelated to swallowing. The film taken through the open mouth is the best single procedure for visualizing the styloid process. Figure 6–30 provides examples of the unexpected diagnosis of Paget's disease of the lateral mass of the atlas. This lesion was severely symptomatic but responded exceedingly well to specific therapy. Kohler and Zimmer[10] and Keats[11] provide excellent

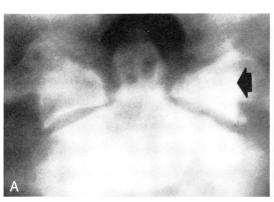

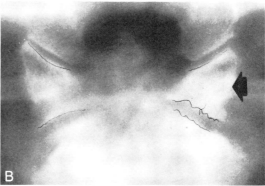

Figure 6–30. *A*, Tomogram showing Paget's disease of the lateral mass of the atlas (arrow). The atlanto-occipital and atlantoaxial joints are well seen. *B*, A clearer tomogram of the bony structures. In this case, diagnostic criteria other than radiologic are required to make the diagnosis of Paget's disease (arrow).

material concerning normal radiologic anatomy of the cervical spine as well as all of its variants.

References

1. Dolan KD: Expanding lesions of the cervical canal. Radiol Clin North Am 15(2):203, 1977.
2. Fielding JW: Dynamic anatomy and cineradiography of the cervical spine. *In* Bailey RW (ed): The Cervical Spine. Philadelphia: Lea and Febiger, 1974, p 29.
3. Bland JH: The reversibility of osteoarthritis. Am J Med 70(Supp 6A): 16, 1983.
4. Bland JH, Van Buskirk FW, Tampas JP, et al: A study of roentgenologic criteria for rheumatoid arthritis of the cervical spine. AJR 95:949, 1965.
5. Bland JH: Rheumatoid arthritis of the cervical spine. A Review. J Rheumatol 1:319, 1974.
6. Gordon SI, Greet RB, Weidner WA: Magnification roentgenographic technique in orthopedics. Clin Orthop 91:169, 1973.
7. Genant HK: Xeroradiography. *In* Resnick D, Niwayama G (eds): Diagnosis of Bone and Joint Disorders. W. B. Saunders Company, 1981, Philadelphia: pp 374–379.
8. Otto RC, Ponliadis GP, Kumpe DA: The evaluation of pathologic alterations of juxtaosseous soft tissue by xeroradiography. Radiology 120:297, 1976.
9. Théron J: Cervicovertebral phlebography: pathological results. Radiology 118:73, 1976.
10. Kohler A, Zimmer EA: Borderlands of the Normal and Early Pathologic in Skeletal Radiology, 3d American ed, 11th German ed. New York: Grune & Stratton, 1968.
11. Keats TE: Atlas of Normal Roentgen Variants that May Simulate Disease. 2nd Ed. Chicago: Year Book Medical Publishers, 1979.

Chapter 7

Craniometry and Roentgenometry of the Skull and Cervical Spine

There are many measurements available, usually done on standard radiograms, that are important and useful in diagnosis and management of disorders of the cervical spine. These measurements often assist in separating the normal from the abnormal. These are various ranges of motion, planes, lines, diameters (sagittal and transverse), angles, and bony landmarks. Their clinical use requires no special roentgenologic training and can be ascertained on standard films of the skull and cervical spine. The goal of this chapter is to bring these measurements together in textual as well as tabular form for clinical use.

RANGES OF MOTION

Motion in the cervical spine is properly divided between two anatomic units, the occipito-atlanto-axial complex and the unit from the second cervical vertebra (C2) through the first thoracic vertebra (T1). The functions and anatomic designs of these two segments are so dissimilar that it is helpful to study each region separately and then consider their combined range of motion capability. A working knowledge of spinal kinematics is necessary to understanding anatomic and pathologic physiology in the diagnosis and management of cervical spine diseases and disorders. Kinematics is a branch of mechanics that examines the motion of bodies without considering the forces that act on them. Elements of kinematics of cervical spine motion are the geometry of the articulating facets and the geometry and relative elasticity of the structures (ligaments and tendons) connecting the vertebrae. I use the terms upper cervical spine to describe the occiput through C2 and lower cervical spine to describe the C3–T1 region.

Occipito-Atlanto-Axial Unit. It is only recently that we have fully appreciated the great range of motion in the upper part of the normal cervical spine.[1, 2] Motion allowed between the occiput and the atlas (atlanto-occipital joints) involves only flexion and extension—no significant lateral flexion or rotation. Between the atlas and axis (atlantoaxial joints), motions permitted are flexion, extension, rotation, and at least measurable lateral gliding.[3] About 15 degrees each of flexion and extension occur in the combined atlanto-occipital and atlantoaxial joints. The odontoid process remains closely bound to the anterior arch of the atlas during flexion and extension. If the distance between the odontoid process and the posterior surface of the anterior arch of the atlas exceeds 3 mm in the adult and 5 mm in a child, there is clearly some abnormality of the transverse ligament of the odontoid process. The odontoid process acts as an eccentrically placed axle for the ring of the atlas; the eccentricity of the odontoid process is at the anterior rim of the ring of the atlas. The atlantoaxial joints coupled with the anterior and posterior joints of the atlanto-odontoid joint permit rotation of at least 45 degrees to the right and 45 degrees to the left. Oblique radiograms of the fully rotated atlantoaxial joint display readily seen offsets between the inferior articular surface of the atlas and the superior articular surface of the axis. Anteroposterior radiograms display narrowing of the joint space or even superimposition of the two surfaces, and the spinous process of the axis is deviated from the midline. The combined vertical height of atlas and axis appears to decrease. With lateral flexion of the head, there is both lateral gliding and rotation, with the rotation being about 10 to 15 degrees. In lateral flexion and gliding, the odontoid process appears to be asymmetrical between the two lateral masses of the atlas, and the facet surfaces seem offset 2 to 4 mm, normally with apparent narrowing of the joint space. These findings, when isolated, may be mistaken for subluxation. Do not assume subluxation is present in anteroposterior open-mouth films showing the odontoid process asymmetrically placed and the atlantoaxial joint surface laterally offset (see Chapter 6, *Radiologic Evaluation*).

Lower Cervical Spine (C3–T1). All four of the classic spinal motions occur between the C3 and T1 vertebrae—flexion, extension, lateral flexion, and rotation. Fielding[1] has demonstrated on cineradiography a smooth, flowing rhythmic, slow movement that is much more apparent in the upper portion of the cervical spine than in the lower portion. Children's cervical spines move much more freely than those of adults and are therefore likely to be misread as being pathological.

In flexion, each upper vertebra glides forward and upward on the articular facets of the vertebra below; the disc spaces widen posteriorly and narrow anteriorly; and the spinous processes separate like a fan. The disc spaces also slide forward perceptibly. Greater shift occurs in children than in adults. In extension, the reverse events occur.

Flexion does not occur as an isolated motion but is associated with accompanying rotation. This is due to increasingly caudally oblique contours of the articular surfaces. In lateral flexion the lower articular surfaces on the concave side glide downward and backward; on the convex side they glide upward and forward, resulting in lateral flexion associated with rotation. The same event occurs in rotation, but it does so to a lesser extent, since about 50% of rotation occurs at the atlantoaxial joint. In rotation and combined lateral flexion, disc tissues narrow on the concave side and widen on the convex side, with an accompanying portion of the intervertebral discs. Discs seem maximally deformed by extreme lateral and forward flexion.

The research data underlying the preceding summary of movement has been collected from plain radiograms, cineradiograms, stereoradiograms, and cadaveric studies.[4, 5, 6] In studying 104 cases, Werne[4] showed that the atlanto-occipital joint has a mean range of motion of 13.4 degrees in flexion-extension and that the atlantoaxial joint had an average range of motion of 10 degrees in flexion extension. This allows a total flexion-extension average at the occipito-atlanto-axial complex of 23.4 degrees. Measurable rotation, to the contrary, occurs only at the atlantoaxial joints. Rotation at the atlanto-occipital joint is prevented by its anatomic design, that is, the extremely firm attachment of the lateral masses of the atlas to the occipital condyles (see Chapter 6, *Radiologic Evaluation*).

Clinical Applications of Normal Range of Motion Data

Knowing that atlanto-occipital rotation does not occur can be useful in studying people with neck pain unrelated to trauma. They frequently hold head and neck in an awkward, "cock robin" position. A true lateral radiograph of the atlas helps in diagnosis. The odd position of the neck with respect to the head suggests that the radiograph will be difficult to obtain. By knowing that there is no rotation at the atlanto-occipital joint, a true lateral view of the atlas is obtained by disregarding the position of the neck and shoulders and placing the film at the lateral side of the skull (Fig. 7–1). Contrary to the atlanto-occipital joint, there is a major axial rotation at the atlantoaxial joint because the articular surfaces of the atlantoaxial joint are convex with a horizontal orientation. This mechanical design permits maximum mobility, that is, 40 to 48 degrees in either direction. This rotation constitutes 40% to 50% of the entire rotation of the neck in the axial plane, whereas the entire lower cervical spine contributes 50% to 60%. This seemingly extreme rotation at the atlantoaxial joint may have very significant clinical consequences.[7] Remember, the vertebral artery enters the transverse foramen at C6, ascends vertically to the offset area, and shifts farther laterally to the transverse foramen of the C2 vertebra (axis). It then deviates farther laterally to enter the transverse foramen of the atlas. Next, it makes a complete U-turn around the lateral mass of the atlas, goes up to the clivus, and joins the opposite vertebral artery to become the basilar

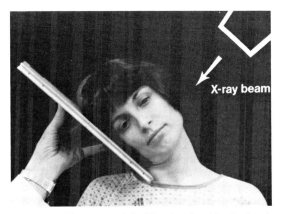

X-ray beam

Figure 7–1. The patient is holding her head in the "cock robin" position, presumably because of rotary subluxation or dislocation of C1 on C2. To get a true lateral view of the atlas, the cassette is held parallel to the lateral aspect of the skull. The x-ray central beam is then directed perpendicular to the plane of the cassette. This technique takes clinical advantage of the anatomic fact that there is no rotation at the atlanto-occipital joints, C1 and the skull.

Table 7–1. AVERAGE RANGE OF MOTION OF THE OCCIPITO-ATLANTO-AXIAL COMPLEX

Upper Cervical Spine	Type of Motion	Degrees
Atlanto-occipital joints (occipital condyles and atlas)	Flexion-extension	13
	Lateral flexion	8
	Rotation	0 (negligible)
Atlantoaxial joints (C1–C2)	Flexion-extension	10
	Lateral flexion	0 (negligible)
	Rotation	47

Adapted from references 1, 4, 5, 6, 9, 14.

artery. At about 30 degrees of rotation, there is normal kinking and stretching of the contralateral vertebral artery. The artery normally becomes rapidly more kinked and stretched as the angle of rotation is increased. At 45 degrees of rotation, the ipsilateral artery is also normally kinked (see Chapter 2, *Anatomy and Biomechanics*). With compromise of blood flow in both vertebral arteries, ischemia of the brain stem and posterior fossa contents may produce a broad spectrum of symptoms (see Chapter 4, *Clinical methods*).

Such clinical circumstances may be associated with calisthenics, yoga, gymnastic performances, simple overhead work, or therapeutic cervical traction.[8, 9] Chiropractic manipulation of the head and neck has been associated with spinal cord and brain stem stroke[10, 11, 12] Schellhas et al reported vertebrobasilar injuries, angiographically proven, following chiropractic maneuvering.[8] Similar complications have been reported in patients who have no medical problems.[9] Thus, such events may occur for normal anatomic reasons in the absence of clinically evident cervical spine or vascular disease. Miller and Burton[10] reported the occurrence of symptoms such as nausea, visual disturbances, vomiting, and vertigo early in the course of such events, suggesting that if the manipulation is stopped, irreversible brain damage is avoidable. Clinically, the wise and informed physician will formulate that patients with cervical osteoarthritis or chronic vascular disease are even more likely to experience serious and catastrophic events from both normal movements as well as cervical spine traction or therapeutic manipulation of the cervical spine.

Werne[4] in cadaver studies noted an average of 11.9 degrees of lateral flexion at the atlanto-occipital joint. Other authors have not agreed with his findings. Fick[13] in 1904 reported 30 to 40 degrees of lateral flexion. This has never been confirmed, though Fick is revered as one of the greatest students of the cervical spine. Perhaps technologic advantages have borne fruit!

Jackson[14] studying 50 adults and 25 children radiologically, concluded that the distance between the posteroinferior margin of the anterior arch of the atlas and the anterior surface of the odontoid process was a maximum of 2.5 mm in adults and 4 mm in children. These results are in agreement with those obtained by Fielding.[1] A measurement greater than 3 mm clinically suggests threatened rupture of the transverse ligament.

Table 7–1 summarizes average range of motion of the occipito-atlanto-axial complex. The occipito-atlanto-axial complex is surely the most complicated set of joints in the body, serving as a transition area between the standard vertebral column joint structures and the grossly different, solid bone of the skull. This joint complex supports the head but permits relatively massive ranges of motion while also protecting the spinal cord and adjacent vital structures during the extremes of movement. Cervical spine mobility is thought to be influenced by aging, biomechanical factors, and pathologic developments. Blanchard and Kottke[15] studied a group of male students, ages 15 to 29 years. They noted an inverse relationship between age and range of motion, that is, as age increases, mobility decreases. The oldest student studied was 29, an age at which one does not expect significant osteoarthritis. Since overall physical fitness and physical performance are associated with maintenance of suppleness and general mobility, it may be that as the students examined entered their second decade they were less active physically. Schoening and Hannan[16] did a goniometric, in vivo study of factors affecting cervical mobility and also found that age was important (decreased mobility with increasing age) but that pain in the upper trunk, neck, and arm, tenderness over the joints and spinous processes, pain with even passive neck motion, and increased muscularity (mesomorph body type) are associated with reduced range of motion. Strangely enough, they further noted that the degree of intervertebral disc space narrowing at one level had no influence on mobility, whereas narrowing at several levels was associated with decreased motion.

Lysell,[2] in cadaveric studies, examined the relationship between intervertebral disc osteoarthritis and mobility by measuring range of motion in a functional spinal unit, and then removing the intervertebral disc of that unit and grading it for osteoarthritis. There is no correlation between the magnitude of intervertebral disc osteoarthritis and loss of mobility, even applied to all directions of motion at all interfaces. This finding is certainly contrary to clinical formulations!

In the flexion-extension movement in the lower cervical spine there is more motion in the central region, as the C5–C6 interspace usually is considered to have the greatest range of motion in the sagittal plane. Lateral flexion and rotation range of motion progressively diminish as one moves lower on the spine. Lower cervical spine range of motion is useful in clinical decision making about cervical spine stability. The maximum sagittal plane of motion in the cervical spine under usual loads has an upper limit of a measured 2.7 mm vertebral offset in well-standardized circumstances. White et al[17, 18] suggest that 3.5 mm is the absolute upper level of normal, considering that the adult cervical spine is unstable when there is 3.5 mm or more horizontal displacement of one vertebra in relation to an adjacent vertebra as measured on the lateral radiograph. White et al[18] worked out a means of clinical evaluation termed the "stretch test." Figure 7–2 illustrates the rationale of the test and its monitoring. The test actually measures the displacement pattern, that is, the change in distance between two cervical vertebrae on cervical spine traction initially and after applying up to 33% of the subject's body weight. The spinal cord can tolerate considerable displacement in the axial direction; so in an acute clinical situ-

Table 7–2. CHECK LIST FOR DIAGNOSIS OF CLINICAL INSTABILITY IN THE LOWER CERVICAL SPINE

Element	Point Value
Anterior elements destroyed or nonfunctional	2
Posterior elements destroyed or nonfunctional	2
Relative sagittal plane translation	2
Relative sagittal plane rotation	2
Positive stretch test	2
Spinal cord damage	2
Nerve root damage	1
Abnormal disc narrowing	1
Dangerous loading anticipated	1
Total of 5 or more = unstable	

From White AA III, Southwick WO, Panjabi MM: Clinical instability in the cervical spine: A review of past and current concepts. Spine 1:15, 1976.

ation, a properly monitored test employing displacement in the axial direction is not as dangerous as a test of horizontal displacement. They studied eight normal subjects and concluded that an abnormal stretch test occurs if an interspace separation is greater than 1.7 mm. If there is excessive relative axial displacement at the interspace in question (compared with other interspaces), one should suspect structural damage. The investigator's check list (Table 7–2) is used to make a diagnosis of clinical instability in the lower cervical spine.[19]

Interestingly, in lateral flexion the spinous processes move toward the convexity of the curve (rather than toward the concavity). In lateral bending to the left, the spinous processes tend to go to the right, and in lateral bending to the right, they go to the left. The clinical significance is that in cervical spine zygapophyseal joint dislocation a traumatic force usually carries a joint well beyond its normal range of motion. If there is exaggeration of this physiologic coupling between lateral bending and axial rotation (neither occurs purely), the facets of the joint on one side go too far caudad and on the other side too far cephalad, resulting in dislocation of the joint. Analysis and understanding of this pattern aid in the manipulative reduction of a unilateral zygapophyseal joint dislocation. Axial rotation is always coupled with lateral bending in varying magnitude. It is generally believed that the incline or "pitch" of the zygapophyseal joint surfaces in the sagittal plane increases from above downward, possibly explaining the relative frequency of unilateral zygapophyseal joint dislocation at C5 and below. Table 7–3 shows the limits and relative values of range of rotation in the lower cervical spine. Much of the work presented in this section is based upon study of the published papers and monographs of the authorities on kinematics listed at the end of this chapter.

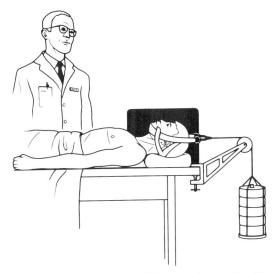

Figure 7–2. The "stretch test." A person knowledgeable about the pathophysiology involved is present. Pretest neurologic examination data are required, and neurologic monitoring of signs and symptoms is done in process. Loads in the traction apparatus are increased up to 33% of the subject's body weight or 65 lbs, whichever comes first. Lateral radiograms are taken before each incremental increase in the load. Results of a stretch test are considered abnormal if an interspace separation of more than 1.7 mm occurs (see Table 7–2). Any excessive relative axial displacement of the interspace in question suggests structural damage.

Table 7–3. LIMITS AND REPRESENTATIVE VALUES OF RANGE OF ROTATION OF THE LOWER CERVICAL SPINE

Interspace	Flexion-Extension (X Axis Rotation)		Lateral Bending (Z Axis Rotation)		Axial Rotation (Y Axis Rotation)	
	Limits of Range (degrees)	Representative Angle (degrees)	Limits of Range (degrees)	Representative Angle (degrees)	Limits of Range (degrees)	Representative Angle (degrees)
C2–C3	5–23	8	11–20	10	6–28	9
C3–C4	7–38	13	9–15	11	10–28	11
C4–C5	8–39	12	0–16	11	10–26	12
C5–C6	4–34	17	0–16	8	8–34	10
C6–C7	1–29	16	0–17	7	6–15	9
C7–T1	4–17	9	0–17	4	5–13	8

From White AA III, Panjabi MN: The basic kinematics of the human spine. Spine 3:12, 1978.

PLANES, LINES, DIAMETERS (SAGITTAL AND TRANSVERSE), ANGLES, AND BONY LANDMARKS

Drawing lines between various anatomic landmarks of the planes of pertinent structures is very useful clinically. The planes of the foramen magnum, the atlas, and the axis, when drawn on a radiograph, give the clinician a clear concept of the anatomic inter-relationships and any existent pathologic change. The plane of the foramen magnum is in a line drawn from the anterior lip of the foramen (basion) to the posterior lip (opisthion). If these anatomic sites are not quite clear, an approximation of the line can be drawn by connecting the lowest point of the occipital bone to the starting point of the anterior margin of the occipital condyle. The plane of the atlas runs through the center of the anterior arch and the posterior arch (tubercle). The plane of the atlas also runs in a line from the lower margin of the radiographic outline of the transverse process to the lowest point of the end line of the posterior arch, the spinolaminar line. The position of the atlas is described by noting whether its anterior arch is horizontal, superior, or inferior to the remainder of this vertebra. With the head erect (normal cervical lordosis), the anterior arch of the atlas is in the superior position, making an open angle of about 6 degrees posteriorly. The plane of the axis is nearly parallel to the plane of the foramen magnum.[20] Movements in the upper cervical spine must be assessed in terms of atlanto-occipital level and atlantoaxial level. Movement occurs in a smooth, rhythmic, coordinated motion, and if a part of the unit remains fixed, an abnormality is present. Midcervical spine kyphosis compensates for this type of abnormality. In all movements between the occiput and the axis, the intervening atlas functions much like a meniscus or a disc, that is, it provides a screwing motion in rotation and lateral flexion and a tilt in anterior flexion and hyperextension. Because of this tilt of the atlas, the planes of the foramen magnum and the axis may be parallel in all positions. The atlanto-occipital joints are very tight, and the atlantoaxial joints are quite loose. In fact, in lateral flexion one can see a normal 2 to 3 mm offset of the lateral mass of the atlas on the facets of the axis (Fig. 7–3). The axis rotates in the direction of the tilt (see Chapter 6, *Radiologic Evaluation).*

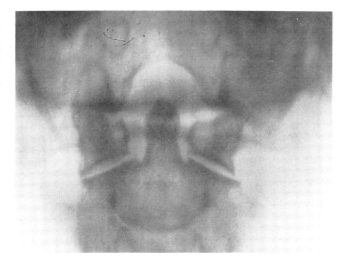

Figure 7–3. Open-mouth, anteroposterior view of the upper cervical spine. The patient is making an effort to abduct the upper cervical spine to the viewer's left. Note that the distance between the odontoid process and the lateral mass of the atlas is smaller on the viewer's right than on the left—an offset of 2.5 mm—a normal finding, not a subluxation.

Atlanto-Odontoid Measurement

Measurement of the distance between the anterior surface of the odontoid process and the posterior surface of the anterior arch of the atlas is of great importance clinically. A number of pathologic states, such as rheumatoid arthritis, retropharyngeal infection, trauma, hereditary absence or defect of the odontoid bone itself, and mongolism, lead to widening of the atlanto-odontoid space. The anterior atlanto-odontoid space can be measured in a lateral film of the cervical spine in two ways. (1) The upper atlanto-odontoid distance, which is the space between the posterior border of the anterior arch of the atlas and the anterior edge of the odontoid process, is measured at the level of the middle plane of the atlas. (2) The lower atlanto-odontoid space is measured between the lower pole of the articular surface of the anterior arch of the atlas and the anterior edge of the odontoid process. These measurements may have the same value. Normally it is 1 to 2 mm, but the value is a function of the thickness of the articular cartilage, which is variable. In adults the average value has been shown to be 0.93 mm, with a standard deviation of 0.36. It does not vary with sex but does vary with age (the space decreases with increasing age). Sharp

and Purser[21] measured the upper atlanto-odontoid distance in 1292 people. In 99.4% values up to a maximum of 3 mm were found. Jackson[14] studied the relationship between maximum flexion and hyperextension of the cervical spine and the lower atlanto-odontoid space. Dislocation can be identified on radiographs that are taken at extreme ranges to produce maximum widening of the anterior atlanto-odontoid space. In 50 adults, the value of the lower atlanto-odontoid distance was unchanged in both positions, never measuring more than 2.5 mm. In 95% of normal adults, the value of the distance in various positions was lower (0.3 to 2.2 mm). Greater movements are physiologic in children, owing to the general laxity and suppleness of their ligamentous and capsular structures. Two to 5 mm is the normal value of the atlanto-odontoid distance usually noted for children. A value of 5 mm is surely the extreme upper limit. There are no significant differences related to age or sex in children.

Frequently more important than the anterior atlanto-odontoid space measurement is the posterior measurement between the posterior surface of the odontoid bone and the anterior margin of the posterior arch—normally the widest sagittal diameter in the cervical spine. If the anterior atlanto-odontoid space measurement is equal to

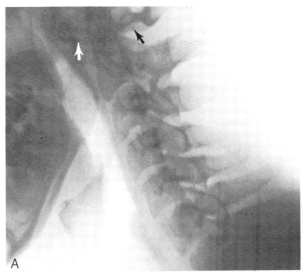

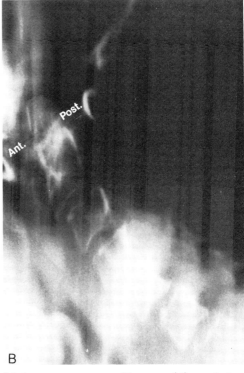

Figure 7–4. *A*, A case of atlantoaxial subluxation. Note the small white arrow pointing to the anterior space between the posterior surface of the anterior arch of the atlas and the anterior surface of the odontoid process, an 8-mm subluxation. Note the bulging superior pharynx pushed forward by the subluxating atlas. The posterior (and more important) space (black arrow), measures 13 mm from the midposterior surface of the odontoid process to the anterior margin of the posterior arch of the atlas. *B*, The anterior space (**Ant.**) shown in this tomogram measures 16 mm, and the posterior space (**Post.**) is only 9 mm—a clear-cut case of spinal cord compression at the level of the foramen magnum. Remember the rule of thirds for the sagittal diameter of the spinal canal at the level of the atlas: the odontoid process and the spinal cord occupy one third each, and there is one third free space at the level of the atlas.

the posterior, a very major subluxation exists, almost always compromising spinal cord function by pressure. The posterior measurement should always be taken. It can be performed readily but seldom is. It constitutes a major guide to surgical intervention (along with many other criteria for surgical management) (Fig. 7–4).

The Spinal Canal Diameter (Anteroposterior and Lateral) and the Retrotracheal and Retropharyngeal Spaces

The lateral cervical spine view by x-ray allows measurement of the width of the prevertebral soft-tissue shadow at the lower edge of the axis (C2) (Fig. 7–5). The retrotracheal space is the soft-tissue distance from the level of the sixth cervical vertebra to the tracheal shadow. The diameter of the spinal canal is measured at the narrowest distance between the posterior edge of the vertebral body and the anterior edge of the vertebral arch. At the level of the atlas this diameter is identical with the retro-odontoid space. The transverse diameter (interpedicular distance) is measured at the widest

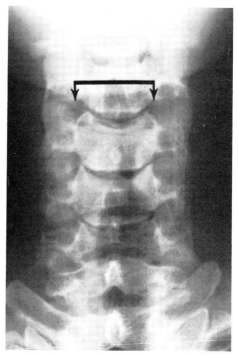

Figure 7–6. Arrows point to the transverse diameter, the interpedicular distance.

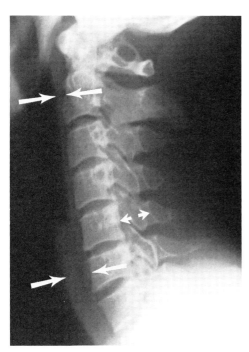

Figure 7–5. Note the prevertebral soft-tissue shadow, the pharynx, at the lower edge of the axis (retropharyngeal space) (upper arrows). Retrotracheal space at level of C6 (lower arrows). Sagittal diameter, the narrowest distance between the posterior edge of the vertebral body and the anterior edge of the vertebral arch (middle arrows).

point between the pedicles in the spinal canal (Fig. 7–6). The retropharyngeal space may be grossly widened by pharyngeal and tonsillar infection (Grisel's syndrome) and the cold abscess of tuberculosis and tumor; trauma may result in hematoma and gross edema. The retropharyngeal space can be narrowed or seen bulging in anterior atlantoaxial subluxation of rheumatoid arthritis (see Fig. 7–4A), trauma, or fractured odontoid process in which the anterior arch of the atlas pushes the superior pharynx into the throat.

Craniometry

Some measurements of bony landmarks about the skull are useful in the diagnosis of platybasia, superior migration of the odontoid process in rheumatoid arthritis, basilar impression and pseudobasilar impression, and condylar hypoplasia. Parts A and B of Figure 7–7 show the usual measurements made between bony landmarks in the skull in lateral and coronal views respectively. Parts C and D illustrate the lines drawn directly on the radiographic film. Parts E, F, and G show how the lines and angles are drawn in standard films. There are certain clinical problems in the use of these measurements because the planes are not fixed—they vary within a normal range. The mastoid processes (for the bimastoid line measurement) may be asymmetric. The hard palate and sometimes the shape of the posterior fossa

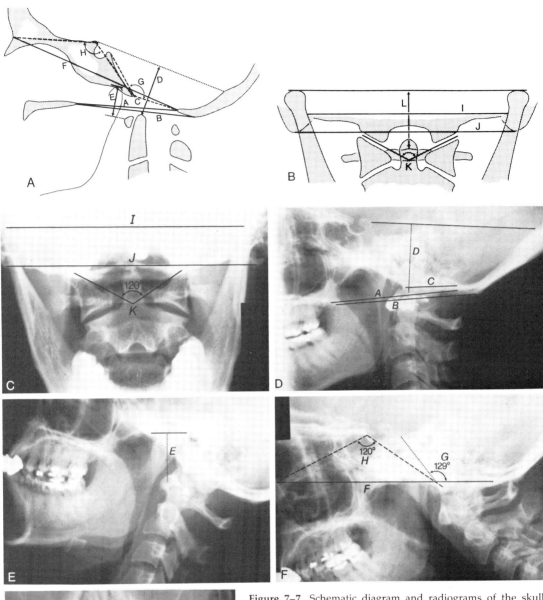

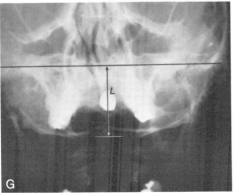

Figure 7–7. Schematic diagram and radiograms of the skull and upper cervical spine illustrating sagittal and coronal views of diagnostically useful craniometric lines and angles. *A*, Lateral view showing Chamberlain's line (**A**), McGregor's line (**B**), McRae's line (**C**), height index of Klaus (**D**), the distance between the mandibular joint level and the arch of the atlas (**E**), Boogaard's line (**F**), angle of Boogaard (**G**), and angle of Welcker (**H**). *B*, Coronal view showing biventer line (**I**), bimastoid line (**J**), angle of atlanto-occipital joint axes (**K**), and the distance between the mandibular joint level and the arch of the atlas (**L**). *C*, Measurement of bimastoid (**J**) and biventer lines (**I**) in a radiogram. **K** is the angle of the atlanto-occipital joint axes. *D*, Measurement of Chamberlain (**A**), McGregor (**B**), and McRae (**C**) lines on radiogram. **D** is the height index of Klaus in the lateral view. *E*, Distance between the mandibular joint level and the arch of the atlas (**E**) in the lateral view. *F*, Boogaard's line (**F**), angle of Boogaard (**G**), angle of Welcker (**H**) in the lateral view. *G*, Distance between the mandibular joint level and the arch of the atlas in the anteroposterior view.

are not constant in morphology. The shape and height and length of the odontoid bone are variable. However, the aggregate of several measurements will identify pathologic change. All these measurements are maximally useful only within the context of all other historical, physical, and radiologic data collected. Of clinical diagnostic use are the anteroposterior view of the bimastoid and biventer lines, the lateral films of McGregor's line (basal line), McRae's line of the foramen magnum, and the palato-occipital line of Chamberlain. The basal angle of Welcker is useful in assessing the degree of flattening of the clivus (platybasia characteristic). Condylar hypoplasia is measurable indirectly by the angle of the temporomandibular joint axes[22] (see Tables 7–4, 7–5, and 7–6). McRae's line relates the top of the odontoid bone to the plane of the foramen magnum. Protrusion upward here is interpreted as a neurologic sign of basilar impression.

Wholey et al[23] measured the distance between the top of the odontoid process and the basion (anterior lip of the foramen magnum) and found an average of 5 mm in adults and 10 mm in children. They suggest that small increases (1.0 to 4.0 mm) in these average measurements are of more important practical use than the relationships of the odontoid process to the lines of Chamberlain and McGregor. I recommend using all three measurements.

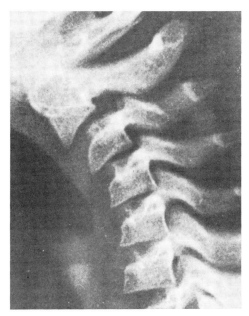

Figure 7–8. Pseudosubluxation in a four-year-old child. Note the seemingly gross slip forward of the axis on the third cervical vertebra and the lesser slip of the atlas on the axis—normal characteristics at this age.

UPPER CERVICAL SPINE IN CHILDREN

The upper cervical spine in children is variable and likely to have special and poorly understood features such as incomplete ossification of the atlas and the axis, variable presence of ossification centers in the upper portion of the odontoid bone (ossiculum terminale), and overall hypermobility due to children's suppleness and general ligamentous and capsular laxity (see Chapter 14, *Cervical Spine in Infancy and Childhood*). "Pseudo" dislocation at C2 to C3 is a common observation and may result in unnecessary therapy (Fig. 7–8). Cattell and Filtzer[24] studied a random sample of 160 children, ages 1 year to 16 years, and noted that 24% had an anterior pseudosubluxation of the atlas on maximal forward flexion. Their assessment of the age group under 8 years revealed that 40% showed the tendency. Fourteen per cent of 22 children showed pseudosubluxation between the third and fourth cervical vertebrae, and in 20 of these children pseudosubluxation was combined with a forward subluxation between the axis and the third cervical vertebra. Fifty per cent of children under 7 years of age show a shift of the distal posterior edge of the axis measuring 3 mm or more. In hyperextension, dorsal subluxation of the axis occurs in 14% of cases, though this shift is relatively small. Twenty per cent of children under 8 years of age show that in hyperextension more than two thirds of the height of the anterior arch of the atlas lies over the tip of the odontoid bone, though there is no evidence of hypoplasia of the odontoid bone. Hypermobility of the axis is secondary to joint, capsular and ligamentous laxity, which appears to become tighter with growth. It is not found in young people over 16 years of age. The absence of development of the joints of Luschka (which appear between ages 10 and 20 years) may also contribute to this laxity (see Chapter 2, *Anatomy and Biomechanics*). A definite kink occurred in approximately the middle of the neck in forward flexion in 16% of children studied. The kyphosis that usually appears does not do so between C2 and C6–C7 in flexion in children. Clinical observation of this absence may lead to a false diagnosis of injury to the posterior longitudinal or the interspinous ligament. The cervical spine in 14% of children is straight in the neutral position. The physician is apt to mistake this posture for muscle spasm and protective behavior consequent to injury. Table 7–4 lists the sagittal (lateral) diameter measurements (average and range) and the widths of the retropharyngeal and retrotracheal spaces. Table 7–5 describes the various lines and angles taken in the lateral view. Table 7–6 lists average values for the craniometric lines and angles in an anteroposterior radiograph.

Table 7–4. SPINAL CANAL DIAMETERS AND WIDTHS OF RETROPHARYNGEAL AND RETROTRACHEAL SPACES

	Measurements			
	Children up to 15 Years		Adults	
Location (see Fig. 7–5)	Average (mm)	Range (mm)	Average (mm)	Range (mm)
Diameter of Spinal Canal at				
C1	21.9	18–27	21.4	16–30
C2	20.9	18–25	19.2	16–28
C3	17.4	14–21	19.1	14–25
C5	16.5	14–20	18.5	14–25
C7	16.0	15–20	17.5	13–24
Retropharyngeal space	3.5	2–7	3.4	1–7
Retrotracheal space	7.9	5–14	14.0	9–22

From Wholey MH, Bruwer AJ, Baker HL: The lateral roentgenogram of the neck (with comments on the atlanto-odontoid-basion relationship). Radiology 71:350, 1958.

Table 7–5. CRANIOMETRIC LINES AND ANGLES IN LATERAL VIEWS (SAGITTAL)

Nomenclature* (Synonyms)	Definition	Normal Measurement
(A) Chamberlain's line (palato-occipital line)	Joins posterior pole hard palate with posterior edge of foramen magnum (opisthion)	Average, tip of odontoid process 1 mm + 3.6 mm below this line
(B) McGregor's line (basal line)	Joins upper posterior edge hard palate with lowest point of occipital squama	Tip of odontoid process no more than 5 mm above this line
(C) McRae's line (foramen magnum line)	Joins anterior (basion) and posterior (opisthion) edges of foramen magnum	Tip of odontoid process does not exceed this line
(D) Height index of Klaus	Distance between tip of odontoid process and tuberculocruciate line (from sellar tubercle to cruciform eminence of internal occipital protuberance)	Average 40–41 mm; between 36 and 40 mm uncertain pathologic implication; below 30 mm indicates basilar impression
(E) Mandibular joint arch of atlas	Distance between horizontal line through mandibular joint and upper edge of anterior arch atlas	Average 30 mm; range 22–39 mm
(F) Boogaard line	Joins nasion and opisthion	Basion below this line
(G) Angle of Boogaard	Plane of foramen magnum to plane of clivus (dorsum sellae to basion)	Average 122 degrees; range 119–135 degrees
(H) Angle of Welcker	Nasion-tuberculum, sellae-basion	Average 132 degrees; sigma 6.2 degrees

From von Torklus D, Gehle W: The Upper Cervical Spine. New York: Grune & Stratton, 1972, p 14. © 1972 by Georg Thieme Verlag.
*Letters correspond to labels of lines and angles in Figure 7–7.

Table 7–6. CRANIOMETRIC LINES AND ANGLES IN ANTEROPOSTERIOR VIEW (CORONAL)

Nomenclature* (Synonyms)	Definition	Normal Values
(I) Biventer line	Joins the origins of the biventer muscles at the medial bases of mastoids	Not passed by tip of odontoid process
(J) Bimastoid line	Joints the tips of the mastoid processes	Tip of odontoid process up to 10 mm above; runs across centers of atlanto-occipital joints
(K) Angle of atlanto-occipital joint axes	The limbs run across the center of the atlanto-occipital joints, about parallel to facets of condylar joints	Average 124 degrees–127 degrees in tomograms measurable only in "slice" of odontoid process
(L) Distance between mandibular joint and anterior arch of atlas	Distance between horizontal line through mandibular joints and upper edge of anterior arch of atlas	Average 30 mm; range 22–39 mm

From von Torklus D, Gehle W: The Upper Cervical Spine. New York: Grune & Stratton, 1972, p 13. © 1972 by Georg Thieme Verlag.
*Letters correspond to labels of lines and angles in Figure 7–7.

References

1. Fielding JW: Cineroentgenography of the normal cervical spine. J Bone Joint Surg 39A:1280, 1957.
2. Lysell E: Motion in the cervical spine. Acta Orthop Scand [Suppl] 123:1, 1969.
3. Hohl M: Normal motion in the upper portion of the cervical spine. J Bone Joint Surg 46A:1777, 1964.
4. Werne S: Studies in spontaneous atlas dislocation. Acta Orthop Scand [Suppl] 23:232, 1957.
5. Penning L: Normal movement of the cervical spine. AJR 130:317, 1978.
6. Selecki BR: The effects of rotation of the atlas on the axis. Med J Aust 1:1012, 1969.
7. Barlow JW, Marjollis MT: Rotational obstruction of the vertebral artery at the atlanto axial joint. Neuroradiology 9:117, 1975.
8. Schellhas KP, Latchow RE, Wendling LR, et al.: Vertebrobasilar injuries following cervical manipulation. JAMA 244:1450, 1980.
9. Ford FR: Syncope, vertigo and disturbances of vision resulting from intermittent obstruction of the vertebral arteries due to defects in the odontoid process and excessive mobility of the second cervical vertebra. Bull Johns Hopkins Hospital 91:168, 1952.
10. Miller RG, Burton R: Stroke following chiropractic manipulation of the spine. JAMA 229:189, 1974.
11. Daneshmeno TK, Hewer RL, Bradshaw JR: Acute brain stem stroke during neck manipulation. Brit Med J 288:189, 1984.
12. Robertson JT: Neck manipulation as cause of stroke. Stroke 13:260, 1982.
13. Fick R: Handbuch der Anatomie und Mechanik der Gelenke. Jena: Verlag von Gustav Fischer, 1911.
14. Jackson H: The diagnosis of minimal atlanto-axial subluxation. Br J Radiol 23:672, 1950.
15. Blanchard RS, Kottke FJ: The study of degenerative changes in the cervical spine in relation to age. Bull of the University of Minnesota Hospital 24:470, 1953.
16. Schoening HA, Hannan V: Factors related to cervical mobility. Part I. Arch Phys Med Rehabil 45:602, 1964.
17. White AA III, Panjabi MM: Clinical Biomechanics of the Cervical Spine. Philadelphia: J. B. Lippincott Company, 1978.
18. White AA III, Johnson RM, Panjabi MM, et al: Biomechanical analysis of clinical stability of the cervical spine. Clin Orthop 109:85, 1975.
19. Scher AT: Anterior cervical subluxation. AJR 133:275, 1978.
20. Von Torklus D, Gehle W: The Upper Cervical Spine. New York: Grune & Stratton, 1972, p 8.
21. Sharp J, Purser DW: Spontaneous atlanto axial dislocation in ankylosing spondylitis and rheumatoid arthritis. Ann Rheum Dis 20:47, 1961.
22. Schmidt HE, Fischer E: Über okzipitale Dysplasie. Stuttgart Thieme: 1960.
23. Wholey MH, Bruwer AJ, Baker HL: The lateral roentgenogram of the neck (with comments on the atlanto-odontoid-basion relationship). Radiology 71:350, 1958.
24. Cattell HS, Filtzer DL: Pseudosubluxation and other normal variations in the cervical spine in children. J Bone Joint Surg 47A:1295, 1965.

Chapter 8

Electrodiagnosis in Differential Diagnosis

Nerve conduction velocity was first measured in 1852, and electromyography was first performed in 1907; both were then used experimentally. During World War II, the great increase in nerve injuries resulted in research with these "old" methods. Utilization of new knowledge of electronics resulted in marked improvement in instrumentation. Now the procedures are predictable and the results reproducible.

Two measurements can be made: (1) a recording of bioelectric potentials from muscles and nerves, (2) the response of nerves and muscles to electric stimulation. These techniques permit detection of abnormal physiologic involvement of the motor unit, and if there is an abnormal response to electric stimulation or abnormal bioelectric potentials recorded, anatomic localization of the lesion is possible.

The motor unit is made up of four basic parts: (1) the motor neuron cell body (anterior horn cell), (2) its axon, (3) the myoneural junctions, (4) all muscle fibers supplied by the terminal branches of the axon. The cell body, its axon, and all terminal branches constitute the lower motor neuron (Fig. 8–1). If functional impairment of any of the components of the motor unit causes abnormal results of one or more of the electrodiagnostic tests, anatomic localization of the lesion is possible at any one of or a combination of six sites: anterior horn cell, ventral nerve root, plexus, peripheral nerve (motor or sensory components), myoneural junction, and muscle fibers. Figure 8–2 illustrates the myoneural junction.

The clinician is often uncertain of whether weakness or other motor abnormality is due to disease of the motor unit or is entirely a consequence of pain, hysteria, conversion reactions, malingering, or unidentified disease. Occasionally the disease is in an early stage that is so mild that objective clinical findings of abnormal motor units are absent. Electrodiagnostic techniques in this circumstance may be of great value.

CLINICAL IMPLICATIONS

The principal clinical symptoms and signs of skeletal neuromuscular disease are pain and tenderness, hypotonia, fatigue, weakness, paresis and atrophy, limitation of motion or deformity, sense of stiffness, muscle spasm, contracture, cramps, and sensory loss. Because weakness is the main symptom bringing the patient to the doctor in diseases of the motor unit, the electrodiagnostic procedures are useful in the differential diagnosis of fatigue, weakness, hypotonia, paresis, and atrophy. Since these tests assess only functional status of the motor unit, they cannot provide specific etiologic diagnosis. They do assist the clinician in the diagnosis in that, here as elsewhere, the electrophysiologic data must be integrated with historical data and findings on physical examination. In fact, it is very important that the electrodiagnostic procedures be done by a physician, because the assessment, the specific tests chosen, and their interpretation require that the person know all relevant clinical data, or the interpretation is compromised.

ELECTRODIAGNOSTIC TESTS

Three clinical electrodiagnostic tests are available. (1) The electromyogram, generally regarded as a screening procedure, detects abnormalities of all divisions of the motor unit. Usually it is not very selective, that is, lesions of the anterior horn cell, the ventral roots, the nerve plexus, and the peripheral nerves often result in identical electromyographic findings. (2) The nerve conduction test, motor and sensory, is the most effective method for assessing the functional status of pe-

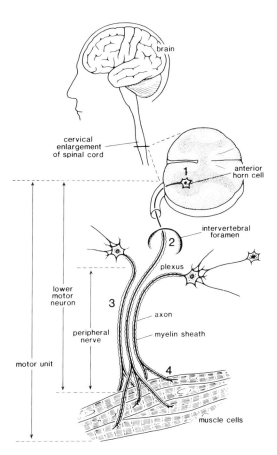

Figure 8–1. Motor unit concept: The human figure depicts the role of the motor unit in the organism as a whole. The will (signal) to induce voluntary muscle contraction starts in a Betz cell in the brain and travels down the corticospinal tract to the first element of the motor unit, the anterior horn cell (motor neuron cell) body. The lower motor neuron is made up of the anterior horn cell, its axon, the peripheral nerve, and the neuromuscular junction where the terminal elements of the axon synapse with the muscle fibers proper (whole muscle also shown). The sarcomere is made up of the actin-myosin filament, contractile elements of the muscle fiber. The axon from the anterior horn cell passes through the intervertebral foramen, joins many other axons from other segmental levels in the plexus, and becomes the peripheral nerve finally reaching the muscle.

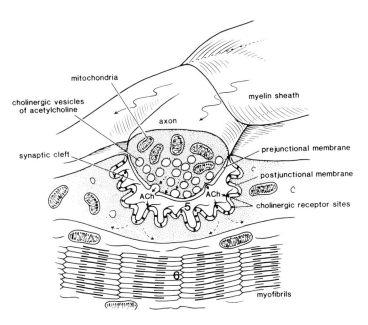

Figure 8–2. Schematic diagram of the skeletal neuromuscular junction and its normal physiology. The electric pulse arrives at the terminus of the nerve and stimulates the synthesis and release of acetylcholine (ACh) from the presynaptic membrane into the synaptic cleft. Here the electric pulse is converted to chemical transmission. The ACh receptors change ionic conduction across the postjunctional membrane, resulting in the development of an electric potential that propagates the impulse into the muscle fiber membrane, and the muscle fiber contracts.

ripheral nerves, distinguishing conditions affecting axons from those affecting anterior horn cells. (3) Repetitive nerve stimulation. The main value of this test is in assessing suspected abnormalities of the myoneural junction.

Clinical reasons for electrodiagnostic studies are to (1) determine the presence or absence of motor unit disease and identify the site of physiologic abnormality in the motor unit; (2) determine the stage and extent of the lesion for prognosis and recovery from muscular weakness; and (3) determine anatomic site of the lesion within the motor unit once functional damage is established. There are classically six anatomic sites along the motor unit pathway where pathologic processes may result in electromyographic abnormalities: (1) anterior horn cell, (2) ventral root, (3) nerve plexus, (4) peripheral nerve (sensory and motor components), (5) myoneural junction apparatus, and (6) muscle fibers (muscle cells themselves). At least two, sometimes more, electrodiagnostic tests are required for identification of the anatomic site. The standard electromyography often can distinguish primary neuropathic disorders of the lower motor neuron from primary myopathic disease. Not so predictable is sorting out lesions affecting the anterior horn cell, nerve root, nerve plexus, and peripheral nerve.

INTERPRETATION OF ELECTRODIAGNOSTIC TEST RESULTS

Although these tests cannot determine etiologic diagnoses or separate classic myopathic and neuropathic lesions, most disorders can be put into clinical symptom-sign combinations that are often reasonably specific for clinical purposes. The clinician can determine whether the symptom of fatigue or the clinical sign weakness is due to disease in the motor unit or to pain, conversion reaction, hysteria, malingering, disuse, or lastly a lesion of the upper motor neuron. A peripheral nerve palsy can be shown to be due to neurapraxia, axon stenosis, axonal cachexia, or axonotmesis, and the anatomic site often can be identified.

BASIC NEURAL PHYSIOLOGY

The electromyograph (EMG) is a sophisticated voltmeter adapted to measure electric activity of muscle. Like nerve, muscle is a polarized tissue with a large resting membrane potential, ready for discharge. The resting membrane potential is maintained by the ionic imbalance across the muscle fiber membrane (cell membrane) maintained by the energetically active, coupled sodium-potassium pump. With an electric stimulus, membrane conductance for these ions is altered. With brief, rapid migration of the ions, the resting electric potential is lost with a slight overshoot—depolarization. With this short change in the electric

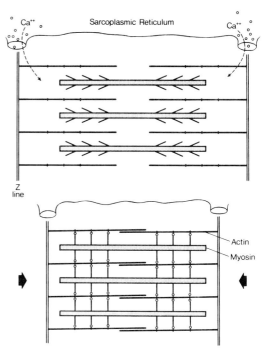

Figure 8–3. The mechanical event of the sliding together of the contractile actin and myosin protein filaments is depicted. Schematic diagram of a sarcomere. The sarcomere contracts, and protein filaments of actin are drawn over the myosin by a chemical linkage between the two molecules. They may overlap in extreme contraction. The reaction is mediated by calcium ion (Ca^{++}) released from the sarcoplasmic reticulum. After contraction, the Ca^{++} is "pumped" from the intracellular to the extracellular space. (From Sokoloff L, Bland JH: The Musculoskeletal System: Structure & Function in Disease. Baltimore: Williams & Wilkins, 1975, p 45.)

environment surrounding the muscle fiber, an electric action potential can be recorded. This is not a localized phenomenon, and once triggered it is transmitted as a wave of depolarization over the full length of each muscle fiber. The triggering for this electric activity originates at the skeletal neuromuscular junction, responding to an electric stimulus traveling down the nerve. The stimulus is converted at the neuromuscular junction into a chemical stimulus (acetylcholine) and recovered to an electric stimulus as it enters the muscle fiber itself (Fig. 8–3).

The origin of a "willed" impulse for contraction of a muscle is in the motor area of the brain, where depolarization of the motor cell in the cortex is transmitted down the axons of the pyramidal (corticospinal) and extrapyramidal tracts to the anterior horn cell. These are conducting systems carrying the signal to the next relay station in the anterior horn cell at the appropriate segmental level.

In clinical practice the electric activity of muscle

is determined by the insertion of fine-needle electrodes directly into the muscle. The resulting signal is displaced visually on an oscilloscope or other recorder and acoustically on a loud speaker. The parameters evaluated are amplitude, duration, frequency, and configuration of the waves. The measurements are made under three conditions: at rest, minimal voluntary contraction (enough to detect only a single motor unit), and maximal voluntary contraction (Fig. 8–4).

There is a brief burst of insertional activity on introduction of the needle, followed by normal resting muscle and electric silence (see *a* in Fig. 8–4). Tense muscle has no tonic contraction, the "tone" of muscle at rest is in the viscoelastic properties of its connective tissue components and myofibers.

Normal spike duration is 5 to 12 msec, and the amplitude is on the order of 2 mv (see *d* in Fig. 8–4). The amplitude is a function of the number of myofibers being excited in the motor unit. Frequency of firing increases with the magnitude of muscular effort (see *e* in Fig. 8–4). Additional motor units are recruited. Each unit spike has a constant appearance at any given position of the

sensing electrode. It is distinguished from additional motor units by conformation, appearances, and frequency. The least number of spikes caused by minimal contraction is termed recruitment frequency for that muscle. Maximal rate of activation of motor units is 50 per second, with the intervals between them being the refractory period of the fibers. Overlay of spikes at high frequency with recruitment of multiple motor units normally leads to complete interference patterns (see *i* in Fig. 8–4). The number of motor units is reduced by denervation, that is, during voluntary contraction. About 2 to 3 weeks after loss of the nerve supply, muscle becomes very irritable. Associated with this are three interpretable EMG changes. (1) Fibrillations, spontaneous contractions of isolated myofibers, occur, appearing electrically as low, short, infrequent spikes under conditions of rest (see *b* in Fig. 8–4). Fasciculation is a coarser, more obvious spontaneous contraction of muscle than fibrillation, and it reflects discharge of motor units rather than individual myofibers. It is characteristic of amyotrophic lateral sclerosis and other anterior horn cell diseases but occurs occasionally in peripheral neuropathy or even extreme fatigue.

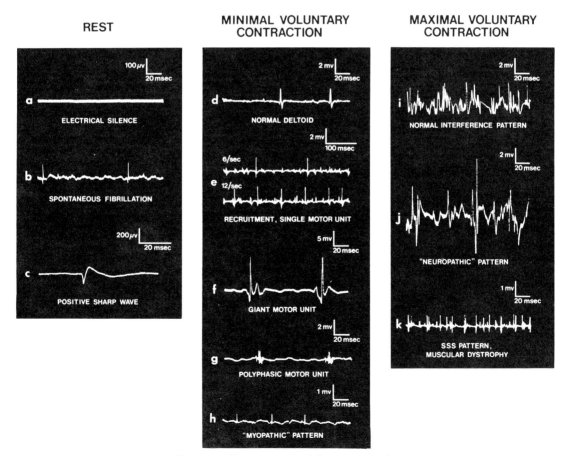

REST

MINIMAL VOLUNTARY CONTRACTION

MAXIMAL VOLUNTARY CONTRACTION

Figure 8–4. Basic patterns of electromyography.

(2) Insertional activity is rather markedly increased. (3) Fortuitous penetration of the sensing needle into a damaged myofiber results in a sharp, positive, downward first wave (see *c* in Fig. 8–4). With partial denervation or loss of a portion of the myofibers in the motor unit, polyphasic spikes (spikes having more than 2 to 3 waves) result because fewer individual fiber potentials are available to summate into a smoother wave form. Reinnervation of muscle results in other types of EMG abnormality, determinable by histochemical differentiation of fiber types. Injured muscle fibers can regenerate, but they cannot do so without benefit of a nerve supply; muscle cells are totally functionally dependent upon their nerve supply. In time however, new axonal fibers proliferate, twig, and migrate to regenerating myofibers creating new myoneural junctions. The differentiation of myofibers into the new types is determined always by the lower motor neuron that resupplies them. This presumably is regulated by the trophic factors synthesized by the neuron. Reinnervating fibers may or may not come from the original neuron. If not, they do impart a new differentiation of regenerating muscle fibers, that is, a previous slow twitch muscle fiber type can become a fast twitch type. Muscle fibers may be reinnervated in two ways: from the original or from some collateral neighboring axon. If the pathologic mechanism does not cause extensive disruption of the nerve, the original axon or its twigs regenerate, and sprouts grow down their own endoneurial tube to the muscle. Conductivity as well as growth rate of these twigs or sprouts is variable and thereby causes the spike to be prolonged and more polyphasic (see *g* in Fig. 8–4). This is called the nascent motor unit. In collateral reinnervation the nerve sprouts grow from an adjacent healthy axon, which must therefore supply an even larger number of myofibers, resulting thus in an increased amplitude of the spike (giant motor units) (see *f* in Fig. 8–4). Thus the classic "neuropathy" EMG under maximal voluntary contraction is characterized by decreased motor units (incomplete interference patterns), high amplitude, and long-lasting spikes (see *j* in Fig. 8–4).

The only disease category in which the EMG pattern is pathognomonic is myotonia. High-frequency discharges of undulating amplitude follow a muscle contraction (Fig. 8–5). The most frequently affected muscle sites are the thenar, forearm, and deltoid muscle.

The electromyograph may also measure conduction velocity in peripheral nerves. Surface electrodes are placed at two points on a motor nerve and stimulated in sequence across the skin while action potentials in the muscles are recorded. Dividing the difference between the latencies (intervals between the stimulation and the muscle spikes) of the two points on the nerve by the difference between them yields the motor nerve conduction velocity. This varies from nerve to

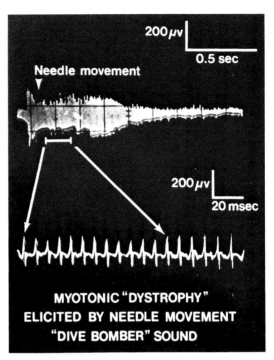

Figure 8–5. Protracted and undulating excitation following slight stimulation is characteristic of myotonia.

nerve and individual to individual. The range is 46 to 66 meters per second. Such values are of course decreased in demyelinating lesions of the axon, and no conduction occurs when both axon and myelin sheath are destroyed. Sensory nerve conduction velocities are more sensitive indicators of peripheral neuropathy than are the motor values. Conduction velocity of muscles is much slower than that of nerves (1.3 to 4.7 meters per second). Disparity between the time that elapses between stimulation of the distal end of the nerve and the time actually required for muscle activation is called residual latency, and it is equivalent to the synaptic delay at the myoneural junction (normally 1.52 msec). Muscle can be stimulated to contract following complete denervation if very strong currents are employed. This procedure has some continuing usefulness in clinical evaluation of the reinnervation of muscle. Alternating (sporadic) current is less effective than direct (galvanic) current, since the stimulus is constantly interrupted and the individual pulses of the electric signal short-lived. Thus the disparity between the response to sporadic and galvanic stimulation is called the reaction of degeneration.

The size of motor units is highly variable, ranging from 100 to 200 muscle fibers per single axon for the intrinsic muscles of the hand to as many as 1500 to 2000 muscle fibers per axon in the very large muscles such as the gastrocnemius.

GENERAL AND SPECIFIC CONSIDERATIONS FOR CERVICAL SPINE SYNDROMES

Though partial injury to a nerve may involve either motor or sensory function, both fibers types are more commonly involved. The magnitude of denervation is the deciding factor regarding motor conduction velocity, since undamaged motor fibers can conduct normally. The amplitude of the response is usually decreased with prolonged duration. The nerve fibers diminish in diameter from proximal origin in the spinal cord to peripheral axon. When large-diameter fibers are injured or diseased, a slower conduction rate is found over the damaged segment and sensory response is usually abolished.

Most commonly, nerve compression is caused by a stenosing or an inflammatory process usually confined to the section of nerves restricted in a fibrosseous, inelastic state, notably in the intervertebral foramina in the cervical spine, the median nerve in the carpal tunnel, or between the two heads of the pronator teres muscle; the ulnar nerve in the cubital tunnel or under the pisiform-hamate ligament; and the radial nerve compression in the axilla, the spiral groove on the humerus or the proximal forearm. If segmental involvement is suspected, several points along the involved nerve should have conduction velocity measured.

When peripheral nerves are involved, there are various magnitudes of involvement of the nerve fibers. Neurapraxia describes a local interruption of nerve fiber conductivity in which stimulation below the block produces a normal motor reaction. Axonal stenosis refers to local attenuation in axon caliber, and the conduction velocity is reduced over the involved portion but normal or near normal below it. Axonal cachexia is a reduction of caliber of the axon over the entire distal segment of the nerve, and a fall in conduction velocity is recorded over the entire involved portion. Neurotmesis is complete discontinuity of the nerve, with no response to nerve stimulation. Of course, when a nerve is severed, the distal portion undergoes wallerian degeneration.

Many systemic diseases affect peripheral nerves, resulting in abnormal nerve conduction in early polyneuropathy of many mechanisms. These diseases include alcoholism, lead poisoning, carbon monoxide poisoning, Guillain-Barré syndrome, diabetes mellitus, porphyria, uremia, amyloidosis, myxedema, rheumatoid arthritis, systemic lupus erythematosus.

Table 8–1 outlines the many mechanisms by which muscle function may be compromised by injury or disease. The many disc syndromes of cervical osteoarthritis constitute the clinical condition for which EMG and nerve conduction times are most commonly required. This condition is an entrapment neuropathy, since the nerve root is compressed by the herniated intervertebral disc,

Table 8–1. MECHANISMS OF COMPROMISE OF MUSCLE FUNCTION

Upper motor neuron	Cerebrovascular accidents; brain injury or disease; spinal cord injury or disease (paraplegia, quadriplegia); cervical osteoarthritis with myelopathy; central nervous system degenerative diseases
Lower motor neuron	Intervertebral disc protrusion; spinal cord trauma; syringomyelia
Cell body in the anterior column of the spinal cord	Poliomyelitis and spinal muscle atrophies
Axon	Nerve trauma; entrapment neuropathies; systemic peripheral neuropathies
Neuromuscular junction	Myasthenia gravis; electrolyte disorders; curare or other blocking agents; poisonings; botulism
Divisions of muscle function	
Sarcolemma and T tubules	Myotonia
Excitation (contraction coupling mechanism, sarcoplasmic reticulum)	Hyperthermia; myxedematous myopathy
Contractile elements (actin and myosin, sarcomere)	Primary myopathic diseases
Aerobic and anaerobic energy supply in the muscle fiber	Mitochondrial and metabolic myopathies
Vascular supply to nerve and muscle	Arteriole-capillary-venule vasculitis (rheumatoid arthritis, lupus erythematosus, scleroderma periarteritis nodosa) Large vessel block (thrombosis, atherosclerosis, cervical spine osteoarthritis with partial or complete vertebral artery occlusion)

osteophytes from the vertebrae proper, joints of Luschka, or zygapophyseal joints as the nerve exits through the intervertebral foramen. It is a truly segmental lesion, with abnormal findings localized to a specific myotome. For example, involvement of the C7 nerve root studied by EMG would disclose fibrillation and positive sharp wave potentials in the triceps brachii, the extensor carpi radialis, and the flexor carpi radialis. Two of these muscles are innervated by the radial nerve but one by the median nerve. Because other muscles innervated by the median nerve are normal, the lesion must be of the C7 nerve root or the middle trunk of the brachial plexus. To localize the lesion more fully, the erector muscles of the spine are examined. If these muscles are abnormal on the involved side but not on the asymptomatic side, the lesion must be at or proximal to the intervertebral foramen. The most common condition would be entrapment of the C7 nerve root by herniated disc or osteophyte.

It is sometimes difficult to determine which nerve root or roots are actually irritated, because the segmental distribution of cervical nerves is not confined strictly to the corresponding sclerotome, myotome, or dermatome. Often at least one fiber of a nerve root fails to continue in that particular nerve root but descends to join the adjacent distal nerve root. For instance, one fiber of the fourth nerve root leaving the cord at that level may actually leave the spinal canal with the fibers of the fifth nerve root. There is overlap of the peripheral sensory distribution also, so that no one area of skin is supplied by any one nerve root. Stimulation of the sympathetic supply adds further confusion to determining the exact location of the site of involvement.

The fifth nerve root is involved more frequently than any other, and the general order of frequency of involvement is fifth, sixth, fourth, third, second, and seventh roots. The first eight entries in Table 8–2 illustrate the segmental distribution of the fifth nerve root, showing that all areas supplied by this nerve root receive innervation from at least one other nerve root. Remember that irritation or compression of a nerve root may cause pain or sensory changes anywhere along its distribution, including myotome, sclerotome, and dermatome. Thus localized areas of tenderness and muscle spasm will be found at the site of

painful areas. Some areas of segmental tenderness of which the patient is unaware are found. Myalgic areas are detected by deep palpation, since hyperalgesia or superficial tenderness is not present.

Study of muscles listed in Table 8–2, which show peripheral nerve distribution and myotomes for the cervical spine and upper extremity, may be needed in order to separate involvement in the brachial plexus from involvement of peripheral nerves or spinal nerve roots. If there is a lesion of the upper trunk of the brachial plexus, all muscles innervated by the fifth and sixth cervical myotomes (except for the rhomboid muscle and erector muscles of the spine) would be abnormal. The erector muscles of the spine are spared because the lesion is distal to the division of the spinal nerve into its anterior and posterior primary divisions. The rhomboid muscles are spared because the dorsoscapular nerve to this muscle is formed at root levels higher than the levels at which the fifth and sixth roots combine to form the upper trunk of the brachial plexus. Brachial plexus anatomy is quite constant, and many muscles can be studied in the upper extremity; this is not the case with the lower extremity. The process of elimination is useful if surgery is planned, localizing the level of the lesion in the brachial plexus.

All peripheral nerves may suffer entrapment, but some, as noted previously, are much more likely to do so than others.

CAUTIONARY NOTES

There are many pitfalls in the interpretation of electromyograms. For example, a person who has had a laminectomy may show partial denervation that could be either a new development or the

Table 8–2. PERIPHERAL NERVE DISTRIBUTION AND MYOTOMES FOR THE CERVICAL SPINE AND UPPER EXTREMITY

Muscle	Myotome	Peripheral Nerve
Rhomboideus	C4, C5	Dorsascapular
Infraspinatus	C5	Suprascapular
Supraspinatus	C5, C6	Suprascapular
Deltoideus	C5, C6	Axillary
Teres minor	C5, C6	Axillary
Biceps brachii	C5, C6	Musculocutaneous
Brachioradialis	C5, C6	Radial
Supinator	C5, C6	Radial
Triceps brachii	C6, C7, C8	Radial
Extensor carpi radialis	C6, C7, C8	Radial
Flexor carpi radialis	C7, C8	Median
Extensor digitorum communis	C7, C8	Median
Flexor digitorum superficialis	C7, C8, T1	Median
Flexor digitorum profundus	C7, C8, T1	Median and radial
Flexor carpi ulnaris	C8, T1	Ulnar
Thenar	C8, T1	Median
Dorsal interossei	C8, T1	Ulnar
Hypothenar	C8, T1	Ulnar

residual consequence of previous root damage. Or the signs in a patient with a history of carpal tunnel decompression might reflect recent nerve compression, incomplete surgical management of their previous condition, or residual median nerve damage. The same is true of motor and sensory nerve root compression in the cervical spine.

An issue about muscle that always must be taken into account is the fact that wallerian degeneration shows no electric signs until at least 3 weeks before the onset of nerve damage. This delay is one of the several disadvantages in diagnostic electromyography.Thus the electromyographer should be a physician well trained in clinical neurologic anatomy as well as electromyography. Lesions in the brachial plexus or peripheral nerves can be differentiated from root compression in the intervertebral foramina by analysis of a pattern of electromyographic abnormalities in muscle. In acute cervical nerve root compression (herniated disc) with a partially denervated muscle at rest, fibrillation and positive waves are found in both the anterior and posterior myotomes. If denervation evidence is limited to the supraspinous and infraspinous muscles, the nerve injury is suprascapular rather than partial compression of the fifth or sixth cervical root. Also, a dorsoscapular nerve injury can be distinguished from a fifth cervical root injury by denervation signs found in the rhomboid muscles only. Classic electromyographic signs of denervation, fibrillation, and positive waves do not appear until after about 3 weeks regardless of the cause of wallerian degeneration. Such electromyographic abnormalities are more often a consequence of acute cervical root syndromes than of cervical osteoarthritis. In chronic nerve root disorders, the osteophytes develop so gradually as to permit the nerves to adjust to the narrowed foramina (i.e.,

no acute injury). Acute injury to C2–C3 or C4 may injure the C2, C3, and C4 cervical nerve roots and cause denervation activity in the trapezius and sternocleidomastoid muscles. Delayed nerve conduction is more reliable than electromyographic denervation patterns in the diagnosis of neuritis and nerve compression distal to the root. Delayed nerve conduction is not always detectable in compression symptoms that can be caused by scalene, claviculocostal, pectoralis minor, and cervical rib syndromes.

Electromyographic examination for cervical rib syndrome is needed only occasionally in the muscles supplied by C8 and T1 nerves. Symptoms may occur only when traction is placed on the brachial plexus (abduction or elevation of the shoulder). Results of electromyographic examination and nerve conduction velocity are usually negative in thoracic outlet syndromes. The reason for this is unclear. It seems likely that the patient's tendency to relieve pain by changing the position of neck and shoulder may relieve the compression, preventing wallerian degeneration.

Intermittent root compression is thought to occur and may result in insufficient pressure to cause compression, and wallerian degeneration is incomplete. With partial nerve destruction, the distribution pattern in cervical myotomes may allow diagnosis; however, this pattern does not necessarily suggest the vertebral level of root damage. Such level depends on the magnitude of the pressure mechanism. A posterolaterally extruded nucleus pulposus between C5 and C6 may compress the sixth root, but a more centrally extruded nucleus at the same level may affect C7 or even C8. Electrodiagnostic procedures are certainly well established and have proved to be of value in the differentiation of neck and arm pain. They are often essential in planning any surgical approach.

Chapter 9

Laboratory Studies

Laboratory studies in diagnosis and management of cervical spine syndromes generally play a minor role. They may confirm diagnoses, especially of systemic diseases involving the cervical spine, such as rheumatoid arthritis or malignant disease with cervical spine metastases. Examinations most important in the study of cervical spine syndromes are those of blood, urine, cerebrospinal fluid, synovial fluid, biopsy specimens for histologic study, immunofluorescent studies of blood, tissue, and aspirated fluid from collection in soft tissues, bursae, abscesses, or swellings of unknown etiology, and biochemical and enzymatic tests of muscle function.

GENERAL BASELINE STUDIES

A urinalysis and a complete blood count (CBC) should be done routinely on every patient. The CBC includes hemoglobin level, hematocrit, red blood cell count, white blood cell count, differential leukocyte count, platelets per high-power field on microscopic examination, and erythrocyte sedimentation rate. The presence of anemia strongly suggests a systemic disease that either is primarily of hematologic pathophysiology or is a secondary anemia associated with some other disease.

Primary Hematologic Diseases. Hemophilia has been shown to involve the cervical spine, though this involvement is rare. Historical data and genetic inquiry usually strongly suggest this diagnosis. Sickle cell anemia and sickle cell trait may be identified in the blood count. During crisis, leukocytosis is usual. The characteristic sickling of red cells is diagnostic. Thalassemia major and thalassemia minor (forms of β-thalassemia) rarely involve the cervical spine. Musculoskeletal manifestations in the cervical spine occur in leukemia and may be an early mode of presentation, with arthritis being more common in children who have acute leukemia.[1] Lymphoma with bone involvement has been shown at autopsy in up to 50% of patients with Hodgkin's disease.[2] Compression fractures and osteoporosis in the cervical spine can result from lymphomatous as well as multiple myeloma bone involvement. An abnormal CBC aids in the diagnosis of infections, inflammatory arthritides, and some tumors and is an excellent screening test. An elevated erythrocyte sedimentation rate provides strong evidence for evidence for some more systemic disorder, such as the presence of an immunologic event in process, and aids in identifying significant magnitude of inflammation of any primary cause. A routine urinalysis may suggest such disorders as systemic lupus erythematosus, vasculitis, scleroderma, or periarteritis nodosa. The diagnosis of rheumatoid arthritis, which so commonly involves the cervical spine,[3] should only rarely be made in the absence of a clearly elevated erythrocyte sedimentation rate.

BLOOD BIOCHEMICAL STUDIES

Calcium. Abnormalities in calcium metabolism are reflected in phosphorus metabolism, neuromuscular function, osteoporosis, and osteomalacia of many pathophysiologic mechanisms, most of which may involve bone, joint, and other connective tissue structures of the cervical spine. Ninety-nine per cent of calcium is in bones. To remain in calcium homeostasis, adults require 10 to 15 mg per kg of body weight, and children require 45 mg per kg of body weight. The calcium electrolyte is absorbed in the intestine and regulated by vitamin D, fat, soluble salts, and a normal pH. Total plasma calcium is composed of ionized (diffusible) calcium and nondiffusible calcium bound to plasma proteins in about equal amounts. The parathyroid hormone regulates this equilibrium. Normal serum calcium concentrations vary from 8.5 to 11.5 in the adult and are slightly higher in children. Studies of calcium in blood and urine are essential to the diagnosis of hyperparathyroidism, hypoparathyroidism, the hypercalcemia of many malignant diseases, chronic renal insufficiency with secondary hyperparathyroidism, the whole spectrum of malabsorption syndromes as well as the infrequent, but not uncommon, rickets.

Phosphorus. Phosphorus is a necessary buffer in the blood as it is reciprocally involved in calcium-phosphorus metabolism with the electrolyte calcium. Eighty per cent of body phosphorus is in bone matrix, complexed as an insoluble calcium salt. Like calcium, phosphorus is regulated by parathyroid hormone at the kidney level and by calcium mobilization from bones at the skeletal level. Phosphorus is influenced by vitamin D, growth hormone, the spectrum of kidney diseases, and the serum concentration of calcium. Hyperphosphatemia occurs in acromegaly (which may involve the bones and joints of the cervical spine) and also in most renal diseases after renal function is compromised. Hypophosphatemia occurs in certain rare hereditary disorders. Determinations of calcium and phosphorus concentration in the urine may be necessary in studies of calcium and phosphorus metabolic disorders. A spot urine calcium concentration measured on a random specimen of urine in midmorning allows general assessment of the estimated calcium excretion per 24 hours—a useful screening test.

Alkaline Phosphatase. Alkaline phosphatase is an enzyme occurring in osteoblasts of bone and in renal tubular cells, adrenal glands, leukocytes, intestinal mucosal cells, and seminiferous tubules. The serum alkaline phosphatase level is elevated in any disease of bone involving increased osteoblastic activitity. We have seen Paget's disease involving the cervical spine—a disease in which the highest levels are seen. Though nonspecific for bone disease, high levels of alkaline phosphatase arouse suspicion. The alkaline phosphatase level is strikingly elevated in obstructive diseases of the liver and bile ducts. The enzyme's application occurs in all metabolic bone diseases, in Paget's disease, and occasionally in primary or metastatic malignant disease of bone.

Acid Phosphatase. Acid phosphatase is synthesized primarily in the acinar cells of the prostate gland; smaller amounts are synthesized by red blood cells. Acid phosphatase is also produced by carcinomatous cells of the bladder, bronchi, bones, and stomach, particularly metastatic lesions. An elevation of acid phosphatase level in a patient over age 50 is strong evidence of metastatic prostatic carcinoma.

Blood Glucose. There are ten rheumatic syndromes associated with and directly or indirectly related to the metabolic defect in carbohydrate metabolism of diabetes mellitus, occasionally involving the cervical spine.[4]

Serum Uric Acid. The measurement of serum uric acid concentration is useful in any patients with rheumatic symptoms and signs. Though only one person in ten with an elevated serum uric acid level has gout, the serum uric acid level reflects all purine (nucleoprotein) metabolism occurring in all cells of the body. Though clinical gout manifestations are concentrated in the lower extremities, the deposition of monosodium urate crystals may occur in the cervical spine. Many diverse disease states that may involve the cervical spine are associated with hyperuricemia. These disease states include myeloproliferative and lymphoproliferative disorders such as lymphomas, multiple myeloma, polycythemia vera, chronic hemolytic anemia, psoriasis, chronic renal failure, hyperparathyrodism, hypothyroidism with myxedema, and Paget's disease. A variety of drugs can cause secondary elevation of serum uric acid level—chlorothiazide, hydrochlorothiazide, furosemide, ethacrynic acid, low-dose salicylate, levodopa, pyrazinamide, and ethambutol. Concentrations of serum uric acid are measured by the uricase method (uric acid levels [optical density] determined both before and after uricase digestion, eliminating the number of compounds that may also be measured by colorimetric methods). The serum value is generally standardized between 7 and 8 mg per 100 ml. Serum uric acid level is influenced by diet and is subject to mild to moderate variation, such as diurnal fluctuation. Serum uric acid concentrations also differ at various times of the year. This necessitates repeating serum acid determinations at least three times before one can be secure that the level is elevated.

The rate of uric acid excretion for people on a very low purine diet should not exceed 600 mg per 24 hours. For people on an average daily diet, the uric acid excretion rate should not exceed 900 mg per 24 hours. A person whose rate exceeds either limit may be regarded as an overproducer of uric acid. Less than 40% of a whole gouty population is considered to overexcrete uric acid, however, so a normal excretion level does not exclude the diagnosis of gout. The abnormal metabolic enzymatic transport lesion is in the kidney in 80% of people with gout.

Total Cholesterol, Triglyceride, and High-Density Lipoprotein (HDL). Since atherosclerosis occurs very commonly in the carotid and vertebral arteries in the cervical spine, the determination of the levels of these fatty components of serum in atherosclerosis may be diagnostically useful. Elevated levels of HDL indicate that atherosclerosis is not as severe and that such a person is "protected" against myocardial infarction. Hypercholesterolemia and hypertriglyceridemia constitute evidence of the greater probability of atherosclerosis and hence may contribute data in the formulation of cervical spine syndromes associated with carotid and vertebral basilar artery insufficiency.

Serum Muscle Enzymes. The measurement of muscle enzymes in serum is essential in the diagnosis of muscle disorders, many of which may involve the musculature of the cervical spine. The muscle enzyme values commonly are elevated in primary muscle diseases. Such an elevation is quite unusual in neuropathic muscle atrophy.

Serum Glutamic-Oxaloacetic Transaminase (SGOT), Aldolase, and Creatine Phosphokinase (CPK). These three enzymes are the most sensitive measures of muscle disease. Levels of all three may be elevated in certain patients with severe primary myopathy, or elevation of one or two may occur. All three enzyme measurements are recommended. The CPK measurement is the most sensitive, and the SGOT is the least sensitive. The SGOT level is elevated in myocardial infarction and liver cell necrosis, and the serum aldolase level may be elevated when hepatic cell damage is present. Elevation of the CPK level may occur in myocardial infarction or even after very frequent intramuscular injections or prolonged exercise.[5, 6]

Increases in concentrations of these enzymes reflect diffusion of enzyme into the blood from damaged muscle cells or escape of enzymes through increased muscle membrane permeability. Thus, increased concentrations may add to evidence of diagnosis for myopathy, but normal levels do occur in the presence of active muscle disease.

Creatine-Creatinine Ratio. Creatine, synthesized in the liver, is converted into creatinine by muscle metabolism. In muscle disease, creatine conversion decreases and creatine excretion in the urine increases. To assess the ratio of urinary creatine to creatinine, a 24-hour urine specimen is collected and the quantitative creatinine excretion rate is measured. Urinary creatine is converted to creatinine, and the analysis is repeated. The result reflects total urinary creatine plus creatinine. The first creatinine value subtracted from the total gives an absolute measure of creatine excreted. The following formula provides the result:

$$\% \text{ Creatinuria} = \frac{\text{Creatine (mg/24 hr)}}{(\text{Creatine} + \text{Creatinine mg/24 hr}) \times 100}$$

Percent creatinuria for men and for women who are not pregnant should not exceed 6%. It is somewhat higher in pregnant women. Children have physiologic creatinuria values of up to 40% at age 3 years and 20% at age 8. They have normal adult values by age 15. Two 24-hour urinary determinations are necessary for accurate information. Creatine-creatinine ratios are elevated in primary myopathic disease but also in the atrophy of disuse and in neuropathic muscle atrophy. The increase in this value does appear far earlier in primary muscle disease than in neuropathic muscle atrophy. The study is used as a diagnostic method and also to monitor disease during therapy.

Immunologic Measurements

Rheumatoid Factors. This antibody appears in the serum of about 70% of people with rheumatoid arthritis. Actually there are many "rheumatoid factors," and these circulating proteins, very heterogeneous, are classified as antibodies on the basis of physical, chemical, and behavioral characteristics. They are really antibodies against an antibody, that is, they are immunoglobulins. Most clinically measured rheumatoid factors are IgM (19S [sedimentation constant] macroglobulin). Less commonly, rheumatoid factors are IgG or IgA types. Rheumatoid factor reacts with IgG (7S gamma globulin), and the reaction is the basis of most tests for rheumatoid factor. The most common test is the latex fixation test in which latex particles are coated with slightly denatured IgG. Sera being tested are heated to block prozone reactions and then added to a suspension of globulin-coated latex particles. The test is positive (rheumatoid factor is present) if the serum reacts with the IgG and causes agglutination of the latex particles. In general, the test is regarded as positive if there is agglutination in a serum dilution of 1:40 or more. In early rheumatoid arthritis, only 40% to 50% of patients have positive test results, but later this figure may rise to as much as 85%. The rheumatoid factor tends to persist in the serum irrespective of the course of the disease.

Because rheumatoid factor occurs in such a broad spectrum of other circumstances (2% to 4% of the normal population, relatives of rheumatoid arthritis patients, 10% to 20% of healthy people over 65 years of age, lupus erythematosus, sarcoidosis, a variety of liver diseases, syphilis, acute viral infections, vaccination, subacute bacterial endocarditis, diabetic patients on insulin therapy, and multiple blood transfusions), its presence does not strongly support the diagnosis of rheumatoid arthritis except when occurring in quite high titer. In most of the clinical circumstances listed above, the concentrations of rheumatoid factor are low. Thus in certain obscure problems in the cervical spine, such as inflammatory disease of the cervical spine with relatively little involvement elsewhere, the diagnosis of rheumatoid arthritis may be confirmed by a high titer of rheumatoid factor.

Complement. There are nine discrete protein substances (C1–C9) intimately related to both immune and inflammatory processes. The complement fixation is generally regarded as activated by antigen-antibody complexes beginning at the C1 site (the first complement protein). It is apparent now that later components may be directly activated. Changes in the concentration of the serum complement components occur in certain connective tissue diseases, such as systemic lupus erythematosus and rheumatoid arthritis, and their study is useful in diagnosis and assessment of ongoing disease activity. Low serum complement levels are characteristic of an exacerbation of systemic lupus erythematosus, particularly when the kidney is involved. Decrease in complement levels also occurs in people with rheumatoid arthritis when the concentration of serum rheumatoid factor is very high. Optimally, the whole hemolytic complement activity, CH50, is measured. However, C3 and C4 do constitute useful measurements and are readily available in most clinical laboratories.

Synovial fluid complement is occasionally important in differential diagnosis. Low concentrations occur in systemic lupus erythematosus, whereas the synovial fluid complement levels in rheumatoid arthritis may be low, normal, or slightly elevated. Synovial fluid complement is characteristically high in concentration in many patients with Reiter's syndrome. Since approximately 80% of people with Reiter's syndrome have the HLA-B27 antigen, and since this disease, ankylosing spondylitis, and psoriasis involve the axial skeleton—particularly the cervical spine—this measurement may be useful.

Antinuclear Antibodies and Lupus Erythematosus (LE) Cell Measurements. Antinuclear antibodies are seen in a variety of chronic diseases; however, these antibody proteins react with nuclei and with molecular structural components of nuclei, nuclear protein, DNA, RNA, and histone and are strongly positive in as much as 90% of patients with systemic lupus erythematosus. Thus a positive test confirms the clinical diagnosis, and a negative test is strong evidence against SLE. Antinuclear antibodies are IgG (7S) in the main, but IgM (19S) antibodies do occur. These are a heterogeneous family of antibodies with widely varying specificities for nuclear components.

The fluorescent antibody technique is utilized and comprises a two-stage procedure. The unknown serum is applied to tissue sections (spleen or liver of mouse) containing nucleated cells. The test is positive if the serum contains antinuclear antibody and binds to nuclei or nuclear component. Fluorescein-labeled antiserum to human gamma globulin is flooded over the slide, and the antihuman gamma globulin reacts with the antinuclear antibody, causing nuclear fluorescence. Various patterns are useful in diagnosis. A homogeneous pattern is the least specific; the peripheral rim pattern suggests SLE; the nucleoli or speckled pattern suggests either scleroderma or Sjögren's syndrome. Mixed connective disease results in a speckled pattern most commonly. Accurate diagnoses on the basis of patterns cannot be depended upon.

Purified, native, double-stranded DNA antibody is most specific for SLE and occurs much less frequently and in far lower titer in all other connective tissue diseases.

The LE cell test, not as commonly used today, measures interaction between antinuclear antibodies, nuclear components, and phagocytic white blood cells.

Antinuclear antibodies occur also in rheumatoid arthritis, scleroderma, dermatomyositis, Sjögren's syndrome, 25% of healthy women over age 60, chronic liver disease, infectious hepatitis, chronic pulmonary fibrosis, and pneumoconiosis. A broad spectrum of drugs may result in formation of antinuclear antibodies—hydralazine, procainamide, isoniazid, certain antibiotics, anticonvulsant drugs, methyldopa, oral contraceptive pills, quinidine, and D-penicillamine—thus their specificity is not great.

HLA Typing. The HLA antigen was first noted to have a 95% incidence in the HLA-B27 type of ankylosing spondylitis. Thus, it has diagnostic capability, but clinical methods of diagnosis are just as good and in some instances are even better. Rheumatic diseases with strong HLA association are ankylosing spondylitis (89.8%), Reiter's syndrome (78.2%), Yersinia arthritis (79.4%), Salmonella arthritis (66.7%), and psoriatic arthritis (40.2%).[7] Since the seronegative spondyloarthropathies, juvenile rheumatoid arthritis, Reiter's syndrome, and anklyosing spondylitis are primarily axial rheumatic diseases including the cervical spine, HLA typing may occasionally be useful. The clinical diagnosis however can be made on the basis of historical and physical data plus radiographic study of the sacroiliac joints.

Quantitative Immunoglobulins (IGG, IGA, IGM). Measurement of these main antibody types may only occasionally be useful, as they are almost never specific in diagnostic capability. An increase or a decrease that is clearly well out of normal concentration range may put the clinician on the alert for some as yet unidentified immunologic rheumatic disease involving the cervical spine.

Cryoglobulins, CIQ Binding Study, and Raji Cell Assay. These three studies plus measurement of serum complement levels are clinical methods of identifying circulating immune complexes and are rarely indicated in disorders of the cervical spine.

BODY FLUID ANALYSES

Cerebrospinal Fluid. Although the cerebrospinal fluid is seldom examined in diseases of the cervical spine, in extensive and advanced cervical osteoarthritis (cervical spondylosis) the spinal fluid protein is increased to moderate or even extreme levels. Examination of cerebrospinal fluid is rarely necessary in diagnosis, since the diagnosis is established so readily.

In a study of patients with systemic lupus erythematosus, 32% of 37 patients having neuropsychiatric episodes had abnormalities of the cerebrospinal fluid.[8] Protein elevation was noted in about half the fluids, and some had an increase in protein as well as numbers of white blood cells. Protein elevation may be associated with papilledema and has some prognostic significance. Deaths occurred in patients with cerebrospinal fluid abnormalities, whereas none died who had normal cerebrospinal fluids.

Synovial Fluid. Synovial fluid is almost never obtained from joints in the cervical spine. In our studies of anatomic and pathologic specimens of the cervical spine, we found that the joints universally contained fibrofatty menisci capable of proliferation (especially on immobilization) and certainly serving the function of lubrication under circumstances.

Synovial fluid analysis (synovianalysis) is essential to the evaluation of rheumatic diseases, just as urinalysis is essential to the detection of renal disease. The finding of monosodium urate monohydrate (MSU) crystals permits the precise and secure diagnosis of the disease gout, requiring little other confirmatory data—that is, the finding is absolutely pathognomonic. Shortly after the rediscovery concerning MSU, McCarty and workers discovered that calcium pyrophosphate dihydrate (CPPD) crystals were present in the joint fluid of patients experiencing acute goutlike attacks (pseudogout).[9, 10] This discovery led again to a mechanism for precise diagnosis of a very common, broad spectrum of diseases, including CPPD crystal–induced arthritis as well as disorders caused by crystal deposits in periarticular soft tissues. This constitutes the rare instance in medicine in which a single diagnostic test is pathognomonic.

Synovianalysis presently is so firmly established in the clinical assessment of rheumatic disease that it is of great importance to make a careful search for even a very small joint effusion in order to identify those who have joint fluid for examination. In cervical spine disorders, more precise diagnosis may be forthcoming by examining the synovial fluid from joints far removed from the cervical spine. For example, asymptomatic first metatarsal phalangeal joints when aspirated may confirm the presence of MSU and CPPD crystals in patients with gout as well as in those with pseudogout.[11]

Routine synovianalysis includes gross evaluation and inspection for volume, viscosity, color, and clarity; a microscopic examination for total white blood cell count and differential white blood cell count—particularly polymorphonuclear leukocytes, lymphocytes, monocytes, macrophages, and synoviocytes; assessment of a wet preparation for crystals and other pathologic material by compensated, polarized light microscopy; mucin clot test; culture; occasional immunologic studies; latex fixation test, quantitative immunoglobulins, or immunoelectrophoresis; staining of synovia for routine differential white blood cell counts—gram stain particularly and, occasionally, Ziehl-Neelsen's stain for acid-fast bacilli, Congo red for amyloid deposits, alizarin red S for calcium (hydroxyapatite clumps), von Kossa's stain for CPPD (hydroxyapatite crystals), alcian blue for intracellular proteoglycans, Sudan black for large monocytes or large lymphocytes (immunoblasts) or synovial lining cells; joint fluid cultures for *Neisseria gonorrhoeae*, anaerobic bacteria, fungi, mycobacterium tuberculosis, or viruses.

A newer method for rapid identification of septic arthritis is the use of gas-liquid chromatography, revealing that elevated lactic acid levels in the range of 150 mg per 100 ml are found in synovial fluid compared with 2 mg per 100 ml in inflammatory arthritis and 23 mg per 100 ml in noninflammatory arthritis. The test is of value even if antibiotic therapy has been started, and the sequential data are useful in assessing therapeutic response.[12, 13] In gonococcal infection, the lactic acid, strangely, is not high. True glucose measurement in synovial fluid compared with blood may help differentiate infection from inflammation. The blood and joint glucose must be simultaneously obtained following a fast of 8 hours. The autoanalyzer method (ferricyanide method) is effective. In noninflammatory (normal) synovial fluid the differential between blood and synovial fluid is less than 10 mg per 100 ml. In inflammation it may be be up to 40 mg per 100 ml, and in infection the differential is greater yet, but the area between 20 and 60 is an overlap zone dependent on the intensity of the inflammation or the infection. When synovial fluid true glucose is below 20 mg per 100 ml, infection is very likely. Rheumatoid arthritis of great chronicity in the involved joint also is associated with low glucose levels and constitutes the most puzzling differentiation.

TISSUE BIOPSY

Tissue Study Biopsies. Any fluid collection in any area of bone, soft tissue, or bursae in the musculoskeletal system (certainly including the cervical spine) should be examined grossly and microscopically by aspiration or, if a tumor is suspected, by open biopsy. For bone marrow study, specimens may be aspirated from the sternum or the iliac crest. A punch biopsy may be performed in the event of suspicion of either metabolic bone disease or, in particular, multiple myeloma, which frequently involves the cervical spine. If a tumor is suspected clinically and radiologically identified, an open biopsy in a surgical operating room is the best course. Bone marrow studies are essential in the ultimate diagnosis of multiple myeloma.

Indication for tissue biopsy should always follow extensive clinical and laboratory assessment, after which the detection of the discrete tissue lesion may make the diagnosis obvious. Many tumors, inflammations, metabolic or biochemical diseases, or even hereditary diseases require tissue diagnosis before secure diagnostic conclusion can be reached.

Obtaining specimens from joint tissues themselves, including those in the cervical spine, may be necessary. Open biopsy carried out under local anesthesia may be preferable in order to obtain adequate samples of tissue and to be certain that the tissue is taken from the site of the lesion. A biopsy of gouty tophi may be performed, ultimately resulting in precise diagnosis. Skeletal muscle biopsy is useful in a group of disorders for demonstration of arteritis, rheumatoid arthritis, and inflammatory lesions of muscle in periarteritis nodosa, dermatomyositis, and polymyositis. Biopsy of peripheral nerves is not often indicated; however, when it is, the sural nerve is the nerve of choice. Rheumatoid subcutaneous nodules may be present, and since they constitute the one specific characteristic of rheumatoid arthritis, they should almost always be sampled to confirm their precise histologic traits. Lymph node biopsy is usually nonspecific, but in cases of lymphoma or Hodgkin's disease, results of the biopsy may confirm the diagnosis. Diagnosis of amyloidosis may be confirmed by needle punch biopsy of liver, spleen, kidney, gum, or rectal mucosa.

Occasionally frozen sections and section fixed in formaldehyde may be obtained. Frozen sections allow detailed enzymatic studies, which are rarely done but sometimes very useful. Biopsy study by electron microscope is valuable in the more unusual disorders. One should not hesitate to perform a biopsy of cervical spine tissues when the diagnosis is critical and has not been solidly confirmed by less invasive techniques.

Synovial Biopsy. Synovial biopsy is most useful in the differential diagnosis of monarticular and oligoarticular arthritis. In more widespread or diffuse joint disease, results of the biopsy are more likely to be nonspecific owing to similarities in pathologic findings in a spectrum of diseases. Special needles for closed synovial biopsy are available and can be used safely. The most commonly performed biopsies are those of the knee, since it is the most accessible joint. Closed biopsy is generally successful and should be considered before opening a joint for biopsy. Synovial fluid is always removed in the greatest quantity possible at the time of biopsy. Local anesthesia is almost always sufficient.

SKIN TESTS

Occasionally skin tests may be necessary in diagnosing some of the infectious diseases affecting bone, including the cervical spine. Tuberculosis, coccidioidomycosis, and histoplasmosis may, on specific testing, reveal a diagnosis. Further investigations by microscopy, sputum smears, and gastric washings may be necessary.

SUMMARY

The many laboratory indications of rheumatic disease appear in ever-increasing numbers year by year. It is urgent to stress that in the great majority of instances the clinical diagnosis can be achieved readily outside the laboratory. In other words, clinical diagnosis can be reached by proper study of the patient's symptoms, signs, radio-graphic features, and data obtained through sophisticated historical elicitation and physical examination.

Occasionally a laboratory test is essential to complete diagnosis, for example, gout with bizarre cervical spine manifestation or sepsis elsewhere with reflected cervical spine symptoms or signs. Much more commonly, however, the nonessential laboratory test is performed. It either confirms or fails to support a suspected diagnosis. It may suggest to the clinician the severity, extent, and therapeutic response of the disease. A highly selective utilization of the broad spectrum of tests is urged. The tests should never replace the skilled clinical approach to the individual patient, whose historical data and physical signs give the most precise reflection of the underlying disease process. It is noteworthy that several types of laboratory testing have contributed to the basic formulations of joint physiology and pathophysiology in the identification and categorization of rheumatic disease, thus leading to more precise treatment methods.

References

1. Emkey RD, Ragsdale BD, Ropes MW, et al: A case of lymphoproliferative disease presenting as juvenile rheumatoid arthritis diagnosed by synovial fluid examination. Am J Med 54:825, 1973.
2. Reimer RR, Chabner BA, Young RC, et al.: Lymphoma presenting in bone. Ann Intern Med 87:50, 1977.
3. Bland JH: Rheumatoid arthritis of the cervical spine. J Rheumatol 1:319, 1974.
4. Bland JH, Frymoyer JW, Revers R, et al: Rheumatic syndromes in endocrine disease. Semin Arthritis Rheum 9:23, 1979.
5. Demos MA, Gitin EL: Acute exertional rhabdomyolysis. Arch Intern Med 133:233, 1974.
6. Cacace L: Elevated serum CPK after drug injections. N Engl J Med 287:309, 1972.
7. McDevitt HO, Engleman EG: Association between genes in the major histocompatibility complex and disease susceptibility. Arthritis Rheum 20:59, 1977.
8. Feinglass EJ, Arnett FC, Dorsch CL, et al: Neuropsychiatric manifestations of systemic lupus erythematosus: Diagnosis, clinical spectrum and relationship to other features of the disease. Medicine 55:323, 1976.
9. McCarty DJ, Hollander JL: Identification of urate crystals in gouty synovial fluid. Ann Intern Med 54:452, 1961.
10. McCarty DJ, Kohn NN, Faires JS: The significance of calcium phosphate crystals in the synovial fluid of arthritis patients. The pseudogout syndrome. I. Clinical aspects. Ann Intern Med 56:711, 1962.
11. Weinberg A, Schumacher HR, Agadelo CA: Urate crystals in asymptomatic metatarsal phalangeal joints. Ann Intern Med 91:56, 1979.
12. Manshady BM, Thompson GR, Weiss JJ: Septic arthritis in a general hospital 1966–1977. J Rheumatol 7:523, 1980.
13. Riordan T, Doyle D, Tabaqchali S: Synovial fluid lactic acid measurement in the diagnosis and management of septic arthritis. J Clin Pathol 35:390, 1982.

Part II ○ CLINICAL MANAGEMENT

Chapter 10

Problem-Oriented Approach

Disorders of the cervical spine, like all other medical and health problems, should never be approached in isolation—the whole patient must be considered. The problem-oriented medical record (POMR) devised by Dr. Lawrence L. Weed[1] allows the patient to utilize all medical advances successfully without becoming lost in the monolithic medical system. The POMR consists of (1) the "data base," which includes the patient's history, physical examination findings, some laboratory tests, and radiographic study, (2) the "problem list," which includes all medical problems, past and present, (3) the "plan of action," and (4) the "progress notes," or evaluation of the plan. The doctor carefully observes and re-evaluates the treatment plan, reinterviews and re-examines the patient, assesses the response to management, alters plans as indicated, and continues evaluation until the best possible result is reached.

Ideally the patient should have his or her own POMR and update it with the help and advice of the doctor. The medical record should be the property of the patient, as are other vital documents, such as birth certificates, insurance papers, deeds, and tax records. Modern patients need much coordination, organization, and discipline in their basic health care, often in conjunction with the highly focused methods and techniques of specialists.

Symptoms and signs in the cervical spine arise from any involvement of the specific segmental levels C1 to C7–T1, with trauma, inflammation, infection, tumor (benign or malignant, primary or metastatic), or change (metabolic, biochemical, or endocrinologic) or from any rheumatic lesions in the area. Identification of the pain-sensitive structure can be made if one knows the distribution patterns of neural and somatic pain perception, the differences between deep structure and superficial structure pain, and the separation of neural pain from connective tissue structure pain.

Clinical Signs Indicating Origin of Cervical Pain. (1) Tenderness on pressure upon transverse processes, particularly the sixth, strongly suggests involvement of intervertebral articulations, as in zygapophyseal or facet joint osteoarthritis. (2) Supraclavicular tenderness in the lower portion of the posterior triangle indicates involvement of the brachial plexus. (3) Suboccipital tenderness between mastoid process and midline indicates involvement of the greater occipital nerve, C2. (4) Deep tenderness of the shoulder girdle suggests involvement of the trapezius, levator muscle of scapula, or rhomboid muscles either directly or by radiation from the cervical spine, neural structures, or connective tissue structures. (5) A trigger point at the upper, inner scapular angle suggests the fibrositis syndrome or a syndrome of the levator muscle of scapula. (6) Specific tenderness of spinous processes suggests some instability of the vertebral bodies due to intervertebral disc disease or herniation.

Clinical Signs Elicited by Resistance to Movement. (1) Pain on resisted cervical spine extension is characteristic of cervical osteoarthritis and intervertebral disc disease. (2) Free side-bending (lateral flexion) with pain on resisted rotation suggests involvement of the atlanto-occipital and atlantoaxial joints. (3) Pain on resistance to forward flexion suggests spinous process disease and possible fracture. (4) Unilateral pain on resistance to lateral flexion with pain on the resisted side suggests involvement of zygapophyseal joints or foraminal impingement on that side. (5) Unilateral resistance to rotation with induced pain suggests some subluxation in the contralateral zygapophyseal joints.

Symptoms in the cervical spine conveniently fall into five principal groups. (1) Involvement of nerve roots and peripheral nerves, with radicular symptoms—acute and transient, chronic and permanent. (2) Involvement of connective tissue structures—bone, joint, ligament, tendon, muscle, meninges, blood vessels. (3) Involvement of the spinal cord—myelopathy. (4) Headache. (5) Vascular insufficiency—vertebral, basilar, carotid, or all three.

CERVICAL OSTEOARTHRITIS (SPONDYLOSIS)

Cervical osteoarthritis is the most common disorder of the cervical spine and serves as the best model of the broad spectrum of clinical reflections that occur with involvement of most structures in the cervical spine. Cervical spondylosis is actually osteoarthritis involving amphiarthrodial joints (intervertebral discs), uncovertebral joints (joints of Luschka), and zygapophyseal joints, though the involvement of each varies in degree and incidence. Cervical spondylosis has many bizarre, unexpected, and secondary clinical reflections in the cervical spine nerve roots, the intervertebral and the transverse foramina, the spinal cord, the esophagus, and the vertebral artery. Most patients with cervical osteoarthritis also have osteoarthritis elsewhere, frequently asymptomatic. The pathology and pathogenesis of osteoarthritis is not considered here, but the clinician should be familiar with the recent great advances in our understanding of the basic process. The new concepts in etiology and pathogenesis have as much clinical pertinence in diagnosis and management of cervical osteoarthritis as they do in diagnosis and management of osteoarthritis elsewhere.[1a] It is no longer acceptable to regard cervical osteoarthritis as a degenerative disease, an integral part of the aging process, or a simple "wear and tear" consequence.

Clinical Aspects of Cervical Osteoarthritis

There is a high incidence of cervical osteoarthritis in the second half of life, increasing in severity with advancing age and becoming universal beyond age 70.[1, 2] Cervical spondylosis is commonly silent, and asymptomatic, that is, the radiologic evidence varies from mild to severe without subjective symptoms or objective signs referable to the neck. Past episodes of pain, stiffness, or paresthesia may be elicited and may be termed "part of growing old," "rheumatism," or a result of having "slept in a draft." Pallis et al[2a] studied 50 patients over age 50 years who entered the hospital for reasons unrelated to the spine or nervous system and found that 75% had very significant radiologic evidence of cervical spondylosis; 75% showed narrowing of the intervertebral foramina due to uncovertebral and apophyseal joint osteophytosis; 50% had objective physical signs of cord involvement. The signs were impaired vibration sense at the ankle, brisk knee and ankle jerk, positive Babinski's reflex, and positive Hoffmann's sign. Few had complaints. Forty per cent had signs of root involvement, and 60% had abnormalities of the neck on clinical examination.

Symptomatic cervical osteoarthritis includes stiffness, limitation of movement, crepitus, local pain and tenderness, and rather considerable muscle spasm. Lateral flexion, rotation, and extension are more limited than forward flexion. Pain is worse with movement, usually is in the upper to middle cervical spine, and may be referred to the occiput or shoulder. The osteoarthritic spine is especially vulnerable to trauma. The site and mechanism of pain are probably ligamentous, tendinous, or capsular. Upper cervical disc pain is perceived in the head and upper neck; pain arising in the lower discs is perceived lower in the neck and into the shoulders and proximal arm, forearm, and hand.

Radiographic Changes. The most obvious findings are alterations in curvature of the spine, with straightening or reversal of lordosis; narrowing of the intervertebral disc spaces mainly from C4 through C7, with anterior and posterior osteophytes (known to have a 1- to 3-mm layer of radiolucent fibrocartilage on their surface); osteophytes on the uncovertebral joints; osteophytes situated laterally on the vertebral bodies; deformity of vertebral bodies; and encroachment on the intervertebral foramina by osteophytes on the apophyseal and uncovertebral joints as well as from the vertebrae themselves. There may be sagittal diameter narrowing with consequent cord compression. Figure 10–1, a sagittal section through five vertebrae, shows the gross lesion and illustrates the classic findings.

Radiculopathy. Root involvement may be single or multiple, unilateral or bilateral, symmetric or asymmetric. There is no predictable pattern. Both the sensory and the motor roots may be involved, with symptoms of irritation or paralysis or both. Autonomic involvement is common. Sensory symptoms are more common and more obtrusive than motor symptoms; they include pain, paresthesia, hypesthesia, and hyperesthesia. Pain may be referred to the neck, upper limbs, head, scapular and suprascapular areas, pectoral muscles, humeroscapular area, deltoid muscle, arm, forearm, hand, and fingers. So-called neuralgic pain

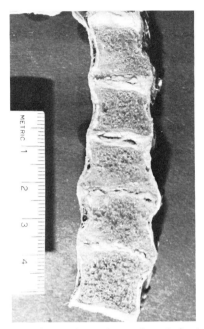

Figure 10–1. Anatomic specimen of cervical spine sagittal section illustrating narrow discs, extensive fissures, osteophytes—anterior and posterior—remodeling, hypertrophied ligamentous structure, and marked increased density of subchondral bone.

from the posterior root is shooting, stabbing, severe, and intermittent. It is referred via the dermatome or sclerotome distribution and reaches its greatest intensity at the periphery. Myalgic pain is referred to the appropriate myotome; the pain is proximal and continuous, with a deep, nagging quality that is associated with deep muscle tenderness in muscles of the neck, shoulder, and arm. The presumed mechanism is that ventral root irritation (efferent pathway) initiates muscle spasm, stimulating sensory fibers in muscles. The afferent pathway involves dorsal roots if and when anterior motor roots cease to function.

Paresthesias. Root pains are proximal, rarely extending below the elbow, whereas paresthesias are often distal. Paresthesias are described as "pins and needles", "going to sleep", creating a cold or hot sensation, a sense of prickling, swelling, numbness, or a clumsy feeling, with reduced dexterity.

Myalgic Spots. Tender areas over muscle about the neck, shoulder girdle, or arm are common and represent local muscle spasm, which is often relieved for long periods by injection of a local anesthetic.

Sensory Changes. Despite common sensory symptoms, objective sensory loss is unusual. Neck movements aggravate sensory symptoms, which may be reproducible through flexion, extension, rotation, lateral flexion, or axial compression of the neck (Spurling test). Motor changes are those

of the lower motor neuron, weakness, atrophy, hypotonic muscles, and, early on, fasciculations. Muscles are innervated from more than one root, and thus extensive paralysis comes only when multiple roots are involved. Depression or absence of reflexes is the most common single objective sign of cervical osteoarthritis.

Dysphagia. Anterior osteophytes from the cervical vertebrae, particularly C5, C6, and C7, may compress the posterior wall of the esophagus, with irritation of tissues and smooth muscle. The symptom may be either dysphagia or simply an annoying awareness of swallowing.

Autonomic Disturbances. Autonomic disturbances seem more likely to be caused by secondary scalene muscle spasm than by primary autonomic nervous system involvement. Such spasm could compress sympathetic fibers in the brachial plexus, mediating vasospastic phenomena in the upper limb, blanching, cyanosis, flushing, altered temperature of or swelling and edema of the hand—a secondary reflex sympathetic dystrophy.

Radicular Syndromes. Radicular syndromes are many and varied, and common complaints, which were previously poorly understood, are now understandable. Cervicobrachial neuralgia has a broad differential diagnosis, but cervical osteoarthritis is its most common etiology. Headache and occipital neuralgia are very common in later life and are mostly due to root compression, vertebral artery and sympathetic nerve pressure, autonomic nervous system instability, and posterior nuchal muscle spasm. Acroparesthesia, wasting of intrinsic hand muscles, lower motor neuron lesions, scalenus anticus syndrome, pseudoangina, frozen shoulder, and reflex sympathetic dystrophy (shoulder-hand syndrome) all occur in either primary or secondary cervical osteoarthritis.

SEQUENCE OF EVENTS IN OSTEOARTHRITIS OF THE INTERVERTEBRAL DISC JOINTS

(1) Young people (more men than women) in the late teens to early 20s have episodes of acute torticollis, severe unilateral pain in the neck, often beginning on waking in the morning. There is visible deformity; pain is constant and severe for 48 to 72 hours, with spontaneous relief in 7 to 10 days. Acute torticollis occurs about once per year, with repeated episodes expected. This seems the analogue of the same event occurring in the lumbar spine—a sudden, relatively small movement of a portion of the intervertebral disc. (2) People in their late 20s and 30s experience intermittent aching in the scapular area. The pain is unilateral but not always on the same side, and it lasts for weeks. Recovery is uneventful. (3) People between 50 and 60 years of age are less likely to experience the intermittent episodes. The pain becomes constant, probably reflecting a swollen disc, with some shift of disc material no longer

returning to its original site. (4) For people 60 years of age and older the scapular ache becomes worse; unilateral, moderately severe cervical root pain appears and is worse at night, often with paresthesias in the hand in variable distribution—most commonly along the ulnar nerve; arm pain increases, remains severe for 6 to 8 weeks, and gradually subsides. If the nerve root loses function (paralysis), the pain is lost in about 3 months. People may experience these events any time after age 35, although their occurrence is uncommon in individuals between 35 and 60 years of age.

(5) The involvement of both upper extremities, with paresthesias in all digits of both hands, probably reflects manifestations of early myelopathy. (6) Central intraspinal intervertebral disc protrusion at the posterior ligament occurs, stretching the dura mater and inducing a fibrotic response with adhesions of the dura mater and the posterior longitudinal ligament. Clinical reflection is constant bilateral aching from occiput to scapulae. Most people with this syndrome are 65 years of age or older. (7) Myelopathy, paresthesias, "pins and needles" in hands as well as feet, claudication pain in the lower extremities, and bilateral aching in upper and lower limbs imply onset of both upper and lower motor neuron manifestations. (8) Myelopathic symptoms occur, as does possible infarction of the spinal cord, with paraplegia secondary to compression of the anterior spinal artery.

Clinical Characteristics of the Previous Sequence

(1) The most common and the earliest site of pain is the scapular area, reflecting C5–C6 and C6–C7 involvement, sometimes with radiation to the ear. Rarely, pain occurs in the pectoral area or in one axilla. (2) Cough, sneeze, and Valsalva's maneuver usually do not affect the pain as they do in thoracic or lumbar disc lesions. (3) Dysphagia may be troublesome. (4) The sternoclavicular or shoulder joint, primarily involved in an inflammatory process, may be associated with referral of pain to the root of the neck. (5) Suprascapular or long thoracic neuritis (serratus anterior muscle) is associated with scapular pain and belongs in the differential diagnosis. (6) Headache of polymyalgia rheumatica or of temporal (giant cell) arteritis is not especially characteristic. Suspect these diseases if headache is very severe and occurs without previous episodes of neck ache in a patient 60 years of age or older. Cervical spine shows no rheumatic signs sufficient to cause the degree of pain manifest. (7) Capsules, synovial membranes, and ligaments of the occipito-atlanto-axial complex commonly cause headache and head pain in patients 65, 70, and 80 years of age. The pain is usually a morning headache that improves as the day goes on. The pain is not severe but is unaffected by the usual analgesics. (8) Unilateral neck pain in the elderly is most commonly caused by intervertebral disc protrusion, with displacement of a fragment of cartilage in the osteoarthritic joint (Luschka or apophyseal). The displacement produces the pain. (9) Ankylosing spondylitis commonly causes pain and stiffness in the neck, radiating to the head, but in younger patients a long history of low back pain is common. Younger patients may however develop ankylosing spondylitis painlessly in the lower spine, with the initial symptoms appearing in the neck. Limitation of motion and quite severe pain occur more rapidly in ankylosing spondylitis—that is, they occur week by week rather than year by year as in the very gradual onset of osteoarthritis in the cervical spine. Careful examination gives the examiner the typical end feel of muscle spasm.

NERVE ROOT ORIGIN OF PAIN

Dorsolateral Disc Protrusion. Abrupt onset of severe radicular pain over minutes, hours, or days, reaching a maximum intensity in a few days, with no history of previous neck or arm pain, is usually due to dorsolateral disc protrusion. The nerve root is compressed against vertebral laminae or by an intraforaminal protrusion just posterior to the uncinate process (the Luschka joint). The pain is severe, aching, shooting, or "electric," with radicular distribution corresponding to the nerve root level involved. Because each spinal nerve has its dermatome, myotome, and sclerotome distribution, the pain may radiate widely depending on the volume of tissue involved (i.e., nerves innervate muscle, bone, joint, tendon, ligaments, and blood vessels). Pain is typically perceived in the neck, shoulder, arm, forearm, and hand, with the fingers receiving the nerve supply from the root or roots involved. The pain may involve both anterior and posterior parts of the chest, particularly if the usual C5, C6, C7 nerve roots are affected. The larger the volume of tissue in the herniation, the greater the area of radiation and the more severe the pain. Changing position of the neck through active or passive rotation or flexion, extension, or tilting the head exaggerates the pain. The position of head and neck most likely to bring out or exaggerate the pain or paresthesia or both is cervical spine extension followed by the combination of lateral flexion and rotation. Such patients cannot lie on the affected side; they are most comfortable in the supine position. Cough and sneeze may worsen the pain. Paresthesia, numbness and tingling, severe muscle spasm, hypesthesia, and anesthesia in the dermatome affected occur frequently, but the pain dominates the clinical picture. Dorsolateral disc protrusion is much more common in young people than it is in older people.

If muscle weakness occurs in the course of acute radiculopathy, the anterior root or motor root has become involved. If the disc protrusion is at C5, the infra- and supraspinous muscles, the deltoid muscle, the biceps muscle, and the brachioradial muscle become weak or even paralyzed. If the protrusion is at C6, the triceps muscle, the greater pectoral muscle, the latissimus dorsi, and the wrist and finger extensors become weak, resulting in rapid atrophy of these muscles in 10 days to 2 weeks. Deep tendon reflexes are diminished to absent.

Peripheral Neuropathy. This radiculopathy is less severe but much more common and of more gradual onset than dorsolateral disc protrusion. Brachial neuropathy is also characterized by pain, but the pain is more limited in area and more likely to be caused by disturbance of a single nerve root. Pain may be perceived in the neck, arm, and shoulder; a broad distribution of muscle spasm is uncommon. Numbness and tingling, dysesthesia, paresthesia, and spotty anesthesia occur in the distribution of the involved root. Muscle wasting and hypotonia are common, but gross muscle weakness is rare. The triceps muscle is most likely to be weak. Deep tendon reflexes are diminished and sometimes absent. So-called "frozen shoulder," carpal tunnel syndrome, and tennis elbow are frequent accompaniments.

Such radiculopathies may occur as a series of acute attacks over several years, finally becoming chronic. Sensory symptoms are the most prominent. If the radiculopathy occurs at C6, the index finger and thumb lose light touch sensation, and if it occurs at C7, the index finger does not feel things well. This handicap impairs a person's ability to perceive small objects, handle money, pull up zippers, or button buttons. Tactile discrimination is compromised and pain sensation decreased, particularly distally at the fingertips.

CERVICAL OSTEOARTHRITIC MYELOPATHY

Myelopathy of cervical osteoarthritis is surely the most common disease of the spinal cord during and after middle age and probably is the true etiology of such syndromes as "idiopathic" primary lateral sclerosis and progressive paraplegia of middle life. Its onset is insidious, and diagnosis is made only after several years, if then! Onset may be as acute as trauma or as an obstructive vascular lesion. The neurologic symptoms and signs are extremely variable and difficult to classify, because they depend on the nature and number of lesions, the site, the rate of evolution, and the extent of disease—all totally variable and unpredictable. In general the symptoms and signs can be classified as either local (cervicobrachial and cervicocephalic) or distant (referred to distal parts).

Motor Changes. Table 10–1 lists motor disturbances commonly seen.

Reflex Changes. In the arms deep tendon re-

Table 10–1. SYMPTOMS AND SIGNS OF MOTOR CHANGES IN CERVICAL MYELOPATHY

First (predominantly lower limbs)
  Spastic paraparesis
  Stiffness and "heaviness", scuff toe, difficulty climbing stairs
  Weakness, spasms, cramps, easy fatigue
  Decreased power, especially of flexors (dorsiflexors of ankles and toes; flexors of hips)
  Hyper-reflexia of knee and ankle jerks, with clonus
  Positive Babinski's sign, extensor hypertonia
  Decreased or absent superficial abdominal and cremasteric reflexes
  Drop foot, crural monoplegia
Later
  Various combinations of upper and lower limb involvement
Later
  Mixed picture of upper and lower motor neuron dysfunction
Later
  Atrophy, weakness, hypotonia, hyper-reflexia to hyporeflexia, and absent deep tendon reflexes

flexes may be increased, decreased, or absent. The reflex arc may be compromised at the root as well as at the cord level. The inverted radial reflex is common, indicating a lesion of the ipsilateral cord at the C5–C6 level (decreased or absent jerk of biceps muscles replaced by finger or wrist flexion or both; triceps muscle reflex is brisk, and finger jerks occur). With abnormal upper extremity deep reflexes, an increase in ipsilateral deep reflexes occurs at the knee and the ankle. The jaw jerk is generally normal.

Sensory Changes. Though motor changes predominate in the lower extremities, sensory changes are most marked in the upper extremities. Table 10–2 lists the sensory changes expected.

Table 10–2. SYMPTOMS AND SIGNS OF SENSORY CHANGES IN CERVICAL MYELOPATHY

Headache and head pain
Neck, eye, ear, throat, or sinus pain
Sensory symptoms in the pharynx and larynx
Paroxysmal hoarseness and aphonia
Rotary vertigo
Tinnitus synchronous with pulse or continuous whistling
Deafness
Oculovisual changes: blurring, photophobia, scintillating scotomata, diplopia, homonymous hemianopia, nystagmus
Autonomic disturbance: sweating, flushing, rhinorrhea, salivation, lacrimation, nausea, and vomiting
Weakness in leg or legs, drop attacks with or without loss of consciousness
Numbness on one or both sides of the body
Dysphagia or dysarthria
Myoclonic jerks
Hiccups
Respiratory changes: Cheyne-Stokes respiration, Biot's respiration or ataxic respiration

They are subject to extreme variability, and they occur in varying degrees.

Autonomic visceral changes are uncommon. However, bladder symptoms, such as urgency, hesitancy, retention, frequency, and incontinence, do occur occasionally but not as commonly as in osteoarthritis in the lumbar spine. Spinal fluid is usually of normal pressure and cell count, but there is frequently a moderate increase (less than 100 mg per 100 ml) in protein concentration. Combined radiculopathy and myelopathy are common, as is occasional vertebrobasilar arterial insufficiency with either or both.

The differential diagnosis may be quite easy or very difficult, since cervical osteoarthritis is a common and frequently an asymptomatic occurrence in the aging spine. Evidence of neurologic disease above the foramen magnum (such as positive jaw jerk) casts doubt on osteoarthritis as a cause. The differential diagnosis includes soft disc protrusion, intracranial tumor, spinal cord tumors, multiple sclerosis, subacute combined degeneration of the cord, peripheral neuropathy, drop foot, motor neuron disease, cerebellar disease, syringomyelia, tabes dorsalis, and hysteria.

Cervical Spinal Cord Compression

Cervical myelopathy is a consequence of the pressure, tension, and torsion of the spinal cord, usually resulting in degeneration of the various elements within the anterior cord. It is secondary to the large osteophytes at the disc levels—bulging intervertebral discs, so-called spondylotic bars. Hypertrophic ligamenta flava may compress the posterior cord. The variables in producing cervical myelopathy are legion. The consequent clinical picture is that of an incomplete lesion of the spinal cord, with neural elements involved in a patchy pattern that is sometimes limited to a single level but more often involves several levels to varying degrees. The time interval between onset of symptoms and identification and treatment of disease varies from 1.5 to 4 years. There is usually a history of radicular symptoms, including attacks of brachial radiculopathy. Dysesthesia, awkwardness, weakness an clumsiness of the hands, and weakness of the lower limbs constitute the principal initial symptoms. Numbness and tingling in the tips of the digits and wasting of muscles in the upper extremity are variable in extent and degree, and their distribution, with resultant patchy ischemia, depends on which segments of the spinal cord are compressed. If the upper part of the cervical enlargement is involved, the muscle atrophy occurs in the infra- and supraspinatus muscles, the deltoid, biceps, and triceps muscles, and the greater pectoral muscle. Dorsiflexors of wrists and fingers may be affected. Muscular fasciculation is present but inconspicuous, never occurring to the degree chacterizing motor neuron disease.

Spastic weakness occurs in the lower extremity, with one leg usually more severely involved than the other. Tendon reflexes are often exaggerated, tending in late stages to diminish and ultimately disappear. If the corticospinal tracts of the anterior cord are compressed, exaggeration of the reflexes is expected.

The jaw jerk is a very useful diagnostic test. A normal jaw jerk associated with exaggerated tendon reflexes in the upper limbs suggests a lesion below the foramen magnum, whereas an exaggerated, diminished, or absent jaw jerk in these circumstances is evidence of a lesion above the level of the pons.

The inverted radial reflex is characteristic. If the fifth cervical level is involved, the normal radial reflex is decreased, but when the corticospinal tract is compressed, the flexor finger jerk occurs. Hoffmann's reflex is also often positive and the triceps jerk exaggerated in such cases. Abdominal reflexes are usually diminished but not completely lost. Lower limb spasticity causes exaggeration of knee and ankle jerks, sometimes with clonus; the plantar reflexes are more likely extensor. Decrease in light touch, vibratory sense, tactile discrimination, and pin prick are usual but not striking. Sphincter control is almost always normally maintained. If the posterior columns are severely involved, subacute combined degeneration or amyotrophic lateral sclerosis may be mimicked. See Chapter 4, *Clinical Methods.*

Pain in the back and legs, simulating lumbar zygapophyseal joint disease or intervertebral disc disease, is common and should be suspected because it can be distinguished clinically from lumbar spine disorders. Pain caused by cord compression tends to be diffuse, involves both legs, and is burning or aching in quality. Lumbosacral nerve root compression produces a sharp, radiating pain in the distribution of the involved root. Neurologic examination may be normal when cord compression is sufficient to produce severe pain. The mechanical signs of lumbar disc herniation—limitation in back mobility and positive reaction to the straight leg raising test—are absent in patients with pain in the back and legs that is caused by cervical cord compression.[3]

A variety of sensory symptoms of pain and temperature perception occur, such as feelings of pain, odd sensations of heat or cold, dysesthesias, and perverted pain or temperature sensibility. Paroxysms of pain are reported that start in the toes and run up the anterior legs, with a dull ache in both legs between paroxysms. Unusually, such obscure pain in the legs is the initial symptom in patients with cervical cord compression, and it is often exaggerated or aggravated by neck movement. Nonetheless pain is far more common with radiculopathy than with cord lesions.

Another painful sign in cervical cord compression is a momentary sensation of shock, "electricity,' and paresthesia, with severe pain and with tingling running down the spine or into arms and legs on one or both sides, especially upon flexion, only rarely upon extension of the neck, and sometimes upon cough or sneeze. This sign has been variously titled electric sign of Lhermitte, neck bending sign, and barber's chair sign by British neurologists.[4] A posterior column lesion seems most likely responsible.

Vertebrobasilar Artery Insufficiency, Constant or Intermittent

Rotation of the neck to one side normally decreases the circulation in the atlantoaxial portion of the contralateral vertebral artery. Such movement, if there is kinking of the artery, atheromata, and osteoarthritis, reduces the circulation even more.[5] Other mechanisms that could alter the blood supply to the brain stem in osteoarthritis of the cervical spine are carotid sinus compression, surgical collar, neck manipulation with release of emboli from atheromatous plaques in the great vessels, or thrombosis with infarction of the cerebellum or brain stem.

The vertebrobasilar system when compromised results in a spectrum of temporary, sometimes permanent, changes that may occur in the distribution of the vertebral artery. The symptoms are as variable as the functions of the structures that become ischemic. Turning or extending the neck may result in any of the following responses: weakness in a leg or legs or drop attacks as described by Kremer[6] (descending motor tract); paresthesia, numbness, tingling on one or both sides of the body (long ascending sensory tract); dysphagia or dysarthria (bulbar structures associated with swallowing or speech); tinnitus or vertigo (auditory and vestibular nuclei in the brain stem or inner ear, Meniere's syndrome); pain or other sensory perceptions in the face, tongue, or throat (trigeminal or glossopharyngeal connections in the brain stem); diplopia or gaze paralysis (ocular motor nuclei and their connections), blurred vision or blindness and homonymous hemianopsia; a visual anosognosia or photopsia via the calcarine and neighboring cortices; ataxia or nystagmus (cerebellum); hiccupping or disturbances in respiration, Cheyne-Stokes respiration, Biot's respiration, or ataxic respiration (vegetative centers in the brain stem); akinetic mutism and sensory loss (globus pallidus and thalamus); tremor and rigidity (substantia nigra); impaired memory and disorientation (temporal lobe); headache from compensatory dilation of occipital branches of the external carotid artery (migraine). Brain[5] studied 100 cases of cervical osteoarthritis with neurologic complications and found vertigo in 17, attacks of unconsciousness in 4, drop attacks in 3, and other evidence of vertebrobasilar ischemia in 5. Such symptoms are often reproducible by rotating the neck, but this involves some

Table 10–3. SYMPTOMS AND SIGNS OF VERTEBROBASILAR ARTERY INSUFFICIENCY*

Dizziness	Myotonic jerks
Giddiness	Tremor and rigidity
Drop attacks	Disorientation
Syncope	Vertigo
Stroke	Photophobia
Diplopia, blurred vision	Numbness and tingling
Visual hallucination	Quadriparesis
Auditory hallucination	Dysphagia
Tinnitus	Dysarthria
Flushing, sweating, lacrimation, rhinorrhea	Photopsia
	Visual anosognosia
Scotomata	Nystagmus
Hiccups	Ataxia

*These paraspinal symptoms result mainly from rotation and extension of the neck, although they sometimes occur upon flexion. The spectrum of neurologic symptoms and signs is as broad as the structures potentially involved. The clinical conclusion is that in a complex, bizarre, and poorly explained neurologic syndrome, vertebrobasilar artery insufficiency should be suspected.

risk.[7, 8] Table 10–3 summarizes the symptoms and signs of vertebrobasilar artery insufficiency.

Vertebral angiography often discloses the tortuous course of the artery and compression by osteophytes of the vertebrae or uncovertebral or zygapophyseal joints. These attacks may result in complete stroke and infarction; such people are at risk during manipulation or positioning of the neck during anesthesia. The attacks may sometimes be difficult to distinguish from labrynthine disturbances.

Sympathetic Nervous System Syndrome of Barré-Liéou—A Pain Syndrome

In 1926 Barré studied and established a syndrome, which was further described by his student Liéou in 1928.[9, 10] So diverse and widespread is the combination of symptoms and signs that some no longer regard it as a disorder associated with the cervical spine.[11, 12] Rather, it has been shown to be caused by vertebral artery insufficiency and its multivariant characteristics. The combination of symptoms is based mainly upon the autonomic innervation of the cervical and cranial vessels and their anatomic connections between the somatic and sympathetic nervous systems of the cervical spine. Barré[11] thought that osteoarthritic change was responsible for the symptoms. The symptoms include pain in the head, neck, eye, ears, face, sinuses, and throat as well as sensory disturbances in the pharynx and larynx, paroxysmal hoarseness and aphonia, tinnitus synchronous with the pulse, various auditory hallucinations (such as whistling and humming), deafness, oculovisual disturbances—blurring, scintillating scotomata, photophobia, blepharospasm, sensations of squinting, a peculiar pulling at the "back of the eyes"—flushing, sweating, salivation, lacrimation, nausea and vomiting, and rhinorrhea. The Barré-Liéou syndrome is said to be due to gross compression and irritation of the posterior cervical sympathetic system. The pain is described as throbbing, burning, stinging, searing, and either continuous or paroxysmal. Steindler[13] divided the syndrome into four major categories, (1) a pharyngeal and laryngeal syndrome, with pain in paranasal sinuses, tonsils, and tongue, causing hoarseness and dysphagia, a facial syndrome with sweating, lacrimation, and salivation, (2) an aural and vestibular syndrome with tinnitus, whistling, and vertigo; (3) an ocular syndrome characterized by defective accommodations of pupils (not rare in cervical spine injuries), (4) a pseudocardiac syndrome.

Surely some of these sensations, such as pulling at the posterior pole of the eyeball, would be currently attributed to psychoneurosis. Rotes-Querol et al[12] studied 64 patients with the syndrome and found very few physical or radiographic abnormalities or abnormalities apparent through laboratory tests. They also found that many of the patients had personality and emotional disorders and responded beneficially to psychotherapy. It seems likely that the Barré-Liéou pain syndrome could be ascribed to vertebral basilar artery circulation more rationally than completely to compression of sympathetic nerve fibers.

Symptoms, Signs, and Syndromes Associated with Cervical Osteoarthritis

Dysphagia

Anterior osteophytes occasionally grow to such magnitude as to compromise swallowing function by pharyngeal compression.[14, 15] Pharyngeal paresthesias have been described.[16]

Noise in the Neck

Normally there is crepitus on movement of the cervical spine at all ages. This is due to the shearing of the planes of tissue and is more apparent following immobilization. The magnitude and intensity of "noise" increase in the patient with cervical osteoarthritis or in the immobilized patient. Calcific, retropharyngeal tendonitis and calcific periarthritis in the cervical spine have been reported.[17] The normal cervical venous hum is continuous and is heard above the medial end of the clavicles and along the anterior border of the sternocleidomastoid muscle. This, according to Fowler and Gause,[18] can be produced in 75% of children and young adults. The hum is louder when the patient is sitting, and turning the head away from the side where auscultation is performed may bring out the hum or give it a higher pitch. Valsalva's maneuver may eliminate it, as may pressing the thumb across the cervical veins. The hum may be misinterpreted as being due to a carotid bruit.

Valvular aortic stenosis murmur may be transmitted into the carotid arteries, decreasing in intensity as it is transmitted up the neck. The murmur of ruptured chordae tendineae of the mitral valve and the consequent systolic ejection murmur may be transmitted into the neck, as may the murmur of severe aortic regurgitation.

The origin of the left subclavian artery may be obstructed by atheromata and produce a noise—a murmur suggesting occlusive carotid artery disease. The prognosis is generally good, even with complete obstruction of the left subclavian artery.[19, 20]

Various bruits originating in the cervical arteries are due to atherosclerosis—rarely to fibromuscular hyperplasia or arteritis. A bruit may be heard in the unusual case of periarteritis nodosa.

Angiography is the best way to study extracranial carotid arteries as well as vertebral arteries. The incidence of cervical arterial bruit is 4.4% in one study.[20] Arterial venous fistula in the neck is an unusual but not unheard of lesion.[20]

Cervical Migraine

A syndrome indistinguishable from usual migraine has been described in patients with demonstrated vertebral artery insufficiency. The characteristic feature is its intermittent nature. Cervical migraine is more likely to occur after standing for a prolonged period with head and neck in a flexed position. The episodes come in "attacks," with no prodrome, nausea or vomiting, visual symptoms, or vertigo.[22]

Headache

Headache is a very common symptom in cervical osteoarthritis. It is located in the occiput on one or both sides, spreads frequently to the parietal, temporal region and to the eye, worsens on awakening in the morning, and tends to improve during the day. The headache may occur when the osteoarthritic changes involve the lower cervical discs as well as when the upper zygapophyseal joints are involved. The mechanism of headache has been attributed variously to nerve root compression, pressure on the vertebral artery and sympathetic nerves, autonomic disturbance in the Barré-Liéou syndrome,[9, 10] and posterior nuchal muscular spasm. Brain[5] believes the pain of headache comes from the osteoarthritis in the zygapophyseal joints of the upper cervical spine. Clinically the headaches are associated with pain in the neck and upper limbs, which is sometimes accompanied by occipital or vertex paresthesias that fluctuate in severity with the brachial and neck pain. The following information is of diagnostic importance: the headache is invariably occipital, may be unilateral or bilateral, is annoying and nonpulsating, is aggravated by head and neck movements, strain, and cough, occurs in the morning, and may wake the patient in the night, raising the question of brain tumor. Headaches that do not occur in the occipital region are unlikely to be due to cervical osteoarthritis.

Cervical Vertigo

Disease of the neck is a fairly common cause of vertigo, and Ryan and Cope[23] suggest that the syndrome be called cervical vertigo. There are three groups of patients who have the syndrome: those with cervical osteoarthritis, patients treated by neck traction, and patients with certain types of neck injury. They usually have pain in the posterior neck and occipital region, accompanied by stiffness and diminished range of motion. After a varying latent interval, recurrent postural vertigo occurring on lying down and on bending the neck in certain positions appears. The symptom is reproducible, and nystagmus is induced by flexing the neck but not by merely positioning the head in space. The prognosis is good, hence precise diagnosis is of some importance.[23]

Pseudoangina

At the level of C6 and especially C7, severe radiculopathy may result in pain in the neck and left precordium, with radiation into the left arm. The myalgic pain and tenderness in the precordium are due to continuous and sustained muscle spasm secondary to very irritable motor (ventral) nerve roots. The scapular region also may be quite painful. The chest pain is constricting in quality and may be aggravated by effort. True angina pectoris tends to be referred to the ulnar border of the arm, forearm, and hand, but this is not true of pseudoangina. The clarification may be enhanced by finding further clinical signs and symptoms of radiculopathy or by excluding cardiac disease. Pseudoangina is aggravated by neck movement, and such movement increases cervical muscle spasm and induces torticollis-like results. In pseudoangina there is no shock, fever, elevated sedimentation rate, or leukocytosis, and the electrocardiogram is normal.[24, 25]

It is easy to err in both directions, leading either to unnecessary alarm if pseudoangina is mistaken for true angina or to unwarranted cervical operation if true angina is overlooked. True angina and pseudoangina may coexist.[26]

Lower Motor Neuron Syndromes

A lower motor neuron syndrome may occur in cervical osteoarthritis, making it difficult to know whether the lesion is radiculopathic or myelopathic. Wasting of muscle, weakness, and muscle fasciculation commonly involve the C6 or C7 myotome and dermatome. Such a radiculopathy may be confused with peripheral palsy of the proximal radial nerve. In a C7 radiculopathy of the musculocutaneous nerve and in a C6 radiculopathy with C8 and T1 root involvement, there may be wasting of the small hand muscles, and the wasting may have to be distinguished from various forms of muscular atrophy.

Paresthesias in the Upper Extremity

Paresthesias, hypesthesia, and dysesthesia are very common in cervical osteoarthritis and are certainly common causes of this symptom in middle aged and older people. Likewise, carpal tunnel syndrome or brachial plexus compressions and cervical rib or scalenus anticus syndrome may confuse the clinical picture. In carpal tunnel syndrome, the differential diagnosis is made by using any of the following methods: finding local tenderness to pressure or percussion over the wrist (Phalen's sign);[27] performing Gilliatt and Wilson's tourniquet test[28] in which symptoms are reproduced by inflating a blood pressure cuff around the forearm to a pressure above arterial systolic, measuring conduction time in the motor and sensory fibers; or injecting corticosteroid into the carpal tunnel.[27] The scalene muscles may develop sufficient spasm to produce neurovascular symptoms—an epiphenomenon of cervical osteoarthritis. Thus, a vascular change in the hand or sensory symptoms could be explained on the basis of nerves compressed by scalene muscle spasm rather than on the basis of the radiculopathy of C4–C5 and C6 anterior scalene muscles. Likewise scalene muscle spasm may compress the vertebral artery and compromise blood flow.

Frozen Shoulder

The lesions about the shoulder, rotator cuff disease, supraspinatus tendonitis, and the shoulder-hand syndrome may be difficult to separate clinically from cervical osteoarthritis. However, precise clinical study, historical elicitation, and physical examination should successfully separate these various syndromes. There seems little question that rotator cuff shoulder syndromes, reflex sympathetic dystrophy, frozen shoulder, epicondylitis (tennis elbow), carpal tunnel syndrome, and Dupuytren's contracture are in a definite but obscure cause and effect relationship with cervical osteoarthritis—the latter being the precipitating or triggering mechanism. Their associations are far too frequent to be due to chance alone.[29]

References

1. Weed LL: Your Health and How to Manage It. Promis Laboratory, University of Vermont. Essex Junction, VT: Essex Publishing Co, 1975.
1a. Bland JH, Cooper SM: Osteoarthritis: A review of the cell biology involved and evidence for reversibility; management related to known genesis and pathophysiology. Semin Arthritis Rheum 14:106, 1984.
2. Elias F: Roentgen findings in the asymptomatic cervical spine. NY State J Med 58:3300, 1958.
2a. Pallis C, Jones AM, Spillane JD: Cervical spondylosis: Incidence and implication. Brain 77:274, 1984.

3. Langfitt TW, Elliott FA: Pain in the back and legs caused by cervical spinal cord compression. JAMA 200:381, 1967.

4. Brieg A: Biomechanics of the Central Nervous System. Chicago: Year Book Medical Publisher, 1960.

5. Brain WR: Some unsolved problems in cervical spondylosis. Br Med J 1:771, 1963.

6. Kremer M: Sitting, standing and walking. Br Med J 2:63–67 and 121–126, 1958.

7. Biemond A: Thrombosis of the basilar artery and the vascularization of the brain stem. Brain 74:300, 1951.

8. Taplow WFT, Bammer HG: Syndrome of vertebral artery compression. Neurology 7:331, 1957.

9. Barré JA: Le syndrome sympathique cervical postérieur et sa cause frequente, l'arthrite cervicale. Rev Neurol (Paris) 33:1246, 1926.

10. Liéou YC: Syndrome sympathique cervical postérieur et arthrite cervicale chronique. Etude clinique et radiologique. Strasbourg, Schuler and Minh, 1928.

11. Kovacs A: Subluxation and deformation of the apophyseal joint: a contribution to etiology of headache. Acta Radiol 43:1, 1955.

12. Rotes-Querol J, Crespi PB, Puiggros AC: Studies on locomotor syndromes of possible psychogenic origin. II. The so-called Barré-Liéou syndrome. Med Clin (Barc)33:235, 1949 (in Spanish).

13. Steindler A: Lectures on the Interpretation of Pain in Orthopedic Practice. Springfield, Illinois: Charles C Thomas Publisher, pp 249–250.

14. Bauer F: Dysphagia due to cervical spondylosis. J Laryngol Otol 67:615, 1953.

15. Bettmane EH, Neudorfer RJ: Cervical disc pathology resulting in dysphagia in an adolescent boy. NY State J Med 60:2465, 1960.

16. Terracol J: Les troubles segmentaires sensatifs et trophiques du pharynx et l'ostéoarthrite dé formante de la colonne cervicale. Arch Int Laryngol 33:1025, 1927.

17. Sarkozi I, Fam AG: Retropharyngeal tendinitis: An unusual cause of neck pain. Arthritis Rheum 27:708, 1984.

18. Fowler NO, Gause R: The cervical venous hum. Am Heart J 67:135, 1964.

19. Hurst JW, Hopkins LC, Smith RB: Noises in the neck. New Engl J Med 302:862, 1980.

20. Wardrop PA, Shapera R, May M: An unusual cause of pain in the neck. Hosp Pract 13:131, 1978.

21. Heyman A, Wilkinson WE, Heyden S, et al: Risk of stroke in asymptomatic persons with cervical arterial bruits. New Engl J Med 302:838, 1980.

22. Dutton CB, Riley LH: Cervical migraine not merely a pain in the neck. Am J Med 47:141, 1969.

23. Ryan GMS, Cope S: Cervical vertigo. Lancet 2:1355, 1955.

24. Brain WR, Northfield DWC, Wilkinson M: The neurological manifestations of cervical spondylosis. Brain 75:187, 1952.

25. Knight GC: Discussion on rupture of the intervertebral disc in the cervical region. Proc Soc Med 41:511, 1948.

26. Northfield DWC: Diagnosis and treatment of myelopathy due to cervical spondylosis. Brit Med J 2:1474, 1955.

27. Phalen GS, Kendrick JF: Compression neuropathy of the median nerve in the carpal tunnel. JAMA 164:524, 1957.

28. Gilliatt RW, Wilson TG: Ischemic sensory loss in patients with peripheral nerve lesions. J Neurol Neurosurg Psychiatry 17:104, 1954.

29. Murray-Leslie CF, Wright V: Carpal tunnel syndrome, humeral epicondylitis and the cervical spine: a study of clinical and dimensional relations. Br Med J 1:1439, 1976.

Chapter 11

Differential Diagnosis and Specific Treatment

Diagnosis

I knew what was the matter with him
as soon as he walked in the room
Don't ask me how
I knew.
Before he said a word or asked a question.
Before I examined him.
The look on his face, the way he walked.
It must have been something,
because I knew at once.
But don't ask me how.
Tests, x-rays, scans
help.
The pattern that mimics the textbook
helps.
But there is no substitute for having been there before.
If you have seen the beast you will recognize him.

ROBERT RAY MCGEE, M.D.

This is a practical chapter, which is designed not for reading and study but for rapid, accurate, and precise consultation. The goal is presentation of a large volume of information in a format that allows it to be perceived at a glance. This chapter is not written in textbook style.

How is a diagnosis made? The human mind works like a computer. It has been "programmed" with historical data, symptoms, signs, and other clinical characteristics of patterns of presentation of diseases. We learn certain clinical characteristics of diseases and fit the presence or absence of clinical features with the patient at hand, and with such "programming," we make a correct diagnosis. It is necessary to know as much about the most unusual disease or disorder as about the most common. This chapter is designed to provide such information. The physician who has had very broad previous experience has done a great deal of "programming" and is far more likely to reach a correct diagnosis in a short time than one whose mind has not been extensively "programmed." Sometimes the diagnostic process is like an algorithm, that is, some characteristic is identified, and the mechanisms of the mind trip instantaneously from one characteristic to another until the diagnosis is reached. The physician who has seen many instances of a given disease process with all of its variations is more likely to make an accurate diagnosis than one who has not. The "textbook" picture is the exception, not the rule. An accurate diagnosis is like the hidden face in the picture. Once you have seen it, it leaps out at you—but until you have, it remains hidden.

This chapter is organized according to an arbitrary classification of diseases, disorders, and syndromes of the cervical spine. The specific diseases and syndromes are classified under the following broad etiologic and pathogenetic headings:

1. idiopathic disorders;
2. heritable disorders—genetic and congenital;
3. inflammatory disorders;
4. osteoarthritis;
5. neoplastic lesions—benign and malignant;
6. trauma;
7. vascular diseases and syndromes;
8. endocrine and metabolic disorders;
9. disorders of the cervical spinal cord.

The information pertaining to each syndrome is organized along the following lines: (1) key references, preferably recent reviews; (2) definition of disease or syndrome, including etiology (when known) and genetic implications; (3) epidemiology, incidence, and prevalence, including age and sex, family history, and specific predisposition; (4) tissue involved; (5) symptoms, precipitating factors, order of development, and rapidity of onset; (6) signs; (7) radiologic characteristics; (8) laboratory data; (9) special studies, including electromyography, cerebrospinal fluid examination, electrocardiography, cineradiography, computed tomography, and magnetic resonance imaging, (10) treatment and management; and (11) prognosis. In some cases, additional categories of organization have been inserted, and in others, categories not relevant to the syndrome under discussion have been omitted.

IDIOPATHIC DISORDERS
Torticollis—Congenital and Acquired[1–5]

Table 11–1 presents a classification of torticollis.

Congenital Torticollis—Postural and Muscular

Definition. A rotational deformity of the head and neck; sternocleidomastoid muscle is contracted, spastic, and fibrotic.

Etiology and Pathogenesis. Unknown. Genetic predisposition; precise heritable details unknown. Possible birth injury; possible mysterious sternocleidomastoid tumor; possible organized hematoma with fibrous contracture; ischemia of the sternocleidomastoid muscle.

Incidence and Epidemiology. Largely unknown, 507 cases were seen over a period of 27 years in one large center.

Tissue Involved. Sternocleidomastoid muscle.

Symptoms. Ten days post partum, a hard lump appears in the sternocleidomastoid muscle; head tilts toward the side of the contracted and spastic muscle; chin has rotated away to the opposite side, facial asymmetry with ocular disturbance (due to change in horizon of vision) occurs in 2 to 3 years.

Signs. Palpable fibrous tissue mass midportion of the affected sternocleidomastoid muscle; gross asymmetry of external facial features; muscle hard and tight; scoliosis later; compensatory thoracic curve to the opposite side.

Radiologic Characteristics. Scoliotic cervical and thoracic spine.

Laboratory Data. None pertinent.

Special Studies. None pertinent.

Treatment and Management. Conservative treatment successful in majority of cases; if organic contracture develops, surgical division of the tight muscle necessary at age 2 to 3 years.

Prognosis. Excellent for congenital postural torticollis; guarded in congenital muscular torticollis.

Acute Torticollis in Children

Definition. Acute torticollis occurring in children ages 5 to 10 years.

Etiology and Pathogenesis. Etiologic considerations include trauma, infection, tonsillitis, severe chicken pox, and tuberculosis of the upper cervical spine.

Incidence and Epidemiology. Related only to trauma, infection, or other inflammation.

Tissue Involved. Connective tissue about upper cervical spine.

Symptoms. Cervical spine pain, dysphagia, chills, fever, sepsis, severe illness.

Signs. Head tilted to the side of the taut sternocleidomastoid muscle; chin pointed in opposite direction; painful, tender muscle.

Radiologic Characteristics. Unilateral atlantoaxial rotatory change, sometimes with subluxation in trauma; asymmetry of the lateral joints between axis and atlas.

Laboratory Data. Elevated sedimentation rate and leukocytosis.

Special Studies. Results of blood culture positive.

Treatment and Management. Therapy should be directed at the consequence of trauma or at the infectious process.

Prognosis. Usually excellent.

Spasmodic Torticollis

Definition. Wryneck with rare, involuntary movements of the cervical musculature causing tonic deviation of the head and neck. Both sexes are affected equally; familial cases occur occasionally. Associated with benign essential tremor; regarded as a variety of segmental dystonia.

Etiology and Pathogenesis. Little known.

Incidence and Epidemiology. No available data.

Tissue Involved. Cervical spine musculature.

Symptoms. Head uncontrollably drawn toward the shoulder; head flexion and later hyperexten-

Table 11–1. CLASSIFICATION OF TORTICOLLIS

Congenital Torticollis
  Congenital postural torticollis
  Congenital muscular torticollis
Acquired Torticollis
  Skeletal disorders
    Trauma to cervical spine, bone, joints, and
      discs
    Inflammatory lesions of the cervical spine
  Neurologic and psychologic disorders
    Spasmodic torticollis
    Ocular torticollis
    Habit
    Paralytic (peripheral or central nervous
      system lesion)
    Reflex (from lymph glands in the neck)
  Soft-tissue contracture

sion; painless. Early head tilt may be corrected by light pressure on deviated chin. Later stages involve fixed, painful contracture with tonic spasm of several neck muscles and high incidence of secondary cervical osteoarthritis. There is a high incidence of physical and mental effort aggravating the condition. Symptoms disappear during sleep.

Signs. Spasmodic jerking of the head, relieved by counterpressure; sometimes intermittent; chin rotated to the side; trapezius muscle prominently involved.

Radiologic Characteristics. Radiologic torticollis.

Laboratory Data. No pertinent findings.

Special Studies. No pertinent findings.

Treatment and Management

1. Rule out other less serious forms of torticollis.

2. Educate patient regarding the prognosis, which is usually guarded and variable. Treat psychologic factors—no specific routine management; review variety of standard surgical procedures.

3. Heat as hot shower, hot, moist pack, Hubbard tank.

4. Stretching and range of motion exercises.

5. Analgesic drugs.

6. Passive exercises to patient's limit of tolerance.

7. Occasional cervical spine traction.

8. Local rest—soft collar rarely required.

9. Massage.

Prognosis. Guarded and variable.

Acute Torticollis in Adults and Adolescents

Definition. Occurrence is rare before age 21. It occurs equally in both sexes and is probably an early manifestation of osteoarthritis (cervical spondylosis).

Etiology and Pathogenesis. May be related to trauma; awkward postural position over many hours; no specific genetic or environmental factors other than the universality of cervical osteoarthritis.

Incidence and Epidemiology. No pertinent data.

Tissue Involved. Muscle, ligament, tendon, and probably joint in cervical spine.

Symptoms. Patient (age 15 to 35) wakes up with a crick in the neck; neck is fixed in side flexion sometimes toward, sometimes away from, the painful side, without rotational deformity. Marked limitation of only one lateral and only one rotational movement; pain is unilateral.

Signs. Limitation of one lateral and one rotational movement; very tender sternocleidomastoid and trapezius muscles; joint blocked by intraarticular displacement. Sometimes progressive bulging occurs, owing to constant angulation of the joint; bulging worsens when patient sits up, causing neck to bear weight; pain is constant and

severe for several days and usually resolves completely within 7 to 15 days.

Radiologic Characteristics. Cervical spine straightening due to muscle spasm.

Laboratory Data. No significant findings.

Special Studies. No significant findings.

Treatment and Management. Rest, analgesics, passive exercises, physical therapy as heat and gentle stretching exercises; resolves itself.

Prognosis. Excellent.

Hysterical Torticollis

Definition. Patient contracts scapular muscle. Scapula is hunched, with neck flexed toward that side. Other signs of hysteria are present.

Etiology and Pathogenesis. Obscure mental mechanism.

Incidence and Epidemiology. No known significant factor.

Genetic and Environmental Factors. Unknown.

Tissue Involved. Soft tissues of the neck, including muscle, ligament, tendon, joint, and capsule.

Symptoms. Severe pain, hysteric behavior; elevation of the scapula resulting in the head held fixed in side flexion (see Chapter 21, *Malingering, Psychoneurosis, Hysteria, and "Compensationitis"*).

Signs. No movement in any direction is possible (no other disorder compromises movement in all directions). Muscle contraction is overcome easily by applying sustained, passive pressure during persuasion. Passive range of motion is much greater than active range of motion—the principal clue.

Differential Diagnosis. Parkinsonism in which the neck may become gradually stiff and painful owing to muscle rigidity.

Radiologic Characteristics. Because the radiograph virtually always shows cervical osteoarthritis, the true diagnosis is often obscured.

Laboratory Data. No pertinent findings.

Special Studies. Psychologic testing; psychiatric consultation.

Treatment and Management. Manage the problem of hysteria. Inspection of the facies is confirmatory.

Prognosis. Variable and guarded.

Hyoid Bone Syndrome[6]

Definition. Pain and tenderness at the site of the greater cornu of the hyoid bone. A form of insertion tendonitis, an enthesopathy.

Etiology and Pathogenesis. Unknown.

Incidence and Epidemiology. Unknown.

Tissue Involved. The tendon and the site of its insertion in the greater cornu of the hyoid bone.

Symptoms. Early discomfort and aching on either or both sides of the neck at the level of the hyoid bone.

Signs. Tenderness in the area previously described, hoarseness, and dysphagia on initiating the act of swallowing.

Radiologic Characteristics. None established. Radionuclide scan possibly useful.

Laboratory Data. No information.

Special Studies. No information.

Treatment and Management. Injection of the area with corticosteroid and procaine in very tiny amounts. Use a low concentration of the corticosteroid (triamcinolone hexacetonide [Aristospan] preferred). Diagnosis is made by exclusion, and if the symptoms become severe and troublesome, excision of the greater cornu of the hyoid bone is an option. It has been done in 18 patients, resulting in permanent relief of head and neck pain.

Prognosis. Good to excellent.

Neck-Tongue Syndrome on Sudden Turning of the Head[7]

Definition. Unilateral upper nuchal pain and numbness or occipital pain and numbness or both, with paresthesia of tongue on the same side.

Etiology and Pathogenesis. Compression of the second cervical nerve root in the atlantoaxial space on sharp rotation of the neck. Pathogenesis unknown.

Incidence and Epidemiology. Unknown.

Tissue Involved. C2 nerve root and atlantoaxial space.

Symptoms. High nuchal and occipital pain on abrupt turning of the head.

Signs. Tenderness on pressure or percussion of the spinous process of the axis.

Mechanism of Production. Afferent fibers from the lingual nerve travel via the hypoglossal nerve to the second cervical nerve root, whose compression provides anatomic explanation for numbness of one half of the tongue, with pain in the neck and occiput.

Radiologic Characteristics. None.

Laboratory Data. None.

Special Studies. None.

Treatment and Management. Stretching exercises; avoiding abrupt turning of the head.

Prognosis. Good. Generally resolves spontaneously.

Calcific Retropharyngeal Tendonitis[8, 9]

Definition. Tendonitis and tenosynovitis of the longus colli muscle and tendon.

Etiology and Pathogenesis. Unknown.

Incidence and Epidemiology. Unknown.

Tissue Involved. The longus colli muscle and the tendon and its sheath, located on the anterior surface of the vertebral column and extending from the atlas to the third thoracic vertebra.

Symptoms. Gradually increasing anterior cervical spine pain, dysphagia, and increasing "throat" pain. Pain aggravated by head and neck movement.

Signs. Tenderness (extreme and out of proportion to clinical findings) in the anterior cervical spine area from C1 to C4. Marked tenderness of the transverse process of C1.

Radiologic Characteristics. Prevertebral soft-tissue swelling from C1 to C4 and amorphous calcific density in the longus colli tendon anterior to the body of C2 and inferior to the anterior arch of C1.

Laboratory Data. No findings.

Special Studies. No findings.

Treatment and Management. Condition is self-limited. Nonsteroidal anti-inflammatory agents; moist heat applied to the neck 20 minutes twice daily; gentle stretching exercises. The differential diagnosis is very important. It includes retropharyngeal abscess, meningitis, infectious spondylitis (osteomyelitis and post-traumatic muscle spasm).

Prognosis. Good.

Psychiatric Clinical Syndromes in Patients with Osteoarthritis[10]

Definition. Specific, identifiable psychiatric disorders in the context of cervical spine disease.

Etiology and Pathogenesis. Probably the same mechanisms as those that occur without osteoarthritis of the cervical spine.

Genetic and Hereditary Factors. No specific data.

Incidence and Epidemiology. No specific data.

Tissue Involved. Tissues of the cervical spine with or without relationship to the psychiatric syndrome.

Symptoms. The Barré-Liéou syndrome is so thoroughly subjective as to raise doubts in the mind of the average examiner.* Differential diagnosis is required for any precision in management decisions. The clinical mixture of a certain degree of objectivity and so much subjectivity taxes to the utmost one's clinical skills. In sequence, the symptoms and signs follow: pain, severe pain, pain interrupted by frequent paroxysms, constant base-level pain, pain precipitated by change of position, sudden movements of head and neck, sneezing, sighing, or coughing; vertigo, tinnitus, pharyngolaryngeal paresthesias, aphonia, ocular symptoms, blurred vision, loss of vision; corneal hypesthesia (validly demonstrated), slow or absent pupillary responses—direct and consensual (valid); recalcitrant and recurrent corneal ulcers,

---

*The Barré-Liéou syndrome may be purely psychiatric in nature, but the clinical symptoms and signs can be produced by vertebrobasilar artery insufficiency. The differential diagnosis is extremely difficult and is sometimes made only by exclusion of the latter.

miosis or mydriasis, pain within the eye and retro-orbitally, photophobia, sense of necessity to squint; vasomotor paroxysmal disturbance, flushing, heat flash, paresthesia, hypesthesia and anesthesia, lacrimation, rhinorrhea and salivation, tongue paresthesia and hypesthesia. Severe attack may last 5 to 10 minutes and is easily mistaken for trigeminal neuralgia.

Differential Diagnosis. Patient's description of pain and symptoms is extremely functional and includes a great excess of bizarre metaphors. Pain and radiations are neurologically atypical; they fail to follow the dermatome, myotome, and sclerotome distribution patterns. Pain precipitation occurs with only mild emotional state. Complaints are recited with great flourish.

It is always possible for the true syndrome of Barré-Liéou and psychiatric disease to coexist in a patient.

Signs. As noted in *Symptoms*, with relatively few objective signs.

Radiologic Characteristics. Only those of cervical spine osteoarthritis.

Special Studies. Psychiatric consultation, specific eye-ear-nose-throat studies of vertigo, vestibular apparatus, and gait, possible presence of agoraphobia. Great urge for bedrest; withdrawal, hypochondria, and gross neurosis; permanent or temporary relief of all symptoms by some therapeutic maneuver.

Treatment and Management

1. Apply methods recommended under *Osteoarthritis* in this chapter.

2. Patient education. Approach clinical problem with sympathy and empathy along with discipline. Consider psychologic and psychiatric consultation. Prognosis is dependent upon the prognosis of the psychiatric disorder, which requires precise diagnosis.

Involutional depressive reaction, agitation, hysteria, pseudohysteria, and psychomotor neurosis have been well identified. Antisocial psychopathic behavior, alcoholism, drug addiction, suicidal attitudes, attempts at work avoidance, and claustrophobia may be encountered and are useful in more precise diagnosis.

Prognosis. Dependent upon the prognosis of the psychiatric disorder.

Thoracic Outlet Syndrome

Note: Broad diagnostic categories also include *Neoplastic Lesions* and *Vascular Diseases and Syndromes*.

Definition. Thoracic outlet syndrome comprises a spectrum of disorders of the brachial plexus, not the nerve roots. The compression phenomenon may be neural or vascular, arterial or venous. Thus, symptoms are not perceived at the base of the neck, which is the location of the lesion, but are referred to the distal part of the upper extremity. The syndrome almost always involves the nerves from C8 and T1, affecting the lower trunk of the cervical plexus. Hence neurologic signs reflecting the C7 nerve root or nerve roots at higher levels exclude the thoracic outlet syndrome. The two types of pressure are that associated with a cervical rib and that associated with the first rib.

Etiology and Pathogenesis. The pressure phenomena from a variety of mechanisms acting on the lower trunk of the brachial plexus cause the symptoms. An abnormality of the muscle, tendon, or bone may be causative. A long transverse process of the seventh cervical vertebra, large cervical ribs, or strong fibrous bands in the position of the cervical rib, with and without ossification, may cause the syndrome.

Thoracic outlet syndrome is a classic example of the release phenomenon. Pressure on the trunk elicits paresthesias but not hypesthesia or anesthesia. These paresthesias are release phenomena, that is, faint tingling and numbness appear momentarily when a nerve trunk is irritated, then nothing is perceived until the pressure on the nerve is released, when painful paresthesia occurs for some time after the pressure on the nerve trunk ceases. The interval has a close relationship to the duration of the original pressure. After 5 minutes of the pressure, the paresthesia appears in about 30 seconds; after release from 12 hours of compression, the patient may not feel the paresthesia for 2 to 3 hours. For example, pressure on the sciatic nerve while sitting causes no symptoms; the pins and needles feeling occurs when the subject relieves the pressure by standing. Active movement of affected fingers or stroking of the hyperesthetic area of skin brings on a "shower of pins and needles."

Genetic and Hereditary Factors. The inheritance of a cervical rib, a congenital anomaly, is a genetic factor.

Incidence and Epidemiology. No firm data available.

Tissue Involved. The structures in and about the clavicle, the neurovascular bundle, the lowest trunk of the cervical plexus, and axillary artery and vein are involved.

Symptoms. Distal symptoms are more often related to nerve pressure than to pressure on the subclavian artery or vein. Paresthesia and some dysesthesia and anesthesia in median and ulnar distribution (more often ulnar) occur. The distribution is commonly bilateral but is more severe on one side than another. In young people 20 to 30 years of age, carrying a heavy bag or a heavy overcoat brings on paresthesia. Dependent upper extremity causes aching in the hand and sometimes causes Raynaud's phenomenon (subclavian artery compression).

Subclavian vein pressure causes edema of the hand and cyanosis for hours or days; painless wasting of the short abductor muscle of the thumb and of the thenar eminence occurs.

Signs. Scapular elevation; arms are often held up, with shoulders shrugging; approximation of scapulae pulls clavicles back and compromises radial pulse. Passive depression of scapulae by the examiner has no effect. Having patient carry a weight may increase or exacerbate symptoms. Palpation at the root of the neck may cause unilateral increase in subclavian pulses. Cervical spine usually has a full range of free and painless movement, as do the shoulder, elbow, and small joints of the hand.

Clinical Variations. *Acute Onset.* Thoracic outlet syndrome rarely occurs abruptly. Occasional onset with sense of threatened fainting, pain in the chest and upper limb and hand, and blanching of hand and forearm may occur. Breathing may be painful, pleuritic, and shallow; suspicion of spontaneous pneumothorax is common. Radial pulse may be diminished to absent; warmth and color return to the upper limb in a few hours. Severe momentary pectoral pain caused by sudden compression of the clavicle against a costochondral junction of the first rib may occur.

Gradual Onset. Characteristically, a middle-aged woman awakens in the night with ''pins and needles'' in all fingers of both hands; when she sits up, the symptoms disappear; when she wakes up in the morning, both hands are ''numb'' for a few minutes. During the day there are no symptoms. Etiology is that of drooping of the pectoral girdle; poor postural mechanism leads to compression of the lower trunk of the brachial plexus, which is in contact with the first rib. With the arm supported by a mattress, resilience of the tissue lifts the plexus trunk off the bone, and paresthesias appear. The trunk recovers at night as fast as it is compressed by day, hence there are no neurologic signs.

Thus, diagnostic characteristics are nocturnal appearance of symptoms, normal results of examination of head and neck and upper limbs, and causing ''pins and needles'' (paresthesias) by keeping the scapulae elevated for minutes (with the arms raised). The woman usually experiences no difficulty during the day unless she carries a heavy weight. After months or years the nocturnal pain appears in hands and forearms, finally involving the shoulder. It may be noted that the amount of pain felt at night increases with the amount of exertion expended during the day. After a few days in bed with a minor illness, the nocturnal symptoms disappear. No color change occurs in the hands.

Examination of all movements of neck and upper limb discloses the ranges of power and of painlessness; sustained elevation of the scapulae and the arms causes the symptoms. These two postures should be maintained for several minutes to determine whether paresthesias appear. If these two tests are negative, the physician should have the patient lie supine with arms above the head for 5 to 10 minutes; the symptoms usually appear.

Radiologic Characteristics. Cervical rib and long transverse process of C7 vertebra may be noted by radiograph. Note that a strong fibrous band or an uncalcified cartilage may cause the syndrome, but neither is radiologically visible.

Laboratory Data. Not pertinent.

Special Studies. Angiogram, electromyogram.

Treatment and Management

1. Use conservative measures for the majority of patients.

2. Use surgical intervention for those with objective signs who are failing to respond satisfactorily or who show critical arterial, neural, or venous impairment on initial study.

3. Prescribe postural exercises, avoiding positions that increase pressure; treat specific clinical signs—neuritis, myositis, chronic strain, and pain syndrome.

4. For patients who sleep with upraised arm, tie a length of gauze about the wrists and attach it to the foot of the bed, with enough slack to permit bringing the arms as high as the shoulder.

5. Assess magnitude of emotional tension involved in any relationship to job, workers' compensation, and secondary gain.

6. Encourage use of an arm chair.

7. Prescribe exercises involving scapular elevation.

8. Consider prescribing a brace. It may retrain the patient posturally, raising the trapezius muscles.

9. Prescribe very specific exercises designed to correct the formulated mechanism of production of symptoms.

10. Consult a surgeon regarding cervical rib resection and scalene muscle section. Search for long transverse process of C7 vertebra; strong fibrous band or uncalcified cartilage may cause syndrome and not be radiologically visible.

Differential Diagnosis. Protrusion of the seventh cervical disc.

Prognosis. Generally good.

Double Crush Syndrome[11]

Note: The syndromes discussed here also apply to the following other sections of this chapter: *Idiopathic Disorders, Heritable Disorders, Inflammatory Disorders, Osteoarthritis, Neoplastic Lesions, Trauma, Vascular Diseases and Syndromes,* and *Endocrine and Metabolic Disorders.*

Clinical syndromes of the cervical spine, arm, forearm, and hand overlap a great deal both clinically and pathologically. The syndromes have been attributed to nerve root involvement, syndromes of the brachial plexus, cervical rib, and scalene muscle, fibrous bands, drooping shoulder, intervertebral disc protrusion, and fibrosis of the dural root sleeve, all of which have been associated with syndromes of shoulder rotator cuff inflammation, nerve entrapment syndromes, superficial and deep heads of the pronator teres syndrome, and the syndrome of the anterior interosseous nerve and transverse carpal ligament (carpal tunnel syndrome). These associations have been reported in frequency greater than could occur by chance. Ulnar, median, and radial nerve entrapment syndromes all have been noted. In recent years some interrelationship among all of these syndromes has been suspected. Several clinical nerve entrapments have been reported as occurring simultaneously in the same patient, and it is not unusual to find no visible evidence of compression upon exposing peripheral nerves that have a valid clinical reflection and positive neurologic symptoms and signs. A polyneuropathy may be suspected in such clinical circumstances.

The double crush hypothesis has been proposed to explain these unusual clinical observations.[11] Upton and McComas propose a hypothesis based on the phenomenon of axoplasmic flow. The key features are that a normal motor neuron has special trophic messenger substances synthesized within its cell body and then transported along the axon to the muscle fibers. These substances are required for normal physiology and function of the muscle fibers and of the motor axon and its terminal, that is, they will not function normally without the continuing synthesis of these compounds. If there is a surplus of trophic material, enough will be delivered beyond areas of minimal constriction to the muscle fiber, and the nerve will not regenerate. This circumstance will change dramatically if the axon is damaged at another point. Some neural tubules and neural filaments within the axon will be destroyed, and others will be damaged. Thus, failure of delivery of trophic material beyond a point of constriction results in neural damage and damage at two or three locations.

This hypothesis provides an explanation for the high incidence of peripheral nerve entrapment syndromes in people with diabetes mellitus, chronic renal insufficiency, and hereditary neuropathies. It seems reasonable to assume that the cell body of the motor neuron is affected and is not able to synthesize the required amount of trophic material, and if so, minor degrees of axon compression become critical and result in the denervation phenomenon. McComas[11] coined the term "double crush," recognizing that in some instances nerve fibers might be affected at two or more levels and that the lesion could result from damage of sudden stretch as in whiplash.

This explanation further fits cervical osteoarthritis, in which most patients have injury to several roots, particularly at the C5–C6, C6–C7, and C7–C8 levels. Thus such patients would be predisposed to developing multiple syndromes, such as carpal tunnel syndrome, shoulder lesions, and cubital entrapment syndromes. If upper cervical roots are damaged, peripheral nerve lesions may cause weakness of the trapezius induced by a C2–C3–C4 lesion, allowing shoulders to droop. When this happens, further stretch and pull on nerve roots initiate even more abnormal function, with clinical reflections. The theory also provides similar explanations for brachial plexus lesions and for those occurring in the lower extremities, such as spontaneous peroneal nerve palsies associated with a lumbosacral root lesion. A "slowing" of axoplasmic flow has been confirmed recently by isotopic studies.

Syndromes of the Nerve Plexuses

Note: These syndromes also apply to the following other sections of this chapter: *Inflammatory Disorders, Osteoarthritis, Neoplastic Lesions*, and *Trauma*.

Disease and disorder of the cervical plexuses (cervical and brachial plexuses) cause changes in sensory, motor, and autonomic function, differing somewhat in distribution from those changes resulting from peripheral nerve involvement and from those resulting from radicular lesions.

Cervical Plexus. The cervical plexus is formed by the anterior primary rami of the upper four cervical nerves, which connect with the superior cervical sympathetic ganglion and two cranial nerves—the spinal accessory nerve and the hypoglossal nerve. Anatomically, the plexuses lie on the side of the neck behind the sternocleidomastoid muscle but anterior to the levator muscle of the scapula and the middle scalene muscle. Cutaneous branches go to the skin on the lateral occipital portion of the scalp, the greater part of the ear, the angle of the jaw, the neck, the supraclavicular region, and the upper thorax through the greater and lesser occipital, greater auricular, cutaneous, cervical, and supraclavicular nerves. Muscular motor branches supply the scalene muscles, levators, diaphragm, and the vertebral muscles as well as the sternocleidomastoid, trapezius, and infrahyoid muscles. There are intercommunications with tongue muscles and with suprahyoid muscles. Cervical plexus injuries are uncommon, but any individual nerves may be compromised by wounds, operative trauma or disease, or trauma to cervical vertebrae. Cervical occipital neuralgia and headache are clinical events; abnormality of motor branches cause weakness, paralysis, and muscle atrophy; irritation may result in spasm of muscles of the neck or diaphragm, and rigidity of the neck occurs in meningitis and in diseases of the cervical vertebrae and muscles—a protective reflex mechanism.

Brachial Plexus. Brachial plexus lesions result in motor and sensory syndromes of muscles of the upper extremities. The brachial plexus is made up of the anterior primary rami of the four lower cervical nerves, C5 through C8 and the greater part of T1. The C5 and C6 rami form the upper trunk; the C7 ramus forms the middle trunk; and the C8 and T1 rami form the lower trunk. Trunks are placed in the supraclavicular fossae distal to the anterior scalene muscle. Each trunk splits into an anterior and a posterior division, with derivation of the three cords from them. The lateral cord is formed by the anterior division of the upper and middle trunks, the medial cord by the anterior division of the lower trunk (C8 and T1), and the posterior cord by the posterior divisions of all of these trunks and nerves. The upper trunk branches to the supraclavicular nerve, innervating the supraspinatus and infraspinatus muscles as well as the subclavius muscles. The lateral cord branches to the lateral anterior thoracic nerve, innervating the greater pectoral muscle. The medial cord gives rise to the medial anterior thoracic cord, which goes to the pectoral muscles and the medial antebrachial and brachiocutaneous nerves. The posterior cord branches to the subscapular nerve, innervating the subscapular muscle and teres major, and the thoracodorsal nerve innervates the latissimus dorsi muscles. Terminal branches of the posterior cord are the axillary and radial nerves, and terminal branches of the lateral cord are the musculocutaneous (biceps) component and the lateral component of the median nerve. Terminal branches of the medial cord are the ulnar nerve and the medial component of the median nerve.

Upper-Arm Type of Brachial Plexus Palsy (Erb's Palsy or Duchenne-Erb Paralysis)

Injury to the C5–C6 cervical roots, the upper trunk, and sometimes the upper and middle trunk is caused by severe traction, injury or blow to the head or shoulder, stab wounds, or obstetric injury. Paralysis of the deltoid, biceps, brachial, and brachioradialis muscles and occasionally of the supraspinatus, infraspinatus, and rhomboid muscles occurs. The arm hangs limp in adduction and internal rotation at the side of the body and the forearm is in extension, pronation, and medial rotation. The patient cannot abduct or externally rotate the arm or flex or supinate the forearm. Biceps reflex is absent; little sensory change occurs, owing to peripheral nerve distribution overlap.

Lower-Arm Type of Brachial Plexus Palsy (Dejerine-Klumpke Syndrome)

Injury to the C8 and T1 roots, the lower trunk, or the medial cord may be caused by tumors, disease of the pulmonary apex, fractured clavicle or cervical rib, aneurysm of the arch of the aorta, fracture or dislocation of the humeral head, or usually abrupt, severe, traumatic upward traction on the arm. The syndrome may be caused by traction on the arm or shoulder or by hyperabduction both with and without dislocation. The syndrome involves paralysis of muscles supplied by the ulnar and, to a lesser degree, the median nerves; sensory changes in the distribution of these nerves (inner border of arm, forearm, and hand), C8–T1; loss of flexion of wrist and fingers; weakness of small muscles of the hand; weak grip; edema and trophic changes ultimately; Horner's syndrome; and paralysis of wrist and finger flexors (claw hand).

Middle-Arm Type of Brachial Plexus Palsy

This syndrome is rare, and it involves weakness of extensors of forearm, wrist, and fingers and sensory changes in the distribution of the radial nerve.

Syndromes of the Peripheral Nerves

Note: These syndromes also apply to the following other sections of this chapter: *Inflammatory Disorders, Osteoarthritis, Neoplastic Lesions, Trauma* and *Endocrine and Metabolic Disorders*.

Typical peripheral nerves have mixed function—sensory, motor, and autonomic. Motor components of a peripheral nerve arise in the anterior horn cells of the spinal cord and proceed in converging fibers to the ventral spinal root, ultimately reaching striated muscles. Sensory components arise in receptors or end-organs all over the body, but their cell bodies are in the dorsal root ganglia, entering the spinal cord through the dorsal spinal roots. Ventral and dorsal roots unite to form the mixed spinal nerve, which, after passing through the intervertebral foramina (in the cervical spine in this instance), divides into anterior and posterior primary rami, which subdivide to supply muscular or sensory structures. Autonomic components of the 12 thoracic and upper 3 lumbar segments (sympathetic system) arise from cells in the intermediolateral column, exiting with the ventral roots of the segmental nerves and traversing the mixed spinal nerve to reach the anterior primary ramus. Here they separate from the proximal part of this ramus as finely myelinated fibers (white rami communicantes) entering the ganglionated sympathetic chain. Postganglionic fibers are unmyelinated (grey rami communicantes), which, on reaching the anterior primary ramus, split into two groups—the anterior primary ramus and the posterior primary ramus. The posterior primary rami are smaller than the anterior and supply the dorsal structures of the body, the skin, the longitudinal muscles, and the axial skeleton.

Most peripheral nerves are myelinated. A cut nerve sustains wallerian degeneration distal to the point of section. The myelin sheath swells, retracts, fragments, and breaks down into lipid material. Neurofibrillae of the axon are swollen and fragmented. Neurilemmal cells of Schwann mitose and multiply. The sheath hypertrophies and fills up the space occupied by myelin, and its cells become phagocytic. In 1 to 3 months the fibers and the myelin have disappeared and motor end plates have degenerated. Neurilemmal sheath and connective tissue septa of the nerve remain. The proximal segment of the nerve degenerates for just a short distance, with injury close to the cell body; it may sustain chromatolysis regeneration proceeding distally from the central stump, and growing fibers penetrate the scar tissue entering the empty sheath. Functional maturation of an axonal pathway, that is, myelinization and restoration of fiber diameter, goes more slowly than regrowth of the axis fiber. Regeneration is accelerated by nerve suturing. Rate of growth varies with different nerves, and atrophy of muscle has an adverse effect on restoration of function. There is no regeneration within the central nervous system. Tissue interposed between the nerve ends blocks regeneration. A neuroma may develop at the site of a nerve injury.

Etiologies of peripheral nerve injury are trauma, pressure, chemical or toxic substances, injury, anoxia, infection, and deficiency diseases of substances necessary to nerve metabolism. There are considerable differences in the diameters of nerve fibers as well as a variability in conduction rate of impulses and their refractory periods. So-called A fibers carry motor, proprioceptive, pressure, and tactile impulses and are most vulnerable to pressure and anoxia. The B fibers are smaller and carry localized, fast pain impulses as well as heat perception. The C fibers, which are the smallest and are mainly unmyelinated, carry less well-localized, second, or slow pain impulses along with vasomotor impulses.

Clinically, diagnosis and localization of peripheral nerve lesions involve recognition of changes in function. Sensory and motor examinations as well as study of autonomic nervous system function (sweating, vasomotion, skin temperature) must be done. It is important to test deep and superficial reflexes and to recognize syndromes with interruption of, compression of, and irritation of the peripheral nerve.

Radial Nerve (Musculospiral Nerve). It is the largest branch of the brachial plexus and the continuation of the posterior cord. It is derived from the fifth through the eighth cervical segment of T1. Anatomically, it winds about the humerus in the musculospiral groove. At the antecubital fossa it divides into terminal deep and superficial branches supplying the biceps, anconeus, and brachioradial muscles, the long and short radial wrist extensor muscles, the ulnar wrist extensor muscle, the extensor muscles of the fingers (including index and little fingers), the long and short extensor muscles of the thumb, the long abductor muscle of the thumb, and the supinator muscle. Sensory impulses are tested from the

dorsal aspect of the lower forearm, wrist, hand, and radial fingers.

Radial nerve paralysis is the most frequent of all peripheral nerve palsies; the nerve may be affected anywhere along its course. It may be injured by pressure in the axilla by crutches, the back of a chair, or by shoulder dislocation. It may be involved in fractures of the humerus or radius or in perforating wounds, or it may be compressed by a callus or by pressure above the wrist.

Clinical Reflections. Clinical findings include loss of extension and adduction of wrist, fingers, and thumbs and wrist drop; finger flexors remain intact, but weakness of grip occurs, since the patient cannot flex fingers with the wrist in flexion, owing to weakness of synergistic muscles. Interphalangeal joint extension is preserved. Forearm is pronated; thumb is adducted, flexed, and opposed; wrist and fingers are flexed; deformity is most apparent with forearm flexed at the elbow.

Median Nerve. The median nerve arises from two roots—the medial cord and the lateral cord of the brachial plexus; the fibers derive from C5–C6 and T1–T2. Motor fibers supply the pronator muscles, the radial flexor muscle of the wrist, the superficial flexor muscle of the fingers, the radial half of the deep flexor muscle of the fingers, the long palmar muscle, the long flexor muscle of the thumb, the short flexor muscle of the thumb, the short abductor muscle of the thumb, the opposing muscle of the thumb, and the two or three radial lumbrical muscles. Sensory impulses are supplied to the radial half of the palm of the hand and of the palmar surfaces of thumb and index and middle fingers, the palmar aspect of the radial half of the ring finger, the dorsal aspect of the middle and distal phalanges of index and middle fingers, and the radial half of the ring finger.

Clinical Reflections. Clinical manifestations of loss of function include paralysis of wrist flexion and of thumb and radial finger flexion, poor grip, loss of pronation, inability to oppose or approximate the thumb and fingertips. *Inability to flex distal phalanx of index finger is pathognomonic*; wrists are supinated and drawn toward the ulna. Pronator syndrome results from compression of the median nerve as it passes between the two heads of the round pronator muscle just below the elbow. More common is carpal tunnel syndrome, which is caused by compression of the nerve under the transverse carpal ligament of the wrist. Causes of compression include synovitis, tumor, trauma, thickened ligaments, rheumatoid or gouty arthritis, and myxedema. Men experience these syndromes more frequently than women. Compression of the median nerve is often bilateral and is the commonest cause of hand paresthesias.

Ulnar Nerve. The ulnar nerve originates from the medial cord of the brachial plexus and receives fibers from C7–C8 and T1. It innervates the ulnar flexor muscle of the wrist, the ulnar half of the deep flexor muscle of fingers, the adductor muscle of the thumb, the medial head of the short flexor muscle of the thumb, the short palmar muscle, the interosseous muscles, the ulnar lumbrical muscles, and the muscles of the hypothenar eminence. Sensation goes to the dorsal and palmar aspects of the ulnar side of the hand, the little finger, and the ulnar half of the ring finger.

Clinical Reflections. Flexion and adduction of wrist and fingers are compromised; hand is turned toward the radius; extension of distal phalanges and flexion of proximal phalanges are lost; adduction and abduction of fingers are impaired, and thumb adduction is lost. Grip of the two ulnar fingers is weak; hypothenar atrophy occurs—less so in the thenar eminence. Palm is "hollowed"; interosseous spaces are deeply grooved; hyperextension of fingers occurs at the metacarpophalangeal joints, and flexion occurs at the interphalangeal joints (claw hands). No useful reflex abnormalities and no trophic changes occur. Combined median and ulnar nerve paralysis may occur, with consequent complete claw hand. Volkmann's ischemic contracture simulates combined median and ulnar nerve paralysis.

Axillary Nerve (Circumflex). The axillary nerve receives fibers from C5–C6 through the posterior cord of the brachial plexus. It winds around the neck of the humerus and supplies the deltoid and teres minor muscles. Sensation is tested from the surface of the upper and outer aspects of the arm. Etiology of injury includes pressure in the axilla, fracture, dislocation of the head of the humerus, and perforating wounds or direct blows to the shoulder. It is commonly involved in peripheral neuritis.

Clinical Reflections. Clinical reflections include failure of abduction, weakness of external rotation of the arm, inability to raise the arm to a horizontal plane, with some weakness of flexion, extension, and internal rotation. Anesthesia of a small area on the outer surface of the upper third of the arm also occurs.

Musculocutaneous Nerve. It is derived from C5–C6 and C7 and the lateral cord of the brachial plexus. It innervates the biceps, brachial, and coracobrachial muscles. Sensation is supplied to the lateral aspect of the forearm from the elbow to the thenar eminence. It is rarely involved in syndromes.

Clinical Reflections. Clinical reflections include weakness of flexion of the forearm and marked weakness of supination. Semipronated forearm is still flexed by brachioradial muscle; that is, it is functionally serviceable. Small area of anesthesia of lateral surface of forearm occurs; biceps muscle reflex is absent.

Long Thoracic Nerve. It is derived from C5–C8 and supplies the serratus anterior muscle. It may be injured by continuous heavy effort with the arm above the shoulder or through the pressure

of carrying heavy objects on the shoulder or by supraclavicular or axillary wounds; paralysis of the serratus muscle results, with winging of the scapula.

Phrenic Nerve. It is the principal respiratory nerve and is derived from C3 through C5. It supplies motor fibers to the diaphragm and sensory fibers from the diaphragm, pericardium, points of the costal and mediastinal pleurae, and extrapleural and extraperitoneal connective tissues.

Clinical Reflections. The phrenic nerve may be involved by neoplasm, penetrating wound, and unilateral or bilateral paralysis. Unilateral paralysis results in no symptoms, whereas bilateral paralysis causes dyspnea (on even slight exertion), abdomen scaphoid (does not protrude on expiration), retraction of the epigastrium on deep breathing, and overactivity of accessory respiratory muscles. Symptoms include uncomfortable cough or sneeze.

Syndromes Due to Postural Faults, Muscle Strain, and Muscle Imbalance[12, 13]

This section is concerned with clinical problems caused by muscle imbalance, strain, or faulty posture as they relate to painful syndromes of the upper thoracic and cervical portions of the spine. Painful syndromes in the lower back, pelvis, and legs are closely related, as are pain syndromes in the upper trunk, upper thoracic spine, neck, and arms. Abnormalities of posture and alignment of the pelvis and lower back also may require correction of abnormal alignment of the upper trunk, where the painful symptoms are noted. Postural pain in the upper trunk is quite characteristically different from that of lower back postural pain. Muscles are commonly overdeveloped in the lower back and demonstrate the adaptation of shortening; management is that of heat, massage, and stretching of the contracted muscles. Overdevelopment of muscles is usually due to a disparity between lengths of agonist and antagonist muscles. In the case of the upper trunk the muscles are weakened and stretched, and management entails correction of overstrain and increasing the strength of the muscles.

Trapezius Muscle Strain

Definition. The lower and middle portions of the trapezius muscle become painful owing to chronic and continual tension. This is a common condition that sometimes becomes constant and chronic. Rarely is the onset acute, although the pain may become quite disabling.

Etiology and Pathogenesis. Continuous and sustained contraction, often due to habitual forward positioning of the shoulders and a round upper back (or some combination of these postural faults), results in stretch weakness and chronic muscle strain. Shoulders may be pulled forward chronically by overdevelopment and shortening of the muscles of the anterior shoulder girdle. Heavy breasts that are inadequately supported sometimes contribute to faulty upper back and shoulder position. Excessive compression of the anterior surfaces of the thoracic vertebral bodies occurs.

Genetic and Environmental Factors. The syndrome is commonly related to particular jobs. For example, drawing, using a microscope, and working at a desk or from a high stool are all commonly causative.

Incidence and Epidemiology. No specific data; related to postural abnormalities of specific job.

Tissue Involved. Middle and lower trapezius muscle.

Symptoms. Soreness and fatigue, sometimes ultimately resulting in a "burning" pain along the course of the lower and middle trapezius; symptoms usually not constant. Lying down or changing the sitting posture provides relief. Symptoms may become severe and acute owing to an element of traction by the muscle on its enthesis, the site of tendon-bone junction.

Signs. Focal points of marked tenderness (sore spots) often at sites of attachment of the trapezius to the dorsolumbar spine; pectoral muscles and tendons tight and tender. Chronic fatigue common; adaptive shortening of the pectoral muscles; symptoms and signs seen much more commonly in older people than in young adults. In the presence of rounding of the upper back, pain and tenderness in the posterior neck occur; with thoracic spine kyphosis the head is carried forward to preserve the erect position of the head; cervical spine hyperextension.

Radiologic Characteristics. None specific.

Laboratory Data. No findings.

Special Studies. No findings.

Treatment and Management

1. Heat and massage to the upper back over the area of painful muscle strain.

2. Various supports of the shoulders to bring them back in a position that relieves trapezius tension.

3. Postural training in preserving normal lumbar and cervical lordosis and thoracic kyphosis.

4. A brassiere that lifts and supports.

5. Postural correction of "forward shoulders."

6. Taylor brace sometimes useful.

7. Change of occupation.

8. Exercises: With back to the wall, 1) abduct both shoulders to 80 to 90 degrees; press both elbows against the wall; hold for 6 to 10 seconds; release; repeat 6 times, 2 to 3 times daily; 2) extend both arms forward, with palms facing each other; with elbows in extension, arms straight, move arms slowly backward against wall; hold for 6 to 10 seconds; release; repeat 6 times, 2 to 3 times daily; 3) pull arms back against the wall in a diagonal overhead position (strengthening of the trapezius).

Prognosis. Generally good.

Strain of the Upper Trapezius Muscle

Definition. Strain of the upper trapezius, the portion extending from the occiput to the acromial process of the scapula. Strain in this portion of the trapezius causes pain—commonly an acute syndrome—in the posterolateral portion of the neck.

Etiology and Pathogenesis. Acute or chronic contraction of the upper trapezius muscle. Strain experienced when reaching for something while holding the head tilted in the opposite direction may be the initial event. Arm abduction requires trapezius contraction with the scapula fixed; lateral head tilt tenses the muscle.

Genetic and Environmental Factors. Specific movements associated with activity, sports, and job.

Incidence and Epidemiology. No specific factors.

Tissue Involved. Upper trapezius muscle.

Symptoms. Pain in the posterolateral portion of the neck; excessive spasm and contraction, with tenderness of this portion of the muscle.

Signs. Tight, tense, and tender upper trapezius muscle along its insertion, from occiput to acromion.

Radiologic Characteristics. None.

Laboratory Data. None.

Special Studies. None.

Treatment and Management. Massage and kneading, gentle and increasingly firm as muscle allows the pressure; note relaxation occurring; direct pressure upward to relieve tension of the muscle above (downward stroking is irritating). Soft collar is useful; overall vigorous application of heat is not effective.

Prognosis. Generally good. Expect pain to last from days to a week, with eventual complete relief.

Postural Cervical Spine Pain Syndrome

Definition. Pain in the posterior neck associated with either muscle tightness or muscle strain or both; very common; usually gradual onset of symptoms, with chronic strain symptoms becoming constant.

Etiology and Pathogenesis. Continuous and sustained muscle spasm in the cervical spine, with no specific underlying causative disease; faulty posture of the cervical, thoracic, or lumbar portions of the spine; faulty mechanics due to excessive compression of the zygapophyseal joint facets posteriorly and of the posterior surfaces of cervical vertebral bodies; stretch weakness of anterior vertebral neck flexors (muscle imbalance between agonist and antagonist); tight cervical spine extensors, upper trapezius, splenius capitis, and cervical erector muscles; consequent compression or impingement of the suboccipital nerves emerging through fascial and muscular structures at the occiput; occipital headache associated with the pain.

Genetic and Environmental Factors. Postural imbalance of various types; sometimes job related.

Incidence and Epidemiology. No pertinent factors.

Tissue Involved. Extensor, flexor, lateral flexion, and rotator muscles of the cervical spine.

Symptoms. Pain in the posterior neck; weakness of anterior cervical flexor muscles; occipital headaches; sense of tension in the back of the neck.

Signs. Extensor muscles tight on palpation; cervical spine movements limited except in hyperextension; less pain in recumbent position, but when syndrome is severe, the pain is troublesome in any position.

Radiologic Characteristics. Sometimes a "straight" cervical spine; otherwise normal radiogram.

Laboratory Data. No specific findings.

Special Studies. None.

Treatment and Management

1. Daily heat, massage, and stretching exercises; massage should be gentle and relaxing, with deep kneading.

2. Stretching of tight muscles is accomplished only very gradually with active and assisted movement; patient performs stretching exercises by "flattening" the cervical spine, with chin down and in ("chin on chest"). (*Note*: This is comparable to pelvic tilt in efforts to flatten the lumbar spine in cases of excessive lordosis.) Exercises should be performed in supine and sitting positions, never in prone position. Hyperextension exercises are contraindicated.

3. Faulty head position compensates for dorsal kyphosis, which may be due to postural defects in the lower back or pelvis. Thus, it may be necessary to treat the neck pain by correcting postural abnormalities in the lumbar spine with, for example, abdominal muscle strengthening exercises.

4. Abdominal support occasionally useful.

Prognosis. Generally good.

Coracoid Pressure Syndrome

Definition. Arm pain with clinical symptoms and signs of compression or irritation of the brachial plexus; associated with muscle imbalance and faulty posture; occurs at attachment of the smaller pectoral muscle to the coracoid process of the scapula. The three cords of the plexus and the axillary artery and vein pass beneath these structures and the rib cage; forward depression of the coracoid process follows in some faulty postural alignments, narrowing the space. Forward depression of the shoulders with tilt of the coracoid process down and forward can occur from tightness or strain of muscles pulling in that

direction; the tilt may be due to weakness of other muscles, allowing the coracoid process to ride into that position. Principal specific muscle is the smaller pectoral; the rhomboid muscles and the levator muscle of scapula pull up, shifting the scapula upward but with forward depression; tightness of the latissimus dorsi muscles indirectly depresses the humeral head, as does tightness of the greater pectoral muscle; treatment of the biceps and coracobrachial muscles (also originating on the coracoid process along with the smaller pectoral muscle) may be effective.

Etiology and Pathogenesis. Multiple causes related to the previous formulations of muscle function.

Genetic and Environmental Factors. None.

Incidence and Epidemiology. No specific factors.

Tissue Involved. See muscles previously noted as resulting in forward shoulder depression.

Symptoms. Muscle weakness of the lower trapezius; constant pain due to tightness of the smaller pectoral muscle; strikingly tender pressure over the coracoid process, with radiation of pain down the arm; pain in the anterior chest; may be confused with cardiac or breast disease; paresthesia, numbness, weakness, poor grip in the hand; puffiness of the hand, sometimes slow emptying of veins of the hand; rarely cyanosis.

Signs. Tenderness over the coracoid process; tightness of the muscles involved, particularly the smaller pectoral muscle; neurologic signs when the problem is extreme; tenderness of the upper trapezius muscle distribution; protective spasm.

Radiologic Characteristics. None.

Laboratory Data. None.

Special Studies. None.

Treatment and Management

1. Early in an acute episode, a sling to support the weight of the arm (relieving the weight on the shoulder) is symptomatically useful.

2. Heat and massage to the upper trapezius.

3. Stretch of the pectoral muscles.

4. With patient in a supine position with knees flexed, the involved arm is placed in as much overhead extension as tolerated.

5. Heat as infrared, electric pad or hot, wet compresses applied to the tight pectoral muscles.

6. Massage: gentle and relaxing, progressing to kneading and stretching.

7. Sometimes excessive pressure by brassiere straps in woman with large breasts may be a factor. An appropriate brassiere is needed.

8. Strengthening exercises.

9. Correction of the specific faulty posture, such as shoulder girdle faults.

10. Avoid head and shoulder exercising from a supine position (movement increases compression in the anterior shoulder region); shoulder adduction which depresses the humeral head and coracoid process is to be avoided.

Prognosis. Good.

Teres Muscle Syndrome

Definition. Arm pain in axillary or radial distribution due to posterior brachial plexus cord pressure at a level above the pain site.

Etiology and Pathogenesis. Axillary nerve emerges between teres major and teres minor, supplying the deltoid muscle; radial nerve goes under the teres major and long head of the triceps muscle, spiraling around the humerus, supplying extensor muscles of elbow, wrist, and finger; teres major, an internal rotator, is tight or strained, holding the humerus in internal rotation; teres minor, an external rotator, is tight by being in tension due to internal rotation; syndrome is due to compression of nerve trunk around the humeral head.

Genetic and Environmental Factors. None specific.

Incidence and Epidemiology. No specific factors.

Tissue Involved. Teres major and teres minor muscles, axillary and radial nerves.

Symptoms. Pain in the distribution of the radial and axillary nerves; pain worsens with active motion, suggesting irritation to the axillary nerve by teres muscle movement.

Signs. Pain increased by active motion; specific internal or external rotation actively or passively very painful; external rotation limited; active abduction movements painful since the humerus does not rotate outward normally as it should during abduction; may simulate subacromial bursitis; tenderness over the triangle between the teres major and teres minor causes sharp pain radiating into the deltoid area. Palpation over the long head of the triceps muscle and elbow extension against resistance are painful; arm hangs in a position of internal rotation, that is, the palm of the hand faces more posteriorly than toward the side of the body (as is normal).

Radiologic Characteristics. None.

Laboratory Data. None.

Special Studies. None.

Treatment and Management

1. Heat and massage to the under portion of the arm and pectoral areas.

2. Stretching exercises for internal humeral rotators; stretching of arm in overhead extension and in external rotation accomplished very gradually over several days. An assistant should hold the scapulae back to localize stretching to the scapulohumeral muscles rather than to the muscles that attach the scapulae to the spine—that is, the trapezius and rhomboid muscles, which are often already stretched by abducted scapulae.

Prognosis. Good.

Cervical Nerve Root Syndrome

Definition. Though cervical nerve root compression is basically a part of the syndrome of cervical osteoarthritis, particularly with zygapophyseal and Luschka joint involvement, faulty posture of the cervical spine may either contribute to cervical nerve root compression or be primary in etiology.

Etiology and Pathogenesis. Postural production of hyperextension of the cervical spine, with a forward head position and consequent compression on the zygapophyseal and Luschka joints and on the posterior surfaces of the bodies of the cervical vertebrae.

Genetic and Environmental Factors. None.

Incidence and Epidemiology. No specific factors.

Tissue Involved. Cervical spine nerve roots.

Symptoms. Pain and paresthesias similar to syndromes described for cervical osteoarthritis.

Signs. Signs of anterior and posterior nerve root compression.

Radiologic Characteristics. Hyperextension of the cervical spine; may see radiologic characteristics of cervical osteoarthritis with the additional postural causative factors operating.

Laboratory Data. No specific findings.

Special Studies. None.

Treatment and Management

1. Cervical spine collar, intermittently used.

2. Correcting postural defects in alignment and muscle balance.

3. Avoid hyperextension of the cervical spine; support the weight of the head by transmitting its weight to the shoulder girdle (if the collar exerts slight traction, an upward lift will result).

Prognosis. Generally good.

Cervical Rib Syndrome

Definition. Though a more specific description of cervical rib syndrome appears elsewhere in this chapter (see *Vascular Diseases and Syndromes*), it is important to recognize that postural abnormalities may render a cervical rib (otherwise quite asymptomatic) symptomatic. Malalignment secondary to posture often helps determine whether painful syndromes will occur. The occurrence of symptoms and the presence of a symptomatic cervical rib in adult life are due to postural defects in most instances. Gradual loss of normal cervical, thoracic, and lumbar alignment changes the relationship of the rib and the adjacent nerve trunks, with resultant symptoms. Faulty alignment causes forward head position, and postural correction may be all that is needed, obviating surgical intervention.

HERITABLE DISORDERS—GENETIC AND CONGENITAL

Congenital Disorders

This section deals with congenital anomalies of the cervical spine. They are often painful and first appear in adult life. They are treated here as a group (see Chapter 15, *Congenital Anomalies*, for more detail). The onset of clinical manifestations in adulthood, the differential diagnosis, and an awareness that congenital anomalies present primarily in adult life are important. These disorders include the previously noted basilar invagination, occipitalization of the atlas to the occiput, Arnold-Chiari malformation, and anomalies of the atlantoaxial vertebrae—with and without subluxation. There is a major association of vascular as well as neurologic anomalies in the adult with these bony abnormalities. For example, aplasia of one vertebral artery may result in cerebral ischemia or central nervous system anomaly.

Clinically, congenital cervical defects are most often diagnosed in the asymptomatic adult after a trauma because, at that time, the patient has symptoms, and radiograms are obtained.

Definition. See Chapter 15, *Congenital Anomalies*.

Etiology and Pathogenesis. Based on the embryonic, transitional, unstable nature of the upper cervical spine—mainly the atlas, axis, and occiput.

Incidence and Epidemiology. Precise data not available.

Tissue Involved. Bone, capsule, ligament, spinal cord, nerve root, nerves, joints, and blood vessels in the cervical spine.

Symptoms. Pain in occiput and neck, dizziness, vertigo (usually related to movements of the head), unsteady gait, paresis of the limbs, paresthesia, hoarseness, diplopia, auditory noise, dysphagia, and speech disturbance.

Signs. Abnormality of gait, nystagmus, abnormal reflexes with asymmetry, hypesthesia, bowel and bladder disturbances, and hypalgesia increasing distally. More uncommonly, signs of raised intracranial pressure, somnolence, and organic psychologic changes. Also, short, broad neck, high scapula, low hairline, deformed skull, kyphosis or scoliosis, dwarfism, funnel chest, pes cavus, or equinovarus with partial syndactyly.

Radiologic Characteristics. See Chapter 15.

Laboratory Data. See Chapter 6, *Radiologic Evaluation*, and Chapter 7, *Craniometry and Roentgenometry of the Skull and Cervical Spine*.

Special Studies. See Chapters 6 and 7.

Treatment and Management
1. Be certain of accurate diagnosis and precise defects present.
2. Consult with neurologist, neurosurgeon, or orthopedic surgeon.
3. Consider neurosurgical procedure if threatening neurologic signs are present.
4. Physical therapy as moist heat, ultrasonography, and gentle active exercises—range of motion and strengthening within the constraints of symptom production.
5. Congenital anomalies may be discovered in adult life and require no treatment if they are not clearly symptomatic or are not threatening disability.

Prognosis. Generally good; dependent on severity of lesion.

Congenital Stenosis of the Cervical Spinal Canal

Definition. Congenital narrowing of the sagittal diameter of the spinal canal to 13 mm or less.

Etiology and Pathogenesis. Due to developmental errors.

Incidence and Epidemiology. Little definitive data available.

Tissue Involved. The cervical spine, particularly the upper portion.

Symptoms. Cervical spinal cord endangered later in life with development of cervical osteoarthritis and intervertebral disc protrusions, which further compromise spinal canal diameter. Individuals within this population are at risk if involved in sports or trauma. This disorder is frequently not recognized. Early spinal cord compression, ataxia, spasticity, weakness of the extremities, sense of heaviness, "marble" sensation, cervical spine pain, legs "don't feel right."

Signs. Narrow intervertebral canal at atlas level—sagittal diameter less than 18 mm; difficulty with gait; decreased cervical spine mobility; hyperactive reflexes, pathologic reflexes, positive Hoffmann's sign, positive Babinski's sign; gross weakness; and sensory loss. In adults a sagittal diameter measuring less than 13 to 15 mm between C4 and C7 is an ominous sign because it implies spinal cord compromise at some time by trauma or cervical osteoarthritis. Klippel-Feil syndrome and Arnold-Chiari syndrome usually are not recognized until adult life.

Radiologic Characteristics. See Chapter 6, *Radiologic Evaluation* and Chapter 7, *Craniometry and Roentgenometry of the Skull and Cervical Spine*.

Laboratory Data. See Chapters 6 and 7.

Special Studies. See Chapters 6 and 7.

Treatment and Management. Generally neurosurgical procedure.

Prognosis. Variable and individualized.

Note: Cervical ribs as congenital lesions are far more commonly recognized in adult life than in childhood.

Genetic and Congenital Disorders

Syndrome of Occipital Neuralgia (C2 Nerves) in Adolescents and Young Adults[14–16]

Note: See *Trauma* in this chapter.

Definition. This syndrome is distinctive in the age group in which it is seen and consists of the clinical signs of a C2 occipital neuritis.

Etiology and Pathogenesis. This syndrome has a wide variety of etiologic and pathogenetic mechanisms, notably trauma. Previously undiagnosed, usually common congenital anomalies are brought to light by the syndrome. Genetic implications are often those of heritable defects in the upper cervical spine (see Chapter 15, *Congenital Anomalies*).

Incidence and Epidemiology. No specific data available. Over a 3-year period, the author has seen 13 patients in this age group with the syndrome.

Tissue Involved. Joints, ligaments, tendons, and structures in and about the foramen magnum and the second occipital nerves.

Symptoms. Cervical and occipital headaches, occipital neuralgia with scalp pain and tenderness, paresthesia in the distribution of the second cervical dermatome, loss of normal cervical lordosis, and neurologic signs—usually mild but definite. Reflex spasm of the posterior neck muscles, occipital tension, a tense and anxious adolescent or young adult.

Signs. Tenderness over the posterior scalp on one or both sides; temporal and retro-orbital pain in more severe cases, with scalp tenderness; loss of light touch sensation in the distribution of C2 posterior root over the scalp; shoulder higher on one side than the other (sometimes); clinical evidence of a cervical rib; low hairline; clinical suggestion of platybasia; cardiac murmurs; scoliosis and kyphosis; short or very long neck; occasional loss of consciousness.

Radiologic Characteristics. Plain films may show cervical rib; congenital malformations of first and second cervical vertebrae; deformity of occipital condyles, platybasia; cervical or thoracic hemivertebrae (limitation of motion of the cervical spine); eight cervical vertebrae with fusion of some of the bodies; slight rotary subluxation at the atlas level; palpable transverse processes that are tender; odontoid abnormality.

Laboratory Data. No specific abnormalities noted.

Special Studies. CAT scan very useful; tomogram; biopsy rarely indicated.

Treatment and Management

1. Be certain of precise diagnosis of the syndrome, which is distinctive in adolescents and young adults.

2. Thomas collar often promptly effective.

3. Consider appropriate management of a congenital anomaly if found—physical therapy, heat application, and gentle stretching exercises.

4. Reassure the patient regarding the nature of the problem.

5. Anesthetic blocking of the C2 nerve may be useful.

Patient may show other signs of seemingly unrelated congenital and genetic physical defect, such as body asymmetry, left handedness, evidence of muscular imbalance, talipes equinovarus, or some historical evidence of mild neurologic lesion dating back to early life. Minimal trauma antedates the headache, usually leading to proper

identification of a cervical spine lesion. The distribution of the second cervical segment immediately calls attention to atlantoaxial joint disorders that can produce this type of sensation along the perivertebral regions and in the arms or even the legs.

The disorder generally results from instability of the atlantoaxial joint, with resultant signs of high cervical or brain stem lesion. Early recognition and treatment are very important.

Prognosis. Variable; a function of the specific lesion.

Long Neck [17]

Definition. On clinical observation of the cervical spine in slight extension, the neck appears long in comparison with an average neck of normal length.

Etiology and Pathogenesis. A clinically insignificant congenital anomaly characterized by the location of more than seven cervical vertebrae above the clavicle (65 cases reported).

Incidence and Epidemiology. Unknown.

Tissue Involved. Cervical vertebrae varying in location.

Symptoms. Usually asymptomatic; increased range of motion in the cervical spine compared with an estimated normal range of motion; may show other congenital anomalies, which will influence the clinical presentation.

Signs. An apparent long neck.

Radiologic Characteristics. Lateral films of the cervical spine show more than seven vertebrae above the clavicle.

Laboratory Data. None.

Special Studies. CAT scan may be useful and interesting; full ordinary radiograph of the cervical spine, including the AP, lateral, neutral, flexion, and extension views, both oblique views, and the open-mouth view.

Treatment and Management. Usually nothing required.

Prognosis. Excellent.

Cervical Spine in Fibrodysplasia Ossificans Progressiva [18, 19]

Definition. A hereditary mesodermal disorder characterized by progressive ossification of striated muscles, tendons, ligaments, and fasciae.

Etiology and Pathogenesis. Classified as hereditary disorder on the basis of two lines of evidence: (1) two sets of homozygous twins with the disease; (2) high association of congenital digital anomaly—bilateral microdactyly of the first toes with thin cortices of the phalanges.

Genetic and Hereditary Factors. Pattern of inheritance unknown; probable autosomal dominant trait with a wide range of expressivity. Most reported cases are spontaneous mutations. No known sexual predilection.

Incidence and Epidemiology. No specific data available.

Tissue Involved. Potentially all mesodermal structures; formation of true bone in connective tissues. Figure 11–1 shows a patient, age 14, with fibrodysplasia ossificans progressiva.

Symptoms. Onset usually occurs in the first decade. Ossification is not present at birth. Torticollis is the most frequent presenting symptom and is due to the painful mass within the sternocleidomastoid muscle. The disease progresses with ossification from the shoulder girdle to the upper arms, spine, and pelvis. Distal extremities are involved late in the course. Heart, diaphragm, larynx, tongue, and sphincters are spared, as are all smooth muscle structures. The natural history of the disorder is one of remissions and exacerbations. New episode of ossification is precipitated by minor trauma, with the first symptoms being heat, edema, and a painful mass. These are followed by fever. As the pain decreases, the mass gradually hardens as new bone.

Signs. Clear evidence of ossification of the soft tissues, abdominal wall, and particularly the cervical spine. Limitation of cardiac and pulmonary

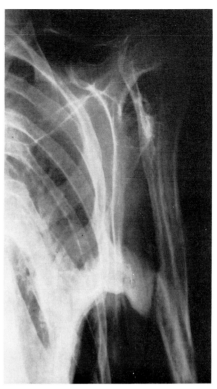

Figure 11–2. Fibrodysplasia ossificans progressiva. True bone in soft tissues, muscle, ligament, tendon, and, in some places, even skin.

function, although these structures are normal. Swelling, heat, and redness in an area of newly developing ossification. Crippling and deformity are consequences of contractures of the areas of involvement (Fig. 11–2).

Radiologic Characteristics. Digital anomalies at birth (see Fig. 11–3). Bony abnormalities seen in all patients. Small cervical vertebral bodies with enlarged pedicles in early childhood; variable fusion of the vertebrae apparent in all patients; fusion first noted between adjacent neural arches in late childhood, but it also involves the vertebral bodies in some adult patients; often associated with ossification of adjacent neck muscles as well as the dermis in the skin. Very important cause of serious and disabling neck stiffness and immobility. Radiologic changes readily confused with Still's disease (juvenile polyarthritis) or the Klippel-Feil syndrome (Fig. 11–3).

Laboratory Data. No specific findings.

Special Studies. Many special examinations may be needed and are useful, depending on the specific mechanical problems arising from the rigidity produced by ossification throughout.

Treatment and Management. No satisfactory treatment; clinician deals with the problems as they arise.

Prognosis. Poor.

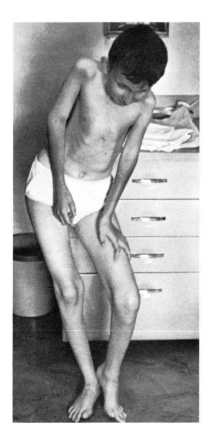

Figure 11–1. A 14-year-old patient with fibrodysplasia ossificans progressiva. True bone has formed in most soft tissues, with gross rigidity and postural deformity.

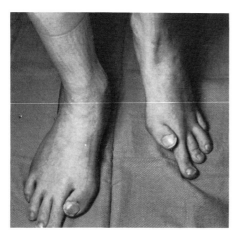

Figure 11–3. Digital anomalies of fibrodysplasia ossificans progressiva.

Tophaceous Gout [20–22]

Note: See *Endocrine and Metabolic Disorders* in this chapter.

Definition. Gouty arthritis of the cervical spine, though unusual, does occur. Symptomatic gout initiated by monosodium urate (MSU) crystal deposition in the cervical spine—as elsewhere.

Incidence and Epidemiology. See references 20–22.

Tissue Involved. Bone, joint, tendon, and ligament of the cervical spine.

Symptoms. Cervical spine pain; radicular symptoms; limitation of motion in the cervical spine; neurologic involvement, with occasional loss of power; paresthesias with no known or documented protrusion of tissue into the spinal canal.

Signs. Associated, intermittent podagra, effusions in peripheral joints, and chronic tophaceous gout.

Radiologic Characteristics. Lytic lesions, bony involvement and encroachment, characteristic radiologic findings of gout in the peripheral joints.

Laboratory Data. No pertinent findings other than those relevant to systemic gout.

Special Studies. Tomograms and CAT scans have been useful.

Treatment and Management. The same as for the management of gout generally.

Prognosis. Good.

INFLAMMATORY DISORDERS
Rheumatoid Arthritis [23–26]

Definition. A chronic inflammatory disease, most probably infectious in etiology, with broad immunologic, environmental, and autoimmune underlying mechanisms. The descriptions that follow apply only to the relatively few severe cases.

Etiology and Pathogenesis. Infection—probably viral; metabolic and biochemical abnormalities; autoimmune and genetic mechanisms. The pathogenesis is ultimately that of a severe inflammatory process mainly in and around joints, with final enzymatic destruction of the supporting tissues, including cartilage and bone.

Incidence and Epidemiology. The prevalence rate of rheumatoid arthritis in the United States varies from 0.3% to 1.5%. The prevalence increases with advancing age, up to the seventh decade. Rheumatoid arthritis is clearly associated with HLA-Dw4 and the B-cell alloantigen HLA-DRw4. The incidence is estimated at approximately 3.1% of the population.

Tissue Involved. Includes mainly articular and periarticular tissues, although virtually all tissues of the body may be involved in varying magnitude. The cervical spine, particularly the upper portion, is the second most commonly involved area in the body.

Symptoms. Cervical spine pain—neck, temporal area, and retro-orbital area. Paresthesia, hypesthesia, hyperesthesia, and anesthesia. Weakness of arms and legs, vertigo, nystagmus, loss of consciousness, drop attacks, quadriplegia, transient blindness, hyperparesis, atrophy of peripheral muscles, and death.

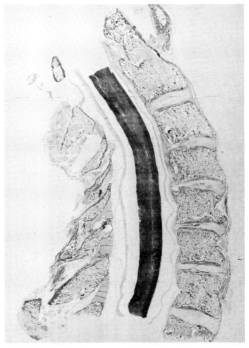

Figure 11–4. Whole human cervical spine in sagittal section. Note spinal cord and meninges; erosion on the posterior odontoid process; narrow discs without osteophytes; severe atlantoaxial subluxation; vertebral erosions.

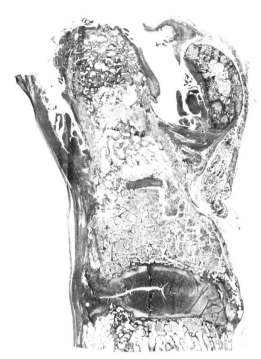

Figure 11–5. Histologic sagittal section of the axis and the anterior arch of the atlas of a patient with rheumatoid arthritis. Note odontoid process and anterior arch atlas erosions; destruction of the transverse ligament; the interesting phylogenetic remnant of the intervertebral disc at the base of the odontoid process.

The clinical symptoms reflect the pathologic process in the cervical spine, most severely at the occiput-atlas-axis complex. Upper and lower motor neuron myelopathic symptoms may occur from compression of the spinal cord at any level.

Signs. Upper and lower motor neuron manifestations, mainly the former; disturbance in gait; loss of sensory perception at the level at which the nerve roots or spinal cord is compromised; bowel and bladder dysfunction; hyper-reflexia, hyporeflexia, and even areflexia; inability to sit or stand; spastic quadriplegia; loss of motor power; "jumping legs"; rheumatoid nodules; radiologic evidence of gross subluxation—vertical, atlantoaxial, and subaxial.

Radiologic Characteristics. See Chapter 6, *Radiologic Evaluation*. Evaluation by computed tomography with multiplanar reconstruction provides an accurate assessment of the magnitude and type of subluxation.

Laboratory Data. High-titer rheumatoid factor concentration in serum; very rapid Westergren sedimentation rate: eosinophilia, thrombocytosis.

Special Studies. Tomogram discloses loss of bony tissue and extensive subluxation. Figure 11–4 shows a whole human cervical spine made

into a single section. Note the erosion on the posterior odontoid process, narrow discs without osteophytes, and the atlantoaxial subluxation. Figure 11–5 is a histologic sagittal section of the axis and the anterior arch of the atlas of a patient with rheumatoid arthritis. Figure 11–6 shows a tomogram of severe dislocation of the atlas on the axis, with the odontoid process situated in the foramen magnum. The odontoid process is eroded; there is subluxation of the axis on C3; the anterior arch of the atlas is to the right, the posterior arch to the left. Note that the space between the anterior surface of the posterior arch of the atlas and the posterior surface of the odontoid process is less than that between the anterior arch of the atlas and the anterior surface of the odontoid process. There is very little space for the spinal cord, and it was involved in a severe myelopathy.

Treatment and Management

1. Educate the patient extensively concerning the natural history of rheumatoid arthritis of the cervical spine.

2. Treat the overall disease. Patients with rheumatoid arthritis of the cervical spine generally have much more severe rheumatoid disease—seropositive, nodular, extra-articular mani-

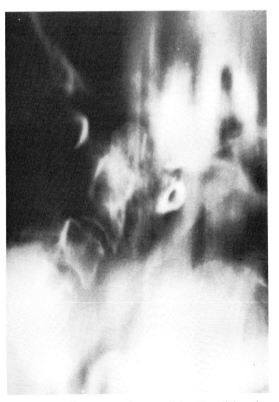

Figure 11–6. Tomogram of severe dislocation of the atlas on the axis, with the odontoid process situated in the foramen magnum.

festations—than those with rheumatoid arthritis of other areas, and their prognosis is usually worse than that for others.

3. Clinically define the precise abnormalities occurring in the cervical spine, such as subluxation of the atlas on the axis, vertical subluxation, pain syndromes and their mechanisms, so that management is directed at the abnormality in question.

4. Prescribe collars, braces, or combinations of the two. All patients with significant subluxation require collar or brace management.

5. Seek neurologic consultation if there are neurologic symptoms and signs.

6. Prescribe systemic, daily rest.

7. Recommend cervical spine (as well as general) exercises to enhance strength and range of motion and to maintain ligamentous, tendinous, and capsular integrity in the joints of the cervical spine.

8. Recommend relaxation techniques.

9. Suggest pillows for the cervical spine—Cervi pillow, Wal-Pil-O, or "Shape of Sleep" pillow.

10. Refer patient to physical therapist, occupational therapist, social worker, or brace maker.

11. Apply heat, with trial of the various modalities; trial of cold therapy is always worthwhile.

12. Prescribe anti-inflammatory drugs (less emphasis on analgesic drugs), immunosuppressive drugs, and remission-inducing drugs depending upon the overall severity of disease and the immediate social, economic, and job responsibilities of the patient.

13. Consider surgery for management of the cervical spine; consult neurosurgical or orthopedic surgeon. Consider cervical spine fusion and release of nerve entrapments. Approximately 5% to 10% of patients with cervical spine rheumatoid arthritis require surgical fusion.

Prognosis. Generally good for 85% of the population with rheumatoid arthritis.

Ankylosing Spondylitis[27]

Definition. An inflammatory arthropathy with a striking predilection for the cartilaginous joints of the axial skeleton. Because 95% of patients with ankylosing spondylitis have HLA-B27, the disease has major genetic implications.

Etiology and Pathogenesis. An inflammatory disease attacking the joints of the axial skeleton, the nonsynovial, cartilaginous synchondroses of the intervertebral spaces, the diarthrodial synovial joints, and the sacroiliac joints. The basic lesion is an enthesopathy.

Incidence and Epidemiology. The prevalence rate is 1.5 to 2 persons per 1000 in a white population; widespread geographic incidence, varying with the presence of HLA-B27 (histocompatibility complex) in the population.

Tissue Involved. Major target tissue is primarily cartilage, especially fibrocartilage; frank osteitis of underlying adjacent subchondral bone, fibrous tissue of joint capsules, and anulus fibrosus occurs. About 25% of patients have peripheral arthritis, but not with the inflammatory intensity seen in rheumatoid arthritis. Men are more clinically involved than women.

Symptoms. Gradual onset of pain and aching in the lower back and both buttocks (bilateral pseudosciatica). Morning stiffness that improves with exercise. Peripheral arthritis found in 15% to 25% of patients with ankylosing spondylitis. Average age of onset is 15 to 30 years. Characteristic features of back pain or discomfort are (1) age at onset below 40 years, (2) insidious onset, (3) duration longer than 3 months, (4) association with morning stiffness, (5) improvement with exercise.

Signs. Diminished motion in the entire spine. Chest expansion reduced to less than 1 inch. Focal points of tenderness: heels, sternum, iliac crest, ischial tuberosity. Peripheral joints may be swollen. Positive result of Schober's test. Forward flexion limited; sacroiliac joint tenderness and pain (Gaenslen's sign). HLA-B27 positive.

Radiologic Characteristics. Sacroiliac joint inflammatory signs, syndesmophytes, squaring of vertebrae, "shiny corners" on vertebrae, evidence of ankylosis in the spine, and loss of normal lumbar lordosis. Root joints more involved than peripheral joints, hips, and shoulders. Radionuclide bone scans show areas of inflammation.

Five per cent of cases have either aortic incompetence or cardiac conduction defects; iritis occurs in 25%. Other characteristics include atlantoaxial subluxation and fractures of the rigid segments of the spine (mainly cervical). Lytic lesions are uncommon; "Bamboo" spine occurs.

Laboratory Data. Erythrocyte sedimentation rate elevated in 80% of cases. Mild anemia. Negative results of latex fixation test. Synovial fluid inflammatory. WBC up to 20,000 per mm^3—mostly polymorphonuclear leukocytes.

Special Studies. Radionuclide scanning in questionable instances of sacroiliitis.

Treatment and Management. The guidelines provided here for treatment and management of ankylosing spondylitis also apply to the following other syndromes: juvenile polyarthritis, psoriatic cervical spine involvement, Reiter's disease, and the seronegative spondylotic arthropathies with involvement of the cervical spine. Management of these syndromes is the same because of their clinical pathologic and radiologic overlaps.

1. Stretching and strengthening exercises. Cervical massage, active and passive exercises, stretching. Postural exercises; hard bed. Extension exercises. Remind the patient that the disorder tends to produce loss of height and anterior curvature; exercises should be performed twice daily.

2. Breathing exercises.

3. Appropriate treatment of primary disease.

4. Patient education. Teach the natural history

of ankylosing spondylitis and the hyperostotic manifestations of the other disorders listed. Prognosis is generally good.

5. Drug therapy—notably aspirin, indomethacin, phenylbutazone, and muscle relaxants, usually recommended intermittently.

6. Hot tub baths, Hubbard tank treatments, hydrocollator packs, heating pads, and infrared lamps.

7. Majority of patients with ankylosing spondylitis may expect a good prognosis and a successful life pattern; disease progresses to severe and total ankylosis in relatively few patients. Patients with ankylosing spondylitis should stop smoking completely because they are at risk of developing pulmonary disease.

8. Swimming is the best routine exercise or sport.

9. Admission to active and vigorous rehabilitation unit should be considered.

10. Application of moist heat prior to exercise.

11. Genetic counseling should be considered.

12. Antibiotic therapy in certain instances of Reiter's syndrome.

13. Surgery is rarely indicated.

Therapy should be carried out if and when the disorders appear. Figure 11–7 illustrates a fracture following a relatively minor fall, with subluxation at the C4–C5 level of the spine. Figure 11–8 shows a fatal, complete fracture in a totally ankylosed spine. Figure 11–9 illustrates a completely ankylosed cervical spine in a patient with ankylosing

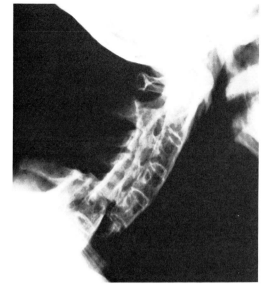

Figure 11–8. Fatal, complete fracture in a totally ankylosed cervical spine shearing through the spinal cord.

spondylitis. Note the anterior arch of the atlas and a missing posterior arch.

Prognosis. Good in the majority of diagnosed patients.

Osteomyelitis

Definition. Infectious spondylitis can be caused by a variety of pyogenic bacteria, too often from

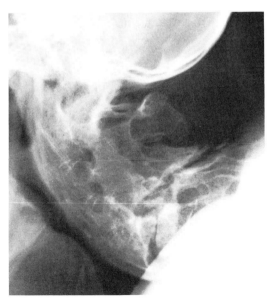

Figure 11–7. A through-and-through fracture following a relatively minor fall, with cord compression injury at the C4–C5 level of the spine.

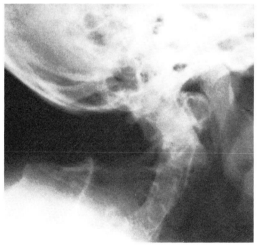

Figure 11–9. Completely ankylosed cervical spine in a patient with ankylosing spondylitis. Note the anterior arch of the atlas and a missing posterior arch.

an iatrogenic source. It is now rarely caused by the *tubercle bacillus*. Cervical spine bone infection can follow scarlatina, measles, whooping cough, and other infectious diseases. The most common organism is still the *staphylococcus*. The cervical spine is relatively immune to infection compared with the rest of the spine. Route of entry is hematogenous unless introduced by extension from the nasopharynx, a puncture, or an open wound. The venous plexus of Batson is valveless and hence may be the site of entry, though nutrient arteries are a much more ready access route.

Etiology and Pathogenesis. Infection in bone.

Incidence and Epidemiology. Rare; preceded by history of injury; possible previous tuberculous or urinary tract infection. Epidemiology dependent on preceding clinical circumstance.

Tissue Involved. Bone and joint, with occasional spread to soft tissues.

Symptoms. Neck pain, referred to shoulder or occiput; limitation of neck movement in all directions; head fixed in a deformed position; fever, chills, and general illness. Symptom severity dependent on virulence of the infectious agent and resistance of the patient. Osteomyelitis usually occurs in children.

Signs. Meningismus; tenderness of the cervical spine; long tract signs late; striking tenderness to gentle percussion over the cervical spinous processes at the involved area.

Radiologic Characteristics. None early. After days to weeks, radiographic changes appear as an increase in the soft-tissue shadow between the anterior vertebral body and the pharynx. Xeroradiography is useful. Destruction of bone and narrowing of disc space and sequestra occur late; difficult to differentiate sepsis from tumor. Radionuclide scanning is useful for showing increased bone activity at the site of infection.

Laboratory Data. Positive results of blood cultures or cultures from direct aspiration of the vertebra.

Special Studies. Radionuclide scan.

Treatment and Management

1. Bedrest.
2. Identify organism and treat with appropriate antibiotics.
3. Consultation concerning infectious disease.
4. Systemic rest and only minimal exercise of the neck.
5. Surgical intervention required in serious neurologic involvement, in instability due to excessive bone destruction, or to drain an abscess if conservative treatment fails.

Prognosis. Generally good.

Bursae of the Cervical Spine[28–30]

Definition. The bursal spaces between the interspinous processes can become clinically involved in rheumatoid arthritis, monosodium urate (MSU) crystal–induced inflammation, calcium py-

rophosphate dihydrate (CPPD) crystal inflammation, and enthesopathic lesions of the spinous processes. An association between intervertebral disc lesions (rheumatoid arthritis and osteoarthritis), spinous process erosion by enthesopathy, and interspinous bursitis is noted. There have been listed 156 bursae in the body.

Etiology and Pathogenesis. Dependent upon etiologic factors present; MSU or CPPD crystals, osteoarthritis, rheumatoid arthritis, osteomyelitis.

Incidence and Epidemiology. It appears these bursae may be involved in many different processes with unknown incidence and little available epidemiologic data.

Tissue Involved. Bursae between the spinous processes in the cervical spine; their presence is a function of the closeness of the spinous processes to one another. They are narrow slits lined with synovium; their function is lubrication.

Symptoms. Tenderness and pain in the interspinous area if the bursae are inflamed. Note they are on the surface of the ligamenta flava.

Signs. The bursae may have rheumatoid granulomatous involvement about or around them in patients with rheumatoid arthritis, though there is no specific rheumatoid granulomatous involvement in the bursae themselves; erosions (radiologic) of spinous processes consequent to an enthesopathy of the posterior interspinous ligaments; occurrence of syndrome in ankylosing spondylitis as well as rheumatoid arthritis. Posterior cervical pain can be explained by these inflamed bursae; congenital anomalies such as myositis ossificans progressiva are also associated with such bursal lesions.

Radiologic Characteristics. None pertinent except the bony spinous process erosions.

Laboratory Data. None specific.

Special Studies. Biopsy of the bursal material.

Treatment and Management. Active inflammation may occur primarily in association with rheumatoid arthritis, osteoarthritis, or ankylosing spondylitis.

1. See Chapter 10, *Problem-Oriented Approach*, regarding necessity for precise diagnosis.
2. May require no therapy other than management of the overall disorder.
3. Anti-inflammatory drugs.
4. Physical therapy; heat; trial of cold therapy is worthwhile.
5. Consider injection of corticosteroid if bursa can be precisely identified.

Prognosis. Generally good.

Otologic Symptoms and Signs in Cervical Spine Syndrome

Note: See *Osteoarthritis, Trauma, Vascular Diseases and Syndromes*, and *Neoplastic Lesions*.

Definition. Dizziness, tinnitus, deafness, and transient loss of vision occurring in the course of a broad variety of cervical disorders.

Etiology and Pathogenesis. EENT symptoms and signs have been observed and reported in poor posture syndromes, acute muscular torticollis, rheumatoid arthritis, occipital neuritis, carotid sinus syndrome, cervical spine syndrome, and acromioclavicular osteoarthritis. Head and neck lesions producing neck or arm symptoms include arteriosclerotic cerebral changes and Meniere's syndrome. Combinations of cervical osteoarthritis and chronic otitis media or subacromial bursitis and chronic sinusitis may result in EENT symptoms. Other etiologies include neck sprain with traumatic rupture of an eardrum, neck sprain with postconcussion syndrome from cerebral contusion, or metastatic tumor to the head and neck. If there is no measurable or identifiable organic disease, psychoneurosis is likely the etiology.

Genetic and Hereditary Factors. No specific data available.

Incidence and Epidemiology. No specific data available.

Tissue Involved. Sympathetic nervous system, large and small blood vessels of the cervical spine, vestibular apparatus, muscle, bone, and joint.

Symptoms. Unilateral or bilateral headache, tinnitus, variable deafness, dizziness, and true vertigo. Tinnitus as ringing, hissing, buzzing, or clicking. Deafness of perceptive type, mild to severe. Dizziness; positional vertigo and some episodes of rotational vertigo; blurring of vision and retro-orbital pain ("eyes being pulled from behind"); dilation of pupil on the same side; pharyngeal sense of tickling and lump in the lower throat; fatigue and anorexia (probably secondary); nausea and vomiting. Either compression of or thrombosis of the vertebral artery is suspected and is either confirmed or ruled out by vertebral artery angiography with catheterization. The symptoms are often reversible by changing position of the head and neck. Some suspect venous congestion in the basilar system, since it has softer vessels and the vertebral venous system is more likely to be compressed.

Signs. Exaggeration of symptoms by changing neck and head position; manual traction may relieve symptoms, and manual compression downward (Spurling test) may produce or intensify symptoms. Relief by cervical collar or brace; reversible audiographic findings on treatment. Successful stellate ganglion block with lidocaine (Xylocaine)—success is demonstrated by presence of Horner's syndrome. Paresthesia, sweating changes, and lacrimation are reversed by simple management procedures.

Radiologic Characteristics. Those of the disorders in which EENT symptoms may occur.

Laboratory Data. No specific data.

Special Studies. Audiometry; extensive neurologic examination; occasionally special radiologic methods, such as tomography. Psychiatric consultation.

Treatment and Management. Apply optimum management as it relates to clinical formulation of mechanism of production of symptoms.

Prognosis. Good.

Syndromes of Flaccid Neck Paralysis

Note: These syndromes may also be related to endocrine and metabolic etiology. See *Endocrine and Metabolic Disorders* in this chapter.

Definition. Paralysis and extreme weakness of the upper cervical spine rotators, extensors, and flexors and of the lower cervical spine extensors and flexors may occur in a variety of diseases—poliomyelitis, myasthenia gravis, polymyositis, dermatomyositis, and long-standing rheumatoid arthritis with severe cervical spine involvement.

Etiology and Pathogenesis. As noted for the diseases previously listed.

Genetic and Hereditary Factors. Genetic implications of rheumatoid arthritis; HLA-DRw4 antigen; no other pertinent data.

Incidence and Epidemiology. No specifically pertinent data.

Tissue Involved. Neural and muscular structures of the cervical spine and occiput.

Symptoms. Head falling about when the patient moves with any speed, restricting the subject to immobility. Note that even rather marked paralysis may be overlooked by the clinician as a reason for a given patient's inactivity; motion of the head not controlled well clinically. Inability to utilize movements of the head to extend the field of vision or to allow more effective use of other senses. Patient has adopted odd postures and measures—seldom workable—to make the head stable. Complaints secondary to compression and collapse of pharyngeal and esophageal structures (difficulty swallowing and talking). Patient may manually hold the head up in position for speaking and swallowing.

Signs. May be wearing brace. Unable to tolerate full weight of the head resting on chin support or forehead strap.

Radiologic Characteristics. Esophageal study may reveal difficulty in swallowing. Etiology of the weakness or paralysis, such as rheumatoid arthritis or myasthenia gravis, may be revealed by radiologic investigation.

Laboratory Data. Muscle enzymes—CPK, LDH, SGOT, SGPT; Westergren sedimentation rate; latex fixation test; HLA typing; neurologic consultation.

Special Studies. Electromyography; immunologic studies for myasthenia gravis.

Treatment and Management

1. Trials of collars and braces, with use of exercises to maintain any minimal strength that may remain; halo apparatus.

2. Spinal fusion between the second cervical and the second thoracic vertebrae (avoid damage

to the capital muscles); fascial transplants have been useful and effective (fascia lata).

3. Neurologic consultation.

Prognosis. Poor.

Acute Suppurative Thyroiditis: Thyroglossal Duct Abscess[31]

Though rare, pain, fever, and marked tenderness of soft-tissue structures in the neck occur in the differential diagnosis of cervical spine pain. Thyroglossal duct septic abscess and acute suppurative thyroiditis have similar symptoms and signs. Appropriate therapeutic application requires their differentiation from other causes of painful thyroid-related neck masses. Ultrasonography and thyroid radioscintigraphy are new techniques used in making this differential diagnosis.

OSTEOARTHRITIS

Osteoarthritis of the Intervertebral Discs[32, 33]

Definition. In young people and in the course of early development of osteoarthritis, the intervertebral discs are involved. In some instances there is acute protrusion of the nucleus pulposus into the spinal canal at several sites about the posterolateral aspects of the vertebra (central, posterolateral, intraforaminal). Because of the anatomic characteristics of the uncinate processes (joints of Luschka), it is nearly impossible for a nucleus pulposus or other cartilaginous disc material to protrude into the lateral foramina at the level of the Luschka joint. The nuclear protrusions constitute a small minority of cervical disc lesions; the great majority proceed to chronic osteoarthritis without acute protrusion, which is usually a severe, temporary, totally disabling syndrome. This section deals with the acute intervertebral disc syndromes, the so-called soft disc lesions; the intervertebral disc syndromes of osteoarthritis, which are much more common, are termed hard disc lesions. Soft disc lesions are more successfully approached surgically than hard disc lesions.

Etiology and Pathogenesis. There are no well-established and secure etiologic mechanisms other than those of the well-known osteoarthritis of the intervertebral discs. The pathogenesis is that of the four cellular and tissue manifestations of osteoarthritis in the intervertebral discs. In this particular instance, it is an acute protrusion of the nucleus pulposus or other disc material into the spinal canal (see Chapter 3, *Pathology*).

Genetic and Hereditary Factors. No firm evidence of contribution by specific genetic factors other than those of osteoarthritis generally.

Incidence and Epidemiology. Relatively common and occurring in a younger age group than that of the usual cervical osteoarthritis patient—most such patients have their lesions at one or, at most, two levels of protrusion rather than at multiple levels.

Tissue Involved. Intervertebral disc material, nucleus pulposus, anulus fibrosus, and fibrocartilaginous pieces protruded into the spinal canal.

Symptoms. Pain in the posterior or lateral portions of the neck, severe in acute disc protrusion. Dull or aching discomfort below the level of severe pain. The discomfort worsens with fatigue, tension, postural factors, and hyperextension of the spine.

Signs. Most common at C5–C6, C6–C7; pain and subjective sensory deficit commonly over the radial aspect of the forearm, thumb, and index finger. Weakness and atrophy of the biceps muscle; biceps reflex exaggerated, reduced, or absent; pain and subjective sensory deficit over the dorsum of the forearm, wrist, and index, middle and occasionally ring fingers, with weakness of the triceps muscle and diminished or absent triceps reflex. Symptoms of cord compression are paresthesias and weakness of the hands, with progressive, spastic paresis; both upper and lower motor neuron signs; spinal fluid may have increase in protein concentration level.

Radiologic Characteristics. May be no abnormality on routine radiogram. Disc height commonly maintained. Evidence of early osteoarthritis—posterior shift of a vertebral body on bending, coupled with flexion beyond the normally parallel end plate; facet overriding on anteroposterior and lateral projection; vacuum phenomenon; may see early cleft formation; traction chondroosteophytes. Filling defect may be seen on myelography in patients with disc disease, depending on location and size of the protrusion. Discography is very rarely indicated, and complications render the risk of the procedure too great relative to its benefit.

Laboratory Data. No specific findings other than the cerebrospinal fluid manifestation.

Special Studies. Myelography (see previous discussion). Special (oblique) views of the cervical spine to show any narrowing of the intervertebral foramina.

Treatment and Management

1. Patient education; most patients treated without surgery.

2. Rest in bed or with limited activity.

3. Cervical spine exercises within the constraints of pain and symptom production.

4. Sedation, muscle relaxant drugs, analgesic drugs.

5. Cervical spine traction—intermittent to assess results in progress.

6. Heat—hot, moist packs, shower, ultrasound.

7. Careful follow-up regarding progression of neurologic signs; neurosurgical consultation.

Intradiscal corticosteroids in the treatment of cervical disc problems have been used with significant success. The success rate is in the magnitude of about 20%.[33] For intractable pain in the neck, shoulder, and arm and posterolateral rupture with extrusion of a soft intervertebral disc fragment, decompression of the involved root and excision are necessary. Acute central cervical disc protrusion, though relatively uncommon, is more serious, since cord compression and transverse myelopathy are possible.

Acute, prolapsed cervical intervertebral disc occurs most commonly in the third to fourth decade of life. Men outnumber women in a ratio of 1.4:1. Associated relatively strongly with prolapsed cervical disc were cigarette smoking and frequent diving from a board. Of borderline significance, but not statistically significant, were operating or driving vibrating equipment and time spent in motor vehicles. Variables that did not affect the risk for a prolapsed cervical disc were participation in sports other than diving, wearing shoes with high heels, number of pregnancies or live births, frequent twisting of the neck on the job, time spent sitting on the job, and cigar or pipe smoking.

Prognosis. Excellent.

Clinical Symptoms and Signs at Specific Cervical Disc Levels

Note: The symptoms and signs discussed here also apply to the following other sections of this chapter: *Idiopathic Disorders, Heritable Disorders, Inflammatory Disorders, Osteoarthritis, Neoplastic Lesions, Trauma, Vascular Diseases and Syndromes, Endocrine and Metabolic Disorders,* and *Disorders of the Cervical Cord.*

The first intervertebral disc is between the second and third cervical vertebrae. Cervical root 1 emerges between the occiput and the atlas, and cervical root 8 is between the seventh cervical and first thoracic vertebrae, thus when a cervical intervertebral disc protrudes, it compresses the root that is one higher in number. For example, a disc protrusion at the level of C6 affects the seventh cervical root.

*C1 **and** C2 Roots.* Neck pain radiates to vertex of skull, temporal area, forehead, and retro-orbitally (C2); pain (usually unilateral) arises in joints of upper cervical spine; pain mechanism is that of dura mater involvement, adhesions, and extrasegmental reference and it is not necessarily due to first and second cervical roots (pain in the head).

Unilateral pain of the upper neck and paresthesias in the occipitoparietal region with decreased cervical spine rotation suggest osteoarthritis of the atlantoaxial joint, with a chondro-osteophyte compressing the C2 root.

C3 Root. Rarely affected. Paresthesia and numbness at the ear, the posterior portion of a cheek, the temporal area, and the whole lateral aspect of the neck. No muscle weakness; unilateral analgesia of skin on portions of the neck. Frequently mistaken for symptoms and signs of psychoneurosis or some undiagnosed disorder; vertebral artery insufficiency is a part of the differential diagnosis. Rule out trigeminal neuritis.

C4 Root. Rarely affected. Pain radiates outward from midportion of neck and is concentrated at the shoulder. Paresthesias are absent. Transverse band of cutaneous analgesia near spine of the scapula and mid-deltoid area. No muscle weakness.

C5 Root. Pain from scapular area to anterior arm and forearm and the radial side of the hand, not involving the thumb. Paresthesia and weakness of the supraspinatus, deltoid, and biceps muscles. Biceps reflex diminished or absent. Brachioradial reflex sluggish, absent, or inverted.

Broad differential diagnosis required: rupture of either supraspinatus tendon, diaphragmatic pleurisy, subclavian artery syndrome; neuritis from long thoracic or suprascapular nerve, herpes zoster, myopathy, axillary nerve neuritis after shoulder dislocation.

C6 Root. Pain down radial side of anterior arm and forearm; paresthesias in thumb and index finger; cutaneous analgesia of tips of thumb and index finger; weak biceps muscle, weak short supinator muscle, weak radial extensor muscle of wrist; atrophy of brachioradial muscle; subscapular and serratus anterior muscles weak; biceps reflex diminished or absent.

Differential diagnosis: carpal tunnel syndrome, thoracic outlet syndrome, biceps tendon rupture (partial or complete), peripheral neuritis, and tennis elbow.

C7 Root. By far the most frequently affected in osteoarthritis. Pain from the scapular area down the posterior arm to the outer arm and the fingertips; paresthesias in index, middle, and ring fingers; pain is sometimes pectoral instead of scapular. Pain may be in the anterior upper thoracic spine; neck movements exaggerate pectoral pain and inhibit thoracic movements, but resisted abduction of the arm does not. Symptom-free upper limb; triceps and radial flexors are weak; much more uncommonly the extensors of the wrist are weak; triceps reflex uncommonly affected even if the muscle is weak. Cutaneous hypesthesia dorsum of the middle and index fingers. In instances of long duration, wasting of the greater pectoral muscle occurs as a triangular depression between the parts of the muscle from the sixth and eighth myotomes; *relief is provided by putting the hand on the head—a posture relieving tension on the root.* Patients advised to use this position in trying to fall asleep.

Differential diagnosis: radial nerve neuritis (crutch), old fracture of humerus, lead poisoning (always bilateral), bronchial carcinoma, tennis elbow, tricipital tendonitis, olecranon fracture.

C8 Root. Pain in lower scapular area of back or medial aspect of arm and inner forearm (paresthesias at third, fourth, and fifth fingers); weak ulnar deviators of the wrist, extensor and adductor muscles of the thumb, and extensor muscles of the fingers. Triceps muscle weak; cutaneous hypesthesia at the fifth finger.

Differential diagnosis: pressure on lower trunk of the brachial plexus (thoracic outlet syndrome), cervical rib, metastatic carcinoma at C7–T1 level, Pancoast's tumor, cardiac angina, ulnar neuritis, subclavian artery thrombosis.

T1 Root. Disc lesions rare at this level; most patients suspected of T1 root disorder have some other problem, such as cervical rib, secondary neoplasm, pressure on median or ulnar nerve, or pulmonary sulcus tumor.

Pain radiates diffusely over lower pectoroscapular area and down medial aspect of arm to ulnar border, where paresthesia is noted. Fingers unaffected. No weakness of the hand; if so consider neoplasm or cervical disc.

First thoracic root can be traumatized by forward movement of the scapula during elevation and abduction of the arm to horizontal plane, followed by stretching the ulnar nerve in elbow flexion. Both movements aggravate thoracic pain, as do coughing and cervical spine flexion.

Cervical Disc Protrusion with Immediate Spinal Cord Compression

Note: See *Trauma* in this chapter.

Signs

Abrupt Onset. Severe, totally disabling pain in the neck, with unidentified mechanism, followed quickly by weakness and paresthesias in both upper extremities or in all four limbs, suggesting that the bulging posterior longitudinal ligament and the dura are causing the severe initial pain.

Was once called syndrome of transverse myelitis; pain in both scapular areas radiates to arms and forearms, may alternate from one arm to the other. Paresthesias of the soles of the feet are increased by cervical spine flexion. Displacement usually central; great limitation of extension; may suggest thoracic outlet syndrome or "sensory stroke"—difficult differential diagnosis. No tendency to spontaneous cure if the protrusion is central to the spinal cord.

Painless, Slow Onset. Slow onset is more common than abrupt onset. Difficulty in gait; upper motor neuron signs affecting both legs; both hands and feet paresthetic; sensation of pins and needles from the anterior knees to all toes; myelography shows protrusions that are often multiple (several sites of compression of the spinal cord); occurrence of both chondro-osteophyte formation and disc herniation, distinguishable only at laminectomy. Posterior longitudinal ligament has adhesions to the dura mater due to proliferative, thick fibrosis; neck flexion causes overstretch and further damage to spinal cord; pressure on anterior spinal artery may cause widespread ischemia and infarction in the cord, with paraplegia.

The signs previously listed may occur in an automobile crash secondary to acute cervical spine fracture. Differential diagnosis includes multiple sclerosis; dragging one leg may not necessarily be caused by pain in the neck; look for upper motor neuron signs; perform myelography to resolve doubt.

Tennis Elbow, Carpal Tunnel Syndrome, Rotator Cuff Tendonitis

Definition. The clinical symptoms and signs of carpal tunnel syndrome, tennis elbow, and rotator cuff tendonitis are well known. In most cases of each syndrome a clear cause for the syndrome is not shown. Idiopathic carpal tunnel syndrome has been noted in association with upper arm and shoulder pain, cervicobrachial pain, neck pain, and tennis elbow. Recent publications[34–36] strongly suggest that the cervical spine is a primary etiologic and pathogenetic source of these underlying conditions. Specifically, it is a reflex localization of painful radiculopathy. Clinical, radiologic, and electromyographic findings support this concept.

Etiology and Pathogenesis. Since the embryonic sclerotome, myotome, and dermatome cellular migrations of the neck, shoulder, anterior and posterior chest, and the entire upper extremity are from the cervical spine, referral patterns of all three may have their clinical origins in structures of the cervical spine from C5 through T1, the general pathophysiologic manifestations of cervical spine osteoarthritis (cervical spondylosis).

Genetic and Hereditary Factors. Only those referable to the evidence for genetic factors responsible for cervical osteoarthritis.

Incidence and Epidemiology. Tennis elbow, carpal tunnel syndrome, rotator cuff tendonitis, and osteoarthritis are all very common. When there is poor or no response to treatment of the first three, treatment directed to the cervical spine will relieve the majority of patients.

Tissue Involved. Connective tissue structures in the cervical spine, the tendons of the rotator cuff, the carpal tunnel, and the lateral and medial epicondyles and extensor structures inserting therein. Muscle atrophy in the appropriate locations in each clinical instance, weakness, tender motor points, muscle spasm, limitation of motion.

Symptoms. Characteristic symptoms of the three syndromes.

Signs. Limitation of motion, marked tenderness in the area of the lateral epicondyle (much less commonly, the medial epicondyle), swelling in the carpal tunnel area, positive results of wrist extension test, of Tinel's test, and of Phalen's test, diminished perception to light touch, muscle atrophy in the thenar eminence, muscular weakness where there is atrophy, autonomic signs (pilomotor and sudomotor), goose pimples (erector pili effect), increased perspiration (unusual), deep tendon reflex changes in more extensive cervical osteoarthritis.

Radiologic Characteristics. Varying degrees of cervical osteoarthritis; calcification of the tendons in the rotator cuff in the shoulder; more rarely, calcification in and about the lateral epicondyle.

Laboratory Data. No specific findings.

Special Studies. Radiologic study; electromyographic study. Special neurologic examination as indicated; identification of specific motor points, the site where muscle twitch may be evoked in response to minimal electric stimulation—a site very close to where the motor nerve enters the muscle. Many motor points of wrist extensors lie about lateral epicondyle of the humerus, where there is a rich supply of sensory nerve fiber endings.

Treatment and Management

1. Mobilization of the cervical spine according to Maitland's grades 1–4.[37]

2. Treat both the cervical spine and the localized disorder, as they are closely interrelated.

3. Cervical traction.

4. Isometric cervical exercises.

5. Heat, ultrasound, moist heat, particularly to zygapophyseal joints if excessive tenderness is noted.

6. Rest.

7. Judicious splinting.

8. Consider local corticosteroid injections followed by strengthening exercises.

Prognosis. Good.

Cervical Osteoarthritis

See *Trauma* in this chapter.

Definition. Modern use of the term cervical osteoarthritis implies the cellular and tissue events occurring in three areas in the cervical spine—the intervertebral discs, the zygapophyseal joints, and the joints of Luschka. The presumed pathophysiologic events in sequence in osteoarthritis in the cervical spine (and in any other joints) are as follows: (1) Some change occurs in the microenvironment of the chondrocyte, resulting in mitosis and overproduction of the elements of cartilage, type II collagen, and proteoglycans as well as of the multiple enzymes of synthesis and degradation known to be produced by the chondrocyte. (2) Activation, presumably by intercellular communication, of the osteoblasts in subchondral bone (the junction of hyaline cartilage and bone) occurs, with resultant increase in the rate of synthesis of the macromolecular components of subchondral bone. There follows thickening of subchondral bone, increase in density, and reduction in compliance. Microfractures follow, with callus formation, followed by more microfracture and more callus formation. (3) At the periphery of the joints, cellular metaplasia occurs (probably in the synoviocytes), and at the periphery of the bone, usually in the path of least resistance, chondroosteophytes are produced. They consist of bone and a mixture of fibrocartilage and hyaline cartilage and are coated with a layer of fibrocartilage.

(4) Pseudocysts form in the marrow just below subchondral bone, presumably secondary to joint fluid's being forced through microfractures in subchondral bone, with resulting cellular reaction about them.

Etiology and Pathogenesis. During the past two decades, the great increase in knowledge of the cell biology of osteoarthritis has allowed identification of considerably more etiologic factors and pathogenetic steps in the evolution of osteoarthritis.[38] Physical or biochemical events in hyaline cartilage that alter the microenvironment of the chondrocyte currently seem to be the initial triggering event. Most obviously, such disorders as ochronosis (homogentisic acid deposits in the cartilage), calcium pyrophosphate dihydrate (CPPD) crystal deposition disease (deposition of an excess of pyrophosphate in the hyaline cartilage), myxedema with an excess of proteoglycan, acromegaly with overproduction of all elements of connective tissue, trauma, any change in the biomechanical relationships within a joint, and genetic factors that alter the relative rates of synthesis of the macromolecular components of cartilage (primary generalized osteoarthritis) may trigger a "final common pathway" as described in the four pathophysiologic events previously outlined. It is not known whether the osteoarthritic process may be arrested or reversed, though there is some evidence to support this position.[38]

Terminology. Brain and Wilkinson in 1967[39] and Wilkinson in 1971[40] made enormous advances in knowledge of cervical osteoarthritis. In coining the term cervical spondylosis to indicate intervertebral disc osteoarthritis, they made the assumption that the remaining localization of osteoarthritis in the cervical spine (Luschka and zygapophyseal joint osteoarthritis) was secondary to the intervertebral disc disease rather than that it was all the same primary process or perhaps even three separate processes.

The position taken in this chapter is to utilize the term osteoarthritis to describe all joint involvement in the cervical spine, including all secondary manifestations in vertebrae, tendons, ligaments, capsules, muscles, and hyaline cartilage, without the overall assumption that the primary disorder begins in the intervertebral disc (see Chapter 3, *Pathology*). My objections to the term spondylosis are several: (1) The Greek derivation, spondylos (vertebra) and osis (an excess of), simply means an excess of vertebrae, whereas osteoarthritis means an excess of virtually all elements not only in but around the joints. (2) Cervical spondylosis as described by Brain and Wilkinson[39, 40] is clinically significant only very late in the course of the disorder, whereas virtually the entire population has "cervical spondylosis" that is asymptomatic. (3) Confusion arises because of the relative exclusion of clinical criteria in favor of reliance on radiologic diagnosis. Cyriax[41] lists 16 different disorders that may be grouped under the term cervical spondylosis:

1. Asymptomatic osteophyte formation radiologically noted at a cervical vertebral body or foramen.

2. Asymptomatic narrowing of one or more joint spaces, indicating erosion of an intervertebral disc.

3. Osteoarthritis causing upper cervical pain or pain in the head, zygapophyseal joints, and Luschka joints.

4. Chondro-osteophytic compression of one or more nerve roots—radiculitis, acute or chronic.

5. Chondro-osteophytic compression of the spinal cord—paresthesia in hands and feet, myelopathy.

6. Chondro-osteophytic compression of the anterior spinal artery—paraplegia.

7. Chondro-osteophytic kinking and tortuosity of the vertebral artery due to pressure from superior facet processes, compromising the vertebrobasilar circulation.

8. Cervical intervertebral disc lesion with unilateral or alternating scapular pain.

9. Cervical intervertebral disc lesion with bilateral cervical spine pain.

10. Cervical disc lesion causing headache by extrasegmental dural reference. (*Note*: The dura does not follow the anatomic segmental reference pattern at all. Extrasegmental reference from the dura is also common in the lumbar spine—a fact too little appreciated).

11. Cervical intervertebral disc lesion with unilateral scapulobrachial pain and without nerve root compression and neuritis.

12. Cervical intervertebral disc lesion with unilateral scapulobrachial pain and nerve root inflammation.

13. Cervical intervertebral disc lesion with bilateral aching in the upper limbs and paresthesia of the hands due to bilateral protrusion.

14. Cervical intervertebral disc lesion causing paresthesia in hands and feet as a consequence of central disc protrusion.

15. Cervical intervertebral disc lesion, compression of the spinal cord with one or more root inflammations in one or both upper limbs, and spastic paresis in the lower limbs.

16. The mushroom phenomenon at a cervical level (rare in the neck); occurs usually in elderly patients. When lying down with head supported on a pillow, patient is perfectly comfortable and can move painlessly. After sitting or standing, patient develops pain in the neck because the cervical joints have supported the weight of the head. If this compression continues, discomfort in both arms and paresthesias in the hands occur. Manual traction lifting the head up symmetrically relieves all symptoms.

Genetic and Hereditary Factors. Primary generalized osteoarthritis has strong genetic implications. Dominant in women; recessive in men.

Pattern of joint involvement is distal interphalangeal (DIP), proximal interphalangeal (PIP), and first carpometacarpal (CMC) joints; cervical spine, lumbar spine, knees, and first metatarsophalangeal (MTP) joint, seemingly skipping most other joints in the body.

Hereditary factors in ochronosis, CPPD crystal disease, gout, and rheumatoid arthritis may play a role in the occurrence of secondary osteoarthritis.

Incidence and Epidemiology. Cervical spine osteoarthritis becomes virtually universal in individuals 50 years of age and older.

Tissue Involved. All structures in and around the joint; intervertebral disc joints, zygapophyseal and Luschka joints, ligament, tendon, muscle, bone, capsule, hyaline cartilage, subchondral bone, and many other cervical and distant tissues secondarily involved.

The clinical syndromes, symptoms, and signs in osteoarthritis of the cervical spine are conveniently divided into the following five general categories, which overlap considerably: (1) involvement of the joints, intra- and extra-articular structures, with consequent clinical reflections; (2) nerve rootlets, anterior and posterior nerve roots, and anterior and posterior rami of the peripheral nerves; (3) compression of the spinal cord, cervical myelopathy; (4) involvement of the vertebral artery by the osteoarthritic process, notably at the atlas-axis-occipital level; and (5) esophageal involvement. The presentation of the remainder of this section of the chapter is organized according to these five categories.

Involvement of Joints—Intra- and Extra-articular Structures

Symptoms. Attacks, occurring approximately once per year, of waking with severe unilateral pain in the neck; neck is sometimes fixed in definite deformity, acute torticollis. Pain is constant, severe, and lasts 2 to 3 days. Recovery occurs in 7 to 10 days. Pain caused by joint involvement is more likely to arise from the upper cervical spine, whereas pain caused by intervertebral disc osteoarthritis is more likely to arise from the lower cervical spine.

Intermittent aching in the scapular area in patients 30 to 40 years of age lasts several weeks and is unilateral, varying from one side to the other. In patients 50 to 60 and even 70 years of age, ache may become constant. At any time after the age of 35 years, the appearance of moderate to severe unilateral cervical posterior root pain may occur. It becomes worse at night, with paresthesias in the hand. The arm pain is at its worst for 2 to 3 weeks but remains for 1 to 2 months, subsiding gradually. If there is root paresis, the pain is lost in about 3 months.

If bilateral disc protrusion occurs, pain is present in both upper limbs, and paresthesia occurs in the digits of both hands. Central protrusion presses on the posterior longitudinal ligament and the dura mater, which becomes adherent, fibrotic, and adhesive, resulting in constant bilateral aching from occiput to scapula. Bilateral disc protrusion occurs mostly in patients 60 years of age and older.

Motion is limited usually in only 1 to 3 of the six classic movements of the cervical spine; flexion is usually preserved, with lateral flexion, extension, and rotation limited. Painless restriction (painless stiffness) is interpreted as osteoarthritis.

Signs. Limited movement of the cervical spine in the capsular pattern (the capsular pattern is little or no limitation of flexion, equal limitation of side flexion and rotation, and either some or striking limitation of extension). Tenderness on manual compression of the zygapophyseal joints; general painless stiffness; osteoarthritis of the zygapophyseal, atlantoaxial, and atlanto-occipital joints causes ligamentous contracture and pain in the occiput and forehead (the pain is usually worse in the morning); difficulty in backing up a car.

Radiologic Characteristics. Zygapophyseal and Luschka joints show increased density of subchondral bone, varying degrees of chondro-osteophytosis, irregular narrowing of the joint spaces, and, somewhat unusually, pseudocysts.

Laboratory Data. Usually no specific findings except in relationship to an underlying, etiologic, pathogenetic disorder initiating the osteoarthritis.

Special Studies. Occasionally need tomography and cineradiography; open-mouth views, computed tomography, xeroradiography.

Treatment and Management

1. Patient education; teach the natural history of osteoarthritis of the cervical spine; the majority of people continue to be functional and effective.

2. Exercises—stretching and range of motion—include cervical, thoracic, and lumbar portions of the spine.

3. Cervical spine traction.

4. Physical therapy, heat, ultrasound. Diathermy, hydrotherapy whirlpool, heating pads. Infrared lamps, hot, wet packs (hydrocollator), hot-tub baths, Hubbard tank.

5. Special pillows (see Chapter 12, *General Management Methods*).

6. Analgesic and anti-inflammatory drugs; muscle relaxant drugs.

7. Special attention to patients with complications of cervical spine osteoarthritis, such as radiculopathy, peripheral neuropathy, myelopathy, esophageal involvement by osteophytes, and vertebral artery compressive syndromes. Neurologic, neurosurgical, or orthopedic consultation; traction in selected instances; hot, moist packs, ultrasound, and diathermy; cold packs in acute injury.

8. Relaxation techniques; relieve the emotional stress that aggravates the symptoms. Surgical procedures on the cervical spine are reserved for the rare patient who does not respond to conservative measures.

9. Cervical massage.

10. Treat shoulder, tennis elbow, and carpal tunnel if such symptoms appear.

Manipulation and manual traction have been used in some instances[42] and are very effective only in skilled hands.

Prognosis. Generally very good.

Syndromes of the Nerve Roots in the Cervical Spine

The clinical manifestations of nerve root involvement are like those of peripheral nerve disease. The distribution of the changes is different. Sensory changes include perversions of function, pain, paresthesia, anesthesia, hypesthesia, and hyperesthesia and are confined to dermatomes (skin areas supplied by specific cord segments, dorsal roots, or ganglia). Symptoms of nerve root origin, termed radicular, are increased by motion, cough, sneeze, strain, nerve root stretching, or any increase in intraspinal pressure. The pain is lancinating in character, usually intermittent, and rarely constant. It may be relieved by nerve root section medial to the dorsal root ganglia, spinal anesthesia, or intraspinal alcohol injection.

Etiologies for nerve root involvement are osteoarthritis, pachymeningitis, extramedullary tumors, protruded intervertebral discs, extradural abscesses, a variety of viral disorders, and active inflammation (nonspecific, noninfectious granuloma of rheumatoid arthritis). Sometimes muscle spasm alone causes nerve root compression.

Herpes Zoster (Viral Disease). Herpes zoster mainly affects dorsal root ganglia. Severe burning pain in dermatome distribution is associated with vesicles in cutaneous distribution of the involved root and ganglia. Residual pain (post-herpetic neuralgia) may remain after vesicles are gone. Motor involvement is rare. Herpes zoster usually accompanies some general debility or loss of immunologic competence. It is associated with systemic infections, leukemia, neoplastic infiltrations, or inflammation of vertebrae and nerve roots.

Tabes Dorsalis. Inflammatory and osteoarthritic changes about the dorsal roots and ganglia and in spinal cord posterior funiculi. Sensory changes, proprioception, delayed cutaneous pain response, autonomic changes, and loss of reflexes with muscle hypotonia but no loss of power.

Polyradiculoneuritis (Guillain-Barré Syndrome). Motor, sensory, and reflex changes as in polyneuritis of many other etiologies; extensive involvement; high protein concentration of the spinal fluid; ascending or axonal degeneration of anterior horn cells.

Refsum's Syndrome. Hereditary ataxic polyneuropathy. Visual and auditory symptoms, electrocardiographic abnormalities, increased protein content of cerebrospinal fluid, ataxia, and peripheral nerve reflections. Thickening occurs with infiltration of peripheral nerves but nerve roots are affected also.

Hereditary Sensory Neuropathy. Profound and superficial sensory disturbances, areflexia, trophic changes but *little motor dysfunction*, primary histologic changes in dorsal root ganglia.

Cervical Radiculopathy of Osteoarthritis. May be single or multiple, bilateral, symmetric or asymmetric, and the magnitude of involvement of each separate root is variable. Also commonly associated with myelopathy. The clinical syndromes are divided into acute, subacute, and chronic radiculopathies.

Acute Radiculopathy. Sudden onset of severe pain and aching in the dermatome distribution of the cervical nerve root involved. The pain perception is supplied to bones, joints, muscles, and blood vessels as well as skin, hence the radiation is wide—neck, shoulders, and down the arm and forearm to the digit. It may extend into the chest anteriorly and posteriorly, particularly with C5, C6, C7 nerve root involvement. Pain is altered by head and neck position. Scalp, retro-orbital, and cervical spine pains worsen with both active and passive rotation—lateral flexion, extension, and rotation are the most painful. The pain is not worsened by coughing unless there is acute intervertebral disc protrusion. Paresthesias occur within the dermatome.

Symptoms. In some patients muscular weakness and diminished or absent reflexes occur, reflecting involvement of the motor as well as the sensory root. Atrophy may occur rapidly, with fasciculations; tendon reflexes are diminished or lost.

Subacute Radiculopathy. Typical "brachial neuritis"; usually more than one root involved; pain in the neck with associated paresthesia and rather severe muscle spasm.

Signs. Mild muscle atrophy and hypotonia. Muscle weakness is uncommon. Frozen shoulder is frequent complication, as are tennis elbow and carpal tunnel syndrome.

Chronic Radiculopathy. Usually following unaccustomed exercise or work in an awkward position; insidious development of symptoms and signs; may only partially clear after an acute attack, with pain lingering.

Signs. See *Subacute Radiculopathy.*

Radiologic Characteristics. Narrowing of intervertebral disc spaces and of zygapophyseal and Luschka joints; chondrosteophytes about these joints; increased density of subchondral bone; loss of normal cervical lordosis; vacuum sign in intervertebral disc spaces.

Special Studies. Electromyography; special radiologic views to identify narrowed intervertebral foramina; tomography; computed tomography.

Treatment and Management

1. Patient education regarding probable ultimate outcome—prognosis is generally good.

2. Physical therapy; heat; occasionally cold therapy; gentle stretching and strengthening exercises; range of motion exercises; intermittent soft or hard plastic collar; anti-inflammatory drugs, occasional analgesic medication (little or no role for narcotic or potentially addictive drugs).

3. Traction judiciously applied, with close follow-up; monitor traction according to specific results obtained.

4. Cervical spine pillows.

5. Massage.

6. Occasional lidocaine (Xylocaine) and corticosteroid injection in areas of pain and spasm.

7. Hydrotherapy.

Cervical Myelopathy

Symptoms. Symptoms are clearly related to ischemia and compression of the spinal cord by spondylotic bars, hypertrophied ligamenta flava, surrounding structures, pressure and tension, and stretching and compression of the cord tissue; hence there is a great spectrum of variability in the clinical symptoms.

Disability increases subtly and is often preceded by a history of radicular symptoms and recurrent attacks of brachial neuritis. Paresthesia and dysesthesia of the hands, weak and clumsy function of the hands, weakness of the lower limbs, and vague, deep pain in the lower extremities. Numbness and tingling in the tips of the digits. The pain is often but not necessarily radicular in distribution. Gross compromise of perception of touch is not a feature in the average case. Vague impairment of light touch and tactile discrimination; pin-prick sensation. Sensory loss may be one or two dermatomes above the upper segmental level of the spinal compression. Vibration sense impaired or lost below iliac crest or costal margin. Some loss over the digits of the hands. Perception of passive movement in fingers and toes may be slightly impaired.

Signs. Atrophy of upper limbs variable; distribution a function of cord segments involved. If upper cervical enlargement is compromised, the supra- and infraspinatus muscles and the deltoid, triceps, biceps, and greater pectoral muscles may be involved as well as the dorsiflexion muscles of the wrists and fingers.

If the lower part of the cervical enlargement is involved, most wasting will be in the flexor muscles of the wrist and fingers and in the intrinsic muscles of the hand; the wasting is variable. Corticospinal tract involvement below the level of other involvement (if there is coexisting motor radiculopathy) causes signs of a lower motor neuron lesion; muscle fasciculation is not conspicuous; spastic weakness of the lower extremity occurs (one leg more than the other); mild general wasting as in paraplegia. Note that muscular wasting and pain may be associated with concomitant osteoarthritis of the lumbar spine.

Tendon reflexes are all of diagnostic importance. Normal jaw jerk with exaggerated tendon reflexes of the upper extremity suggests that the lesion is below the foramen magnum. Exaggerated, diminished, or absent jaw jerk suggests a lesion above the level of the pons.

Tendon reflexes in myelopathy are a function of both upper and lower motor neuron lesions—that is, anterior horn cells and hence lower motor neurons in the myelopathy of the corticospinal tract. Ultimate absence of reflexes with preceding period of exaggeration; inverted radial reflex; exaggeration of flexor finger jerks; positive Hoffmann's reflex; positive Babinski's reflex; abdominal reflexes are diminished but rarely lost; clonus; bowel and bladder control rarely, if ever, disappears.

Rarely, only the corticospinal tract is involved; symptoms are limited to the lower limbs—spastic paraplegia with no upper limb symptoms. Rarely, symptoms are motor only, with muscular wasting of the upper limbs and spastic weakness of the lower limbs, simulating motor neuron disease. Rarely, severe paraplegia or quadriplegia and loss of sphincter control occur.

Cerebrospinal fluid often shows increased protein content (80 to 125 mg per 100 ml). Pressure may be elevated, and the Queckenstedt test result may be positive. Passive extension of the neck may raise the pressure, indicating partial but not complete block.

Radiologic Characteristics. Radiologic changes of usual osteoarthritis; may note decreased sagittal diameter of spinal canal in lateral view.

Laboratory Data. No specific findings.

Special Studies. Narrowing of the sagittal diameter of the spinal canal as measured on standard radiographic film (see Chapter 7, *Craniometry and Roentgenometry of the Skull and Cervical Spine*); myelography; cineradiography combined with myelography; angiography of vertebral artery and venous system.

Treatment and Management. See all the features previously noted, with special adaptations for the problems of cervical cord compression.

Surgical therapy indicated in unusual circumstances only. Extensive laminectomy, foraminotomy, and excision of osteophyte not commonly successful (see Chapter 17, *Indications for Surgery: Trauma, Rheumatoid Arthritis, and Osteoarthritis*). The natural history of cervical spondylotic myelopathy is such that the disability is mild and after an initial period of deterioration, a static period lasting a number of years follows.

Esophageal Compression in Osteoarthritis

Note: See *Endocrine and Metabolic Disorders* in this chapter.

Definition. Esophageal compression by osteoarthritic chondro-osteophytes or compression by subluxated cervical vertebrae (atlantoaxial subluxation or subaxial subluxation in rheumatoid arthritis).

Symptoms. Dysphagia, sense of difficulty in initiating the act of swallowing (atlantoaxial subluxation); perception of discomfort or pain during swallowing; referred pain from the esophagus or the gastroesophageal junction to the chest.

Signs. Evident radiologic esophageal compression by anterior chondro-osteophytes in osteoarthritis. Note that some such lesions may be asymptomatic even though they appear grossly compressive.

Radiologic Characteristics. Demonstration of compression of the esophagus with consequent dysphagia.

Special Studies. Barium swallow studies; lateral view of the cervical spine in neutral, flexion, and extension positions; esophagoscopy and gastroscopy if there is any suggestion of ulceration at sites of pressure by the chondro-osteophytes.

Treatment and Management

1. No treatment indicated unless the patient has symptoms.

2. Apply the many possibly useful therapeutic maneuvers previously listed.

3. Surgical removal of the anterior osteophytes.

Vertebrobasilar Artery Insufficiency

See discussion under *Vascular Diseases and Syndromes* in this chapter.

NEOPLASTIC LESIONS—BENIGN AND MALIGNANT

Horner's Syndrome (Miosis, Ptosis, and Enophthalmos) with Ipsilateral Vocal Cord and Phrenic Nerve Palsies[43]

Definition. Newly recognized cervical spine syndrome. Horner's syndrome, with vocal cord and phrenic nerve palsies secondary to disruption of the sympathetic chain. Compromise of the phrenic nerve and the innervation of the ipsilateral vocal cord is usually due to metastatic carcinoma of the breast and probably occurs with other diseases, such as carcinoma of the lung.

Etiology and Pathogenesis. Metastatic lesions of carcinoma.

Incidence and Epidemiology. Unknown, other than those etiologic factors pertinent to malignant tumors.

Tissue Involved. Sympathetic chain and surrounding connective tissue.

Symptoms. Pain and weakness in the shoulder of the involved side. Intermittent hoarseness of the voice, blurring of vision, cervical spine pain, and weakness of shoulder abduction.

Signs. Supraclavicular adenopathy; ipsilateral miosis, ptosis, and enophthalmos; some hemifacial anhidrosis. Paralyzed hemidiaphragm.

Radiologic Characteristics. Computed tomography allows identification of lymph node infiltration (at the level of the sixth cervical vertebra).

Sympathetic, phrenic, and vagus nerves are in apposition and intimately related to the fifth cervical nerve and the internal jugular lymphatic chain. A metastatic tumor at this level would involve sympathetic, vagus, phrenic, and cervical nerve roots.

Characteristics of Related Syndromes. (1) Horner's syndrome, miosis, ptosis, enophthalmos, and hemifacial anhidrosis—ocular hypotonia, increased facial temperature, alteration of lacrimation, and tendency to cataract formation. (2) Dejerine-Klumpke syndrome—weakness along distribution of first dorsal nerve root; Horner's syndrome. (3) Pancoast's syndrome—pain in the shoulder and down the arm, Horner's syndrome, atrophy of small muscles of the hand, local rib destruction, and vertebral infiltration. Etiology is apical carcinoma of the lung.

Treatment and Management. Symptomatic management and treatment of the malignant disease.

Prognosis. Poor.

Syndromes of the Third Neuron of the Cervical Sympathetic System[44]

Note: These syndromes are also categorized in *Trauma* and *Vascular Diseases and Syndromes* in this chapter.

Definition. Lesions of the cervical sympathetic system at the third neuron level taking origin from the superior cervical ganglion. May involve the intra- or extracranial course, and its interruption may implicate the total system or be confined to one subdivision. Of considerable clinical importance are recognition of these syndromes (unusual though they are), clear delineation of well-defined, recognizable clinical symptoms and signs, and appreciation of their probable pathogenesis and prognostic characteristics.

The clinical syndromes are

  1. paralysis of the cervical sympathetic system;
  2. idiopathic hemifacial hyperhidrosis;
  3. hemifacial anhidrosis;
  4. postsympathectomy facial hyperhidrosis;
  5. the auriculotemporal syndrome (Frey's syndrome);
  6. ophthalmoplegic migraine;
  7. ptosis as a sole manifestation of oculosympathetic disease;
  8. cluster headaches syndrome;
  9. Raeder's syndrome;
  10. oculosympathetic paralysis associated with infective and toxic states.

Table 11–2 lists syndromes of the third neuron of the cervical sympathetic system. Table 11–3 depicts the most common etiologic mechanisms. Incidence and epidemiology are a function of the specific etiology and pathogenesis in each syndrome. Tissue involved is variable but always includes the third neuron of the cervical sympathetic system. Each syndrome will be separately characterized clinically.

Anatomy. The three-neuron pathway of the cervical sympathetic system is entirely undecussated. The first order of neurons relays in the ciliospinal center (Budge's center) in the region of the seventh and eighth cervical segments and the first thoracic segment. Vasomotor and sudorific fibers seem to extend to the upper thoracic cord as low as the level of T6. The second-order preganglionic fibers course through the cervical portion of the sympathetic chain, through the inferior and middle cervical ganglia, synapsing with cells of the superior cervical ganglion. There post ganglionic fibers of the third neuron separate into two divisions. The smaller remains extracranial and runs as a plexus around the external carotid artery to innervate sweat glands, blood vessels, the pilomotor system of the face, and to some

Table 11–2. SYNDROMES OF THE THIRD NEURON OF THE CERVICAL SYMPATHETIC SYSTEM

Hyperfunction
  Main trunk
    Associated with generalized sympathetic overactivity
    As an isolated lesion
  Branch
    Oculosympathetic system; ocular features only
    Facial system
      Hyperhidrosis (not solely of gustatory origin)
      Vasomotor changes
      Pilomoton
      Alteration of lacrimal secretion
Hypofunction
  Main trunk (Horner's syndrome)
  Branch
    Oculosympathetic system
      Total miosis, ptosis
      Pupillary motor division: miosis
      Tarsal division: ptosis
Deranged Function (abnormal innervation via cervical sympathetic system)
  Main trunk injury (e.g., postsympathectomy gustatory sweating)
  Auriculotemporal nerve injury (auriculotemporal nerve syndrome)
  Chorda tympani nerve injury (chorda tympani nerve syndrome)

Table 11–3. ETIOLOGY OF THE SYNDROMES OF OCULOSYMPATHETIC PARALYSIS

Migrainous States
  Migraine
  Ophthalmoplegic migraine
  Cluster headaches
Raeder's Paratrigeminal Syndrome (primary form)
Toxic and Infective States
  Adjacent lesions (e.g., middle ear, sinuses, mastoid, teeth); superior orbital fissure syndrome
  Distant lesions, lobar pneumonia

extent the lacrimal gland. The other division ascends as a plexus around the internal carotid artery. Within the carotid canal the artery is separated from the middle ear by the anterior wall of the tympanic cavity. Here sympathetic fibers separate from the internal carotid plexus and penetrate the very thin anterior wall of the tympanic cavity, forming the caroticotympanic nerve and running below the mucosal lining through the middle ear before re-entering the cranial vault.

Stimulation of the cervical sympathetic system causes lid lag, globe lag, diminished blinking, and retraction of the upper (sometimes the lower) eyelid. Smooth muscles of the upper and lower lids, superior and inferior tarsal muscles, contract with cervical sympathetic stimulation—a spastic form of lid retraction (thyrotoxicosis), with exaggeration of the sympathetic response. Exophthalmos may be intensified in thyrotoxicosis; it is readily produced in animals by sympathetic stimulation, reflecting the well-developed state of the orbital muscle of Müller (rudimentary in man).

Vascular and sudorific effects of stimulation are vasoconstriction and increased sweating homolaterally and increased lacrimation. Fibers subserving these functions are separate from those innervating the pupil. Pupils always dilate in emotional states, and the facial vascular response may be either pallor or blushing.

Paralysis of the Cervical Sympathetic System

Paralysis of the sympathetic chain results in constriction of the pupil. The constriction is striking when the lesion involves the seventh and eighth cervical and the first thoracic nerve roots. It is less striking with removal of the superior cervical ganglion and least striking with division of the intervening nerve trunk. This maximal constriction lasts only a few days, when the pupil becomes larger and more mobile. The pupillary light reflex is unaffected by sympathectomy—in fact, constriction may take place more rapidly and last a longer time. Ptosis is of slight degree and not as extensive as that in levator muscle palsy. A rise in the temperature of the homolateral side of the face is due to loss of vasomotor control. Uncommonly, lacrimation is affected, either decreased or increased. Hemifacial anhidrosis is a characteristic feature of Horner's syndrome, and it indicates the presence of a lesion below the bifurcation of the common carotid artery. It is possible that implication of the sweat fibers after they have left the main trunk may produce a similar effect. The sweat glands of the face are the only ones with an accessory nerve supply, but it is usually relatively inactive and of little clinical consequence. The gustatory sweat fibers are entirely parasympathetic. In an analysis of the pathogenesis of 216 cases of Horner's syndrome, Giles and Henderson[44] showed that the most common site of the lesion was the sympathetic trunk in the neck and in the postganglionic fibers prior to their intracranial course. Upper thoracic and lower cervical nerve roots were affected less than half as often. Intraspinal, intracerebral, and intracranial fibers were rarely implicated. Malignant disease was the most common etiology, whereas trauma and vascular disease were the usual causative agents at the anterior spinal nerve and brain stem levels respectively.

Idiopathic Hemifacial Hyperhidrosis

Definition. Excessive perspiration of one half of the face, occurring spontaneously usually in a warm environment and during eating. The entire side of the face sweats if involved, but the beads of sweat stand out particularly above the forehead and in areas about the zygomatic bone, nose, and upper lip. Spicy foods are provocative. Facial hyperemia may occur.

Etiology and Pathogenesis. Variable; mostly neoplastic lesion.

Incidence and Epidemiology. No available data; commonly associated with malignant disease. No genetic or hereditary implications.

Tissue Involved. Cervical sympathetic chain and the neurologic reflections.

Symptoms. Sweating on one side of the face; hyperemia; an annoyance but no systemic symptoms.

Signs. Flushing of the face; beads of sweat above the forehead and in areas about the zygomatic bone, nose, and upper lip; sometimes enhanced by emotional events; sweating may be blocked by cervical sympathetic anesthesia; sweating initiated by eating. Negative findings—no headache or ocular manifestation.

Radiologic Characteristics. No specific radiologic findings except for those that may be associated with tumor, primary or metastatic, in juxtaposition to the cervical sympathetic chain.

Laboratory Data. No specific findings except those associated with malignant disease.

Special Studies. None, except for specific clinical studies to identify hyperhidrosis.

Treatment and Management. Stellate ganglion block with lidocaine may be effective, though this results in Horner's syndrome. Propantheline bromide (15 mg three times daily) has been effective; avoid spicy foods or other precipitating factors that the patient may identify.

Prognosis. Variable and unpredictable.

Hemifacial Anhidrosis

Definition. Paralysis or excision of the superior cervical ganglion results in anhidrosis of the homolateral portion of the face. The face is anhidrotic above the level of the sudomotor fibers. Oculosympathetic manifestations show little or no influence on facial sweating. Preservation or loss of hemifacial perspiration is useful in localizing a lesion; nevertheless, fibers subserving the function of sweating sometimes accompany other cranial nerves. Certain areas of the face, particularly the forehead, may be supplied by sympathetic fibers that are in the orbital branches of the internal carotid artery. Only in exceptional cases is the functional activity of these subsidiary innervations significant. The occurrence of hemifacial anhidrosis is rare.

Postsympathectomy Facial Hyperhidrosis

Definition. Cervical sympathectomy results in loss of thermal sweating on the homolateral portion of the face; however, gustatory sweating persists and is excessive. Months or years pass, however, before there is an appearance of abnormal sweating. With degeneration of autonomic nerve fibers, neighboring fibers twig out and form connections with the appropriate cholinergic or adrenergic endings. The twigging is thought to be secondary to release of an unidentified humoral substance secreted by the degenerating neural structures.

Etiology and Pathogenesis. Neoplastic, traumatic, or vascular.

Genetic and Environmental Factors. None.

Incidence and Epidemiology. No data available.

Tissue Involved. Cervical sympathetic chains.

Symptoms. Homolateral facial hyperhidrosis; may be due to postsympathectomy manifestations or destruction by neoplastic or infectious processes; gustatory sweating excessive, separable from thermal sweating. Paresthesia accompanies gustatory sweating and is due to pilomotor activity, although it falls short of actual production of "goose flesh."

Signs. Pilomotor activity on the side of the lesion; visible beads of sweat as previously noted; abolition of the sweating by injection of local anesthetics into the cervical sympathetic system (interrupting the final common pathway).

Radiologic Characteristics. None except for those identifying the possible etiologic mechanism.

Special Studies. None.

Treatment and Management. Management of the primary disorder or pharmacologic approach to the suppression of hyperhidrosis.

Prognosis. Variable and unpredictable.

Auriculotemporal Syndrome (Frey's Syndrome)[45]

Definition. Gustatory sweating in the area of sensory distribution of the nerve following injury or operation in the area of the parotid gland. The auriculotemporal nerve has both sympathetic and parasympathetic fibers. The parasympathetic fibers originate from the superior cervical ganglion and proceed around the external carotid artery and its branches. From there they reach the auriculotemporal nerve to supply sweat glands to its cutaneous distribution. Parasympathetic fibers arising in the upper part of the medulla oblongata pass in the glossopharyngeal nerve. They leave the glossopharyngeal nerve to form the superficial petrosal nerve, relaying in the otic ganglion from which the postganglionic fibers run to join the auriculotemporal nerve.

Etiology and Pathogenesis. Neoplastic, traumatic, or vascular lesions.

Genetic and Hereditary Factors. None.

Incidence and Epidemiology. No data available.

Tissue Involved. The parotid gland and the auriculotemporal nerve. Commonly a consequence of surgical approach to the parotid gland (i.e., mixed parotid tumors).

Symptoms. Gustatory sweating in the area of sensory distribution of the auriculotemporal nerve. Symptoms are abolished by anesthetic block of the otic ganglion (but not the cervical sympathetic chain). Sometimes unilateral submental sweating appears during meals in the chorda tympani syndrome (analogous in origin to the auriculotemporal syndrome).

Signs. Sweating in the area previously noted.

Radiologic Characteristics. None.

Laboratory Data. No specific data.

Special Studies. None.

Treatment and Management. Anesthetic block of the otic ganglion; section of the glossopharyngeal nerve in its intracranial course (presumably by division of the parasympathetic fibers); heating the patient in a hot-air cradle results in converse production of thermal salivation (demonstrating the effects of sympathetic fibers entering the parasympathetic pathway in the auriculotemporal syndrome).

Prognosis. Variable and unpredictable.

Ophthalmoplegic Migraine[46–48]

Definition. Severe, recurrent headaches, often with prepubertal onset, unilateral, involving ophthalmoplegia, oculomotor nerve, and abducent nerve.

Etiology and Pathogenesis. Oculosympathetic paralysis (requires exclusion of an intracranial aneurysm—pupil always dilated in aneurysm and in only one third of the cases of ophthalmoplegic migraine[47]); pupillomotor fibers affected in seven of eight cases studied by Friedman et al[46]—syndrome generally regarded as a vascular reaction, and contiguous neural structures are compressed by dilated, thickened, edematous arterial segment with periarterial edema (a segment of the internal carotid artery in its intracranial course presses on the third nerve as it emerges between the posterior cerebral artery and the superior cerebellar artery); third, fourth, fifth, and sixth cranial nerves in close anatomic relationship to the internal carotid artery and its branches; third nerve to the posterior cerebral and posterior communicating arteries is also contributory and understandable in this formulation.

Genetic and Environmental Factors. As in the migraine syndrome generally.

Incidence and Epidemiology. Incidence very

low; only eight examples observed in a series of 5,000 cases of migraine.[46]

Tissue Involved. Cervical sympathetic chain, portions of the carotid artery, dilated, thickened, edematous arterial segments, and periarterial edema.

Symptoms. History of recurrent headaches; onset before puberty; antedates ophthalmoplegic state; ophthalmoplegia occurs in the course of a headache, commonly after 6 to 10 hours, when it is tending to subside; intense, continuous, orbital pain invariably caused by the oculomotor nerve with its pupillomotor fiber but often by the abducent nerve. Sympathetic involvement also occurs but is readily overlooked, because it is overshadowed by the features of a third nerve palsy.

Signs. Patient in inordinate distress with third nerve palsy; dilated pupil (homatropine test blocks the parasympathetic system, allowing the sympathetic system to function unopposed). If oculomotor nerve is partially paralyzed, homatropine causes further dilation of the pupil when sympathetic fibers are functioning normally. Such dilation will not occur in conditions of total third nerve palsy or total loss of sympathetic activity. Absence of ptosis and optic nerve damage—a point against compression within the orbit.

Patients with ophthalmoplegia tend to recover completely in a few days; rate of recovery directly related to degree of oculomotor nerve palsy; recurrent attacks of ophthalmoplegic migraine may take place in some instances, and ophthalmoplegia may endure for consecutively longer periods. It rarely endures permanently.

Radiologic Characteristics. No data available.

Laboratory Data. No data available.

Special Studies. Angiography sometimes diagnostically useful.

Treatment and Management. In early stage, intravenous norepinephrine as a pure vasoconstrictor may be helpful. Disturbance of function of fibers of the third neuron of the cervical sympathetic system may be the only neurologic manifestation of vascular headache.[48] Unilateral headache can be induced by inhalation of amyl nitrite or subcutaneous injection of histamine.

Prognosis. Variable, generally good.

Cluster Headaches Syndrome (Cluster Headaches, Horton's Headache, Histamine Cephalalgia, Ciliary Neuralgia, Erythromelalgia of the Head, Periodic Migraine Neuralgia)[49, 50]

Definition. Unilateral headaches occurring in groups of attacks.

Etiology and Pathogenesis. Internal and external carotid arterial vasodilation by unknown mechanisms.

Genetic and Hereditary Factors. Those of general migraine syndromes.

Incidence and Epidemiology. No available practical information.

Tissue Involved. Cervical sympathetic third neuron, internal and external carotid arteries, and third cranial nerve (unusually).

Symptoms. Unilateral headache occurring in groups of attacks; young men especially affected; severe pain behind or close to the eye, extending to the cheek and occipital area; ipsilateral nasal congestion; suffusion of the eyeball; excess lacrimation; facial redness and swelling precede or accompany the headache; duration less than two hours, commonly less than 30 minutes; often appears during sleep, with a characteristic tendency to occur in recurrent clusters of one or more attacks in a 24-hour period or over a period of several days, with intervening periods of freedom from attacks extending from months to a few years, nausea and vomiting unusual.

Signs. Ipsilateral nasal congestion, injection of the eyeball, lacrimation, facial redness; 20% to 25% of cases have oculosympathetic paresis;[49] miosis and ptosis are very unusual; repeated dilations of the internal carotid artery probably cause oculosympathetic paresis, with the dilation occurring in the area of the carotid siphon; rarely, homolateral pupillary dilation associated with feeling of weakness of the legs and tremor and a high pulse rate.

Absence of visual and auditory prodromata and nausea and vomiting; short attacks and peculiar grouping, with predilection for young men and unilaterality, contrast with characteristics of migraine.

Radiologic Characteristics. No specific manifestations.

Laboratory Data. No data available.

Special Studies. No data available.

Treatment and Management. Prescribe a general program of treatment appropriate to the overall migraine syndrome (cluster headaches syndrome is surely a migraine variant).

Prognosis. Generally good.

Raeder's Syndrome (Incomplete Horner's Syndrome)[51, 52]

Definition. Raeder's syndrome is divided into two groups: (1) Those cases with associated involvement of related parasellar nerve, in which location of pathologic process is merely indicated, with no evidence of its nature (that is, there are no distinctive features except those attributable to its site distinguishing it from other intracranial lesions of a localized type). (2) Those in which patients have features of a distinctive nature, that is, paratrigeminal syndrome. The latter form is the primary form of Raeder's syndrome.

Etiology and Pathogenesis. Although no evidence of a specific etiology exists, clinical behavior suggests a local inflammatory process that later always undergoes resolution. An inflammation of the internal carotid artery occurs at the site of a lesion located at the base of the middle fossa of the skull. Involvement of the arterial wall alone produces severe pain along the first division of the trigeminal nerve. The first division of the trigeminal nerve and the oculosympathetic system become damaged, as they lie in the immediate vicinity of the diseased artery.

Genetic and Hereditary Factors. None identified.

Incidence and Epidemiology. A rare cervical sympathetic third neuron syndrome; fewer than 30 examples in the literature.[52]

Tissue Involved. Internal carotid artery at the base of the middle fossa of the skull, arterial wall inflammation, trigeminal nerve, and oculosympathetic system.

Symptoms. Almost always a man in early or late middle life; no previous vascular headaches; abrupt, severe pain behind or around the orbit, with varying local radiation; no systemic symptoms or signs; pain severe; patient very distressed by the severity of the pain. Deep, nagging, continuous pain; only periodic increase in severity; aggravated by vasodilation (alcohol). Oculosympathetic nerve paralysis with ptosis and miosis occurs after days to weeks and is easily overlooked unless eyes are examined under a bright light.

Subsequent course is benign and complete resolution. Pain may continue for months or clear in weeks, but permanent remission is an essential characteristic. Ptosis and miosis also improve and vanish, only rarely persisting indefinitely.

Signs. Ptosis and miosis—bright light required for detection because ensuing contraction of the unaffected pupil may equalize the sizes; lid and pupillary changes vary in degree—they are less evident than in classic Horner's syndrome; pupillary dilation in response to cocaine instillation absent, but present with adrenaline instillation; facial sweating unimpaired (except small area above the eyebrow); localized anhidrosis occurs owing to innervation of the area by sympathetic fibers, which become involved as they course through the supraorbital and supratrochlear arteries.

Variable Features. Increased lacrimation, conjunctival injection, facial flushing on the ipsilateral side; decreased sensitivity to pin prick in the sensory division of the trigeminal nerve.

Radiologic Characteristics. Apparently none.

Laboratory Data. No abnormal data.

Special Studies. None indicated and no data available.

Treatment and Management. Syndrome in its primary form subsides without treatment. Prednisone (30 to 60 mg daily for 3 to 6 weeks) is very worthwhile as a trial. Since etiology is unknown, nonsteroidal anti-inflammatory agents may be indicated—it is very probably a localized arterial inflammation. After precise identification, reassurance to the patient is the essence of optimum management.

Prognosis. A self-limiting, benign process, frightening though it is.

Oculosympathetic Paralysis Associated with Infective and Toxic States

Definition. Retro-orbital pain, miosis, and ptosis.

Etiology and Pathogenesis. Syndrome is recognized complication of an area of sepsis, such as otitis media. Five cases reported in children with unilateral, purulent, draining otitis media.[53] No evidence of mastoiditis or meningitis and no enlargement of the cervical lymph glands.

Two possible mechanisms: (1) In the carotid canal, internal carotid artery becomes separated from the middle ear by the anterior wall of the tympanic membrane, so that its surrounding nerve plexus could be damaged easily by toxins or by pressure of abscess. Variation in the structure of this wall from bony to nearly membranous is pertinent. (2) Caroticotympanic nerves from the internal carotid plexus within the carotid canal; fibers separate to pierce the anterior wall of the tympanic cavity and pass to the tympanic plexus; not certain if all or only some fibers leave the arterial wall; oculosympathetic paralysis has followed mastoidectomy.[54] Other infections in skull and jaws, sinusitis, dental root infection, osteomyelitis, and lobar pneumonia have been implicated.

Genetic and Hereditary Factors. None recognized.

Incidence and Epidemiology. No data available.

Tissue Involved. Carotid artery in the carotid canal, anterior wall of the tympanic cavity and the artery's surrounding plexus of nerve, cervical sympathetic third neuron structures, mastoid process, high cervical spine, skull and mandible bone, dental roots.

Symptoms. Retro-orbital pain, sometimes cranial nerve involved, miosis and sometimes ptosis. Responds very favorably to specific treatment of the infectious or toxic process.

Signs. Commonly in children; ptosis and miosis; oculosympathetic paralysis.

Radiologic Characteristics. Radiologic manifestations of mastoiditis, lobar pneumonia, dental sepsis, or osteomyelitis.

Laboratory Data. Elevated sedimentation rate and leukocytosis; evidence of systemic infection with localized manifestation.

Special Studies. Otolaryngologic consultation.

Treatment and Management. Treatment of the specific infection; sometimes requiring otolaryngologic consultation.

Prognosis. Usually good.

Subset. Superior orbital fissure syndrome, a seeming subset of oculosympathetic paralysis with infective or toxic state. Pain has a more severe, nagging quality and is usually the initial symptom but may appear after the neurologic signs. Neurologic signs confined to the third nerve, but the fourth, sixth, and fifth (in its first division) nerves may be involved. Sympathetic fibers and optic nerves involved in the cranial nerve defect; resolution occurs in days or weeks and is not always complete.

Regarded as consequent to an inflammatory process within the cavernous sinus or to a pachymeningitis in the vicinity of the superior orbital fissure. Exclusion of a neoplasm is required, but differential diagnosis is clarified by spontaneous recovery.[55, 56]

Physiologic Summary of Mechanisms of Third Neuron Syndromes of the Cervical Sympathetic System[44–46]

In the orbit, sympathetic nerves supply pupillary dilator muscle, muscles of the upper and lower lid, the smooth muscle fibers of the retroocular muscle of Müller, and the blood vessels. Müller's muscle is vestigial in humans, and sympathetic innervation plays a relatively minor role in pupillary dilation, hence the insignificance of exophthalmos and mydriasis on stimulation of the cervical sympathetic nervous system. Lid retraction and associated phenomena represent essential clinical features of oculosympathetic stimulation—bilateral in a generalized form and unilateral with localized, irritative lesion.

Skin of head and neck is supplied by postganglionic fibers of the third neuron of the cervical sympathetic system. Sweat glands receive functional cholinergic fibers (thermoregulatory); parasympathetic pathways have fibers controlling gustatory sweating. Overactivity of cholinergic fibers causes excessive thermal sweating in the region of the face and neck. Vasodilator and vasoconstrictor fibers innervate facial blood vessels, which on cervical sympathetic stimulation cause blushing or pallor (both being independent of sweating). Adrenergic fibers in the sympathetic nerves supply pilomotor function (erection of hair, "goose flesh"), which exhibits increased activity with nerve stimulation. Overfunction of the third neuron of the cervical sympathetic system may be a part of a general increase of sympathetic activity or reflect a localized phenomenon.

Diminished or absent function of the third neuron of the cervical sympathetic system (Horner's syndrome) is characterized by loss of function of cutaneous and ocular nerves, resulting in hemifacial anhidrosis and homolateral ptosis and miosis. Hemifacial anhidrosis alone could reflect loss of function of that segment, leaving the common trunk to innervate the sweat glands. The lesional level in separate paralysis of the oculosympathetic segment must lie above the point of separation of the sudomotor nerve supply. This paralysis could involve the entire trunk or be limited to the division passing to the pupillary dilator or to the division that goes to the tarsal musculature. Ptosis and miosis may be present, but because the lesion may result in incomplete

separation, the distinctive feature is allocated to involvement of pupillary fibers. Solitary occurrence of sympathetic ptosis means an affection limited to the nerve supply of the eyelid.

"Abnormal activity" of the cervical sympathetic system demands further explanation. As used here, the term means an altered and abnormal function of the system because of a change in its anatomic composition and behavior. Such alterations follow injuries or diseases of any part of the system that ultimately promote growth and entry of nerve twigs from the adjoining autonomic (sympathetic-parasympathetic structures). After penetration of disrupted sympathetic pathway, connection is established with the appropriate cholinergic or adrenergic endings. Such states are represented in the postsympathectomy, auriculotemporal nerve, and chorda tympani nerve syndromes.

TRAUMA
Neck Sprain[57]

Definition. Simple, uncomplicated, musculoligamentous neck sprain (the most common of all neck injuries). The majority of cases follow automobile collision from the rear, sports injury, or employment injury.

Etiology and Pathogenesis. Minor ligamentous, capsular, or tendinous tears; muscle injury by overstretch or contusion or both. For all practical purposes, tissues are functionally intact though injured.

Genetic and Hereditary Factors. No direct hereditary forces involved.

Incidence and Epidemiology. Certain emotional factors relate to duration of symptomatology. There is commonly a long history of nervousness and tension, a history of taking sedatives and tranquilizers, of being under pressure at work or at home, of being under emotional stress, a history of one or more serious injuries, of operations and illnesses of self, spouse, or children, of being responsible for the constant care of an invalid, mentally retarded child, or an invalid parent, of suffering from the recent death of a spouse, child, or parent, or a previous history of psychiatric care. Our emotional resources are often not adequate to deal with these ordinary—sometimes very severe—life situations. We all have our limits!

The epidemiologic factors are the same as those that govern accidental injury.

Tissue Involved. Tendon, ligament, muscle, and joint of the cervical spine.

Symptoms. Cervical spine pain, headache, occipital pain, limitation of movement of the cervical spine; pain in the shoulder, arm, forearm, and hand is rare; transient paresthesia. The initial symptoms are mild and appear slowly (days after the traumatic event), gradually becoming progressive and increasing in intensity. They are persistent in duration.

Signs. Limitation of movement; facial appearance of being in pain; active cervical spine motion more diminished than passive cervical spine motion (provided relaxation of muscles can be achieved); tenderness of spinous processes of cervical vertebrae and muscle spasm about the shoulders, neck, scalp, arm, forearm, and hands. Completely negative physical signs of spinal cord involvement, subluxations, nerve root compression, or any other neurologic signs reflecting organic disorder. Patient is reluctant to be examined for range of motion, muscle spasm, tenderness, induration, swelling, deformity, and guarding. Range of motion of the shoulders is normal. Patient is fearful of moving neck but with encouragement is able to do so. Many patients arrive wearing neck collars that have been worn for many months. Many have a full range of passive movement (when complete cooperation is obtained) but very limited active motion (with residual of an injury, the clinician expects symptomatic response in both active and passive motion).

Radiologic Characteristics. "Straight" cervical spine secondary to muscle spasm (normal cervical lordosis is absent); no evidence of bone injury, joint trauma, fracture, or subluxation—tissues are radiologically normal.

Laboratory Data. Results of all tests are negative—normal sedimentation rate, blood count, muscle enzymes (SGOT, SGPT, CPK, and LDH).

Special Studies. Psychologic testing in the study of personality structure and general emotional resources to deal with ordinary life situations; Minnesota Multiphasic Personality Inventory (MMPI) and other psychologic tests. Psychiatric consultation.

Treatment and Management

1. Patient education. Special attention to problems of anxiety, conversion reaction, emotional consequences of pending litigation, psychologic, or psychiatric care.

2. Analgesic and nonsteroidal anti-inflammatory drugs.

3. Rest, gentle massage, active and passive exercises; cervical spine collar, intermittently utilized.

4. Cervical spine traction.

5. Manipulation is sometimes useful.

6. Massage techniques.

7. Hot, moist packs, ultrasound, diathermy; in acute injury, cold packs often more helpful.

8. Treatment and management is a function of the magnitude of the sprain.

See Chapter 20, *Disability Determinations* and Chapter 21, *Malingering, Psychoneurosis, Hysteria, and "Compensationitis"* for details. Cervical spine sprain and so-called whiplash syndromes represent a continuum, with the latter having a worse prognosis concerning ultimate cure.

Duration of symptoms is clearly increased in patients who have used a neck collar, neck traction, manipulation, or chiropractic adjustments. It is difficult to determine whether more treatment results in longer symptom duration or whether longer duration of symptoms leads to more treatment. I believe both play a pathogenetic role.

Prognosis. Excellent in 85% of cases, presuming absolute optimum management of all contributing factors occurs.

Summary. These syndromes deal with very ordinary neck sprain, not the more extensive circumstance usually diagnosed as "whiplash." I regard ordinary neck sprain and so-called whiplash syndromes as elements of a continuum, and I deal here with those elements of lesser clinical significance.

There is an enormous disparity in duration of symptoms after sustaining uncomplicated neck sprain. In most patients, symptoms disappear promptly, whereas others with seemingly identical injuries have prolonged symptoms, usually with symptoms appearing days after the traumatic event. These syndromes have been and continue to be a subject of great controversy.

The following four factors are most closely associated with increased duration of symptoms (9 months to 1 year or longer): (1) strong emotional factors; (2) extensive medical history; (3) prolonged and frequent treatment, particularly treatment involving neck collar, neck traction, manipulation, or chiropractic adjustments, and (4) litigation. The single most significant factor is the emotional component. A knowledge of these factors before undertaking management of patients with neck sprain constitutes a helpful and effective guide in management and prognostication.

Curiously, the only factor of treatment that has not been, perhaps could not be, measured is the attitude, ability, sensitivity, and experience of the physician in charge. In a trauma of this minimal degree an expected favorable result in a reasonable period of time requires the physician's recognition and analysis of the patient's personality, basic emotional status, medical history, recovery pattern from other illnesses, motivation, and overall resources to deal with life's ordinary problems. We must be aware of the patient's reaction to treatment and utilize tact, wisdom, care, sympathy, empathy, discipline, and lots of patient education. Settlement of litigation, including financial settlement, is almost always very therapeutic, particularly after a year or longer—a common circumstance.

Unilateral or Bilateral Atlanto-occipital or Atlantoaxial Dislocation— Atlantoaxial Rotary Fixation— A Rare but Significant Entity[58–60]

Definition. Dislocation, unilateral or bilateral, of the atlanto-occipital or atlantoaxial joint or both. Dislocation of the atlantoaxial joint is the more common of the two.

Etiology and Pathogenesis. The subluxation or dislocation may be secondary to an upper respiratory tract infection, minor trauma, or major trauma, or it may be a spontaneous dislocation of unknown cause.

Genetic and Hereditary Factors. Patients with an undiagnosed anomaly of the occipito-atlanto-axial complex are more susceptible to these dislocations.

Incidence and Epidemiology. Generally unknown and regarded as rare but very important, since the management is so effective. *Striking features are delay in diagnosis and persistent clinical and roentgenographic abnormalities.*

Tissue Involved. Upper cervical spine, occipital condyles, atlantoaxial joints, and the atlanto-odontoid joints.

Symptoms. Onset abrupt, sometimes spontaneous; cervical spine pain; characteristic "cock robin" position of rotary fixation—tilt to one side with rotation toward the opposite side and slight cervical spine flexion. Figure 11–10 provides an instance of subluxation with locking at the atlanto-occipital joint.

In one report, delay in diagnosis varied from no delay to 28 months, with an average of 11.6 months.[60] Onset followed application of an orthodontic device in one patient, surgical repair of a cleft palate in another, and removal of a body cast during treatment of scoliosis in a patient with neurofibromatosis. In two patients the lesion was accurately diagnosed at onset, but in others a multitude of diagnoses were made and many

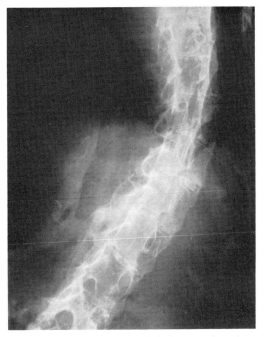

Figure 11–10. Subluxation with locking at the atlanto-occipital joint.

treatments were attempted before the cause was correctly identified as an atlantoaxial rotatory fixation.

Signs. All patients have torticollis and a decreased range of motion; facial flattening; mild to severe pain produced by any effort to correct the deformity. Active use of cervical muscles increases the clinical deformity but corrects the dislocation only to the neutral position or just beyond it; neck extension was decreased by 50%. Characteristic head position is 20 degrees of tilt to one side, 20 degrees of rotation to the opposite side, and slight flexion (position likened to that of a robin listening for a worm—the cock robin position). Weakness of lower extremities may occur; positive Hoffmann's sign, positive Babinski sign, clonus, radiculopathy of a cervical nerve root (usually C2–C3). Sternocleidomastoid muscle spasm, muscle very tender.

Radiologic Characteristics. May be confusing owing to problems in patient positioning as well as radiographic interpretation. Difficulties enhanced by considerable normal variation in the upper cervical spine and slight malalignment of the head or the x-ray beam. Many congenital and developmental anomalies occur in this region.

Positive Findings. (1) Open-mouth anteroposterior projection; (A) Lateral mass of the atlas rotated forward appears wider and closer to the midline (medial offset); opposite mass appears narrower and farther away from the midline (lateral offset). (B) On the side where the atlas is rotated backward (right side on right rotation and vice versa), joint between lateral masses of the atlas and axis is obscured owing to overlapping. Normally the spinous process of the axis is not deviated from the midline until rotation of more than 50% of total normal rotation occurs, that is, deviation to the left with slight rotation, and vice versa. If any lateral flexion (tilt) is noted, with rotation of the cervical spine below the atlas, the spinous process of the axis appears markedly deviated from the midline, that is, deviated to the right with left tilt, and vice versa. Thus, if the spinous process of the axis, the best indicator of axial rotation, is tilting in one direction and rotated in the opposite direction, rotatory fixation, or torticollis, is present. The chin and spinous process are on the same side of the midline. (2) Lateral projection: If one lateral mass of the atlas has rotated anteriorly to where the oval anterior arch of the atlas normally lies, measurement of the atlanto-odontoid interval is difficult, but lateral tomograms resolve the problem. Tomograms in the anteroposterior projection may show the two lateral masses of the atlas to be in different coronal planes, erroneously suggesting that one lateral mass is absent. Due to the tilt of the atlas, the two halves of its posterior arch are not superimposed on each other on the radiogram, suggesting assimilation of the atlas into the skull if the occiput is superimposed on the posterior arch of the atlas.

The most useful single procedure in a diagnosis of atlantoaxial rotatory fixation is cineradiography in the lateral projection. This study shows the posterior arches of the atlas and axis moving as a unit during attempted neck rotation. Normally the atlas clearly rotates independently on the relatively immobile axis.

Laboratory Data. No significant findings.

Special Studies. Cineradiography. Note that long-standing rotary fixation, like long-standing torticollis of any other etiology, results in facial asymmetry, particularly in young patients.

Treatment and Management. With rotatory fixation, atlantoaxial stability may be compromised. Minor injury may be catastrophic, particularly with anterior displacment. Skeletal skull traction should be applied. The weight for skull traction depends on the age of the patient (3.4 to 3.8 kg in younger children and up to 6.8 kg in adults) and should be increased in increments of 0.5 to 0.9 kg every 3 to 4 days. If the deformity is corrected, the reduction should be maintained by means of some form of immobilization, such as a Minerva jacket, a 4-poster brace, or continued traction for 3 months. If correction does not occur with skull traction up to an arbitrary maximum weight of 6.8 kg in children and 9.1 kg in adults, further increase in weight of traction should be carried out with careful neurologic monitoring.

Recurrence is common (more common with long-standing fixation) and probably best treated by fusion. Manipulation is dangerous. Fusion should always be done when there is neural involvement, even if it is transient neural involvement. Anterior displacement of more than 4 mm also calls for fusion.

Traction should be carried out 2 to 3 weeks preoperatively to get as much correction of the deformity as possible. A halo cast is sometimes necessary. Arthrodesis of atlantoaxial joints limits rotation but usually by only 25 degrees in either direction. Loss of rotation is not a great problem in these patients (most of whom are young) when compensatory motion develops in the lower part of the cervical spine.

Prognosis. Good if there is no gross neurologic change.

Bilateral Facet Dislocations of the Cervical Spine Below the Level of C3[61, 62]

Bilateral locked facets may occur below the level of C3. The most common level involved is C6–C7. This is much more serious than atlantoaxial subluxation and may be associated with complete spinal cord lesions and loss of function below the level of the locked facet. Sonntag[61] studied 15 cases of bilateral locked facets of the cervical spine. Thirteen patients had complete spinal cord lesions, with loss of function below the level of the locked facet. Two had intact dorsal column function. One patient had an ascending spinal cord deficit that did not change after open reduction.

The remainder had no change in spinal cord function after reduction. Closed reduction was accomplished by skeletal traction and weight application, manual reduction under sedatives, and manual reduction under general anesthesia. This report cites various methods of reduction and stabilization.

Posterior Cervical Sympathetic Syndrome—Barré-Liéou Syndrome

Note: This syndrome may also be related to those listed under *Inflammatory Disorders* (specific sepsis), *Osteoarthritis, Vascular Diseases and Syndromes*, and *Idiopathic Disorders*.

Definition. The original description of this syndrome was by M. Barré in 1926. Barré emphasized that the syndrome is almost always exclusively subjective; hence, it has been in and out of favor variably since that time. The most current view is that the apparently nebulous, bizarre, and atypical complaints are explicable on the basis of known neurologic and pathophysiologic events. Clinical appreciation recognizes the interplay between the cervical sympathetic nervous system, the vertebral artery, the scalene muscle system, and a pre-existing degree of arterial sclerosis and collateral circulations—all related to mechanical derangements of the cervical spine.[63] With today's marked increased incidence of acceleration and deceleration injuries, increased geriatric population, and frequent cervical spine injuries, there is need for resynthesis and redefinition in analyzing this syndrome.

Etiology and Pathogenesis. Irritation caused by disease or trauma of the three sympathetic ganglia in the neck and their web of sympathetic fibers and small ganglionic masses following the carotid artery and the vertebral artery in their course through the transverse foramina of C6 to the foramen magnum.

Genetic and Hereditary Factors. No specific application.

Incidence and Epidemiology. Uncommon but without specific data on incidence related to population density or even frequency of occurrence within populations.

Tissue Involved. Blood vessels, neurologic structures—particularly sympathetic fibers—large and small vascular elements of the cervical spine, intervertebral discs, zygapophyseal joints, Luschka joints, and the vertebrae themselves.

Symptoms. Suboccipital headache, vertigo, tinnitus, intermittent aphonia and hoarseness, crepitus of the cervical spine, severe fatigue, bradycardia, precordial distress, temperature changes, and dysesthesias of hands and forearms (provoked by emotion, temperature, humidity, or noise).

Cranial facial syndromes, with pain, sense of eye being "pulled out," corneal sensitivity and absent corneal reflexes, anesthesia of cheek and tongue, dental pain, brachialgia and shoulder pain, lacrimation, tenderness over supraorbital, infraorbital, and occipital nerves, amblyopia, facial numbness, swelling of one side of the face, localized cyanosis of the face, "goose flesh," and abnormal encephalogram, nausea, vomiting, and explosive diarrhea.

Signs. Few objective signs available. Mechanisms by which symptoms as well as signs might occur follow: Cervical osteoarthritis via the sympathetic nervous system, causing hypertonia of the vertebral nerve. The vertebral nerve contains sympathetic fibers joining the carotid plexus and thereby furnishes sympathetic fibers to head and neck. The sixth cervical root contains sympathetic fibers proceeding to the subclavian and brachial plexuses; the seventh cervical root supplies sympathetic fibers to the cardiac, aortic, and phrenic complexes. This tangled web of sympathetic fibers and small ganglionic masses follows the vertebral artery. Thus, disease of the cervical spinal column caused by irritating ventral nerve roots C5 to T1 could irritate their sympathetic fibers, which could reach carotid plexus, external carotid artery, external maxillary, lingual, occipital, postauricular, superficial temporal, and internal maxillary arteries, producing symptoms unrelated to somatic sensation and somatic motor fibers of the nerve root and explaining such symptoms as precordial ache, temperature dysesthesias, cranial facial syndromes, and both deep and dull pain influenced by emotion, temperature, or noise. Relief of symptoms by cervical sympathetic blocks, scalenotomy, periarterial sympathectomy of the subclavian artery, and cervical sympathectomy lends credence to this theory. Inflammation as well as fibrosis of root sleeves tends to perpetuate symptoms and signs.

Radiologic Characteristics. Cervical osteoarthritis; fracture or fracture subluxations; secondary osteoarthritis following trauma.

Laboratory Data. No specific findings.

Special Studies. Angiography of carotid and vertebral arteries. Abundant evidence to support a purely vascular origin: vertebral artery can be completely occluded by turning the head in lateral flexion, extension, and rotation, with production of symptoms; vertebral artery capable of causing a bony excavation or niche by pressure of the artery on bone and on superior zygapophyseal facet and uncovertebral joints (Fig. 11–11); electrocardiographic and electromyographic evidence. Sympathetic spread of excitation from vestibular nucleus to adjacent vagal centers could produce nausea, vomiting, and diarrhea— seemingly far removed symptomatically from the lesion.

Treatment and Management

1. Treat all the underlying problems, such as cervical osteoarthritis, vascular disease, previous trauma.

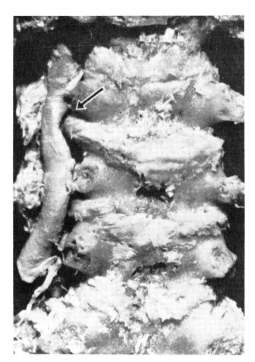

Figure 11–11. Osteophyte from the joint of Luschka compressing the vertebral artery (arrow). (From Frykholm R: Handbuch der Neurochirurgie, Band VII. New York: Springer-Verlag, 1969.)

2. Continue study to attempt to define mechanism; possible intervertebral disc removal.

3. Usual management of cervical spine osteoarthritis, with specific application to the presumed pathophysiologic understructure of this syndrome.

The clinician should try seriously to interpret bizarre and atypical complaints before concluding that any patient is a malingerer or has an hysteric or histrionic personality. Barré formulated the syndrome without any angiographic data, but it has been shown in the past decade to be reasonably correct, not speculative or hypothetical. This should be brought vigorously and dynamically to workers' compensation board hearings, to disability determination proceedings, and to clinical and surgical practice.

Prognosis. Generally good, but not predictable.

Flexion and Extension Injury to the Atlanto-occipital Joint—"High Neck Strain or Sprain"

Definition. Injury to the atlanto-occipital and atlantoaxial joints as opposed to injury at the C4–C5, C5–C6, or C6–C7 level. The high cervical spine is the most vulnerable area, and it is relatively weak. In very severe automobile collisions from the rear, decapitation has occurred at both the atlanto-occipital and atlantoaxial joints.

Etiology and Pathogenesis. Usually severe trauma.

Genetic and Hereditary Factors. None, other than that a patient with undetected congenital anomaly at the atlanto-occipital area is more susceptible to trauma.

Incidence and Epidemiology. With the ever-increasing incidence of automobile accidents, particularly collisions from the rear, these cervical injuries have increased.

Tissue Involved. Occiput, atlas, axis, bone, ligament, muscle, joint, and blood vessel.

Symptoms. Onset of symptoms occurs earlier in atlanto-occipital trauma than in trauma of the lower neck; dazedness or dizziness; headache, frequently occipital, radiating up over the head to retro-orbital areas; blurred vision, lacrimation, impaired balance (caused by reflex sympathetic stimulation); pain and stiffness in muscles of the upper neck exaggerated by any motion or sudden jar; patient may hold own head to turn neck or may turn the whole body instead.

In C4–T1 tissue injury, symptoms are referable to shoulders, chest, and upper extremities; also in lower cervical spine injury, symptoms occur days, weeks, or months after the trauma.

Signs. Simple nodding (yes and no maneuvers) valuable—it is diagnostic if performed hesitantly and with pain; manual traction increases pain, and result of compression test is negative. Anteroposterior distraction test result is positive (supportive hand is placed behind the neck, and the other hand forces either the chin or forehead gently backward as the hand behind pushes the neck forward). Rarely elicits any change in clinical sensory, motor, or reflex pattern of the upper or lower extremities.

It may be difficult to obtain history because of dazed state. Nevertheless, one needs to know position of the patient—driver or passenger, front or back seat. Back-seat passengers have pain higher up in the neck from such injuries than front-seat passengers because of the height of the back part of the seats; back-seat passengers are likely to be thrown forward after the initial extreme hyperextension. Occasionally patient may have been asleep at the time of the accident.

Radiologic Characteristics. Require anteroposterior, open-mouth, or transoral view and supine lateral radiogram.

If the findings of the initial radiograms are negative, more comprehensive study is required—right and left oblique views, lateral action films taken with the head and neck in neutral, full, extreme, forward flexion, and extension positions; tomograms of the atlanto-occipital junction (suspected odontoid fracture). Observe cervical lordotic curve or reversal if long muscles are in spasm. Identify any osteoarthritic changes with osteophytes, foraminal encroachment, and decrease in intervertebral disc space.

Laboratory Data. No specific findings.

Special Studies. See previously listed radiologic studies.

Treatment and Management

1. Prompt, individualized, and conservative management initially; mechanism of headache requires careful analysis and thought; cerebral concussion can occur with extension-flexion injury without striking a blow; vertebral artery irritation may be present from subluxation of the atlanto-occipital joint, with edema and swelling and consequent vasopasm and increase in pain; irritation of the upper two cervical nerves causes occipital pain.

2. Bed rest for 2 days to differentiate headache.

3. Treat symptoms; make decision regarding traction or other occipito-atlanto-axial support.

4. Collars and braces (usually rigid collar is effective).

5. Consider Wal-Pil-O, contour pillow, or cervi-pillow (see Chapter 12, *General Management Methods*); head-tong traction reserved until after acute symptoms have subsided.

6. Conservative management for 10 to 14 days after trauma unless there are changing neurologic or somatic symptoms.

7. Massage, diathermy, ultrasound, and microthermy may be useful; warm bath or shower.

8. Procaine injection combined with one of the tissue enzymes may relieve swelling and tissue congestion.

9. Introduce exercises as early as is feasible, guided by pain induction.

10. Analgesics and nonsteroidal anti-inflammatory agents; muscle relaxants have not been very effective.

Prognosis. Guarded, cautious optimism.

Brief Anatomic Review

High cervical spine most flexible; head is 15- to 20-lb ball perched on the atlas and articulating by just two joints; atlas has no true spinous process but a tubercle, permitting unimpaired extension of the head. Transverse and alar ligaments allow rotatory motion but little anteroposterior motion; vertebral artery function is to supply the cervical segment of the spinal cord and two fifths of the brain. Vertebral vein begins in a plexus of veins in the suboccipital region, surrounding the vertebral artery in its course through the foramina, emerging to the single vein, and ending in the innominate vein. Cervical nerves have sympathetic components, through white rami communicantes of the upper two dorsal nerves and the postganglionic fibers from the cervical ganglia to the anterior primary rami of the cervical nerves. Muscles of the neck are divided into head flexors and extensors and cervical flexors and extensors. Strain and tearing of muscles is as important as injury to ligaments.

Mechanism of Injury. The great majority of injuries are caused by automobile collisions from the rear. The body is accelerated forward suddenly, leaving the head behind because of its inertia. Severe hyperextension of the neck occurs (flexion is limited as the chin strikes the chest, but there is little to stop the extreme hyperextension posteriorly). Anterior muscles and ligaments are strained and torn as deceleration occurs. Flexion follows, and posterior ligaments and muscles are torn.

VASCULAR DISEASES AND SYNDROMES
Vertebrobasilar Insufficiency

Note: See *Osteoarthritis* and *Inflammatory Disorders (Rheumatoid Arthritis)* in this chapter.

Definition. Compromise of function of the vertebral arteries interferes with the cerebral circulation.

Symptoms. Paroxysmal symptoms induced by head movement—mainly rotation, extension, and lateral flexion. Dizziness, diplopia, drop attack, syncope, and spinal stroke increase in frequency and intensity with increasing magnitudes of cervical osteoarthritis, atheromatosis in the vessels, and increasing age; manipulation of the neck in such patients is hazardous.

Signs. Sudden, transient quadriparesis; transient, horizontal, rotational nystagmus on rotation of the head; true vertigo; precipitation of symptoms on looking over the shoulder or up at the ceiling; dysarthria; frequent pathologic plantar reflexes.

A clinical test to identify vertebral artery insufficiency: Patient stands with arms at sides; stretches arms out horizontally in front; keeps very still and rotates the head fully to one side; holds for 1 minute, turns the head in the other direction. Outstretched arms are observed, and any straying of the arm from the parallel position suggests cerebral ischemia induced by cervical rotation. *If the test finding is positive, cervical spine manipulation, stretching, or traction should never be done.* Arteriography may be indicated.

Differential Diagnosis. Differential diagnosis of cervical osteoarthritis includes carpal tunnel syndrome, peripheral neuritis of the ulnar nerve, costoclavicular syndrome, other thoracic outlet syndromes, neuralgic amyotrophy, cardiac diseases, multiple sclerosis, subacute combined degeneration and malabsorption, diabetes mellitus, and atherosclerotic vascular disease. Other differential considerations are acute, nonosteoarthritic torticollis in adults, spasmodic torticollis, hysteric torticollis, migraine syndrome, postconcussional headache, temporal arteritis, metastatic malignant disease, cervical neurofibromatosis, and fracture.

Radiologic Characteristics. Marked involvement of the Luschka and zygapophyseal joints with encroachment on the vertebral artery, principally at the occipito-atlanto-axial level but may occur at any level; atheromatous plaques, with calcification noted in the carotid artery (specifically at the siphon) and in the walls of the vertebral artery; occasional and rare aneurysm of the vertebral or carotid artery in the cervical spine; angiography discloses obstruction in varying magnitudes or complete obstruction by thrombosis.

Laboratory Data. No specific findings.

Special Studies. See radiologic studies previously outlined.

Treatment and Management

1. See previous discussion, with selective use of the various therapeutic techniques. Keep in mind the risks entailed in vertebral and vertebrobasilar vascular insufficiency.

2. Consider anticoagulant therapy.

3. Consider surgical approach to relieving compression of the vertebral artery.

4. Use of collar or brace.

Prognosis. Variable and guarded.

Cervicobrachial Neurovascular Compression Syndromes
Cervical Rib Syndrome (Scalenus Syndrome)

Definition. In scalenus syndrome, the most characteristic of the cervicobrachial neurovascular compression syndromes, hypertrophied anterior scalene muscle creates pressure on the nerve trunks of the brachial plexus and subclavian artery and vein. The superior type involves pressure on the upper trunk of the brachial plexus by tendons of the anterior scalene muscle. The lower type is more common, with compression of the lower trunk by tendons of insertion of the anterior scalene muscle.

Symptoms. The main symptom is pain in the outer anterior shoulder radiating from the supraclavicular area to the arm and hand on either the ulnar or the radial side or both; pain may radiate to the neck, scapula, shoulder, or thoracic wall; pain worsens at night and is *increased by recumbency*; turning head toward unaffected side worsens pain; downward traction on arm and shoulder, retraction of shoulder, or pressure on scalene muscle increases the symptoms; scalene muscle is very tender and painful on palpation, especially at its insertion on the first rib; pain is relieved by abduction of the arm; paresthesias in thumb and fingers with little objective sensory change; motor changes uncommon, weakness of hand and finger muscles; rarely atrophy of interossei, thenar, and hypothenar muscles; sensory motor change mainly in distribution of the ulnar nerve and its muscles; vascular and autonomic changes are power loss, cyanosis, coldness, decreased skin temperature, increased sweating, edema of arm and hand, and rarely thrombosis of digital arteries and gangrene of affected fingers; rarely associated with subclavian artery aneurysm; radial pulse diminished or obliterated by variety of maneuvers noted elsewhere (see Chapter 4, *Clinical Methods*).

Related Compression Phenomena. Other compression phenomena with closely related symptoms and signs are costoclavicular syndrome (between the first rib and the clavicle); subcoracoid smaller pectoral muscle compression (hyperabduction syndrome); paralytic brachial neuritis—sudden onset of pain in the shoulder and extensive paralysis, with consequent atrophy of muscles supplied by certain branches of the brachial plexus. Sometimes brachial plexus neuralgia may be associated with pain but with no objective sensory or motor changes. Its etiology is obscure; possible reflex origin associated with arthritic changes—rheumatoid arthritis, osteoarthritis, periarthritis, bursitis, or myositis.

Shoulder Hand Syndrome

This syndrome may be caused by lung apex lesions, tumors of the cervical portion of the spinal cord, and herniated intervertebral discs.

Cervical Trauma with Vertebral Artery Injury

Note: See *Trauma* in this chapter.

Definition. Traumatic damage to the vertebral artery in extension-flexion injury.

Etiology and Pathogenesis. Usually automobile crash, collision from rear.

Genetic and Hereditary Factors. Lesions will be more severe in the presence of atherosclerosis, tortuous course of the artery, and osteoarthritis in the cervical spine.

Incidence and Epidemiology. Great increase in frequency (though vertebral artery involvement is often overlooked) with increasing number of automobile crashes, particularly collisions from rear.

Tissue Involved. Special areas in the cervical spine, but particularly the vertebral artery and its associated specific symptoms and signs. Commonest site of involvement is in the suboccipital triangle, where vertebral artery is compressed and in spasm by muscles bounding the triangle and by those innervated by the first cervical root.

Symptoms. Headache due to posterior cervical muscle spasm, but dizziness, blurring of vision, unsteady gait, and nausea related to impairment of vertebral arterial circulation.

Signs. Visible and palpable muscle spasm in the posterior upper cervical region; tenderness over one or both suboccipital triangles; frequent diminished perception of touch in the distribution of the posterior division of one of the second cervical nerve roots; tenderness over the spinous process of second cervical vertebra (axis); and striking decrease in the normal range of motion of the cervical spine, especially the nodding (yes and no) movement.

Radiologic Characteristics. Lateral projection may show the posterior arch of the atlas to approximate the occipital bone more closely than is seen in neutral and extension views; films required are flexion and extension in lateral projection—note reversal of normal curve, limitation of range of motion, and hypermobility of vertebral bodies.

Laboratory Data. No specific findings.

Special Studies. With severe vascular symptoms or suspicion of complete obstruction, angiography of the vertebral artery is needed. Obstruction may vary from slight narrowing (due to spasm) to complete occlusion.

Treatment and Management

1. If obstruction and thrombosis are suspected, an anticoagulant regimen may be required. However, reinitiation of traumatic bleeding is always a potential hazard in this situation.

2. Cervical traction on bed.

3. Physical therapy after a few days to include heat and massage to the posterior cervical root.

4. Vasodilator therapy.

5. Analgesia; heating pad kept behind the neck of the patient while on traction; frequent short periods of traction.

Prognosis. Depends on magnitude of trauma.

ENDOCRINE AND METABOLIC DISORDERS

Diffuse Idiopathic Skeletal Hyperostosis (DISH Syndrome)[64, 65]

This hyperostotic disorder has also been called senile ankylosing hyperostosis of the spine, generalized juxta-articular ossification of vertebral ligaments, vertebral osteophytosis, severe spondylosis deformans, and Forestier's disease.

Definition. DISH syndrome is a skeletal hyperostotic disease characterized by alterations in both spinal and extraspinal structures. The disease is characterized by overproduction of bone, particularly in the cervical, thoracic, and lumbar portions of the spine, but it also involves multiple sites throughout the skeleton, particularly at the entheses, the sites of entry of ligament, tendon, capsule, and periosteum into bone. Diagnostic criteria include the presence of flowing calcification and ossification along the anterolateral aspect of at least four contiguous vertebral bodies, with or without associated localized and pointed hyperostoses at the intervening vertebral body. There is relative preservation of intervertebral disc height in the involved vertebral segment, and there is absence of the radiologic changes of osteoarthritis, including the vacuum phenomenon and vertebral body marginal osteophytes. Apophyseal joint bony sclerosis and sacroiliac joint erosion sclerosis are absent.

DISH is a disorder of middle-aged and elderly people—those in whom there is some degree of osteoarthritis already present. The disease is often mistaken for spinal osteoarthritis, though it may mimic osteoarthritis, rheumatoid arthritis, and a number of other hyperostotic conditions, namely acromegaly, ossification of the posterior longitudinal ligament, ankylosing spondylitis, fluorosis, and osteoarthritis deformans.

Etiology and Pathogenesis. The mechanism of overproduction of bone is not well understood. Because approximately 50% of patients with the DISH syndrome have diabetes, the syndrome is thought to have endocrine implication. Peripheral musculoskeletal symptoms are common and may mimic active synovitis, painful localized sites of new bone formation, tendonitis, and osteoarthritis.

Incidence and Epidemiology. DISH is a disease of older individuals and is very common; the mean age is 66 years at the time of diagnosis. There may be relatively few symptoms. DISH occurs predominantly in men. Racial characteristics are little known, though blacks represented fewer than 10% of a referral population.

Tissue Involved. The bony skeleton, particularly the axial skeleton, but peripheral sites are also involved, with special predilection for bony prominences and sites of insertion of ligament, capsule, and tendon into bone, such as ischial tuberosities, elbows, iliac crests, knees, and hips. All dense connective tissue structures of high-tensile strength may be involved.

Symptoms. Characteristic symptoms are morning stiffness, recurring evening stiffness, and stiffness increased by immobilization and activated by cold; dysphagia is rather frequent, particularly when the cervical spine is involved with the hyperostotic state; peripheral bone and joint pain, acute synovitis of a single joint, heel pain, and elbow pain; the stiffness generally is relieved by analgesics or local heat.

Signs. Tenderness over bony prominences; restriction of cervical, thoracic, and lumbar spine motion, though the posterior elements—spinous processes, laminae, and zygapophyseal joints—as well as the intervertebral discs are notoriously little involved.

Dysphagia may be a prominent symptom, whereas back pain and ache are the principal clinical manifestations; tenderness to percussion over the middle portion of the cervical spine as well as over the sacroiliac joints and the thoracolumbar spine also occurs. Active synovitis may be present; Achilles tendonitis and retrocalcaneobursitis and elbow pain are common. Shoulder stiffness is a frequent manifestation of DISH syndrome.

Radiologic Characteristics. The peculiar, predominant ossification of the spine is the primary radiologic characteristic—homogeneous in density, distinct from the anterior margins of the vertebrae, often showing a "curly" type of ossification, with a radiolucent area between the flowing layer of bone and the bony cortex of the vertebra. Fluffy or woolly periostitis at sites of ligamentous attachment; cervical spine involved in about 78% of patients, though the thoracic spine is the most common area involved.

Special Studies. Heterotopic ossification is common at a variety of sites. The unusual overproduction of bone may be more grossly apparent by study of special views of joints and bone. Computed tomography may be useful in assessing the magnitude of the hyperostotic condition in specific locations.

Treatment and Management. Patients with the DISH syndrome may be relatively free of symptoms. Recommend simple stretching exercises, attention to general fitness, and sufficient rest. Prescribe nonsteroidal anti-inflammatory drugs if there is inflammation and evidence of swelling.

Prognosis. Generally good, provided optimum management is achieved.

Calcification of the Ligamenta Flava[66–69]

Definition. Calcifications, ranging from asymptomatic to massive, and consequent cord compression and myelopathy occur in the ligamenta flava. In some cases calcium pyrophosphate dihydrate (CPPD) crystal deposition constitutes the initial and progressive lesion. Monosodium urate (MSU) crystals of gout have been shown rarely. Hydroxyapatite crystals also have been noted in the ligamenta flava but in the clinical context of multiple periarticular deposits of hydroxyapatite, a seemingly more systemic manifestation. There are no known genetic implications.

Etiology and Pathogenesis. See *Definition*.

Incidence and Epidemiology. No data available.

Tissue Involved. The ligamenta flava (note that these ligaments are paired, very large elastic structures).

Symptoms. May be asymptomatic; may be associated with pain on flexion as well as extension of the cervical spine; localized tenderness; a variety of posterior column compressive syndromes in which the symptoms are exaggerated by extension of the cervical spine, with consequent buckling of the ligamenta flava into the spinal canal, compressing the cord.

Signs. Tenderness to deep compression; clinical neurologic signs of posterior column dysfunction; limitation of motion of the cervical spine is present but is not a striking feature.

Radiculomyelopathy is a clinical characteristic—a syndrome simulating meningitis—elevated erythrocyte sedimentation rate, chills, fever, and normal cerebrospinal fluid. Calcifications in atlantoaxial joint and osteoarthritis-like arthropathies have proved to be CPPD crystal–induced.

Radiologic Characteristics. Round, radiopaque nodules seen in conventional radiogram. CAT scan is the single most valuable diagnostic tool.

Laboratory Data. No specific data available.

Special Studies. Computed tomography.

Treatment and Management. Nonsteroidal anti-inflammatory drugs in the case of CPPD crystal–induced deposits; optimum management of gout in MSU deposits; simple stretching exercises for the cervical spine in the maintenance of general fitness; continuing diagnostic efforts and long-term observation seem indicated in further study of this syndrome.

Prognosis. Generally good but variable.

Cervical Spine Anomalies in Fetal Alcohol Syndrome[70]

Definition. The teratogenic effects on the fetus of alcohol ingestion by the mother include certain predictable cervical spine anomalies. Fifty-three per cent show congenital fusion of two or more cervical vertebrae.

Etiology and Pathogenesis. The teratogenic consequences of alcohol ingestion by pregnant women constitute the etiology leading to pathogenesis.

Genetic and Hereditary Factors. Only those pertinent to the heritability of alcoholism.

Incidence and Epidemiology. Largely unknown. See reference 70.

Tissue Involved. Cervical spine, kidneys, skull, heart, and other parts of the cardiovascular system.

Symptoms. Only those of fused cervical vertebrae; usually asymptomatic.

Signs. Some stiffening of the cervical spine.

Radiologic Characteristics. Fusion of two or more cervical vertebrae (53%).

Laboratory Data. No pertinent findings.

Special Studies. No pertinent findings.

Treatment and Management. Usually no therapy indicated.

Prognosis. Prognosis is variable depending on the magnitude of the teratogenic consequences of alcohol ingestion. The fetal alcohol syndrome manifestation in the cervical spine does resemble the Klippel-Feil syndrome, but it is thought that the two syndromes are separate. The patterns of occurrence of the vertebral anomalies are different in the two groups, and the visceral expression of the fetal alcohol syndrome is also different. The major visceral anomaly in the Klippel-Feil syndrome is in the genitourinary system, and in the fetal alcohol syndrome it is in the cardiovascular system. The patterns, however, are close enough to implicate teratogenic event as the etiology in the Klippel-Feil group. The occurrence of neck fusion in fetal alcohol syndrome is common enough to be used in making the diagnosis.

Axial Osteomalacia[71–73]

Definition. A rare osteomalacic bone disorder characterized by axial pain and coarsening of the trabecular bone pattern. Coarsening of the trabecular bone pattern is seen on radiograms of the axial but not appendicular skeleton.

Etiology and Pathogenesis. Etiology is unknown but is postulated as a bone cell defect.

Genetic and Hereditary Factors. Can be familial[71] and may be associated with polycystic kidney and liver disease.

Incidence and Epidemiology. Ten cases, apparently sporadic, have been reported. It does occur in whites and blacks.

Tissue Involved. The axial skeleton.

Symptoms. Moderate to severe bone pain, usually beginning in the cervical spine, later in the middle and lower back and in the lower extremities, aggravated by weight-bearing; may have "shooting" pain in one leg or the other.

Signs. Tenderness over the spinous processes in the cervical, thoracic, and lumbar areas of the spine; cervical spine pain, sometimes with radiation in the general pattern of cervical osteoarthritis, that is, radiculitis. General health is good except in those patients with polycystic kidney and liver disease.

Radiologic Characteristics. All bones of the spine and the pelvis display a coarsened and sponge-like trabecular pattern; the appendicular skeleton is spared. In Figure 11–12, note osteomalacic characteristics—grossly coarsened bony trabeculae, decreased bone density, and increased intertrabecular spacings. Pseudofracture may occur most often in scapulae, ribs, and pubic bones; later rarefaction of the skeleton occurs, causing weight-bearing deformities and pathologic fractures. Radiographic findings may be normal early in the disease.

Laboratory Data. Biochemical changes are inconsistent. Hypophosphatemia most helpful sign; serum calcium may be depressed but is more often normal. Alkaline phosphatase elevated in varying degree, not always correlating well with the degree of skeletal involvement.

Results of bone biopsy show increased numbers and width of osteoid seams per unit volume of bone. Differential diagnosis includes dietary deficiency of vitamin D, calcium intestinal malabsorption syndrome, renal tubular defect, Fanconi's syndrome, phosphaturic diabetes, primary vitamin D resistant osteomalacia, and Paget's disease.

Treatment and Management

1. After complete study to identify possible etiologies, newer metabolites of vitamin D should be used.

2. Adequate calcium intake (1.2 to 2 g per day); ensure absorption of calcium as well as of the fat-soluble vitamins A, D, E, and K.

Prognosis. Good with some reservation.

Food and Drug Combinations Causing Head and Cervical Spine Pain

Note: See *Vascular Diseases and Syndromes*.

Twenty-five syndromes caused by or associated with the ingestion of certain foods and drugs or

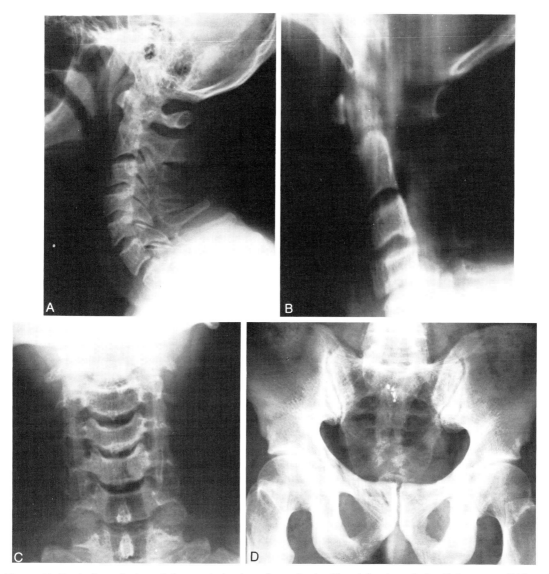

Figure 11–12. *A,* Lateral view of the cervical spine of a patient with axial osteomalacia. Note coarse, thickened trabeculae, rather large intervertebral disc spaces, and the generally bulky appearance of the vertebrae. *B,* Tomogram showing coarse trabeculation and other evidence of axial osteomalacia in the upper cervical spine. Note the anterior and posterior lips of the foramen magnum and C1, C2, C3, and C4. *C,* Posteroanterior view of the cervical spine. A tomogram illustrating the wide trabecular spacings and coarsening characteristic of axial osteomalacia. *D,* Posteroanterior film of the pelvis, illustrating the changes resulting from osteomalacia in the pubic, ischial, and iliac bones. The changes are similar to those brought about by Paget's disease.

combinations thereof have been described.[74] Chronic pain is a major national health problem. A very significant portion of Americans are afflicted with chronic pain of the cervical spine. It is estimated that 75 million Americans are sufferers of chronic pain syndromes; 700 million workdays are lost each year; total expenses, including medications and doctors' and hospital fees, are said to be 57 billion dollars yearly—10% of our national budget and 25% to 30% of total health-care costs.[75]

Food Additives. Monosodium glutamate (MSG) is a monosodium salt of glutamic acid that is widely used as a flavoring enhancer in oriental cooking. Ingestion of MSG may cause Chinese restaurant syndrome (Kwok's disease) in susceptible individuals. The symptoms include severe pain in jaws, neck, or shoulders; a bandlike headache; sharp tightening of muscles of the neck and face associated with numbness; constriction of cervical spine muscles, particularly the trapezius but also the muscles of the back; paresthesia of mucous membranes of mouth and palate, nausea, giddiness, dizziness, palpitations, and weakness.

Recovery occurs in 30 minutes, and the symptomatology is probably based on the fact that glutamate is neurotoxic, causing depolarization of neurons.

Licorice. Licorice is eaten as a confection and is used in the treatment of ulcers, as an expectorant, and as an additive to some alcoholic drinks. It contains glycyrrhizinic acid, a substance structurally and chemically similar to aldosterone, a mineralocorticoid. The ingestion of licorice may result in an excess synthesis of aldosterone. The resulting syndrome is characterized by facial and cervical edema, muscle weakness and tenderness, hypokalemia, and hypernatremia.

Nitrate and Nitrite Compounds. Water and many natural foods contain large quantities of nitrates. These agents are vasodilating, probably histamine-like, and able to induce migraine-like headaches in certain individuals. Pains in the jaw and posterior teeth occur, as do cervical spine pain and headache.

Boron. Boron is used in the form of boric acid as an eye wash, a disinfectant, a buffering agent in ophthalmologic and dermatologic preparations, a gargle, and a urinary antiseptic. Symptoms of toxicity originate mainly from the central nervous system and include weakness, lethargy, severe headache, restlessness, tremors, and convulsion.

Alcohol. Alcohol, a nonspecific vasodilator, produces headaches in susceptible individuals by depressing or altering central vasomotor centers. Cluster headaches may be provoked in certain patients.

Tyramine-Containing Foods. Tyramine is an indirectly acting sympathomimetic amine, a simple phenylethylamine that liberates norepinephrine from sympathetic nerve endings. Such foods as cheeses, canned figs, pickled herring, chopped liver, yeast, and alcoholic beverages (particularly beer) contain tyramine. Cheddar cheese contains the highest content of tyramine. Symptoms resulting from ingestion of tyramine are headache, occipital pain, and pulsating headache secondary to the circulatory vasolability.

Chocolate. Chocolate is probably the most common dietary trigger of migraine headches, which are frequently associated with cervical spine pain, stiffness, and a sense of throbbing.

Fasting. Fasting has been shown to be a precipitating factor in head and neck pain, particularly migraine attacks. The mechanism of hypoglycemia–induced headache is unknown, but it does have a profound effect on the tone of cranial blood vessels. Muscle cramps and twitching and jerking of muscles occur in this circumstance, which is associated with an overall sense of nervousness and depression.

Drug-Induced Torticollis and Other Orofacial-Cervical Dyskinesias. Of all iatrogenic disorders, tardive dyskinesia is one of the most disabling. Orofacial-cervical tremor, myoclonus, tics, dystonia, and chorea are all possible neurologic consequences of a broad spectrum of drugs, including antipsychotic drugs, neuroleptic drugs, and major tranquilizers.

Vitamin A. Excessive intake of vitamin A has become increasingly common with the advent of misguided use of the vitamin. It has been used to treat cancer, skin disorders, and children with learning disabilities. The toxic dose for adults is about 50,000 IU daily for a period of at least a year. Symptoms and signs of excessive intake are thickening of the skin, headache, increased susceptibility to disease, generally increased intracranial pressure and papilledema, cervical spine stiffness, fissures of the lips, glossitis, and stomatitis.

Vitamin D. Vitamin D intoxication is not rare, as the very potent representatives are used increasingly. Symptoms include headache, gastrointestinal disorders, polydipsia, and polyuria.

Caffeine. Caffeinism has not been clearly established as a syndrome. Mood disturbances, however, have been recognized, and anxiety is the most frequent, affective complaint. Irritability, muscle twitchings about the head and neck, headache, rapid breathing, and palpitation occur. Recurrent cervical spine pain and so-called tension headaches occur on caffeine withdrawal, occasionally resulting in repetitive episodes of headache and cervical spine pain. Such headaches tend to occur on weekends because "coffee breaks" are less frequent.

Herbal Teas. Burdock root tea, nutmeg, and other less specific herbal teas have been associated with headache, nausea, and vomiting.

Seafood. Pain, headache, and cervical spine stiffness have been associated with the acute symptoms secondary to shellfish poisoning.

Other. Final considerations in difficult diagnostic circumstances for headache and cervical spine pain are the ingestion of amygdalin (pits of apricot, bitter almond casava beans, cherry, chokecherry, and peach), insecticides, pesticides, and rodenticides.

Treatment and Management. Identification and elimination of offending agent.

DISORDERS OF THE CERVICAL SPINAL CORD
Syndromes of the Cervical Spinal Cord

The spinal cord is an elongated, nearly cylindric portion of the nervous system, with two enlargements—the cervical and the lumbar—accommodating the increased neural traffic from the upper and lower extremities respectively. The spinal cord ends in a conic extremity, the conus medullaris, between the levels of the first and second lumbar vertebrae. The cord is slightly flattened in an anteroposterior direction, and an anterior median fissue and a posterior median sulcus divide it into two symmetric halves. The posterior nerve roots enter the posterolateral sulcus, and the anterior nerve roots exit at the anterolateral sulcus. Spinal cord parenchyma consists of a butterfly-shaped or H-shaped core of gray matter containing nerve cells that are surrounded by tracts of longitudinally arranged nerve processes, mostly myelinated, that carry ascending and descending impulses. A minute central canal runs the entire length of the cord, which is lined by a single layer of ependymal cells.

Lesions of the cervical spinal cord (as elsewhere in the cord) are characterized by sensory, motor, and autonomic clinical reflections, with involvement of the posterior roots or the sensory cells. In the posterior horns of the gray matter, segmental sensory changes occur—either loss of some or all types of sensation in the dermatomes and sclerotomes and myotomes supplied by the involved segment or irritative phenomena, such as pain and paresthesias. If the ascending pathways are abnormal, loss of sensation occurs; pain, temperature, proprioception below the level of the lesion, and dissociation of sensation may be present, with loss of some varieties. With anterior horn cell or anterior root involvement, a lower motor neuron paralysis in the myotomes supplied by the involved segments occurs, with abnormality of the descending motor pathways—corticospinal, extrapyramidal, or vestibulospinal changes in motor power and tone below the level of the lesion. With involvement of the lateral cell groups of the gray matter, the descending autonomic pathways are compromised, and changes in autonomic function occur.

Motor Deficits. A function of the site and extent of the lesion; flaccid paralysis of muscles supplied by the affected segment; flaccid paresis, later becoming spastic below the level of the lesion. Cervical segments C1 through C4 innervate muscles controlling movements of the head and neck.

1. Lesions of C1–C2 cervical cord segments are usually fatal, owing to proximity of critical vasomotor and respiratory centers in the medulla; possible hyperpyrexia.

2. Involvement above the fourth segment causes respiratory abnormality due to diaphragmatic paralysis (patient able to breath only with accessory muscles of respiration). Lesions at the fourth cervical segment allow respiration through diaphragmatic function and accessory muscles of respiration, but paralysis of all four extremities follows. The C4–C5 through T1 segment controls movements of the upper extremities.

3. C5–C6 involvement results in an upper arm type of brachial plexus palsy, with paralysis of rhomboid, supraspinatus, infraspinatus, teres major, teres minor, deltoid, biceps, and brachioradial muscles.

4. Loss of biceps and brachial reflexes, with inversion of the radial reflex; arms adducted and in internal rotation.

5. Involvement of the sixth cervical segment affects the biceps muscle predominantly; deltoid and triceps muscles may both be intact.

6. Seventh cervical segment involvement causes paralysis of triceps muscle and extensor muscles of wrists and fingers, with either loss of triceps reflex or presence of paradoxic reflex of flexion instead of extension of the forearm.

7. C8–T1 involvement results in a syndrome resembling a lower arm type of brachial plexus palsy—atrophic paralysis of flexor muscles of wrists and fingers and of small intrinsic muscles of the hands; arm reflexes are preserved, but wrist and finger flexion reflexes are affected.

Sensory Changes. Usually segmental or dermatomal in distribution; loss or decrease in one or more sensory perceptions, or perversions of either pain or paresthesia; areas of decrease or loss and paresthesia may involve the entire body below the level of the lesion, but pain is usually segmental and affects only the dermatome, sclerotome, and myotome supplied by the lesional level; sensory loss usually is associated—some impaired, others spared; pain, temperature, and proprioception predominate symptomatically; may be difficult to demonstrate most specific level of pain and temperature but not difficult to identify definite level for tactile sense or proprioception; Lhermitte's sign, sudden electric-like shock spreading down the body on flexion of the neck, occurs owing to focal, traumatic, and neoplastic lesions at the cervical level.

Autonomic Nervous System Changes. C8 and T1 lesions cause Horner's syndrome; Horner's syndrome may also reflect a lesion of descending autonomic pathways above this level; transverse spinal lesion causes loss of sweating, vasodilation, piloerection, increased skin resistance, increased skin temperature below the level of the lesion, and later vasoconstriction, with fall in temperature and increase in sweating and pilomotor activity. Interruption of descending pathways disturbs bladder, rectal, and sexual function; lesion at C8–T1 above thoracolumbar outflow can cause disturbance of sympathetic innervation of the entire body.

Lesions of the cervical spinal cord include transverse syndromes (complete interruption of continuity of the spinal cord), syndromes of the gray matter, syndromes of the white matter, systemic disease in the nervous system, complete cord and incomplete cord transection, trauma, neoplasms (extradural, intradural, extramedullary, intramedullary), vascular lesions (thrombosis, meningeal hemorrhage, intraspinal hemorrhage), arteriosclerotic lesions, inflammatory lesions, degenerative processes (progressive spinal muscular atrophy, primary lateral sclerosis), congenital defects, and structural abnormalities of the bony spinal canal.

References

1. Canale ST, Griffin DW, Hubbard CN: Congenital muscular torticollis. J Bone Joint Surg 64A:810, 1982.
2. Hulbert K: Torticollis. Postgrad Med J 41:699, 1965.
3. Forsythe M, Rothman RH: Diagnosis and treatment of infections of the cervical spine. Orthop Clin North Am 9:1039, 1978.
4. Gilbert GJ: Spasmodic torticollis treated effectively by medical means. N Engl J Med 284:896, 1971.
5. Sorensen BF, Hamby WB: Spasmodic torticollis. JAMA 194:706, 1965.
6. Lim RA: The hyoid bone syndrome. Otolaryngol Head Neck Surg 90:198, 1982.
7. Lan JW, Anthony M: Neck tongue syndrome in sudden turning of the head. J Neurol Neurosurg Psychiatry 43:97, 1980.
8. Sarkozi J, Fam AG: Acute calcific retropharyngeal tendonitis: An unusual cause of neck pain. Arthritis Rheum 27:708, 1984.
9. Karasick D, Karasick S: Calcific retropharyngeal tendonitis. Skeletal Radiol 7:203, 1981.
10. Riser M, Gayral L, Neuwirth E: Psychiatric disturbances of patients with osteoarthritis of the cervical spine. Clin Orthop 24:64, 1962.
11. McComas AJ: Neuromuscular Function and Disorders. London: Butterworth Publishers, 1977, p 253.
12. Kendall HO, Kendall FP, Boynton DA: Posture and Pain. Huntington, New York: Robert E. Krieger Publishing Co, 1977.
13. Kendall HO, Kendall FP, Wadsworth GE: Muscles, Testing and Function, 2nd ed. Baltimore: Williams & Wilkins Co, 1971.
14. Dugan MC, Locke S, Gallagher JR: Occipital neuralgia in adolescents and young adults. N Engl J Med 267:1106, 1962.
15. Behrman S: Traumatic neuropathy of the second cervical spinal nerves. Br Med J 286:1312, 1983.
16. Ehni G: Occipital neurologic and C1, C2 arthrosis. N Engl J Med 310:127, 1984.
17. Kes L, Herold HZ: The long neck. Int Surg 65:441, 1980.
18. Connor JM, Smith R: The cervical spine in fibrodysplasia ossificans progressiva. Br J Radiol 55:492, 1982.
19. Bland JH, Kirschbaum B, O'Connor GT, et al: Myositis ossificans progressiva. Effect of intravenously given parathyroid extract on urinary excretion of connective tissue components. Arch Intern Med 132:209, 1973.
20. Miller JDR, Percy JS: Tophaceous gout in the cervical spine. J Rheumatol 6:862, 1984.
21. Kersley GD, Mandel L, Jeffrey MR: Gout, an unusual case with softening and subluxation of the first cervical vertebra and splenomegaly. Ann Rheum Dis 9:282, 1950.
22. Vinstein AZ, Cockerell EM: Involvement of the spine in gout. Radiology 103:311, 1972.
23. Bland JH: Rheumatoid arthritis of the cervical spine. J Rheumatol 1:3, 1974.
24. Pellicee PM, Ranawat CS, Tsairis P, et al: A prospective study of the progression of rheumatoid arthritis of the cervical spine. J Bone Joint Surg 63A:342, 1981.
25. Eulderink F, Meijers KAE: Pathology of the cervical spine: A controlled study of 44 spines. J Pathol 120:91, 1970.
26. Meijers KAE, VanBeusekom GTH, Luyendijk W: Dislocation of the cervical spine with cord compression in rheumatoid arthritis. J Bone Joint Surg 56B:667, 1974.
27. Colin A, Fries JF: Ankylosing Spondylitis. Garden City, New York: Medical Examination Publishing Co, 1978.
28. Bywaters EGL: The bursae of the body. Am Rheum Dis 24:215, 1965.
29. Bywaters EGL: The pathology of the spine. In Sokoloff L (ed): The Joints and the Synovial Fluid. New York: Academic Press, 1980, p 428.
30. Bywaters EGL: Rheumatoid and other diseases of the cervical interspinous bursae and changes in the spinous processes. Ann Rheum Dis 41:360, 1982.
31. Rohn RD, Rubio T: Neck pain due to acute suppurative thyroiditis and thyroglossal duct abscess. J Adolesc Health Care 1:155, 1980.
32. Kelsey JL, Githens PB, Walter SD, et al: An epidemiological study of acute prolapsed cervical intervertebral disc. J Bone Joint Surg 66A:907, 1984.
33. Wilkinson HH, Scherman N: Intradiscal corticosteroids in the treatment of lumbar and cervical disc problems. Spine 5:385, 1980.
34. Gunn CC, Milbrandt WE: Tennis elbow and the cervical spine. Can Med Assoc J 114:803, 1976.
35. Murray-Leslie CF, Wright V: Carpal tunnel syndrome, humeral epicondylitis and the cervical spine: A study of clinical and dimensional relations. Br Med J 1:1439, 1976.
36. Mitchell JD, Reid DM: Reversible neurological causes of tennis elbow. Br Med J 286:1703, 1983.
37. Maitland GD: Vertebral Manipulation, 3rd ed. London: Butterworth Publishers, 1973, p 76.
38. Bland JH, Cooper SC: Osteoarthritis: A review of the cell biology involved and evidence for reversibility; management rationally related to known genesis and pathophysiology. Semin Arthritis Rheum 14:106, 1984.
39. Brain WR, Wilkinson M: Cervical Spondylosis. Philadelphia: W. B. Saunders Co, 1967.
40. Wilkinson M: Cervical spondylosis: Its early diagnosis and treatment. Philadelphia: W. B. Saunders Co, 1971.
41. Cyriax JH: Cervical Spondylosis. London: Butterworth Publishers, 1971.
42. Cyriax JH: Illustrated Manual of Orthopedic Medicine. London: Butterworth Publishers, 1984.
43. Payne CMER: Newly recognized syndromes in the neck: Horner's syndrome with ipsilateral vocal cord and phrenic nerve palsies. J R Soc Med 74:814, 1981.
44. Giles CD, Henderson JW: Horner's syndrome: An analysis of 216 cases. Am J Ophthalmol 46:289, 1958.
45. Glaister DH, Hernshaw JR, Heffron PF, et al: The mechanism of postparotidectomy gustatory sweating (the auriculo-temporal syndrome). Br Med J 1:942, 1958.
46. Friedman AP, Harter DH, Merritt HH: Ophthalmoplegic migraine. Trans Am Neurol Assoc 86:161, 1961.
47. Harrington DO, Flocks M: Ophthalmoplegic migraine. Arch Ophthalmol 49:643, 1953.
48. Jacobsen HH: Unilateral sympathetic hypofunction in migraine. Acta Psychiatr Scand 27:67, 1952.
49. Kunkle EC, Anderson WB: Dual mechanism of eye signs of headache in cluster pattern. Trans Am Neurol Assoc 85:75, 1960.
50. Kunkle ES, Pfeiffer JB Jr, Wilhort WM, et al: Recurrent brief headaches in "cluster" pattern. Trans Am Neurol Assoc 77:240, 1952.

51. Raeder JG: "Paratrigeminal" paralysis of oculopupillary sympathetic system. Brain 47:149, 1924.
52. Minton LR, Bounds GW Jr: Raeder's paratrigeminal syndrome. Am J Ophthalmol 58:271, 1964.
53. Hoefnagel D, Joseph JB: Oculosympathetic paralysis in otitis media. N Engl J Med 265:475, 1961.
54. Berberich J: Pupillary reactions in affections of the ear. Laryngoscope 50:555, 1940.
55. Lakke JP: The syndrome of superior orbital fissure. Arch Neurol 7:289, 1962.
56. Shafar J: The syndromes of the third neuron of the cervical sympathetic system. Am J Med 40:97, 1966.
57. Farbman AA: Neck sprain: Associated factors. JAMA 223:1010, 1973.
58. Fielding JW, Hawkins RJ: Atlanto-axial rotatory fixation. J Bone Joint Surg 59A:37, 1977.
59. Bonna M, Stevenson GW, Tumiel A: Unilateral atlanto-occipital dislocation complication, an anomaly of the atlas. J Bone Joint Surg 65A:685, 1983.
60. Lucas JT, Hungerford GD, Perot PL Jr: Treatment of nontraumatic atlanto-axial dislocation and fibrous fusion. J Neurosurg 56:139, 1982.
61. Sonntag VK: Management of bilateral locked facets of the cervical spine. Neurosurgery 8:150, 1981.
62. Pich RY, Segal N: C7–T1 bilateral facet dislocation, a rare lesion presenting with the syndrome of acute anterior spinal cord injury. Clin Orthop 150:131, 1980.
63. Stewart DY: Current concepts of the Barré syndrome or the posterior cervical sympathetic syndrome. Clin Orthop 24:40, 1962.
64. Resnick D, Niwayama G: Radiographic and pathologic features of spinal involvement in diffuse idiopathic skeletal hyperostosis (DISH). Radiology 119:559, 1976.
65. Resnick D, Schaul SR, Robins JM: Diffuse idiopathic skeletal hyperostosis (DISH): Forestier's disease with extraspinal manifestations. Radiology 115:513, 1975.
66. Inone N, Motomura S, Murai, et al: Computed tomography in calcification of the ligamenta flava of the cervical spine. J Comput Assist Tomogr 7:704, 1983.
67. Iwasaui Y, Hkino M, Tsuru, et al: Calcification of the ligamentum flavum of the cervical spine. J Neurosurg 59:531, 1983.
68. Kawano N, Yoshida S, Ohwda T, et al: Cervical radiculomyelopathy caused by deposition of calcium pyrophosphate dihydrate crystals in the ligamenta flava. J Neurosurg 52:279, 1980.
69. LeGoss P, Penner Y, Houinou P: Articular chondrocalcinosis revealed by acute cervical symptoms simulating meningitis. Sem Hop Paris 56:1575, 1980.
70. Tredwell SJ, Smith DF, MacLeod PJ, et al: Cervical spine anomalies in fetal alcohol syndrome. Spine 7:331, 1982.
71. Frame B, Parfitt AM: Osteomalacia: Current concepts. Ann Intern Med 89:966, 1978.
72. Frame B, Frost HM, Orimond RS, et al: Atypical osteomalacia involving the axial skeleton. Ann Intern Med 55:632, 1961.
73. Whyte MP, Fallen MD, Murphey WA, et al: Axial osteomalacia. Clinical laboratory and genetic investigation of an affected mother and son. Am J Med 71:1041, 1981.
74. Seltzer S: Foods, and food and drug combinations responsible for head and neck pain. Cephalalgia 2:111, 1982.
75. Bonica JJ: The interagency committee on new therapies for pain and discomfort. Report to the White House. U.S. Department of Health, Education and Welfare, Public Health Service, National Institutes of Health, May, 1979.

Chapter 12

General Management Methods

This chapter presents all of the available therapeutic methods and the rationale (known or presumed mechanism of action) used in the general management of disorders of the cervical spine. The information presented includes cautionary notes for procedures, descriptions of undesirable side effects of drugs, varying types of exercise, realistic physiologic and psychologic expectations, the role of rest and exercise, and relaxation techniques. Chapter 11, *Differential Diagnosis and Specific Treatment*, discusses specific diagnoses and treatments.

GENERAL CONCEPTS AND RECOMMENDATIONS

1. The maintenance of optimum overall fitness constitutes a major contribution to the success of management of cervical spine disorders and disease. Sole attention to the cervical spine is doomed to failure. Management and active treatment of disease in process as well as rehabilitation of the cervical spine are strongly linked to the rest of the spine and to the body as a whole—a concept too infrequently promoted. I subscribe to the view of Paul Dudley White, famous cardiologist and exercise enthusiast, who said, "Show me a strong knee, and I will show you a strong heart." This general concept applies directly to the cervical spine.

2. Do all you can to prevent patients from moving into the "sick role," that is, regarding themselves as different, ill, and dependent. Management becomes increasingly ineffective the deeper into the sick role the patient sinks.

3. Patient education constitutes a major contribution to the success of management. Each patient requires additional education about his or her specific health problem. The average person has little knowledge about the cervical spine and its many disorders. The doctor is often the first person to educate the patient concerning disorders. Patient education classes in various kinds of arthritis are available through the Arthritis Foundation. Patient handbooks and educational materials are also useful. Medical consumers clearly have the right to know as much as they can possibly understand about their health care and to have the information presented in familiar, everyday terms. Patients are clearly partners in their own health care. Through questioning, they can become well educated concerning the nature of their problem and the rationale and mechanism for dealing with it successfully.

4. In assessing any therapeutic modality in all clinical areas in medicine, including the cervical spine, one must maintain a keen awareness of the power of the placebo effect. There is overwhelming evidence documenting the major influence of placebo effects in response to any therapeutic method. The color of the pill, the personality and attitude of the doctor, the magnitude of the patient's anxiety, and the patient's perception of the presumed efficacy of the therapy all contribute to the placebo effect. This is not to suggest that the placebo effect is a reflection of psychoneurosis, autonomic lability, ignorance, or an emotional response; it is cited here simply to sound a warning about interpreting the effectiveness of any effort at treatment and management, be it pain relief, improvement in range of motion, or overall increase in performance of functional tasks. Results must be evaluated with full appreciation of the placebo phenomenon.

PHYSICAL THERAPY MODALITIES

The perception of pain is a very complicated experience. Four components have been enumerated: (1) nociception, (2) pain sensation, (3) suffering, and (4) pain behavior.[1] Nociceptors are neuroreceptors that are stimulated by strong impulses or extremes of temperature. On discharge, nociceptors carry the perception of a painful experience to the brain. Pain sensation follows as the central nervous system receives the transmitted impulses. The affective response by the patient is called suffering, and it is a response of the higher cortical centers activated by the lower cortical pain sensation centers. Governing and varying the degree of suffering are mood determinants, fear, depression, isolation, anger, and frustration. Over time, suffering is reflected in the patient's total affect and behavior. Lastly, there follows demonstration of pain behavior.

For abrupt, severe, and acute pain, the physical therapeutic modalities attempt to decrease nociception, the largest component of acute pain. In chronic pain, the physical therapeutic modalities are useful not only in attempting decrease of nociception but also in modifying pain behavior. The same perceptive experience is interpreted in very different ways by each individual. Nociceptors may be more intensely active in some patients, or pain sensation awareness centers in the brain may be more active. Suffering and painful behavior are highly individualized, probably influenced by genetic endowment and previous environmental influences. It behooves us to be very aware of each individual's response to pain; certain physical therapeutic methods may be somewhat painful themselves and will need to be applied below the patient's level of pain tolerance at a particular time. A good example is that of the very capable, enthusiastic, eager athlete who is so intent on returning to the game that there may be absence of pain awareness even though the nociceptor activity is great. Some physical therapeutic modalities may initiate new clinical problems if they are applied to patients who have very high pain thresholds and do not complain.

The modalities of physical therapy may be categorized as follows: (1) cryotherapy, the use of physical cold; (2) thermotherapy (superficial and deep), the use of heat by any method that provides heat; (3) mechanical therapy, the use of massage, whirlpool, and methods that move the tissues about in a variety of ways; (4) electrotherapy, stimulation of nerve and muscle by an electric current.

Cryotherapy

The effects of physical cold on connective tissues are decreased sensitivity of nerve fibers, diminished metabolic turnover, and immediate decreased capillary as well as arteriolar blood flow. The vasoconstriction is a consequence of temperature change, which produces a direct effect on blood vessels and a reflex vasoconstriction through sympathetic fibers. Hemorrhage and edema in acute trauma are clearly diminished with early application of cold, and the effect may last hours to as many as two days. In ischemic tissues, cooling may decrease the metabolic rate further and compromise metabolic waste formation and dispersal. Muscle spasm increases in the presence of waste products, and cooling decreases muscle spasm by decreasing waste product synthesis. Cold renders muscle spindles much less responsive to stretch, decreasing muscle spasm by diminishing the myotactic reflex. Viscosity of interstitial and intracellular fluids is decreased by cold, impairing the muscle's ability to contract. Decrease in skin temperature effectively blocks muscle spasm. *Because of the effect of cold on muscle spasm and the diminished stretch reflex by the muscle spindles, one can gently stretch a spastic muscle after cooling, without triggering the usually instantaneous shortening caused by firing of the muscle spindle.* Such stretching of spastic muscles is quite different from stretching a contracted muscle.

In a contracted muscle, cold increases the distensible properties of collagen, permitting stretched areas of muscle to return to their original length after stretching. Hence, cold is contraindicated if one wishes to stretch long-standing flexion contractures. Conversely, heat increases viscoelastic properties of collagen, permitting greater deformation and longer maintenance of elongation after stretching. With decrease in excitability of free nerve endings as well as peripheral nerve fibers (diminished membrane excitability), the patient's pain threshold rises, and complaints decrease. Hence analgesia, but not real anesthesia, is achieved.

The degree of sensitivity of nerve fibers to cold is a function of the extent of myelination and fiber diameter. Small myelinated fibers mediating light touch and the efferent gamma fibers to muscle spindles are most sensitive to cold. The large myelinated fibers (proprioceptive and alpha motor nerve fibers) are the next most sensitive; unmyelinated fibers (pain and postganglionic sympathetic nerves) are the least sensitive. The clinical perception of coldness is the immediate sensation of cooling, which is followed by a mild aching or burning, and after 5 to 7 minutes of cold application, relative cutaneous anesthesia occurs. Strangely (and importantly), cold application for more than 15 to 20 minutes or a fall in temperature of over 2°C causes vasodilation, with an abrupt increase in blood flow. This response is a reflex that is mediated to prevent excessive lowering of temperatures that could cause cold injury to the tissue. Vasodilation is automatic, occurring intermittently as required, even though cooling is continuous. It continues to occur in sympathectomized muscle but not in denervated muscle, that is, it is mediated by somatic nerves and is probably an axonal reflex. With excessive cooling or total body cooling with lowering of core temperature, the shivering reflex, mediated through the hypothalamus, constitutes an attempt to increase heat production and raise core temperature. The clinical conclusion is that cryotherapy for vasoconstriction in acute trauma should last only 10 to 15 minutes, cooling only the traumatized area. This allows maximal cooling effects in the local area without introducing a fall in overall body temperature.

Cold penetrates more deeply than heat, owing to the convective heat exchange and the concomitant decrease in blood flow. Thus, decreasing temperature occurs in deeper tissues. Cold effects persist longer than heat effects. After removal of an ice pack, skin temperature rises to 25°C and remains there for at least 1 hour before returning to the normal skin temperature of 35 to 37°C.

Cold in the following forms can be used: ice, a frozen gel, a chemical cold pack (commercially available as a compound that produces an endothermic reaction when two components of the package are mixed), or a refrigerant inflatable plastic envelope or bladder. Frozen gels are reusable and can be stored in a deep-freeze unit at home. Since the temperature of the frozen gels is 17°C, a temperature causing frostbite on direct application to the skin, one should place a towel over the area of cooling. McMasters et al[2] found that ice and frozen gel produced faster cooling and gave higher and more prolonged temperature reduction than chemical cold packs or refrigerant inflatable bladders. Ice is the least expensive of all methods. A very satisfactory pack can be made by putting 6 to 20 ice cubes in resealable plastic bags, using the larger bags for a larger area so that more ice is applied. Some chemical cold packs or refrigerant inflatable bladders have precooled elastic bandages or Velcro straps, allowing the cooling bag to be held against the part, in this case the cervical spine.

Cold water baths (hydrotherapy and cryotherapy) can be taken through a broad range of temperatures, the most common of which is 15.5°C. The bath allows cooling of a large area of the body, such as an entire extremity. Immersion is more effective than ice packs because uniformity of temperature is achievable. Spray coolants, such as ethyl chloride, may allow local anesthesia of a small area on the cervical spine. A disadvantage of spray coolants is the relatively brief duration of effect. Cold whirlpool baths or ice massage combine cryotherapy with massage, achieving the lowering of tissue temperature and the massaging effects of moving water. Ice massage can be performed with an ice cube or a disposable Styrofoam cup filled with frozen water. The bottom of the cup serves as a handle. The ice is moved in a circular or stroking motion back and forth over the injured area.

In the cervical spine, any acute musculoskeletal sprain or muscle pull, soft-tissue contusions, hemorrhage, or muscle spasm secondary to injury can be effectively treated with cryotherapy. Range of motion exercises can be initiated sooner following the injury if cryotherapy is used.

Cold should not be applied at temperatures lower than 3 to 4°C unless the skin is shielded by toweling or another insulating method. Frostbite will occur at that temperature. Since relative anesthesia occurs, with peripheral nerves and free nerve endings becoming diminished in response, one can produce cold injury, adding to the problem for which cryotherapy was originally given. Cold allergies also contraindicate the use of cold (giant hives, joint pain, or any history of such a response to cold). Patients with Raynaud's disease, sickle cell anemia, cryoglobulinemia, or anesthetic skin should not receive cryotherapy. In a few patients, hypertension may follow cold immersion.

Thermotherapy

Heat is heat—dry or moist, superficial or deep. Heat energy transfer to tissues occurs by direct contact conduction (hot pack) or by a transferring medium for conduction (infrared lamp) or by energy conversion, transfer of heat from some other energy form (ultrasound diathermy, short wave diathermy, or microwave diathermy). Skin is a poor conductor of heat. Thus when a source of heat is placed on the skin, heat transfer to deeper layers is inadequate; marginal penetration by conductive devices and increased risk of heat damage are caused by lack of heat dispersion.

Physiologic effects of heat are a function of three factors: (1) tissue temperature obtained (40 to 45°C optimal); (2) duration of elevated temperature (5-minute minimum, 20- to 30-minute maximum); (3) the rate at which heating is achieved; and (4) the size of the heated area. Heat effects of the circulatory system are vasodilation and an increase in capillary permeability, promoting absorption and removal of waste products and exudates. With vasodilation, blood flow in the area is augmented, increasing oxygen and nutrient delivery necessary for repair and healing. Vasodilation secondary to heat relaxes smooth muscle of blood vessels directly by activating beta adrenergic fibers and indirectly by accelerating the inflammatory process by heat. With inflammation comes an increase in production of histamine-like substances and bradykinins, both causing vasodilation.

With vasodilation and increased capillary hydrostatic pressure, edema occurs.[3] For this reason heat should not be used immediately after or in the hours following acute injury. Since heat results in vasodilation and augmented removal of waste, it has been thought that hematoma resorption would be promoted by heat therapy.[4] The experimental evidence underlying this clinical assumption is lacking, and further basic control studies are required to identify the role of heat in hematoma absorption.

Cellular metabolism is augmented in biologic systems, but the favorable use of heat in increasing chemical reactions is limited by the temperature at which protein is denatured (46°C). According to van't Hoff's law, a chemical reaction increases by 2 to 3 magnitudes for each temperature increase of 10°C. This basic chemical law has clinical implication. With total body heating (sauna or steam bath), sweating, tachycardia, fall in blood pressure, increase in rate and depth of respiration, and increase in urine production occur. Further physiologic events are loss of water, electrolytes, creatinine, uric acid, and urea. Cervical spine syndromes occur mainly in older patients, so in using heat, one must be aware that for those older patients with edema, increased total body water and electrolyte content, decreased total body fluid content, or a labile cardiovascular system, there are risks in raising core body temperature.

The application of "deep heat" to bone epiphyses through ultrasound, short wave, or microwave diathermy does not affect bone growth if the period of exposure is not prolonged and temperatures above 45°C are not reached; however, with prolonged heating times at low-level temperatures, bone growth is accelerated.[5] The reverse, arrest of bone growth, occurs if heating temperature is raised to levels causing pain even for short periods; this effect is exaggerated if there is circulatory compromise in the tissues involved, preventing heat dissipation. The clinical point here is that deep heat should not be used over and around epiphyses in young people or in the area of healing fractures in the cervical spine or anywhere else in patients of any age!

Heat has been shown clearly to increase viscoelastic properties of collagen, which is useful in flexion contractures. Flexion contractures occur commonly, gradually, and subtly in the cervical spine. At 37°C, collagenous tissues have definite but limited elastic properties, stretching somewhat but returning to their resting length with removal of the stress. Tissue deformation occurs if tension (traction) is applied over a prolonged period, 12 to 15 minutes or more. With increase of tissue temperature to 45°C, the viscous properties of collagen are dominant, and applied loads or stress readily produce irreversible elongations. This has clear application in the cervical spine. Even light loads used at increased temperature over a prolonged time result in greater residual lengthening than either light loads at normal temperature for longer periods or heavy loads (vigorous stretching) at normal or elevated temperature for shorter periods.

Stretch tendon reflexes are decreased by heat through the mechanism of reducing muscle spindle excitability—decreasing gamma fiber activity.

Table 12–1. PHYSIOLOGIC EFFECTS OF HEAT

Increased local temperature
Increased cellular and tissue metabolism
Reflex vasodilation
Sedation
Analgesia
Phagocytosis
Arteriolar dilation
Increased capillary blood flow
Increased oxygen and nutrient supply
Antibody and leucocyte delivery
Increased clearance of heat (itself) and metabolites
Increased capillary pressure
Edema

Thus favorable clinical effects of heat occur by diminishing muscle spasm through using deep heating of muscle and superficial heating of skin and subcutaneous tissue. The superficial heat reaches muscle fiber. Heat reduces ischemia (improves blood flow) by reducing muscle spasm, thus diminishing pain perception. The use of heat as a counterirritant is also effective in the treatment of pain. According to the "gate theory," the heat stimulus floods the "pain gate," blocking painful stimulus reception for central interpretation. Moist heat seems more capable of producing muscle relaxation than dry heat, though precise scientific evidence is lacking.

Application of heat induces some reflex heating. Specifically, heating one extremity increases blood flow on the contralateral side. This "consensual reaction" is a function of the intensity of the local heat. The effect produced on the contralateral side never equals that produced by direct application of heat. Reflex heating occurs in the extremities when heat is applied to the cervical spine.

Table 12–1 lists the physiologic effects of heat, including local, total body, and reflex effects.

Methods of Heat Therapy

Since skin is a poor conductor of heat, conductive heating devices do not heat below a depth of about 1 cm; an ordinary electric heating pad is a simple, conductive, dry heating device. The pads regulate heat delivery by a thermostat; the greatest heat generated is 77°C, with an average temperature range of commercial units between 46 and 71°C. Heat injury is a function of both increased temperature and duration of increased temperature; even lower temperatures over long periods of time (1 to 2 hours) can be damaging. The maximal safe exposure of surfaces to direct heat is for 30 minutes at 45°C. At home, the pad should be placed on top of but not under the cervical spine to be heated, because the pressure of the head and neck may decrease vascularity to the skin exposed to the heating elements, potentially causing thermal damage.

Hot water bottles, usually holding about 1 quart of water, are common and widely available. They are not satisfactory, however, since regulation of temperature is difficult. Application of hot water bottles at a temperature of 48°C for only several minutes can be damaging. Protecting skin with towels prevents such injury. Hot water bottles cool rapidly on exposure to air, making them useful for short periods only.

Hot packs are very effective, and they are available as so-called hydrocollators. These are segmented, flat canvas bags filled with hydrated silicone gel. The gel retains heat for relatively long periods. The gel is heated by placing the pack in water at 65 to 90°C, usually suspending it on racks for even heating. The heating process takes 20 to 30 minutes. If dry, they require 2 to 3 hours of immersion to ensure complete soaking; since the pads are usually heated to a temperature of 65°C or higher, thermal damage to skin is always a risk. Two layers of toweling serve as protective insulation. Commercially available cloth insulators purchased with the canvas hot packs make this technique safe.

Wet compresses are a traditional means of applying moist heat. Towels are placed in a large pan of hot water, allowing them to absorb the moisture. If they are placed in plastic bags immediately after heating, the rapid air evaporation resulting in heat loss is blocked. The now old-fashioned Kenny hot packs used in the management of patients with poliomyelitis are wool or wool-like material heated in hot water to 60°C and wrung out before application. The Kenny hot pack also loses heat rapidly unless precautions are taken.

Total body heating, or immersion heating, is accomplished in hot tub baths, aerated water baths (whirlpools), saunas, steam baths, and paraffin baths for hands, feet, and sometimes the cervical spine. Relatively inexpensive equipment to put a steam bath within most ordinary bathrooms is commercially available. The shower or bathtub must be enclosed to concentrate the steam and moist heat. Placement of a plastic or water- and steamproof stool in the enclosure or tub makes the treatment more convenient.

Saunas and steam baths are very effective and useful in treatment of the cervical spine in those cases in which there is no contraindication to raising total body temperature (see Table 12–1). Saunas use dry heat at temperatures between 54 and 71°C, whereas steam baths are maintained at 41 to 46°C. Both are used from 15 to 30 minutes. Saunas, by their advocates, have been regarded as less tiring than moist steam heat because the tissue is heated at a slower rate, allowing the skin to cool by perspiring.[6] Always consider the consequences of total body heating, vasodilation, tachycardia, hypotension, sweating, and reflex vasodilation.

Paraffin, commonly used as a source of heat for clinical problems with hands and feet, may be applied to the cervical spine. It is painted on with a large paintbrush. Paraffin is prepared as 8 parts paraffin to 1 part mineral oil, commercially heated to 51 to 55°C in a thermostatically controlled metal unit. The mineral oil serves to decrease the melting point of paraffin such that it will liquify at the previously specified temperature. Hands may be dipped 6 to 12 times in the paraffin, which congeals in a few seconds, hardening after each dipping. The result is a 0.25- to 0.5-in layer of hot paraffin covering the surface. After the last dipping, the dipped area is wrapped in plastic for 30 minutes. The effect of heating, soothing, and relaxing the muscle is achieved.

Though paraffin can be painted on with a paintbrush, the immersion method is more soothing and relaxing. Disadvantages of the immersion method are that it is messy and the skin must be well prepared—cleansed of any dirt and debris—prior to immersion. It should be tried in pain problems of the cervical spine along with the number of other potentially usable modalities. I am frequently happily surprised that it is very effective in individual instances.

The many analgesic balms and liniments usually containing such irritants as methyl salicylate (oil of wintergreen), capsicum (red pepper), menthol, various alcohols, and eucalyptol really generate no heat. They irritate the skin and result in capillary dilation, which provides an increase in blood flow to the part, with a pleasant sensation of warmth. Such analgesic balms are simple, safe, and sold in supermarkets and drugstores. The technique involves applying a layer of the balm or liniment over the area, covering the area with an insulator of towel or cloth, and holding the insulator in position with an elastic bandage until the sense of warmth has dissipated, usually 1 to 2 hours. A layer of plastic over the cervical spine following application of the liniment prolongs the period of warmth sensation. This process of counterirritation is thought to so stimulate the nerve endings in the skin that they block or diminish the perception of pain impulses. Their role in cervical spine management is a small one, but they are worth the trial in given instances.

Diathermy or Deep Heat

Diathermy heats by energy conversion. The word is from the Greek *dia*, meaning through, and *thermē*, meaning heat. Short wave or high-frequency current is passed through the tissue involved, in this instance the cervical spine. Each of the three diathermy modalities utilizes a different conversion system to transfer energy deep into tissues. Transfer of energy is by high-frequency current in short wave diathermy, by electromagnetic radiation in microwave diathermy, and by high-frequency acoustic vibration in ultrasound diathermy. Table 12–2 lists the heat transfer system and modalities for each. Each method and

Table 12–2. HEAT TRANSFER SYSTEMS

System	Modality
Conduction	Hot packs
	Paraffin
Convection	Hydrotherapy
	Moist air
Conversion	Radiant heat
	Microwaves
	Short waves
	Ultrasound

technique is different from the other. The goal in therapy is to allow heat energy to reach the tissue presumed involved before the heat conversion occurs, so that the tissue (muscle, ligament, tendon, joint) is heated preferentially, without heating intermediate tissue (burning). Short wave diathermy and microwave diathermy do not penetrate as deeply as ultrasound diathermy. Microwave (frequency 2456 megahertz [MHz]) diathermy penetrates more deeply than short wave diathermy with a condenser plate. However, it penetrates less deeply than short wave diathermy through an induction coil. Both capacitant-coupling short wave and microwave diathermy and induction-coupling short wave diathermy heat skin and superficial muscle while also heating intermediate muscle layers. This occurs because of the induction by applied magnetic fields to a circular electric field caused by eddy currents in the tissue. Microwaves and short waves are particularly absorbed in tissue high in water content, such as muscle, but are also absorbed by fat, which has a water content value higher than that of skin but significantly lower than that of muscle. A physiologic issue involved here is that the magnitude of penetration of short waves and microwaves is a function of the thickness of the subcutaneous panniculus, the fat layer. A 2-cm fat layer blocks energy transmission to underlying muscle. Ultrasonic vibration (acoustic) is not absorbed by fat. Consequently its deep-heating effect is not regulated by the depth of fat. Ultrasound diathermy is more useful than short wave or microwave diathermy in increasing temperatures of joints covered by sizable volumes of soft tissue, such as the hip joint. Ultrasound diathermy is thus very readily and accurately applicable in the cervical spine where ligaments, muscles, bones, and joints are not far from the surface.

The absorption of ultrasound occurs mainly in the proteins of connective tissue. Since sound waves scatter at irregular surfaces, selective absorption occurs at tissue interfaces. High temperatures at such interfaces are achieved 20 to 30 seconds after initiating therapy. A safety factor is that both microwave and ultrasound magnitude can be accurately adjusted and read from the commercial delivery machine. Short wave intensity can only be guessed at, and the therapist

depends on the patient's subjective sensations of discomfort to regulate therapeutic intensity. Short wave diathermy and microwave diathermy require 15- to 25-minute treatment sessions, whereas in ultrasound diathermy, total heating time is 3 to 5 minutes, owing to the speed of penetration. The rise in temperature induced by diathermy lasts only 30 minutes following treatment.

Short Wave Diathermy. The cervical spine is placed between two condenser plates of plastic or glass (capacitant coupling) or is wrapped with a delivery coil (induction coupling). The method involving condenser plates is more commonly used. Current densities produced are related to the application technique and the intensity selected for the particular treatment. When plates are used as condensers, the field between the plates has its greatest density close to the plates, making current density greater near the plates than deep in the tissue. With application, a space of 1 to 2 inches is left between the plates and the skin to prevent the higher currents generated adjacent to the plates from burning the skin. Increased penetration is obtained with the coil. Like the plates, the coil must not be applied directly to the skin, or burning will result. Toweling as insulation is required. Since conductivity of the tissues is a function of water content, the higher the water content, the greater the conductivity, that is, the greater the heating itself. Muscle is selectively heated because of its high water content compared with bone, fat, or skin. As previously noted, a thick, subcutaneous fat layer (2 cm) absorbs much if not all of the energy before it reaches underlying muscle or other connective tissue. Thus, short wave diathermy is best used where muscles or joints treated are beneath minimal soft tissue. Controls on the panel of the commercial instrument allow adjustments of power output (in milliamperes [mA]) and allow for tuning with the power amplifier circuit to bring the patient into resonance. The time of treatment is automatically set on a separate dial. Though sometimes useful, short wave diathermy is less effective than ultrasound diathermy.

Microwave Diathermy. Microwaves lie between infrared and visible light on the electromagnetic spectrum. The wavelength is 3 cm to 3 m, with a frequency of 900 to 2450 MHz. Short waves have a length of 7.5 m to 22 m and a frequency of 13.6 to 40.68 MHz. For microwaves, only the frequency of 2450 MHz has been authorized for medical use. Lower frequencies of microwave energy (900 MHz) cause less conversion of energy in subcutaneous tissues, producing more uniform muscle heating. Microwaves of higher frequency and shorter wavelength are reflected from bone and other surfaces to a greater degree than the microwaves of lower frequency currently in use. The diameter of bone is relatively large compared with short wavelengths of high frequency. Such reflective waves induce "hot spots" that can burn tissue. Since microwaves of lower frequency cause more adequate heating of muscle and less bone reflection (less hot spot burning), many physiatrists would like to change the authorized microwave frequency from 2450 to 916 MHz. A towel should be placed over the skin to absorb any accumulated sweat because sweat droplets absorb microwaves preferentially, potentially resulting in local burning.

Ultrasound Diathermy. The commercial instrument converts electric energy from an ordinary outlet plug to mechanical vibrations delivered through an applicator head. Sound waves are not transmitted well in air and require a coupling medium—water or mineral oil between the applicator head and the patient—to ensure appropriate direction of the sound impulse. The vibrations (sound energy) are converted to heat energy in the tissue. Muscle temperature can be raised 7 to 8° readily. Ultrasound energy propagation is a function of absorption characteristics of the tissue as well as reflection of ultrasound off interfaces. Although this energy is preferentially absorbed by tissue proteins, bone absorbs 10 times more ultrasound than soft tissue. The marketed instrument allows automatic adjustment of time and power output. The latter is usually increased slowly to the patient's tolerance. The dose of ultrasound is expressed in watts per square centimeter (W per cm²). A low-intensity dose ranges from 0.1 to 0.8 W per cm²; one of medium intensity ranges from 0.8 to 1.5 W per cm², and a high-intensity dose ranges from 1.5 to 3 W per cm². Ultrasound diathermy not only produces heat in the tissues but increases the permeability of biologic membranes. Iontophoresis (the driving of chemical substances into the tissue) takes advantage of this increased permeability. Chemicals, placed on the skin prior to ultrasound therapy, are driven deep into the tissue.

In the cervical spine, ultrasound diathermy has been found useful as an adjunct to the many other treatment modalities. It is useful in osteoarthritis of the cervical spine, limited range of motion for whatever reason, general stiffness, and relative immobilization, all of which are basically subacute and chronic inflammatory conditions rather than conditions involving acutely inflamed tissues. An absolute contraindication is the presence of cardiac pacemakers and metallic implants in general. These metals may be heated by the ultrasound, causing local burning. Hot spot formation from metallic reflection does not occur to the same degree with ultrasound that it does with short waves and microwaves. Ischemic vascular disease likewise contraindicates deep heating of all three types. Lack of perception of touch, pain, and vibration in the area to be treated is a contraindication. If the patient cannot note heat intensity, an important safeguard against burning is lost.

Table 12–3 is a summary of the physical thera-

Table 12–3. MODALITIES OF THERMOTHERAPY

Method	Tissue Heated	Depth of Heating
Heat Therapy		
Electric heating pad	Skin and subcutaneous tissue	Superficial
Infrared lamp	Skin and subcutaneous tissue	Superficial
Hot towels	Skin and subcutaneous tissue	Superficial
Hot pack	Skin and subcutaneous tissue	Superficial
Paraffin	Skin and subcutaneous tissue	Superficial
Hydrotherapy	Skin and subcutaneous tissue	Superficial
Sauna	Skin and subcutaneous tissue	Superficial
Steam bath or cabinet	Skin and subcutaneous tissue	Superficial
Diathermy		
Short wave with capacitor plates	Deep subcutaneous tissue	Deep
Microwave at frequency of 2456 MHz	Superficial muscle	Deep
Short wave with reduction coils	Muscle selectively heated	Deep
Microwave at frequency of 915 MHz	Muscle selectively heated	Deep
Ultrasound	Tendons, nerves, ligaments, joints, myofascial interfaces	Deep

peutic heating modalities available, their areas of application, and their depth of heating.

Mechanical Therapy

Massage. Mechanical stimulation of tissues reduces swelling, increases circulation, can mobilize flexion contracture tissue, and is psychologically comforting. Massage is an ancient and venerable method, not used as much today as its effectiveness warrants. The ancient Chinese published and described massage techniques, but because the French translated from the Chinese, French names are widely used for procedures available today, including effleurage (stroking), pétrissage (compression or kneading), and tapotement (percussion). Friction and vibration are also a part of massage. The professional masseur or masseuse, knowing that the therapeutic effect is mechanical as well as psychologic, uses a smooth, rhythmic massage technique, with a lubricant on the patient's skin to allow the hand to glide and flow. Contraindications to massage are infection, boils, acne, skin disease, malignancies, or thrombosis. One may spread these lesions by mechanical stimulation. Certain commercial intermittent compression devices are really only one aspect of massage therapy. There are instruments available that give intermittent compression and circulate water at 0°C around the extremity. This device has been used in horses also. Compression is useful in the prevention of venous stasis in the lower extremities. The cervical spine lends itself well to massage, though it is relatively little used. Most physical and occupational therapists understand and practice the techniques of massage, and I recommend that it be used more often.

Whirlpool. Whirlpool therapy is a combination of massage and hydrotherapy in which immersion in either cold or hot water is accomplished. The effect at a variety of temperatures is that of heat or cold as well as mechanical stimulation of the tissues by the moving water. An aerator maintains water agitation.

The commercial whirlpool tubs are set at 32 to 38°C for total body immersion, 38 to 39°C for the lower extremities, and 41°C for the upper extremities or the cervical spine. Cold water therapy is generally used at 13 to 18°C. Treatment periods in all instances is 15 to 25 minutes. Contrast whirlpools (contrast immersion baths) are thought to be useful in decreasing edema. Presumably this is accomplished through heat-induced vasodilation followed by the vasoconstrictive effects of cold—really a massage action forcing fluid out of interstitial spaces and into the circulation. The part treated is immersed in hot water at 40°C for 4 minutes and in cold water at 13 to 18°C for 2 minutes. Water baths, Hubbard tanks, exercise pools, and whirlpool baths use water buoyancy to decrease stress on joints. It is difficult to apply to the cervical spine but is sometimes rewarding in difficult or long-standing cases.

Electrotherapy

Electrotherapy makes use of the stimulation of nerve and muscle by electric current. Electromyography is used diagnostically. There has been a recent ground swell (probably unjustified) of popularity of electricity as a therapeutic tool. Its uses include the presumed prevention of muscle atrophy secondary to immobilization or denervation, the retraining of surgically transferred muscle or tendon, diminishing spasm, increasing blood flow, preventing phlebitis in immobilized people, decreasing edema, and iontophoresis.

Two types of electric current are employed. The first type, direct (galvanic), is a steady unidirectional flow of current, continuous or interrupted. The other type, alternating (faradic), switches directions of flow rhythmically and in precise timing. Generator terminals alternate from positive to negative polarity. Interrupted alternating current and interrupted direct current can both be regulated, producing different pulse widths and pulse frequencies, measured in cycles per second (hertz [Hz]). High-voltage direct current of short duration clearly stimulates both nerves and muscle. Muscles (denervated and innervated) and nerves (sensory and motor) are all selectively stimulated to measurable magnitude, and each responds to a different pulse frequency and width. Nerves accept electrostimuli better than muscle, and innervated muscle accommodates stimuli more easily than denervated muscle. One can stimulate nerves with frequencies as high as 60 Hz. Nerves can accommodate stimuli of less than 40 Hz and thus do not discharge at this lower frequency. Innervated muscle requires a frequency of 20 Hz or less to respond, because at high frequencies of stimulation, muscle does not have sufficient time to accumulate an effective charge to discharge, that is, to stimulate muscle contraction. Thus, muscle has a higher capacitance than nerve, and denervated muscle must have a pulse frequency as low as 10 Hz to stimulate it to contract.

The idea of pain control with electric stimulation dates back to Greek and Roman times, when live torpedo fish and organs of electric fish were used as afferent stimuli for pain control. Refinement of the stimulation characteristics took a long time, that is, from then to the past decade.

Sensory (afferent) nerve fibers differ from motor (efferent) nerve fibers in accommodation of stimulus, threshold of firing, response to the different wave forms, and length of the refractory period. Motor neurons require pulse frequencies of 25 Hz, with pulse durations of at least 500 microseconds to stimulate them. Though this current activates sensory fibers, motor fibers are preferentially stimulated. Sensory fibers respond maximally to currents of high frequency (100 to 150 Hz) and short duration (100 microseconds or less). Transcutaneous electric nerve stimulation (TENS) units, commonly used with considerable success in controlling acute and chronic pain, utilize current pulses of high frequency and short duration, stimulating sensory fibers in preference to motor fibers. This method has clear application in cervical spine chronic pain syndromes. Much of the increased popularity of this method stems from the work of Melzack and Wall.[7] In their theory, called the "gate" theory, they propose that by bombardment of sensory afferent fibers by electric stimuli, the central "gates" in the spinal cord are flooded and all binding sites occupied, preventing the perception of painful stimuli by myelinated dorsal column fibers. Percutaneous and transcutaneous stimulators were devised. These are small, convenient, battery-powered devices (3 oz, 2 by 2 by 7 in) that can be carried in the pocket or on a belt. There are many instruments on the market. Most have a high-voltage direct current, with two electrodes and an intensity motor. Some control pulse width (0 to 100 microseconds) as well as frequency (10 to 170 Hz). Some have a fixed pulse width and frequency, and various wave forms are used. No single instrument has established itself as the most effective. TENS units stimulate sensory fibers most effectively but can also stimulate motor fibers, with consequent muscle contraction. The patient adjusts the intensity of the unit to the highest possible point of sensory nerve fiber stimulus without muscle contraction, thus it can be comfortably tolerated without the annoyance of twitching muscle. There is much debate and controversy over the most useful placement of electrode plates, that is, determining the location that decreases pain most effectively. Various therapists propose putting the electrodes over the painful area, in the appropriate dermatome of pain, at the trigger points of pain, at the motor points of painful muscles (focal points) or near the peripheral nerves supplying the area of pain. Contralateral nerves have been stimulated, with the hope and supposition that the ipsilateral side will also receive stimuli. Thus, electrode placement remains undecided and usually is a matter of trial and error. The patient and the therapist often use a placement that has been successful for them previously.

An advantage is that TENS units can be rented or purchased, making continuous stimulation available. It is common experience that continuous stimulation for weeks to months controls the pain and can then be stopped without recurrence of pain. Successful pain relief has been achieved through sessions of 30 minutes, 2 to 3 times daily. More recently, TENS units have been used safely in the management of acute pain, and they have a place in the management of cervical spine acute pain syndromes.[8] Since pain results in continuous, chronic, and sustained muscle spasm, effective pain control promotes a more prompt return to full range of motion and strength, a frequent goal in cervical spine disorders. Furthermore, the risks entailed in using TENS units are almost nonexistent (primary skin irritation).

Electric stimulation of muscle retards muscle atrophy caused by immobilization or denervation, aids in retraining surgically transposed muscles, and promotes muscle awareness in regaining voluntary muscle control. Nevertheless, simple exercises—isotonic, isometric, and range of motion—are more effective, and the price is right! There are portable as well as stationary (in physical therapy departments) motor electric stimulation units. A direct or an alternating current can be used and is delivered through the positive pole (hyperpolarization) or through the negative pole (depolarization). Depolarization requires a lower stimulus and is more comfortable. Pulse frequency, 20 to 80 Hz, and pulse width, 40 to 300 microseconds, can be adjusted. There are two electrodes; one is placed over the motor point, and the other is placed anywhere but over the antagonist muscle. Both electrodes can be placed on either end of the muscle to be stimulated (bipolar technique). The muscle's motor point is found by using a small needle electrode to stimulate various sites on the muscle and determine the location of maximal response. The motor point of a normally innervated muscle usually is located in the middle portion of the greatest bulk of the muscle, where motor nerves penetrate before branching peripherally in the specific muscle. For retraining muscle, electric units provide audio as well as visual evidence of muscle contraction and joint response. Thus, by seeing and hearing the contraction, the patient accelerates the process of regaining voluntary control. Electric stimulation is at most an aid; it is not a replacement for optimum musculoskeletal fitness and strengthening programs, particularly in the cervical spine.

A final use of direct current is iontophoresis, the electric means of driving charged chemicals into skin and mucous membranes. Histamine, vasodilators, iodine, salicylic acid, local anesthetics, and hormones can be transferred to interstitial fluid spaces by iontophoresis. The velocity of movement of the drugs (ions) is directly related to the applied voltage. The amount of drug transferred is a function of the duration of current flow but is only estimated because of the many variables. Although iontophoresis has no place in management of the cervical spine, it is used for that purpose.

The methods of physical therapy presented heretofore play a significant role in the management of most conditions in the cervical spine. If applied judiciously, thoughtfully, and scientifically over a sufficient period of time, they can be relied upon to diminish symptoms and, often, to correct the primary problems of pain, swelling, and limitation of motion. All of this occurs by the variable mechanisms described here, an application of the physiology involved. It is of the utmost importance that the physician and therapist comprehend the physiologic action of these modalities, their physiologic effects, and the indications and contraindications in their use.

CERVICAL ORTHOSES

The cervical spine has more than its share of musculoskeletal problems, because it is subject to trauma, osteoarthritis, rheumatoid arthritis, and a broad spectrum of inflammatory, vascular, paralytic, neoplastic, and infectious disorders in addition to supporting and balancing a 15-lb ball, the head. Exercise and movement of the cervical spine is absolutely essential to its continuing function, and immobilization, which is always relative and rarely absolute, is a frequently utilized and effective modality in therapy. Efforts to splint and immobilize the cervical spine are not new. Braces and other devices were used by Hippocrates, and records of brace descriptions date back as far as 2750–2625 BC.[9] Armor makers of the middle ages produced certain cervical spine braces. Today many cervical collars, braces, casts, and other cervical orthoses that immobilize the cervical spine are available. Interestingly, these devices are often named for their originator or the area of the country in which they were designed, for example, the Thomas collar by Hugh Owen Thomas, a Liverpool surgeon (1820–1904); the Guilford brace designed by a Cleveland physical therapist; the Philadelphia collar; and the Yale brace. The reason for prescribing any of the cervical orthoses is to limit spinal motion, reduce pain and muscle spasm, protect vital structures within the cervical spine, correct deformity, support where musculoskeletal structures are inadequate, and take advantage of the physiologic consequences of immobilization. The spectrum of magnitudes of immobilization ranges from approximately 5% to 10% limitation in the soft cervical collar devices to over 90% limitation in the halo devices. For reliable and predictable protection of the spinal cord and nerve roots (as is needed in the case of fracture dislocation), the device must be firmly fixed to structures at both the upper and the lower ends of the neck, that is, the skull and the thorax. The efficacy of any orthosis in immobilization depends upon the security of attachment to these structures.

The range of motion of the normal cervical spine is well known (see Chapter 2, *Anatomy and Biomechanics*), and data on motion of the cervical spine in the various orthoses are available.[10, 11, 12] Johnson et al[13] studied cervical motion and its limitation in normal subjects, with each subject acting as his or her own control except in the cases of the halo vest. The per cent of normal motion permitted by the orthosis is reported in Table 12–4. The soft collar allows approximately 75% of normal motion (restricts 25%), whereas the halo vest allows approximately 4% of normal motion (restricts 96%).

Figures 12–1, 12–2, and 12–3 are composites of all of the types of collars and bracing available.* The soft cervical collar (see Fig. 12–1) is foam rubber in stockinette, comfortable, and well tolerated, but it allows a mean of only about 75% of normal motion (25% restricted motion). The Philadelphia collar (see Fig. 12–2, parts *C, H, I, O*) is constructed of plastizote and reinforced with anterior and posterior plastic struts. The anterior and posterior halves fasten laterally with Velcro. The molded mandibular and occipital supports extend to the upper thorax, allowing a mean of approximately 55% of normal motion. The SOMI (sterno-*o*ccipito-*m*andibular-*i*mmobilizer) brace (see Fig. 12–3*A*) has a rigid anterior plastic chest piece (yoke) to which mandibular and occipital supports are attached. The curved rigid supports extend over the shoulders to the level of the spines of the scapulae. The supports are connected to straps that cross in the back and attach to the bottom of the yoke in the front after passing under the axillae. This arrangement allows the brace to be put on without moving the patient from a supine position, and it has an optional head piece, which snaps on the occipital rest and passes around the forehead, allowing the patient to remove the mandibular support while eating. The four-post brace (see Fig. 12–3, parts *D, J, K*), with molded mandibular and occipital supports, is attached by adjustable struts to anterior and posterior padded thoracic plates. The anterior and posterior sections are connected by leather straps below the ears and over the shoulders. There are no axillary straps. The Guilford brace (see Fig. 12–3*C*) has padded mandibular and occipital supports that are rigidly connected to anterior and posterior thoracic plates. Anterior and posterior

---

*Names and addresses of the manufacturers of the collars and braces pictured follow: AOA Orthopedics Inc., 74 N.E. 75th Street, Miami, FL 33138; Becker Inc., 635 Executive Drive, Troy, MI 48083; Bell-Horn Company, 451 N. Third Street, Philadelphia, PA 19123; Camp International Inc., P.O. Box 89, Jackson, MI 49204; Freeman, 900 W. Chicago Road, Sturgis, MI 49091; LaCal Surgical Supplies, 509 South Flower Street, Burbank, CA 91502; Pope/USM, P.O. Box 5030, Pasadena, CA 91107–0030.

Table 12–4. NORMAL CERVICAL MOTION ALLOWED FROM THE OCCIPUT TO T1

	Number of Subjects	Mean Age (years)	Mean Per Cent of Normal Motion Allowed		
			Flexion-Extension	*Lateral Flexion*	*Rotation*
Normal	44	25.8	100.0	100.0	100.0
Soft collar	20	26.2	74.2	92.3	92.6
Philadelphia collar	17	25.8	28.9	66.4	43.7
SOMI brace	22	25.0	27.7	65.6	33.6
Four-post brace	27	25.9	20.6	45.9	27.1
Rigid cervicothoracic brace	27	25.9	12.8	50.5	18.2
Halo vest	7	40.0	4.0	4.0	1.0

From Johnson RM, Hart DL, Simmons EF, et al: Cervical orthoses: A study comparing their effectiveness in restricting cervical motion in normal subjects. J Bone Joint Surg 59A:332, 1977.

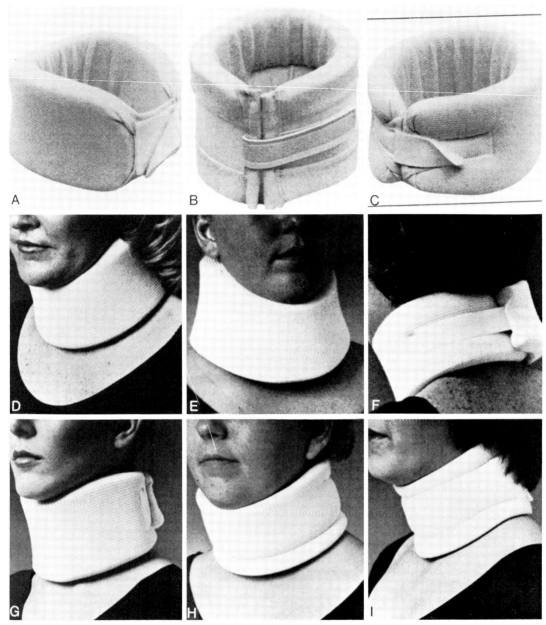

Figure 12–1. Soft Cervical Collars. *A,* Soft foam collar. Sizes range from extra small to extra large, heights from 3 to 4.25 in, lengths from 14.5 to 20.25 in. (Model 830, Freeman.) *B,* Cerv-ease collar. Combines the comfort of soft foam with the more rigid support of plastic collars; Velcro closure. Sizes range from small to large, heights from 3.5 to 4.38 in, lengths from 15.75 to 21.5 in. (Model 815, Freeman.) *C,* Soft foam collar. Contoured. Sizes range from small to extra large, heights from 3.5 to 5 in, lengths from 15.5 to 21.5 in. (Model 825, Freeman.) *D,* Low-contour foam cervical collar. Velcro closure; washable. Sizes range from extra small to extra large. (Model 0701, AOA Orthopedics.) *E,* High-contour foam cervical collar. Velcro closure; washable. Sizes range from extra small to extra large. (Model 0700, AOA Orthopedics.) *F,* Universal foam cervical collar. Velcro closure; washable. Size is universal. (Model 0723, AOA Orthopedics.) *G,* High-contour foam cervical collar. Contoured for chin and mandibular area. Sizes range from small to extra large. (Model 0714, AOA Orthopedics.) *H,* Cervi-foam collar. High-density foam; firm; Velcro closure (flexion position attained by closing in front, and extension position by closing in back). (Model 0704, AOA Orthopedics.) *I,* Serpentine collar. Firm; high-density foam; Velcro closure (flexion position attained by closing in back, and extension position by closing in front). Sizes range from small to extra large. (Model 0705, AOA Orthopedics.)

Illustration continued on opposite page

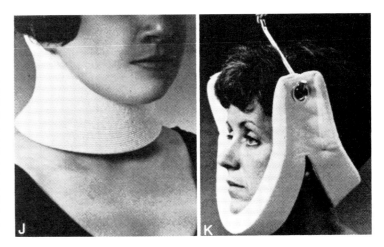

Figure 12–1 *Continued J*, Flexion collar. Medium-density foam; large Velcro closure; cut low in front, high in back to provide maximum support. Sizes range from small to extra large. (Model 0706, AOA Orthopedics.) *K*, Split foam collar. Low-density foam; Velcro closure (flexion position attained by closing in front, and extension position by closing in back). Grommet at each end allows use as head halter. Sizes range from extra small to extra large. (Model 0709, AOA Orthopedics.)

sections interlock to form a rigid metal ring below ear level. Thoracic plates are attached to each other over the shoulders and by a strap under the axillae—a two-post brace.

The cervical thoracic brace (see Fig. 12–3*B*) is like an extended Philadelphia collar. It is made of plastizote, and the anterior and posterior halves are reinforced with plastic struts. The orthosis extends well down the thorax and fastens with straps underneath the axillae. The occipital rest is high.

The halo vest (see Fig. 12–3, parts *N, O, P*) is made of a prefabricated plastic material attached to a halo ring. The halo ring is attached rigidly to the skull. The vest is lined with a soft material (lamb's wool or Kodel). A plaster cast can be substituted for the plastic vest and attached to a similar superstrut. This orthosis, though very effective, provides the most rigid external restriction of cervical spine motion but requires a great deal of experience to utilize.[13]

Flexion and extension are clearly best controlled by the halo vest or halo cast. This degree of motion control is necessary in instances of trauma, dislocations, and fractures but not in most medical cervical spine problems. In the three most useful studies,[10, 11, 13] sagittal plane motion (flexion and extension) was measured at different intervertebral levels in subjects using halo vests. The cervical spine, peculiarly enough, extended at one level and flexed at another level—a motion referred to as paradoxical by Hartman[10, 11] and as "snaking" by Johnson.[13] Thus some levels move more than the cervical spine as a whole. The SOMI brace controls upper and midcervical flexion, C1 to C4, better than the others, whereas the cervicothoracic brace is more restrictive at lower cervical levels, C5 to T1. These more rigid orthoses limit flexion more than extension.

Rotation is less well controlled by the orthoses than flexion-extension. The cervicothoracic brace is the most effective, allowing 18% of normal

rotation. The halo vest controls rotation best, allowing 1% of normal motion.

Lateral flexion is the least well controlled by the orthoses. The cervicothoracic and the four-post braces are the most effective, permitting 46% and 50% of normal motion respectively. The halo vest, with a firm purchase on the skull, limits lateral flexion to a total motion arc of less than 12 degrees.

Though the soft collar does not significantly immobilize the cervical spine, patients uniformly find this collar very comfortable for various reasons. I recommend it whether or not the comfort indicates any degree of support or immobilization—even if the collar simply provides the patient with something to rest the chin on and relax. Some patients report that their head gets so tired that they want to hold it in their hands. They are better fitted with a soft cervical collar, a simple device providing some support. If the muscles of the neck are very fatigued, the head can hang heavy indeed. A patient once reported that her head and neck were so tired that they felt like a pumpkin on the end of a toothpick! The soft collar may function as a reminder to restrict activities and has the psychologic benefit of giving the patient the feeling of being treated and managed.

The Philadelphia collar is almost as comfortable as a soft collar but considerably more effective in controlling neck motion (see Table 12–4). It is well tolerated by most patients and controls cervical spine motion almost as well as the cervicothoracic brace, particularly in controlling flexion in the midcervical level.

The SOMI brace best immobilizes the upper cervical spine, C1–C5, in flexion and is less effective than the four-post and the cervicothoracic braces in controlling the other three basic motions. The SOMI brace is practical in that it can be fitted and adjusted easily and is thus more acceptable to the patient. The patient can be supine when it is put on, and the cervical spine need not be moved—an advantage in the case of acute injury.

Text continued on page 252

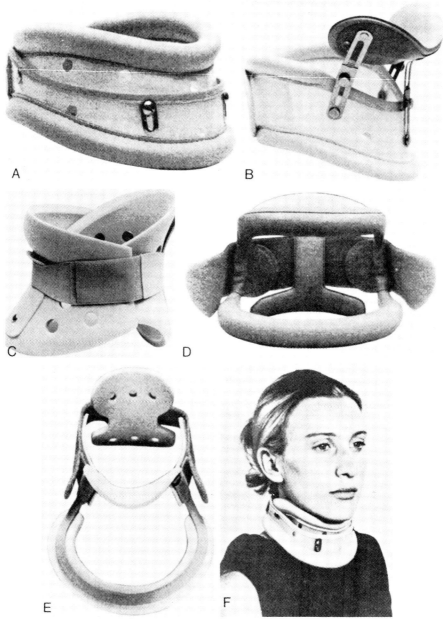

Figure 12–2. Rigid Molded Collars. *A*, Thomas type collar. Two-piece construction; easily adjusted for height and circumference; Velcro closure; ventilated. Heights range from 3.5 to 4.5 in, lengths from 15 to 18 in. (Model 821, Freeman.) *B*, Thomas type collar. Padded adjustable chin rest; ventilated; Velcro closure. Sizes range from small to large. (Model 819, Freeman.) *C*, Philadelphia collar. Lightweight; molded plastizote; double Velcro closures; foam body with rigid plastic occipital and mandibular supports for chin and shoulder contours. Fitted according to neck circumference and height measurement from sternal notch to chin. Sizes include small (10 to 12 in), medium (13 to 15 in), and large (16 to 19 in). (Models 804, 805, 806, and 807, Freeman.) *D*, Wire-frame collar. Open neck construction; adjustable to any height and shape; frame padded with foam rubber. Velcro closure attaches to cushioned back piece; adjustable to circumference of any neck. Size is universal. (Models 792 and 793, Freeman.) *E*, Executive collar. Frame with open neck design. Occipital pad attached to Velcro strap can be positioned to fit circumference of any neck. Size is universal. (Models 792 and 793, Freeman.) *E*, Executive collar. Frame with open neck design. Occipital pad attached to Velcro strap can be positioned to fit circumference of any neck. Sizes range from small to large (4- to 5-in height). (Models 817 and 818, Freeman.) *F*, Adjustable plastic cervical collar. Two set screws in front; fully padded; Velcro closure. Sizes range from extra small to extra large. (Model 1500, Bell-Horn.)

Illustration continued on opposite page

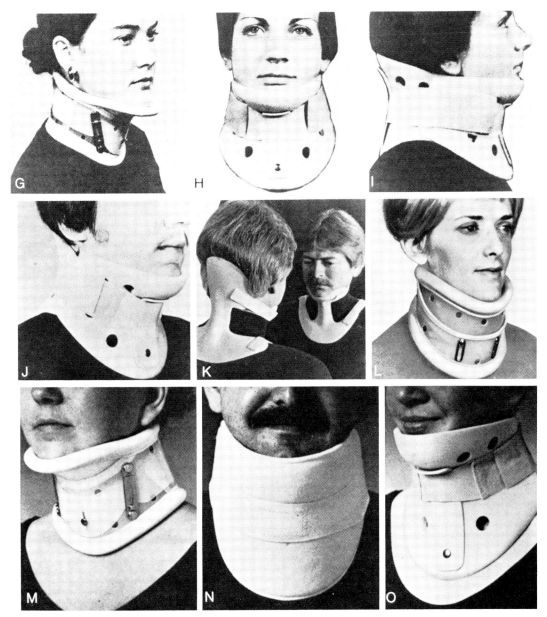

Figure 12–2 *Continued G*, Adjustable plastic cervical collar with chin rest. Contoured deep in front and high in back; flexion with chin tucked in; Velcro closure. Sizes range from small to extra large. (Model 1510, Bell-Horn.) *H*, Philadelphia collar (front view). Molded plastizote; lightweight; adjustable to 3 widths (3.25 in, 4.25 in, and 5.25 in). Molded and shaped to chin; conforms to shoulder contour; double Velcro closure. Sizes include small (10 to 12 in), medium (13 to 15 in), and large (16 to 18 in). Ventilated. (No specific model number, Bell-Horn.) *I*, Side view of Philadelphia collar. *J*, Two-part cervical collar. Adaptable to fit bedridden patients; moldable with heat application; hook and pile closure; polyethylene foam. Sizes include small, medium, and large. (Model C62, Camp International.) *K*, Two-part cervolite collar. Reversible for flexion or extension; hook and pile closure; beige and acrylic-polyvinyl chloride. Sizes include small, medium, and large. Note mirror image for front view. (Model C80, Camp International.) *L*, Complete adjustable collar for immediate (urgent) support. Plastic with vinyl-covered, foam rubber edges; hook and pile closure. Available in narrow or wide width. (Model C56, Camp International.) *M*, Plastic adjustable collar with chin rest. Polyethylene with vinyl-covered, foam-padded top and bottom edges; two screw adjustments for wide-range extension and flexion positions; ventilated; Velcro closure; washable. Chin rest minimizes head movement. Sizes include small, medium, and large. (Model 0502, AOA Orthopedics.) *N*, Cerva-collar II. Molded foam; contoured to head and shoulder; Two-piece construction; chin cups built in; full 360-degree support; double Velcro closure; washable. Sizes include small, medium, large, and extra large. (Model 0787, AOA Orthopedics.) *O*, Philadelphia cervical collar. Polyethylene foam; molded plastic chin support; two-piece construction; four collar heights for each size; rigid plastic occipital and mandibular posts to assure solid support; double Velcro closure, ventilated; washable. Sizes include small, medium, and large. (Model 0758, AOA Orthopedics.)

250

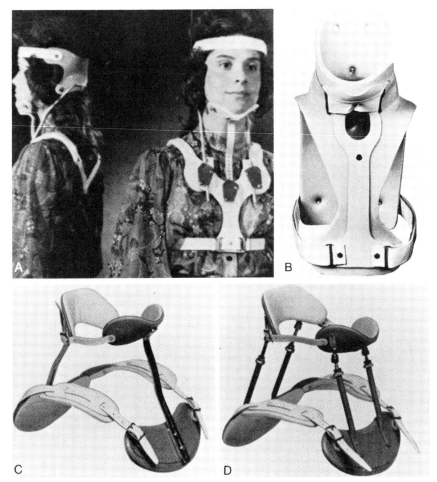

Figure 12–3. Cervical Orthoses and Braces. *A*, Cervical orthosis. Adjustable for sternal, occipital, and mandibular positioning; anterior and posterior adjustments; headband auxiliary support; lightweight, vinyl-coated aluminum. Sizes include small (children), medium (small adult), and large (large adult). (Model 8005, Camp International.) *B*, For patients requiring both cervical and high-thoracic support. Anterior and posterior sections reinforced with Kydex; Velcro closure for neck and chest adjustments; universal application. Sizes include small (Model H9480), medium (Model H9481), and large (Model H9482). (Camp International.) *C*, Two-post cervical brace. Contoured, adjustable, aluminum uprights with padded, vinyl-covered, aluminum chin and occiput pieces. Padded chest and back plates and felt-cushioned, leather shoulder straps allow for wearing under clothing. Sizes include small, medium, and large. (Model 803, Freeman.) *D*, Four-post cervical brace. Steel, swivel-post construction, with locking ball and socket, allows fixation in any position. Four threaded steel rods adjust up or down in tubular aluminum uprights. Aluminum headrests and chest and back plates cushioned; leather shoulder straps cushioned. Sizes include small, medium, and large. (Model 800, Freeman.) *E*, Swivel type neck brace. Four-way swivel type with telescoping. Excellent for any type of cervical trauma. Swivel joint allows complete adjustability. Screw extensions permit any degree of flexion and extension (indications: cervical spine fracture or dislocation, torticollis, cervical Pott's disease). (Model B27, Becker.) *F*, Stationary cervical neck brace. Padded aluminum collar in two parts. Allows easy removal and reapplication. Two horizontal bands, which fit accurately under occiput and chin, are attached to collar by four screw extensions. Easily adjusted; requires measurements around chest, chin, and occiput. (Model 107, Becker.) *G*, Anterior view of rigid APRO (anterior, posterior, rotational orthosis). Semirigid connection bars, which connect the occipital and mandibular supports, allow for flexion-, extension-, and size-range adjustments between chin and occiput. The bars are controlled by adjustable locking discs. Optimum fixation is obtained by extending the orthosis down to the thorax. Straps connect the anterior and posterior sections. Adjustable for patients of nearly any size. Available in one size only. (LaCal.) *H*, Lateral view of rigid APRO. *I*, Posterior view of rigid APRO. *J*, Adjustable cervical brace, four-post model. Immobilizes cervical spine in neck injuries. Aluminum and stainless steel. Back and breast plates have aluminum and felt pads. Foam-padded chin and occiput pieces; fully adjustable; easy to fit. Positive locking device eliminates loosening. Sizes: child and adult. (Model 0790, AOA Orthopedics.) *K*, Standard four-post adjustable cervical brace. Lightweight aluminum; occiput and chin plates padded with leather. Sizes include small, medium, and large. (Model 1060, LaCal.) *L*, Completely adjustable cervical brace. Fits patients of nearly all sizes. Single post with fully adjustable chin plate. Occiput and chin plates padded with special sponge rubber; underarm straps padded. (Model 1061 LaCal.) *M*, Locking ball-and-socket swivel-post cervical neck brace. Adjustable in all directions (up, down, sideways); easy to adjust. Sizes include extra small, small, medium, and large. (Model 5020, LaCal.)

Illustration continued on opposite page

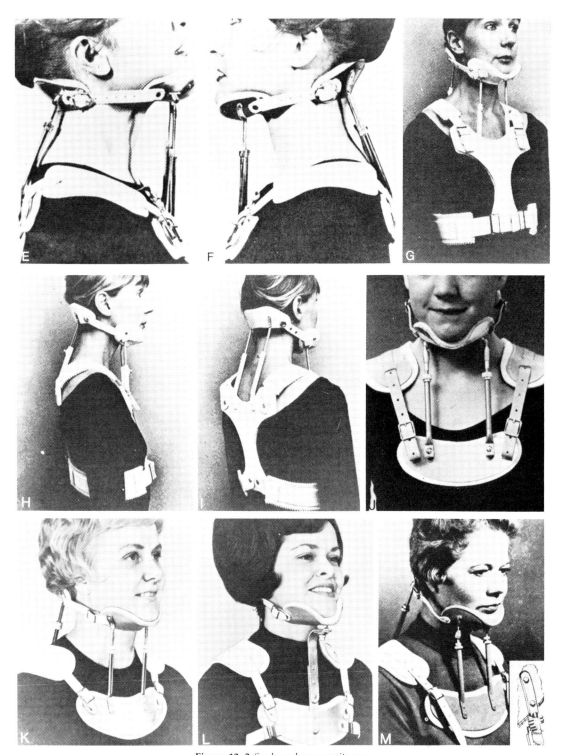

Figure 12–3 *See legend on opposite page*

Illustration continued on following page

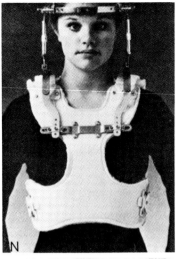
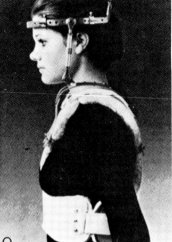
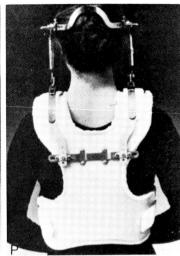
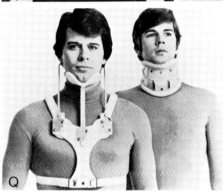

Figure 12–3 *Continued N,* Ambulatory (anterior view). De-signed for preoperative, postoperative, and post-traumatic rigid immobilization of cervical spine. Easy to measure and adjust to fit patient; lightweight, low-profile superstructure. Interlocking tab and Velcro closures at shoulders and sides maintain alignment. Anterior section hinges to allow emergency access to thorax for unobstructed mediolateral and anteroposterior radiographs. Replaceable liner. (No specific model numbers published, Pope/USM.) *O,* Lateral view of ambulatory halo. *P,* Posterior view of ambulatory halo. *Q,* Special model by Camp for a three-post brace with adjustable chin and occiput support; a very adjustable, locking, rigid, plastic collar.

Because the SOMI brace allows more extension, it is not as effective for the injured spine that is unstable in extension. Another disadvantage is that when confined to bed, patients are very uncomfortable because of the posterior plastic yoke pressing into the scapulae. The SOMI brace serves well, however, for ambulatory patients or those using wheelchairs.

The Yale braces (see Fig. 12–3, parts *F, G, H, I, Q*), rigid cervicothoracic immobilization orthoses, are second only to the halo devices in restricting cervical spine motion. Their best control is in flexion and extension, but they are also effective in restricting rotation. They allow up to 50% of lateral flexion.

Halo casts and halo vests for control of cervical spine motion are superior to the other types available. There seems to be no difference between the vest and the cast. A disadvantage of halo orthoses is that their use truly is restricted to doctors who have had a great deal of experience using them, because a keen awareness of the complications that may arise is particularly important.

Patient acceptance of the brace constitutes a major problem, and the doctor prescribing an orthosis must feel confident that the patient has accepted it. The best collar or bracing is ineffective if not used. Areas of skin irritation may constitute a significant complication, making the device intolerable. The halo vest or cast is the only orthosis that safely stops motion between the occiput and C1. Thus a fracture of the atlas or the odontoid process requires such an orthosis if motion is to be prevented. Atlantoaxial motion also is not controlled well by the other orthoses. Of course, the degree of control required varies with the specific clinical circumstance. In cases of trauma, fracture, and fracture-dislocation, control of motion until the acute episode is over is critically important. In instances of trauma in the lower cervical spine, the cervicothoracic, Yale type, and SOMI devices are effective and far better tolerated than the halo devices. The atlanto-odontoid injury requires the more rigid braces.

The most common clinical problems in the cervical spine are those of osteoarthritis involving the intervertebral discs, zygapophyseal joints, and the joints of Luschka. The maintenance of the clinically maximal range of motion short of producing paresthesia or pain is a major aspect of long-term management. Nevertheless, soft collars and plastic collars are important—if only for intermittent immobilization—particularly when the neck is subjected to additional stress, for example, when the patient is driving for long distances or has the neck in unusual extension, lateral flexion, or rotation. The most frequent indication for the collars is in the relief of local or referred pain in the various types of osteoarthritis. This relative immobilization must be balanced against active as well as passive exercises and, often enough, is associated with a program of ''building a better neck'' through isotonic and isometric exercises against resistance. It is common experience that wearing a soft collar or a semirigid plastic collar that holds the neck in a comfortable neutral position or in slight flexion gives symptomatic relief. The real usefulness of the collar in the treatment of osteoarthritis has been challenged.[14, 15] Collars are clearly indicated for the patient with rheumatoid arthritis—the more severe the instability and subluxation, the more rigid the collar must be. The instability, subluxations, and general loss of physiologic motion occur at the atlantoaxial junction and the middle cervical spine. There is no uniform agreement on the effectiveness of collars, but there seems to be no disagreement regarding the symptomatic improvement and comfort these patients derive in using collars and braces.[16]

When prescribing a collar or brace, the physician should always include a program of isometric and isotonic exercises for flexor, extensor, lateral flexor, and rotator muscle groups, since the immobilization results in rapid atrophy of muscles, which causes weak cervical musculature and progression of clinical disability.

Cervical spine immobilization in brace or collar is an integral part of the management of both acute injuries and chronic disorders. Collars and braces are designed to hold the neck in an optimum anatomic position for the healing of injured skeletal, ligamentous, capsular, and joint structures. The neck is held in a relatively straight position, with only slight lordosis, and the chin is tucked in. If the neck is held in hyperextension, it is completely wrong anatomically, wrong in principle, and should not be so used in the management of sprain injuries unless there is clear rupture of the posterior longitudinal ligament. Hyperextension immobilization causes further stretching of the anterior longitudinal ligament, permits posterior ligamentous structures to heal in a shortened position, and results in narrowing of the intervertebral foramina, particularly so if there is instability of the ligamentous and capsular structures.

Most importantly, we must be aware of the connective tissue changes induced in a joint by immobilization in hyperextension. Compression of the articular surface may cause cartilage fibrillation owing to prolonged pressure; the posterior portion of the capsules and the posterior ligamentous structures are ultimately and permanently shortened. If anterior structures are injured, stretched, or sprained, they heal in the extended position, causing anterior instability. Thus, the optimum position for immobilization, partial and complete, is with all anatomic structures relaxed—the principle followed in the management of any other bone or joint injury. Hyperextension decreases the anteroposterior as well as the vertical diameters of the intervertebral foramina, further crowding the nerve roots and inducing radicular symptoms and signs. The position of the relatively straight cervical spine with the chin tucked in is physiologic mechanically and is the position of greatest comfort.

With acute injury, immobilization by collar or brace should be continued for 3 to 8 weeks or longer, though the orthosis should be removed daily, and isotonic and isometric exercises should be done within the constraints of pain and other symptoms or signs. For chronic pain, cervical immobilization is usually for a much shorter time.

CERVICAL SPINE TRACTION

The usefulness and effectiveness of cervical spine traction is well established, since it does cause vertebral distraction. This separation allows alteration of the pathologic relationship between nerve root and compressing disc or between nerve root and zygapophyseal and Luschka joint osteophyte impingement. The plane of the zygapophyseal is also altered. In my experience, 75% to 80% of patients with radicular symptoms receive clear benefit from traction, usually lasting months to years. I prefer intermittent traction initially, and usually that is all that is necessary. The weight applied ranges from a minimum of 15 lb to a maximum of 50 lb (7 to 23 kg) over a period of 15 to 20 minutes. If definite and significant improvement does not occur after 8 to 10 sessions of optimally administered traction, it should be discontinued. Also, if symptoms have clearly worsened, there is little point in continuing, and one should identify precisely why it was not successful.

The amount of weight used is a function of the size of the patient, the presence of neurologic symptoms or signs, the specific lesion for which traction is prescribed, and the patient's general sense of comfort and improvement. One is guided by the results of each traction session. With clear-cut improvements, patients may purchase home traction equipment and continue traction under those circumstances until all symptoms are gone. In those instances, contact should be maintained with a medical authority. Continuous traction does not permit the use of as much weight as that permitted in intermittent traction. Increments of weight are added with each traction session, depending on the degree of the patient's progress. The trial and error method is the best way to deal with such variables as the distance that the patient

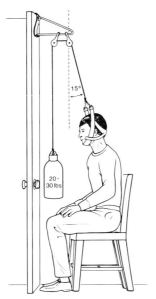

Figure 12–4. Physiologic position for home cervical spine traction. Note the neck is in slight flexion; equal force is exerted from occiput and chin. The angle of the traction rope with the vertical is 15 to 25 degrees. A 20-lb (9 kg) upright is used in the generally healthy patient of average size and body build and without neurologic signs. Symptoms are usually pain and paresthesia of the shoulder, arm, forearm, and hand.

sits from the traction pulley, the direction of traction, and the position of the patient during traction. An average set of circumstances is 20 lb (9 kg) for 20 minutes. The patient is in slight cervical spine flexion, facing the door or apparatus, and the angle of the rope is about 20 to 30 degrees off the vertical. This is the physiologic position (Fig. 12–4). In general, the relief of pain occurs sooner and more completely in the case of radicular symptoms than in that of symptoms arising from the connective tissue structures of the neck itself—ligaments, tendons, muscles, and joints. Symptoms related to the upper extremities are much more likely to be relieved by traction, whereas symptoms related to the cervical spine connective tissue structures are more likely to respond to the use of a collar. In a sense, traction is manipulative therapy, but it is vastly different from adjustments involving rotational and lateral stretches, which pose a greater risk of root irritation.

The patient usually can designate the most effective conditions for traction. If the symptom is produced or exaggerated (either actively by the patient or passively by the examiner) by a certain position of the cervical spine (extension, lateral flexion, or rotation), try traction with the patient in a slightly laterally flexed position. If symptoms arise on one side, the force of the traction should

be in the opposite direction, with the patient in a position of slightly forward flexion. Sometimes though not often, bed traction is superior. In severe disabling pain with neurologic symptoms and signs, hospitalization with more concentrated bed traction may be required. This is better done episodically than constantly. Based on experience, I believe that 95% of patients with symptomatic cervical spine osteoarthritis can be managed with a vigorous, conservative program of sufficient duration, leaving only an estimated 5% to consider for surgical approach.

Traction is one of the most frequently used management tools in disorders of the cervical spine. Nonetheless, it is controversial. Its use arose in antiquity. Hippocrates used traction to reduce dislocation. Archimedes worked out a traction apparatus utilizing levers and pulleys used by doctors in Alexandria in 300 BC. Guy de Chauliac used weights and pulleys for fracture reduction. In our time, traction has been used in reduction of bone deformities, skeletal tuberculosis, spasm of acute poliomyelitis, and certainly in "whiplash" injury of the cervical spine. Controversial aspects involve the following questions: How much weight should be used? Should it be done sitting, supine, even standing? Which head halter is best? Should intermittent or continous traction be used? How long should it be continued? How many times per day, per week, per month should it be performed? At what angle should the traction force be exerted? The physician who is very knowledgeable about the distinctive and unusual anatomy of the cervical spine, the physiology of the structures involved, and the long experience with traction and its history, can, in the presence of precise diagnosis, approach all of these questions objectively.

Methods of Applying Traction: A Review of the Literature

Cervical traction is conveniently divided into three categories: mechanical, manual, and self traction (home traction). Some authors regard manual traction as preferred owing to the immediate sensory feedback to the therapist by the patient and the presumed specificity of treatment. In manual traction, one hand is placed under the chin, with the other under the occiput, or both hands are placed under the occiput (Fig. 12–5). A longitudinal force is exerted at varying angles of cervical flexion, extension, lateral flexion, and even rotation. Degree, direction, and duration of the tractive force are guided by the patient's response, the clinical disorder, and the goal. Prior to starting the traction, relaxation is urged. Sometimes, observing the degree to which a patient relaxes can be used as a method of assessing potential response to mechanical traction. Relaxation can be used also in "unlocking" the apophyseal joint surfaces for reduction of internal derangement, re-establishment or improvement of alignment, or preceding other techniques of manipulation.

Three-dimensional traction is a term used to describe traction in reference to the three cardinal planes—sagittal, coronal, and transverse—dictated by the patient's historical and clinical examination data. Two considerations govern the determination of appropriate positioning: the position should result in the greatest relief of pain, and the degree of force applied should not go beyond the amount that "takes up the slack" in the periarticular tissues.

Cyriax[17] has developed a method of traction manipulation that applies strong manual traction in cervical extension. The goal is reduction of an intervertebal disc protrusion. If clinical signs and symptoms suggest a central lesion (bilateral pain or paresthesia or both), strong traction with manual cervical motion is employed. If symptoms are unilateral—a posterolateral protrusion—strong traction with superimposed cervical motion (manipulation) is used. Cyriax decides on the type of traction to use based on data derived from detailed history, physical examination, and treatment results in process—a well-defined set of clinical findings.

The movements employed in self treatment are repeated axial extension and backward bending (extension). This method is designed by McKenzie[18] and is said to centralize and or abolish the patient's symptoms. In self traction, the pa-

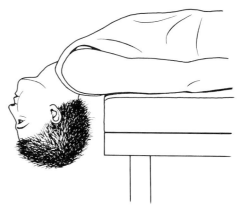

Figure 12–6. McKenzie method of self treatment. In self traction the patient lies in the supine position, with the head, neck, and upper thorax extended over the treatment table. This procedure is repeated for short periods (minutes). It is monitored according to favorable (or unfavorable) results obtained, as interpreted by the patient.

tient lies supine, with the head, neck, and upper thorax extended over the edge of a treatment table. The cervical spine is in extension and distracting in an inverted position (Fig. 12–6). This is repeated for short periods (minutes) if the patient's symptoms are "centralizing" or "abolishing" or both. The patient presumably controls symptoms through this exercise. Education in posture and avoiding aggravating symptoms are used mainly in the correction of a forward head and in the proper control of cervical and lumbar lordosis in sitting, standing, and sleeping.

Stoddard proposes a method called intermittent sustained traction. It involves the use of a head halter attached to a transverse bar, with a traction angle of about 30 degrees cervical flexion. The force is applied and released at a rate of 10 pulls within 10 minutes. It is designed to decrease nerve root irritation by opening intervertebral foramina and presumably improving circulation within the epidural venous-lymphatic system.[19]

Mechanical traction is applied as constant, intermittent, intermittent variable, and progressive. Constant traction is, as implied, continuous traction from 10 to 60 minutes, with a mean of 25 minutes. Rarely, 24 hours of uninterrupted traction is used. Also, continual sessions during the day, with frequent rest intervals and no traction at night are employed. This is accomplished with traction machines set up in physical therapy departments or in a hospital bed. Constant traction is usually reserved for very severe pain or circumstances in which extreme traction forces are required.

Intermittent traction is also done by specific machine. One technique involves traction and release, with a known amount of force applied.

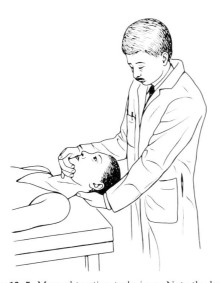

Figure 12–5. Manual traction technique. Note the hands are placed under the patient's occiput and under the chin; traction is exerted with the neck in a neutral to slight flexion position. Force is gradually increased, and the increase is monitored by the patient's response, determined in the process of traction. This is one of the methods of manipulation addressed further on in this chapter.

In another method, the traction force is progressively increased and decreased, with repetitions of an on-off cycle. Advantages of this technique are its effect upon circulation and its stimulation of the mechanoreceptors in capsule, ligament, tendon, and joint. It is ideal for the less acute and less critical cervical diseases and injuries; the instrument used allows a gradual, slow rate of pull and release of the traction.

Intermittent variable traction is done by varying the weight applied, increasing it at one session and decreasing it at the next. The changes are made according to clinical assessment of the result.

Progressive traction involves increasing the weight applied at each session until the clinical result is attained, and continuing traction at that weight for several days. The goal is permanent relief of symptoms.

The most widely used apparatus is a home traction device employing a yoke, an overhead pulley, traction rope, and weight (see Fig. 12–4). Problems in this type of traction are excessive force on the temporomandibular joint, the patient's intolerance of the discomfort involved, and the sometimes advantageous supine position for patient relaxation. A broad range of forces are required for varying problems.

Rath,[20] in an extensive review of the literature on the subject of traction, reported the following list of effects of traction: (1) prevention and freeing up of adhesions within the dural sleeves, nerve roots, and adjacent capsular structures; (2) distraction and separation of articular surfaces of the zygapophyseal joints; (3) relief of nerve root compression and irritation within the intervertebral foramina; (4) decompression of intervertebral joints, with reduction of derangements within the disc; (5) improvement of the circulatory status within the epidural spaces of the spinal and lateral nerve root canals; and (6) reduction of the inflammatory response, pain, and muscle spasm.

Traction is done in either the supine or the sitting position. Ultimately, the clinical response of the patient is the deciding factor in choice of position. The supine position combines the advantages of increased stability and the possibility of relaxation of the muscles. I believe that where greater forces of traction are exerted, the supine position is more effective and somewhat safer than the sitting position. After studying the two positions, Deets et al[21] concluded that the supine position resulted in greater posterior separation, increased relaxation, less muscle spasm, more stability of the patient, less force necessary to overcome the weight of the head, easy alignment of the patient and traction apparatus, and better reversal of cervical lordosis.

The angle of traction is between 15 and 35 degrees. The angle decided upon depends on the clinical response and the patient's interpretation of its efficacy. The type of head halter used affects the angle of traction provided. The perception of force should be about equal under the occiput and the chin. In the great majority of instances, slight cervical flexion is preferred, since it is the position in which posterior zygapophyseal joints are separated, intervertebral foramina are enlarged, and lateral nerve root canals are released. It is most effective in patients with radicular symptoms. Neck flexion between 20 and 30 degrees is appropriate. Using angles of flexion beyond 30 to 35 degrees may negate the ability to distract joint surfaces because the tension created in the posterior ligamentous structures increases the angles of flexion, causing more tensile strain on the spinal cord and its coverings.

Traction in extension is rarely, if ever, indicated. The biomechanical consequences of cervical extension are relaxation of posterior structures, with a decrease in the available space of the spinal canal and lateral nerve root canal, spinal cord compression, and increased radicular symptoms. Traction in extension is generally contraindicated.

The amount of traction force is a most important consideration. In any clinical use of traction, one must understand cervical anatomy and biomechanics in both the normal and the pathologic states and apply sound physiologic principles, using the patient's response to treatment as a guide. An important consideration is that the force adequate for one patient is not proper for another. The weight applied may range from 10 to 50 lb (5 to 23 kg). Some sound scientific rules of thumb are that 8 to 10 lb (4 to 5 kg) provides an anchoring effect, 18 to 22 lb (8 to 10 kg) produces physiologic alignment, and 22 to 62 lb (10 to 28 kg) may be required to correct deformity. Application of these principles is dependent upon individual patient, body size and surface area, sex, and the specific disorder involved.[22] There is a consensus that vertebral separation predictably occurs with the application of traction force between 25 and 45 lb (11 to 20 kg). Less than 20 lb (9 kg)—in the range of 5 to 15 lb (2 to 7 kg)—does no more than partially lift the weight of the head and neck, resulting in relaxation of the paravertebral musculature. Muscle relaxation is essential for optimum results. Even though separation may occur at 25 lb (11 kg) of force, voluntary muscle contraction on the part of the patient can completely negate the separation effect—even at a traction force of 55 lb (25 kg).[23] Therefore, a comfortable treatment position, patient relaxation, and complete patient cooperation are absolutely necessary. Stoddard,[19] in reporting a clinical range at which effective treatment is predicted, suggests that between 24 and 30 lb (11 and 14 kg) of traction is necessary for successful relief of radicular symptoms using the intermittent and sustained manual traction techniques.

The mean duration of traction is 25 minutes. The intermittent technique is generally successful at a rate of 10 pulls within a 10-minute period for radicular symptoms. Judovich[24] uses daily traction for 1 hour on an outpatient basis and, in the hospital, uses continuous traction, with 15 minutes of rest every 1 to 2 hours. Colachis and Strohm[25] suggest that the duration of traction does not influence the degree of vertebral separation; rather, the angle of pull and the amount of tractive force are the important factors.

Prior to seriously considering traction, one should give thought to any forces placed across the mandible and the temporomandibular joint. Abnormal dental occlusion may result in temporomandibular joint dysfunction that is made worse by the traction. Oral plastic splints have sometimes been used to bypass this objection. A resting mandibular splint—as simple as a piece of gauze or a moldable wax—can be used if the patient complains of temporomandibular joint symptoms. Historical inquiry into temporomandibular joint dysfunction is an important consideration.

Contraindications to cervical spine traction are midline intervertebral disc herniation in the presence of acute torticollis, malignant disease with metastasis to the cervical spine, gross inflammatory disease, extensive nuclear prolapse, joint hyperlaxity (hypermobility syndrome), structural scoliosis, marked kyphosis or lordosis, and the presence of nerve root compression (contraindication to rhythmic traction). Further contraindications are malignant disease other than metastatic, clinical symptoms and signs of spinal cord compression, active infectious disease, extensive osteoporosis, serious hypertension and cardiovascular disease, rheumatoid arthritis, pregnancy, and advanced old age.

A general knowledge of the biomechanics and kinematics of the cervical spine is important to the clinician in applying cervical spine traction (see Chapter 2, *Anatomy and Biomechanics*). One must consider the anatomic events occurring in the upper complex (occipito-atlanto-axial) on forward bending and in the lower complex (C2–C3 through C7–T1). On backward bending, the anatomic events of the upper complex and those of the lower complex occur in reverse. Rotational and side bending events are also required assessments.

Before application of cervical traction, the clinical, historical, and physical data are collected, assessed, and analyzed, and the decision for traction is made based upon these data. The two mechanisms by which cervical spine soft tissues can be damaged and fail are a short-duration, high-amplitude loading and a long-duration, low-amplitude loading. The first represents an obvious acute trauma—the classic automobile collision from the rear, with the so-called whiplash injury. The second is a chronic sprain of soft tissues occurring inconspicuously and very gradually, usually with some final event that precipitates a more acute syndrome superimposed on a chronic one. Overuse syndromes are in this category of mechanical onset. Compression packing of vital neurovascular structures in the cervical spine, the upper cervical zygapophyseal joints necessary to body equilibrium, and the contrecoup effect of brain against the inner skull are reasons to be very cautious.

In the hours to days following an acute cervical spine injury, traction is generally contraindicated, since it would tend to aggravate and perpetuate the pathophysiologic event. The patient should get adequate rest and be instructed in the optimum postures for sleeping, sitting, and standing, that is, those positions that promote healing of the involved structures and allow subsidence of muscle spasm and absorption of hemorrhage. Mechanical traction other than simple immobilization is contraindicated in the acute phase of cervical spine injury. In the chronic cervical spine pain syndrome, traction may be utilized. Certainly posterior ligamentous systems suffer fatigue intolerance following prolonged and repetitive loading; a permanent spraining is the clinical result. Such may be seen in the patient who has an abnormally prolonged forward head position caused by sitting, reading, working at a desk or maintaining extensive rotation-extension as a job posture or in a sleeping position. The clinical mechanism by which the pain syndrome developed and the specific diagnostic formulation are the deciding factors in applying cervical traction.

Can cervical spine traction, manual or mechanical, reduce or replace a herniating intervertebral disc? There is some evidence that traction can do this.[26, 27] It is probable that the anulus fibrosus and the posterior longitudinal ligament are pulled taut by traction, resulting in intervertebral separation. This could create decreased intradiscal pressure, allowing enough force to reduce herniation of a nucleus pulposus or a hard piece of disc—a fragment moves about enough to relieve symptoms. Farfan's histologic studies provide impressive support for this position.[28]

In summary, the clinical indications for traction are determined by the goals set, the patient's diagnosis, duration of the disorder, and the capability of the examiner and therapist. Early, following a trauma without neurologic symptoms or signs, traction is contraindicated, because the goals are then to promote rest and relaxation, to allow the healing process to begin, and to assess the overall clinical problem. In gradually acquired disorders, one should begin with low traction weight, either constant or intermittent, and gradually increase it, assessing the progress by the hour or day. In chronic conditions, such as osteoarthritis and intervertebral disc syndromes, the goal is to relax the muscles, unload apophyseal and intervertebral disc surfaces, improve circulation, move any disc fragments to a more favorable location, and encourage cicatrization. If coupled with a global clinical approach to the specific problem, traction can be a successful mode of therapy for many mechanical disorders of the cervical spine. Often neglected is postural instruction (sleeping, sitting, standing, walking) for reduction of symptoms and prevention of recurrence.

Some patients with recurrent or chronic cervical spine disc disorder benefit from short periods of traction at home once or twice daily. This is simple, inexpensive, and worth considering in individual instances. Several types of standing apparatus are available that utilize body weight as the traction force, with no extrinsic friction to overcome. Hanging from a horizontal bar for a few minutes is useful, helpful, safe, and not overly strenuous. Unfortunately, tilt tables for graduated inverted positioning are used. Very recently, special boots clipped to an overhead bar for inverted hanging and thigh platforms for hanging by or kneeling over have been used. I condemn these methods. Such upside-down hanging techniques cause circulatory changes and compress the diaphragm. They should be done only by superb athletes, and even they are at risk! At most, hanging upside down accomplishes whatever stretching in the upright posture accomplishes.

General Indications for Cervical Spine Traction

McKenzie[18] has categorized mechanical disorders in which traction may be indicated and the criteria for making the decision to use traction. He emphasizes educating patients concerning taking responsibility for their own treatment to try to reduce incidence, significance, and recurrence of the disorders. Three mechanical syndromes have been elucidated. (1) Postural syndrome: Mechanical abnormality due to postural defects resulting in pain that is almost always intermittent and occurs when soft tissues surrounding the bony segments are under prolonged stress and consequent strain. Such a patient has no specific restriction of movement or complaint of continuous pain with repeated testing of all motions—active, passive, and against resistance. In such patients traction is not indicated; the patient needs instruction in appropriate posture and preventive exercise only. (2) Dysfunction syndrome: This set of symptoms and signs is caused by poor postural habit, cervical osteoarthritis, abnormal intervertebral discs, and malalignment and is a condition in which adaptive shortening and loss of mobility cause premature pain—the pain occurs before full, normal end range of motion can occur. The condition occurs because movement is inadequately carried out at the same time that contracture of soft tissue is in process. Examination discloses limited range of motion, with pain occurring at the end of whatever range of motion is present. Repeated range of motion study shows no worsening of the condition; pain is suppressed

immediately or in a short period of time after stretching of the adaptively shortened tissue. Treatment is aimed at correcting the restricted movement according to the assessed pathophysiology in progress and the magnitude of irritability of surrounding tissue. An analogy is the restoration of complete knee flexion after acute symptoms of a severe sprain have subsided. Traction is often useful in these circumstances, allowing rest of the involved joints, increasing separation of zygapophyseal and Luschka joints, and improving circulation. Ultimately, however, treatment must be directed at restoring full range of motion. (3) Derangement syndrome: Derangement is defined here as disturbance of the normal, neutral resting position of the zygapophyseal, intervertebral disc, and Luschka joints of two or more adjacent vertebrae. The etiology is cervical osteoarthritis or change in the position of the nucleus pulposus of the intervertebral disc. Change in the position of the nucleus pulposus disturbs anular material, and the change in the joint may affect the ability of joint surfaces to move in normal pathways, from initiating to completing range of motion.

Testing range of motion in the wrong direction (the direction of movement that enhances the derangement) increases symptoms of pain (and sometimes paresthesia), and the symptoms become more peripheral. Repeated motion in the proper direction (the direction of movement that reduces the derangement) tends to make the symptoms more central and to abolish them ultimately. An entire spectrum of disc disorders is included, and those patients capable of cooperation with instruction and having an intact anular wall respond exceedingly well to the cervical spine traction and its consequent reduction of the lesion.

In our practice, cervical traction plays a very important role. The method of traction is specifically designed for the individual patient, and the choice made is based on sophisticated clinical assessment. If nuclear material has breached the anular wall and hydrostatic dynamics is lost, neither traction nor reductive procedures will cure the problem.

BALANCE OF REST AND EXERCISE

It is clear that absolute bed rest has no place in the management of rheumatic diseases generally and of disorders and diseases of the cervical spine specifically. Selective rest or relative immobilization and the overall maintenance of optimum fitness are of great importance in any disorder of the cervical spine. It is further established that immobilization, coupled with both active and passive exercise, even in severe inflammatory joint disease, results in a decrease in the inflammatory process. The gross, disabling, and debilitating physical and psychologic consequences of bed rest are well known and to be avoided. Somewhere between too little and too much of both rest and exercise is the proper amount.

A normal anatomic characteristic peculiar to the cervical spine is that fibrocartilaginous, meniscus-like structures occur in all of its joints (see Chapter 3, *Pathology*). In joints with menisci and fibrofatty connective tissue—and in all joints, for that matter—prolonged immobilization results in a predictable proliferative response of meniscal and fibrofatty tissues to produce a pannus-like structure reminiscent of the rheumatoid granulomatous pannus. A danger of immobilization is that it may cause joint ankylosis. Total immobilization, even of inflamed joints, for as few as 4 weeks, may be carried out without measurable loss of joint mobility, *but muscle power is inevitably much reduced*. Joint immobilization for 3 months or longer is associated with fibrofatty tissue proliferation and threat of ultimate joint destruction; hence the great importance of specifically prescribed and individualized exercise and rest. Mechanical stress resulting from abnormal joints subjected to faulty posture is another major consideration. Preventive rest positions in bed, sitting, and walking are of great importance in prevention of joint damage in rheumatoid arthritis and osteoarthritis of the cervical spine as well as in hip and knee flexion contractures consequent to poor posture (see *Posture, Training and Prophylaxis* in this chapter).

Optimum posture and position are essential to successful accomplishment of relaxation. Stretching exercises are ineffective without relaxation of the muscles crossing and overlying the joints. We live in an imperfect world; tension and anxiety are our daily lot, and the necessity for general muscular relaxation is well recognized. Teaching the emotionally tense person to relax in preparation for stretching exercises and postural training is of great importance.

Exercises

Stretching Exercises. Stretching exercises applied to the cervical spine are used for the same reasons they are elsewhere in the body: to prevent contracture, to increase range of motion if contracture has occurred, and to maintain optimum biomechanical function of the supporting structures in the cervical spine. Stretching in the prevention of joint contractures mechanically stimulates virtually all structures in and about joints—the capsule, synovium, tendons, muscles, and ligamentous structures. Both with and without the inflammatory process present, the capsules, ligaments, tendons, and muscles undergo adaptive shortening in immobilization. The structural characteristics of connective tissue elements change with inflammation and immobilization. The loose, irregular weave of fibrofatty connective tissue differs greatly from the high-tensile–

strength, parallel-array collagen fibers of tough ligaments and the completely parallel-oriented collagen fibers of tendon. The interdigitations in the fabric of fascia, ligament, and capsule constitute sites of adhesion formation when normal movement is restricted. In both rheumatoid arthritis and osteoarthritis, contractures occur in completely uninvolved joints because of disturbed postural mechanisms and failure of maintenance of optimum mechanical stimulation and use of muscle, bone, joint, tendon, and ligament. There is excellent evidence that contractures occur owing to loss of proteoglycans, the water- and salt-rich elements present in varying concentrations of all connective tissues. The proteoglycans are essential to proper cross-linking between collagen fibers in high-tensile–strength structures, such as ligaments, capsules, and tendons. Stretching exercises for the cervical spine include stretching of the thoracic and the lumbar portions of the spine as well.

Flexion, extension, lateral flexion, and rotation are all used in the following exercises: (1) Put the chin on the chest until you feel a stretch in the back of the neck. With the knees stiff and "locked" in extension, reach for the floor, going as far as you can. Hold for 6 to 10 seconds. Return to the first position. (2) Stand in an exaggerated military position and look toward the ceiling. With the knees locked and the shoulders back, extend the spine as much as possible, arching the back and feeling the full stretch. Hold for 6 to 10 seconds. Return to the original position. (3) Again stand and direct your gaze toward where the ceiling meets the wall. Bend the neck sideways, attempting to touch the ear to the shoulder. Then bend sideways as far as you can, with your knees locked and your hand sliding down your thigh. Hold for 6 to 10 seconds. Return to the original position. Repeat the same exercise on the opposite side. (4) Stand in the military position. Turn or rotate the neck as far as you can in one direction, then rotate the entire spine as far as possible, twisting the whole body and keeping the knees stiff. Hold for 6 to 10 seconds and return to the original position. Repeat the exercise, turning in the opposite direction. Repeat all of the above 1 to 4 times daily.

Stretching exercises can be categorized as passive, assisted, and active. In passive exercise, the therapist or member of the family moves the joint through as full a range of motion as possible, with the muscles as relaxed as possible. Assisted exercise is with partial help, but the patient involves him- or herself in motion. Active exercise is without any outside support.

Range of Motion Exercises. To maintain or increase a limited range of motion, exercises must be accomplished in relationship to the intensity of inflammation and the pain induced. Any exercise-induced pain should subside within 2 hours, and any increase in pain that seemingly is associated with the exercise should have disappeared the following day at the latest. In the presence of inflammation, it is important to exercise with the least possible stress on the joints (and still exercise) and with the fewest possible movements made in the least stressful manner possible to accomplish the goal of maintenance of tissue function. It is necessary to "warm up" before performing the exercises. The time of day for exercising is very important. Stiffness in the morning makes it difficult to do the exercises at that time. Thus, the exercise should be done at the time of day when the patient feels "at my best." A hot shower or bath prior to exercising aids in the relaxation of muscle. After anti-inflammatory or analgesic medications are taken, exercise may be accomplished with more efficiency. Immobilization in both osteoarthritis and rheumatoid arthritis is associated with the "gel" phenomenon, and exercise should be done when this reluctance to move is at its least.

Strengthening Exercises. Static (isometric) exercises are those exerting a maximum force against an immovable object. Dynamic (isotonic) exercises are a measure of the heaviest weight that can be lifted by contractions or lowered by lengthening contractions. In isokinetic exercise, the stress is constant throughout the exercise by automatic adjustment of the load throughout the range of motion. This method of using isokinetic exercise with a machine is the single most effective way of building strength.

Power in a muscle is a function of its overall bulk, or cross-sectional diameter. However, strength can increase, both with and without gross muscle hypertrophy, through the mechanism of recruitment. Recruitment of muscle fibers is a function of the nervous system and does not involve the muscles directly. In general, resistance exercises, such as weight lifting, cause hypertrophy of fast-twitch muscle fiber and increased anatomic muscle bulk, whereas low-resistance, repetitive-endurance exercises, such as distance running and rapid walking, stimulate slow-twitch fibers but do not increase muscle bulk.

Strengthening is accomplished by isometric, isotonic, and, more unusually, isokinetic exercises, by relatively high-resistance exercises, and by low-resistance, repetitive exercises, such as rapid walking in the ideal posture, gentle jogging, and distance running. Employment of these exercises depends upon the individual patient's capability. All are very important in prophylaxis. In muscle strengthening, the muscle must be stressed to the point of fatigue so that a training effect will occur. Increased individual muscle tension, an increased number of mitochondria, an accelerated high-oxidative capacity, and an increased synthesis of the contractile proteins will be induced. There is evidence that this capability of achieving the "training effect" in some measurable degree does

not diminish with increasing age; thus, older patients with osteoarthritis should be treated in essentially the same way as younger patients within whatever their tolerance or constraints are.

Exercises for the Cervical Spine. The expected clinical problems in cervical osteoarthritis (intervertebral disc, Luschka joint, and zygapophyseal joint involvement) occur in restriction of range of motion, notably in extension, lateral flexion, and rotation. Flexion remains serviceable. The earliest and the most troublesome restriction is extension of the cervical spine. This is largely because of shortening of the muscles and ligaments and can be treated effectively through stretching, preferably prophylactically. The neck muscles should be as relaxed as possible. Cramping during exercises should be avoided by exerting less effort in the initial stages. The patient generally does not want to extend, laterally flex, or rotate the spine because of pain. Application of heat, moist or dry, is effective in getting maximum results from the exercises.

Figure 12–7 illustrates an excellent exercise for the entire cervical spine that is especially effective in prevention. It is useful in rheumatoid arthritis if there are no grossly abnormal subluxations at the atlanto-occipital joint. Ankylosing spondylitis

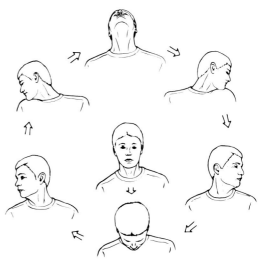

Figure 12–7. Active, gravity-assisted exercises for the neck. In this useful cervical spine stretching technique, the patient, from a standing position, lets the neck flex passively on the chest so that the chin approaches the chest. The patient then rolls one ear to a shoulder, the occiput rolls backward, and the chin rolls to the opposite shoulder and back again to the chest. This exercise is done with the neck and torso as relaxed as they can be. The patient with subluxation of the atlas and axis should exercise caution in performing this technique. The patient should be warned that this exercise may cause vertigo.

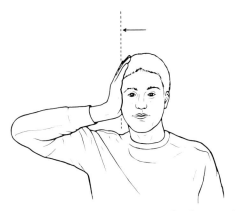

Figure 12–8. Static or isometric strengthening exercise. Place hand on the side of head and exert as much pressure as possible against the resistance for 6 to 10 seconds. The exercise should be repeated 3 to 10 times, 2 to 4 times daily.

can also be favorably affected by these exercises if they are done on a long-term, prophylactic basis.

Rhythmic stabilization exercises apply to acute as well as more chronic torticollis. The patient's head is supported by the therapist and gently turned toward the painful side to the point of intolerance. With the therapist's hands holding both sides of the patient's head, the patient contracts muscles on the painful side by pushing the head against the therapist's hands. The isometric contraction is held for 8 to 10 seconds and relaxed. In relaxation, the head is passively laterally rotated or flexed farther as allowed by the muscle relaxation. The exercise is repeated until maximum stretching has occurred and then is carried out in the opposite direction. Repeat 2 to 3 times daily. The goals are to block painful, restrictive muscle contraction and restore full range of motion. The patient can be taught to carry this out alone.

Cervical isometric exercises preserve and restore muscle power. An important issue is the maintenance of normal agonist-antagonist muscle capability. These exercises are absolutely necessary in patients wearing a brace or collar. Manual resistance with pressure of the palm for 10 seconds against the side of the head, repeated 6 times, 2–3 times daily, is very effective. The same manual resistance to both sides of the head, the occiput, and the forehead, in turn, is a good regimen (Fig. 12–8).

In ankylosing spondylitis, where neck flexion is a major problem and handicap, the patient may stand with back as flat against the wall as possible. With chin pulled in, the patient slides the back up and down the wall by partially flexing then extending both knees, attempting to hold the back of the head against the wall or as close to it as possible. This should be repeated from 5 to 25 times, 2 to 3 times daily.

Figures 12–9 through 12–15 illustrate exercises for the cervical spine that patients can carry out for themselves.

Potential Dangers of Exercise

This section is to sound a cautionary note regarding ill-advised or unsupervised exercise. It is estimated that 36 million Americans exercise regularly and that 38% of all Americans 50 years of age or older exercise regularly. Overall, this "fitness boom" has been of enormous benefit and consequence. Potential dangers should be appreciated, particularly by people with health problems—in this instance, problems with the cervical spine. Many studies are made on the benefits of exercise, but little attention is paid to the potential dangers. Moderate exercise is almost always very beneficial provided it is carried out within the constraints of unusual fatigue and pain, either local or regional, and that it is done under some guidance and supervision relative to any existing health problems and their attendant dangers.

Exercise clearly increases requirements for intake of calories, vitamins, and minerals. A well-balanced diet consists of 1800 to 2000 calories. The over-enthusiastic exerciser is likely to become involved in dietary manipulations. One of my patients, a physician, began a vegetarian diet, and while training and running 50 miles per week, he became quite anemic and generally ill. He was unaware that his dietary change was the causative factor.

An allegedly healthy group of people with inapparent coronary artery disease exists. Such people commonly have cervical spine disorders and become involved in both regional as well as general exercise programs. In such cases, a significant danger is that of induction of cardiac arrhythmias in certain exercise situations. Table 12–5 lists the clinical circumstances that may be associated with exercise-caused arrhythmias. The doctor caring for

Table 12–5. CLINICAL CIRCUMSTANCES FOR EXERCISE-INDUCED ARRHYTHMIAS

Coronary atherosclerosis, pre- and postmyocardial infarction and "bypass" patients
Electrolyte abnormalities
Long QT interval in electrocardiogram
Cardiac drug use—digitalis, quinidine
Excessive intake of caffeine or amphetamine; smoking; addiction to fad diets
Psychotropic drugs
Mitral valve prolapse and variable click-murmur syndromes
Aortic valve stenosis
Cardiomyopathies—congestive, hypertrophic, obstructive
Normal cardiovascular condition in unaccustomed levels of exercise

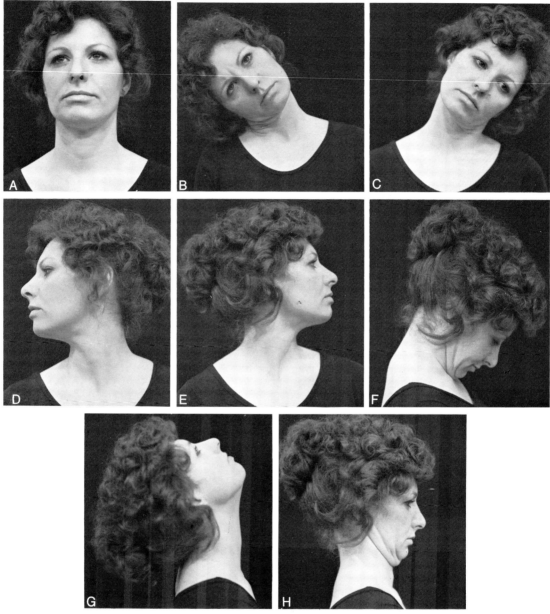

Figure 12–9. Range of motion exercises. To test relaxation and general range of motion, the exercise shown in Figure 12–7 should be done. This accomplishes gentle stretching and muscle relaxation. This exercise is enhanced by doing it sitting or standing in front of a mirror. Even if the range of motion is not grossly limited, it is important to carry out as great a range of motion as is comfortably possible. *A,* The neutral position to start the exercises. Note that the chin is up and the gaze is directed toward where the ceiling meets the wall or toward the horizon. The cervical spine is in normal lordosis and at its most physiologic posture. *B,* Bend the head to the right as far as possible, moving the ear near the shoulder without raising the shoulder. Feel a stretch but not pain; hold for 10 seconds; return to the neutral position. Repeat 3 to 6 times, 2 to 3 times daily. *C,* Bend the head to the left as far as possible, repeat as in *B. D,* Rotate the head as far as possible to the right; keep the chin up and stretch. Hold for 10 seconds; return to the neutral position. *E,* Rotate the head to the left as far as possible; hold for 10 seconds; return to the neutral position. *F,* Flex the neck as far down as possible, placing the chin on the chest in the full range of motion. Hold for 10 seconds; return to the neutral position. *G,* Slowly extend the head and neck, looking at the ceiling. Stretch; hold for 10 seconds; return to the neutral position. *H,* Pull chin in and push back of neck out; raise head slightly.

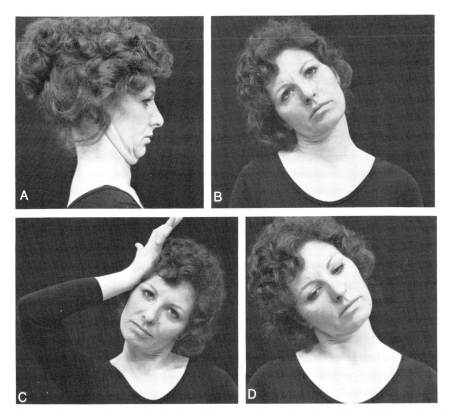

Figure 12–10. Series. Isotonic neck exercises in lateral flexion and side bending. *A*, Start this exercise with the neck in the position shown in Figure 12–9*H*, that is, pull chin in and push back of neck out, raise head slightly. *B*, Laterally flex the neck (bend sideways) to the right as far as can be comfortably stretched. *C*, Place the right hand on the side of the head and press hand against it; hold for 10 seconds. *D*, Relax and again laterally flex the neck to the right as far as possible. Note that the last lateral bend (*D*) is increased over the first (*B*), as muscles are relaxed after the isotonic exercise.

patients with cervical spine disease should be aware of these possibilities. Table 12–6 lists some noncardiac dangers of exercise that should be taken into account when prescribing exercises.

The discussion here should not suppress interest or enthusiasm for exercise. The goal is to have a balanced view of the reasons for and against exercise. The error is much more likely to be made in restricting exercise. Exercise should be prescribed in moderate but gradually increasing levels of intensity and appropriate frequency. The exercise should be prescribed for the individual and his or her specific needs, both regional and general. Prescribing lower to moderate exercise activities promotes compliance with the overall management program.

The patient may need instruction concerning the definition of exercise, that is, that it is not all running and jogging. Dynamic exercises include stationary biking, conventional biking, swimming, tennis, basketball, racquet ball, and any sport that increases oxygen consumption gradually and utilizes muscle, bone, ligament, tendon, and joint. Exercise is not only therapeutic but preventive. In summary, this section is included to stimulate physicians and others in the health field to be aware of their responsibilities with regard to proper exercise.

Table 12–6. POTENTIAL DANGERS OF EXERCISE

Exercise-induced asthma
Precipitation of acute gout
Exercise-induced fainting
Sprains, strains, tendon rupture, stress fractures
Flare-up of rheumatoid arthritis
Exacerbation of localized osteoarthritis
Hematomata into soft tissue
Hemoglobinuria and myoglobinuria
Petechial hemorrhages
Nipple and penile frostbite
Heat stroke and heat exhaustion
Dog bite; auto injury
Diarrhea
Myopathy and paralysis of localized neuromuscular
  groups
Exercise-induced cardiac arrhythmia

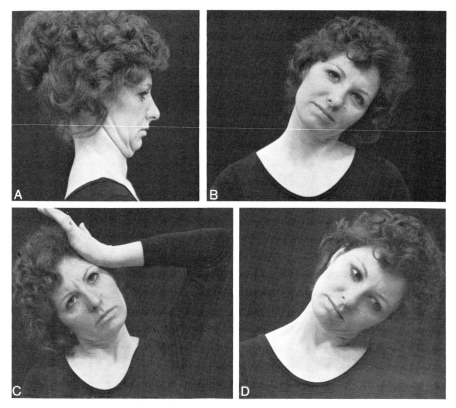

Figure 12–11 *See legend on opposite page*

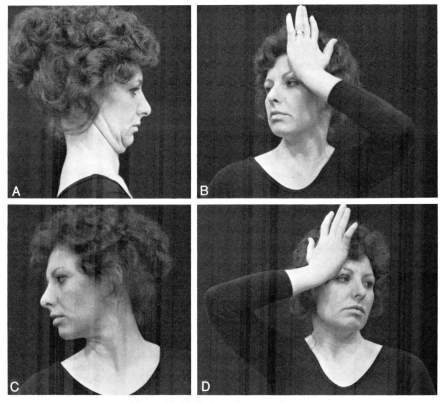

Figure 12–12 *See legend on opposite page*

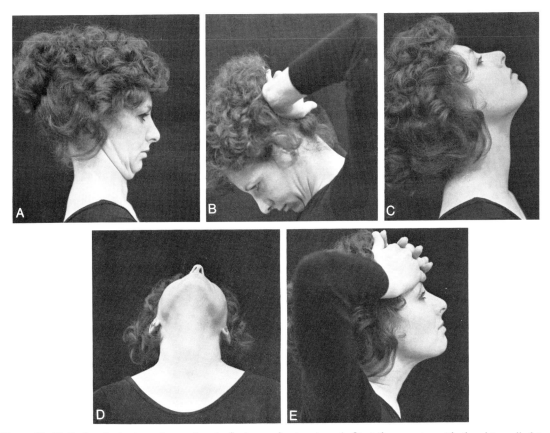

Figure 12–13. Series. Isotonic neck exercises in flexion and extension. *A,* Start the exercise with the chin pulled in, the back of the neck pushed out, and the head up. *B,* Flex the neck so that the chin is on the chest, contacting the breast bone with the chin if possible; feel a stretch; clasp hands behind head and extend the head and neck against the resisting hands; hold for 10 seconds. Release and again flex the chin toward the chest as far as it will go. It flexes farther and more comfortably. *C,* Next extend the neck, look up at the ceiling, and stretch as much as is comfortably possible. *D,* Anterior view of *C. E,* Clasp both hands over the forehead and try to flex forward against the resisting hands; hold for 10 seconds; release. After releasing, extend the head and neck as far as is comfortably possible. Feel a stretch but no pain; the neck extends farther if it was restricted and more comfortably if it was not.

Anticoagulation Therapy

In vertebrobasilar, carotid artery, and vertebral artery syndromes with transient ischemic attacks, threatened stroke, the syndromes of vertigo, relative compromise of proprioception, and visual and auditory symptomatology, anticoagulant therapy is usually indicated. This may be accomplished simply through the administration of 1 to 2 aspirin tablets per day, moderately compromising the aggregating capability of platelets, or it may be done through prescribing a long-term program of sodium warfarin (Coumadin), much as is done following open-heart surgery, recurrent threatening stroke, and other potential disorders of clotting.

Figure 12–11. *A,* Again start with the chin pulled in, the back of the neck pushed out, and the head slightly raised. *B,* Laterally flex the neck to the left until a stretch is felt. *C,* Put the left hand to the side of the head and press head firmly up against the resisting hand; hold for 10 seconds. Release, rest, and laterally flex (*D*) the neck as far as possible to the left side. Note that the final lateral flexion (*D*) is greater than the first (*B*).

Figure 12–12. Series. Isotonic neck exercises in rotation, right and left. *A,* Start the exercise with the chin pulled in, the back of the neck pushed out, and the head up. *B,* Rotate the head toward the right shoulder until it comes to a stop, stretched; place the left hand on the left temple area and rotate the head hard against the resisting hand in the opposite direction; hold for 10 seconds; release. *C,* Rotate the head as far as you can to the right. Note that it rotates 90 degrees without pain. *D,* Repeat the same exercise on the left.

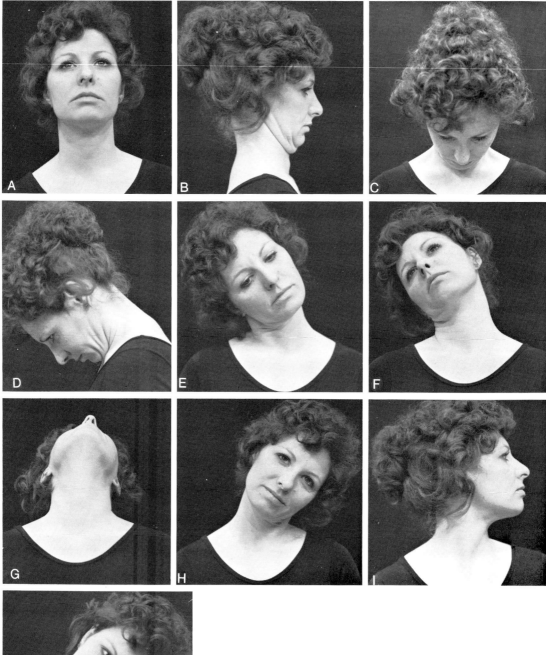

Figure 12–14. Series. Active, gravity-assisted cervical spine exercises. Rotate the head to describe the largest possible circle with the tip of the nose. Rotate first in one direction and then in the other. Repeat 3 to 6 times daily. *A*, Start with chin in, neck back, head up. *B*, Lateral (side) view of starting position. *C*, Maximal flexion, chin on chest (on breast bone if possible). *D*, Lateral view of maximal flexion. *E*, Slowly start to rotate head to the right. *F*, Continue rotation. *G*, Complete extension of head and neck, "rolling around." *H*, Start to flex neck to the left. *I*, Neck is laterally flexed left and fully rotated. *J*, Roll down from lateral flexion toward full frontal flexion again (*C*).

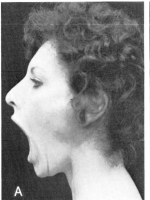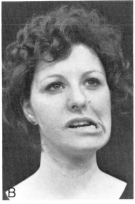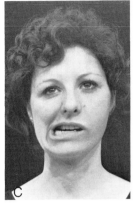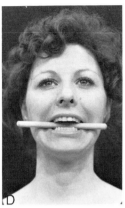

Figure 12–15. Series. Exercises for the temporomandibular joint. *A,* Open mouth as wide as possible without producing pain. Feel a stretch but no pain. Hold for 10 seconds. Release. Repeat 6 times, 2 to 3 times daily. There is no definite anatomic bite distance, but 1 inch between incisors is very serviceable, and 2 inches is not rare. *B,* Slide the jaw sideways and stretch. Hold for 10 seconds; release. Repeat 6 times, 2 to 4 repetitions daily. *C,* Slide the jaw sideways in the opposite direction; stretch. Hold for 10 seconds; release. Repeat 6 times, 2 to 4 repetitions daily. *D,* Bite a wooden stick or wooden spoon; hold for 10 seconds; release. Repeat 6 times, twice daily. You can usually open the mouth farther after biting the wooden spoon. This can be monitored by measuring the distance between incisors. Yawning has a similar effect.

Relaxation Techniques

There is no question that continuing pain—or even the threat and fear of it—limitation of motion, and the reluctance to accept the "sick role," as they all relate to the cervical spine, constitute major life stress. Stress reduction is an important aspect of management of cervical spine disorders. Hence, techniques of reducing stress are of great importance.

Learning relaxation skills is easy, requires no change in lifestyle, is pleasant, simple, and the price is right. The greatest natural resource patients have is their own mind, which requires some training. The priority for learning relaxation is high. The techniques discussed subsequently constitute predictable methods of release of stress, tension, and pain.

The popularity of relaxation methods has resulted in a great increase in ideas, methods, and schools of thought. All relaxation methods are self-administered. General titles given are relaxation training, transcendental meditation, psychocybernetics, biofeedback, self hypnosis, yoga, Jacobsen's progressive relaxation, and the relaxation response. All are strikingly overlapping. Some have specific benefits in special instances, but, by and large, they all have the same ultimate end. Confusion regarding this multitude of choices is unnecessary. One does not have to have biofeedback machines available to learn to relax.

The goal of relaxation is to empty the mind of its thought, preoccupation, fantasy, schemes, memories, worries, responsibilities, hopes, fears, and—in fact—all thought. One "permits" the body to slow down for a period of 15 to 30 minutes. As the mind becomes inactive, the body

relaxes and the muscles release accumulated tension—this includes the clearing of metabolic waste products. The individual stops being work oriented; performance is put out of the mind, and the mind becomes a useful servant rather than a cruel taskmaster. The struggle is halted during this period. It is like taking a 20-minute vacation, and the taut spring of anxiety unwinds.

The instant benefit is the sensation of relaxation and rest. With profound relaxation of mind and body, the perception of pain clearly diminishes as a physiologic event. A sense of well-being comes when the relaxation is truly achieved. Mental depression and anxiety are lessened. There are measurable physical, endocrine, biochemical, and biomechanical changes that occur if proper relaxation is achieved—lower blood pressure, decreasing heart rate, increasing skin temperature, decreasing oxygen utilization, and a decrease in metabolic synthetic activity.

Ziebell[29] suggests a series of "quickies," or techniques that do not require deep concentration. The mind is not really cleared, but the techniques can be practiced anywhere without attracting attention. These immediate methods prevent the accumulation of tension during the day. (1) Deep breathing. Stop, take a deep breath, let the air out slowly, and imagine you are breathing in energy and breathing out tension. Repeat several times. (2) Shrug shoulders. Gently push shoulders up toward the ears, pushing only as far as is comfortable. Hold for 5 seconds. Relax. Repeat 3 times. (3) Stretching. While either standing or sitting, gently stretch, reaching as far up as possible with comfort. Hold the full stretch for 5 to 10 seconds. Relax. Repeat 2 to 5 times. (4) Rag doll. In a comfortable chair, allow the whole body to relax progressively from toes to the head. Be limp and loose—as if bones have been taken away—a "rag doll." (5) Funny face. Make any kind of face, tensing the muscles and relaxing them. Use the face, head, neck, stick out the tongue, open the eyes very wide—use your own creativity. Repeat 3 times. Ziebell lists 200 different things that patients with pain can do to distract themselves from the pain and actually reduce the perception of the painful stimulus.

The best overall synthesis of progressive relaxation techniques is that devised and described by Benson.[30] The relaxation response is a synthesis of all of the other methods, and scientific credibility is given to the process. Anyone using the basic and progressive methods outlined can achieve the relaxation response. There are four basic elements to the relaxation response: (1) A quiet environment. Turn off internal stimuli and all external distractions. (2) An object or mental device to dwell upon, such as repeating a word or sound (the word "one") gazing at a symbol (a flower or a burning candle), or concentrating on a feeling (peace). (3) Passive attitude (the most essential factor), an emptying of all thoughts and distractions from the mind. Thoughts, imagery, and feeling may drift into awareness. Do not concentrate on them, but allow them to pass on. (4) A comfortable position. Be comfortable enough to stay in the same position for 20 minutes.

Technique for eliciting the relaxation response: (1) Sit quietly in a comfortable position, totally alone and free of all distractions, noise, phones, and business. (2) Close your eyes. (3) Deeply relax all your muscles, beginning at the toes and progressing up to the face. Keep them relaxed. (4) Breath in through the nose; become aware of breathing. As you breath out through your mouth, say the word "one" silently to yourself. Continue to empty your mind of all thoughts. (5) Continue for 10 to 20 minutes. Open your eyes to check the time, but do not use an alarm. When finished, sit quietly for a few minutes with eyes closed.

Do not worry that you are not successful in achieving a deep level of relaxation immediately. It requires time and practice. Keep a passive attitude, and allow relaxation to occur. Ignore distracting thoughts—do not dwell on them. Return to repeating the word one.

Practice once or twice daily but not within 2 hours after a meal, because digestive processes interfere with elicitation of the relaxation response. This technique is much like meditation, and meditation provides the principles of the relaxation response. The difference is that one need not spend several hundred dollars to learn to meditate. The entire method is here.

Building a Better Neck

With successful therapy, relief of pain, and achievement of serviceable cervical spine mobility, one may turn to deal with the atrophy and weakening of the cervical musculature. Two goals are to increase strength throughout the neck, rendering it less likely to be injured, and to maintain range of motion and power as well as freedom from stiffness and pain—achieving a super-normal state.

Since cervical spine injuries are common in contact sports, proper conditioning of neck musculature, ligament, tendon, and joint are important in young players and cervical spine osteoarthritis patients alike. In general, very little is done to prevent cervical spine disease and injury. Cervical musculature can be built up and the whole neck strengthened by doing isotonic exercises, such as weight lifting to develop muscle strength and endurance. Neck weight training machines designed to build cervical spine strength have been developed. They consist of a pulley mounted on a wall bracket, and a cord with a head harness on one end and a weight holder with a standard barbell weight on the other. These isometric, neck-developing exercises can be done 3 to 6 times per week and can be monitored by the patient, who can measure neck circumferences and range of motion. These machines are inexpensive and simple to build. There are, however, no such machines presently on the market.

DRUGS APPLICABLE TO DISORDERS AND DISEASES OF THE CERVICAL SPINE

The use of drug therapy constitutes only a part, an estimated 15% to 20%, of a total program of management. The patient should be instructed along this line. Too often the doctor emphasizes drugs as being the entire program of management—a view that is destined to fail. The idea is to use medications intermittently; the goal is to prevent rather than relieve pain, but in instances of very severe pain, analgesics in sufficient amount to control it are indicated. There are three categories of drugs useful in disorders of the cervical spine: (1) nonsteroidal anti-inflammatory drugs, with occasional use of steroids in very acute inflammatory processes; (2) analgesic drugs; and (3) muscle relaxant drugs.

Aspirin. Of the nonsteroidal anti-inflammatory drugs, aspirin remains the drug of choice and is the most effective when it is optimally utilized. It is best not to use aspirin preparations in combination with other drugs, though many of them exist in the over-the-counter market. Osteoarthritis is uniformly an inflammatory process in the cervical spine; aspirin serves both analgesic and anti-inflammatory functions. An analgesic dose of aspirin is 2 tablets taken 4 times per day, whereas an anti-inflammatory dose requires 3 tablets 4 times per day on the average. The total number of tablets may vary from 10 tablets per day to 25 per 24 hours, taken in 3 to 4 divided doses.

The following method has been found effective and is associated with very few side effects: (1) Take the aspirin in food; at breakfast, place 3 tablets in the applesauce, cottage cheese, or yogurt; chew and swallow it. The aspirin is absorbed in 5 to 15 minutes as compared with 1 hour to 3 hours if the tablets are swallowed whole. There is little stomach irritation if the aspirin reaches the stomach in small pieces. The aspirin may be crushed and stirred into milk with a spoon; a drop or two of vanilla also helps. "Buzzing" the milk and aspirin in a blender is helpful. Three tablets are taken in this way at the noon meal, at supper, and at bedtime, for a total dose of 12 aspirin per day on the average. (2) If tinnitus occurs in 3 to 7 days, the aspirin is stopped entirely. It is restarted when the tinnitus has gone completely, assuring one that the mechanism of ringing in the ears is that of aspirin intoxication. (3) Reduce the aspirin by one tablet, and in 3 to 5 days check for the recurrence of tinnitus. If it has not recurred, continue at that dosage; if it has recurred, stop the drug again for 2 to 3 days, and restart the therapy, reducing the aspirin by one tablet again. (4) If tinnitus does not recur in the first week, take one more aspirin and increase (up to no more than three) until tinnitus appears, then reduce appropriately. This will ensure anti-inflammatory concentrations of the aspirin. (5) If an asymptomatic state is achieved over a period of weeks to months, the aspirin is stopped, and the whole program—exercises, rest, relaxation, and physical therapy techniques— is continued. With success in pain relief and symptomatic improvement, the aspirin may be either stopped or used intermittently—1 month on and 1 month off or 1 month on and 2 months off. The ultimate goal is to stop taking the drug.

Analgesic Drugs. The patient shold be educated in the use of analgesic drugs and taught that pain relief is achieved more importantly by other and more reliable and rational methods. The simple analgesics to be used periodically in cervical spine disease are acetaminophen (in its many brands, but the generic acetaminophen is less expensive and is obviously no different); propoxyphene hydrochloride (Darvon, Darvon Compound); propoxyphene napsylate (Darvocet, Darvocet-N); codeine (15 to 30-mg strength); oxycodone hydrochloride (Percodan); phenyltoloxamine citrate (Percogesic); meperidine hydrochloride (Demerol, rarely required, recommended for only very short periods).

Nonsteroidal Anti-inflammatory Drugs. All nonsteroidal anti-inflammatory drugs generally reduce or block the inflammatory process by the same mechanism that aspirin does. Short courses of any may be useful. They are usually used in conjunction with or instead of aspirin. Phenylbutazone (Butazolidin), indomethacin (Indocin), fenoprofen calcium (Nalfon), meclofenamate sodium (Meclomen), naproxen (Naprosyn), tolmetin so-dium (Tolectin), sulindac (Clinoril), and piroxicam (Feldene).

Occasionally a corticosteroid pulse is very effective in the acute and severe inflammatory aspects of osteoarthritis or in the mechanically induced inflammation of intervertebral disc disease. A dose of 15 mg of prednisone in the morning and at bedtime for 5 days, reducing by decrements of 5 mg each 5 days until a baseline dosage of 5 mg daily (each morning) is reached. This may be continued for 2 to 3 months or stopped at any time, depending upon the clinical response.

Muscle Relaxants. Diazepam (Valium), cyclobenzaprine hydrochloride (Flexeril), methocarbamol (Robaxin), metaxalone (Skelaxin), and carisoprodol (Soma) are all muscle relaxants widely used in other conditions and may have an occasional place in the management of cervical osteoarthritis. They are usually worthwhile for a clinical trial period of several weeks, with establishment of effective and valid parameters of drug effect. Their use should be stopped if results are not definitive and striking.

SOME GENERALITIES

It has been shown that skeletal muscle, ligament, tendon, bone, and joint respond with a training effect on very gradual increase of the load in exercises. This was not thought to be so until recent years. Likewise, flexibility in the aging adult is now regarded as treatable and manageable. The loss of flexibility in the great majority of persons age 50 or older is a consequence of increasing immobilization, decreasing exercise, and certain attitudinal behaviors that are associated with chronologic age in the United States. There is no evidence that biologic aging causes the decrease in flexibility, though we need more basic research data on this subject. The physician can educate older people in the maintenance of optimum flexibility. There is reliable evidence that osteoarthritis can be very favorably influenced by maintaining optimum fitness and overall flexibility. Physical activity programming both for persons with arthritis and for otherwise normal older adults is of great prophylactic importance. These goals can be accomplished by simple walking, bicycle riding, gentle jogging, stationary bicycle, isometric and isotonic exercises, stretching exercises, the use of YMCAs and WYCAs by older people, and development of a strong motivating stimulus through the recruitment of interested people—a fraternity of aging colleagues committed to the premise that prudent exercise has a significant positive impact on the quality of life of the elderly. [31]

POSTURE TRAINING AND PROPHYLAXIS

Bad posture is a bad habit that, unfortunately, occurs commonly in otherwise normal people.

Conversely, good posture is a good habit that, once established, requires little voluntary effort to maintain. Postural abnormalities are caused not by structural defects in the normal body but by misuse of the mechanisms provided. If postural defects were of only cosmetic interest, they would not be so important; however, postural faults clearly result in discomfort, pain, and ultimate deformity. The symptoms resulting from postural abnormality range from mild ache and discomfort to thorough incapacitating disability. The symptoms experienced are directly related to the severity of the fault and its duration.

The goals of this section are to define and recognize the concepts of good posture and note how postural faults can add to, exaggerate, and accelerate problems resulting from diseases and conditions in the cervical spine. Underlying chronic postural defects render abnormalities of the cervical spine more symptomatic. Good posture may be compromised by disorders arising in the cervical spine.

To assess postural faults in order to prescribe a means of management requires a standard by which individual postures can be measured. The ideal posture involves a minimum of stress and strain and is conducive to maximal efficiency in the optimum use of the body.

Definition. Posture is defined as the relative arrangement of the parts of the body. Good posture is the state of muscular and skeletal balance that protects supporting structures of the body against injury or progressive deformity regardless of the attitude—erect, lying, squatting, walking, running, or stooping—in which these structures are working or resting. Under such conditions, muscles function efficiently, and the optimum positions are afforded for thoracic and abdominal organs. Poor posture is a faulty relationship of the various parts of the body, producing increased strain on the supporting structures and providing a less efficient balance of the body over its base of support.

Standard posture is concerned with skeletal alignment, since posture is clearly a matter of alignment. There are, of course, variations in body type, size, shape, and proportion, all of which are factors in weight distribution. Still, there is a reasonable standard of skeletal alignment that can fit all individuals. An experienced observer can note the contours of the body and estimate the position of the skeletal structure. The standing position is regarded as a composite alignment of a person from four views—front, back, right side, and left side—and it involves the position and alignment of so many joints and body areas that it is unlikely that any individual meets the standard perfectly in every respect.

In standard body alignment, the center of gravity is in the center of the body's axis. A plumb line from the external auditory meatus transects the lateral tip of the acromion, the greater tro-

chanter of the femur, and the midpoint of the lateral aspect of the knee and reaches just anterior to the lateral malleolus. Dorsal spine kyphosis is present; scapulae are elevated enough to prevent round shoulder; the pelvis is tilted posteriorly to minimize the lumbar lordotic curve. A normal adult should be able to stand with the heels 3 to 4 inches from the wall, rotate the pelvis posteriorly, and tilt so that occiput, dorsal and lumbar spine, and buttocks are touching the wall.[32]

From the front, the observer notes that the head is centered, the shoulders are level, and there is no gross valgus or varus at the knee or of the foot; the medial femoral condyles and the medial malleoli touch. With the center of gravity in the midline, the least stress is exerted to maintain a standing posture, allowing a minimum of muscular strain, fatigue, and stresses on joints, ligaments, tendons, and muscles.

Postural Faults. Each of the postural faults in the following list may be significant in disorders of the cervical spine:

1. *Deviation* describes departure from the standard or accepted form of posture. The term may be modified by use of the words anterior (forward), posterior (backward), right, and left and is used in connection with the plumb line alignment.

2. *Tilt* describes rotation about a horizontal axis, particularly in relation to the pelvis and the head. Anterior pelvic tilt describes anterosuperior spines moved down and forward. A posterior pelvic tilt is one in which anterosuperior spines move up and backward. Lateral pelvic tilt (not a pure tilt) describes the pelvis when it is lower on one side than the other (down on the right or left).

3. *Rotation* describes rotation about a vertical axis. It is used in relation to pelvis, head, trunk, thorax, or extremity. In relation to the head, for example, rotation is right or left by the direction in which the face turns; pelvic rotation or thorax rotation is clockwise or counterclockwise.

4. *Lordosis* is increased anterior curve of the lumbar spine associated with anterior pelvic tilt. Lordosis occurs normally in the cervical spine. Cervical spine lordosis may be exaggerated in the case of a rounded upper back (thoracic spine).

5. *Kyphosis*, increased posterior curve, occurs usually in the dorsal spine and unusually in the lumbar spine. The term generally refers to the thoracic spine when used without qualification, such as dorsal kyphosis. Lumbar kyphosis is associated with a posterior pelvic tilt.

6. *Round shoulders* describes the position of abduction of the scapulae and a forward position of the shoulders. It is associated with "hollow chest."

7. *Rounded upper back* refers to increased posterior curve in the dorsal spine. It is the same as dorsal kyphosis and is associated with deep chest. Round shoulders are considered a curve in the horizontal plane, whereas round upper back is

considered an increased curve in the vertical plane.

8. *Gluteal fold of buttocks* is a horizontal crease between the buttock and the thigh, a gluteofemoral crease.

9. *Gluteal cleft,* or cleft of the buttocks, is the vertical crease between the right and left buttocks. Normally it is in the midline.

10. *Knock-knee;* knees come together while the feet are apart; valgus knees.

11. *Bowlegs;* alignment of the legs in which there is outward bowing of the bones of the leg; varus knees. *Postural bowlegs* describes alignment of the legs in which the appearance of bowlegs results from standing with knees in hyperextension and internal rotation, without true bowing of the bones of the leg.

12. *Pronation* refers to a position of the foot in which the weight of standing is borne on the inner side of the foot—eversion or valgus.

13. *Supination* describes a position of the foot in which the weight of standing is borne on the outer side of the foot—inversion or varus. In assessing posture in cases of cervical spine disorders, all of the elements of posture thus far discussed are pertinent and should be examined, assessed, and treated.

Sleeping Posture. Optimum sleeping position is supine with support to cervical lordosis. Most patients cannot adapt to this and resort to either the side-lying or the prone position; the side-lying position is preferable to the prone. There may be enough support of the lateral cervical region to maintain a neutral position, preventing prolonged lateral bending stretch all night. If the patient sleeps prone, propping up the chest with pillows may allow him or her to lie in this position with minimal rotation of the head (see *Cervical Pillows* in this chapter). A soft mattress causes prolonged stress on muscles and ligaments that becomes even worse if the springs or bedboard sags under the mattress.

Sitting Posture. The key to sitting posture is support of lumbar lordosis. It is also important that the patient avoid soft, overstuffed chairs. The knees should be at the level of the hips, and feet should be flat on the floor, close to the surface upon which the patient is working. Desk height is important; the patient must reach down to the surface to read or write, requiring a sustained forward-head posture. A desk, podium, or mechanical drawing style of desk top may be needed to alleviate a sustained overloading situation.

The tasks to be performed while seated, such as close work over a desk, sitting in a tense posture at a meeting, reading in a relaxed position, working semireclined in a resting position, driving an automobile, or sitting on a stool for kitchen duties, are important determinations of postures. The main issue here is alignment of the spine to minimize skeletal stress. A straight-back chair may not allow room posteriorly for buttock protrusion.

An ill-fitting secretarial chair with a poor lumbar pad position creates a fulcrum that is either too high or too low, exaggerating lumbar lordosis with low back strain, ache, and pain. Other important considerations of the sitting posture are neck position, shoulder and elbow angles, availability of proper light, hip and knee mobility, and the 90-degree angle of the lower leg and the femur. Flexion contractures of the knee render proper sitting, standing, or lying postures difficult— hence the necessity for attention to such a defect. Hip flexion contracture must be compensated for by lumbar lordosis or knee flexion. Attention to a hip flexion contracture—either correcting it or making it as minimally constraining as possible—is an important therapeutic matter.

Standing Posture. The standard, optimum standing posture maximizes the length of the vertebral column and the elevation of the chest, retracts the shoulders, and normalizes lordosis, encouraging an orthostatic posture. Patients must be instructed individually regarding the adaptations necessary for correcting their particular problem. Improper posturing permits sustained loading of the involved soft tissue, perpetuating, if not causing, the problem. It is useless to instruct patients regularly if they spend most of their hours aggravating the problem.

Cervical Spine Postural Problems. The most common muscle problems associated with pain in the posterior neck (the most frequent location) are of two types: those caused by muscle tightness, and those caused by muscle strain. Symptoms and therapeutic methods differ depending upon the underlying fault. With muscle tightness, the onset of symptoms is gradual, whereas with muscle strain, the episode is more acute.

Pain associated with tightness of the posterior muscles is most often found in patients who have a forward projected head and a rounded upper back. The head position is compensatory and is associated with a slumped, rounded upper back, causing relative hyperextension of the cervical spine. Such faulty mechanics results in symptom-producing compression of the zygapophyseal facets and the posterior portions of the bodies of the vertebrae. Stretch weakness of the anterior vertebral neck flexor muscles and tightness of the neck extensor muscles (upper trapezius muscle, splenius muscle of the head, and erector muscles of the cervical spine) occur. Compression and impingement of the suboccipital nerves and the greater occipital nerves result in occipital headache, often occurring with the neck pain. On examination, the muscles feel tense and tight. Cervical spine movements in all directions (except hyperextension) are limited relative to the amount of tightness present. Pain lessens when the patient assumes a recumbent position, but finally it becomes constant in all positions.

Management consists of daily use of heat, massage, and stretching, gradually increasing the latter within the constraints of pain. Massage is gentle and relaxing, progressing to deeper kneading. Stretching of tight muscles requires a gradual therapeutic course with active, passive, and assisted movements. The patient tries to stretch posterior neck muscles by attempting to flatten the cervical spine; the patient pulls the chin down and in—an action similar to the pelvis tilt used to flatten the lumbar spine in lumbar lordosis. These exercises are best done in either a supine or a sitting position, not prone. Any exercises tending to hyperextend the cervical spine are contraindicated.

Faulty head position compensates for dorsal kyphosis, and this also requires attention. Dorsal kyphosis results from postural deviations of the lower back or pelvis, so it is necessary to start treatment by correction of the lumbar-associated faults (a common failure of analysis on the part of the examiner and therapist). Management for neck pain may begin by using abdominal exercises or even a good abdominal support, allowing the patient to assume a better upper back and chest position.

The upper trapezius muscle is often strained, causing pain (usually acute) in the posterolateral portion of the neck. The upper trapezius extends from the occiput to the acromion process of the scapula. The stress causing trapezius strain is a combination of tension on and contraction of the muscle; straining to reach for an object while holding the head tilted in the opposite direction may cause an acute attack. Abduction of the arm demands action by the trapezius for scapular fixation; sideward head tilt causes trapezius muscle tension.

Overall use of heat and massage tends to increase pain because the muscle is sustaining strain. Massage alone is more effective. The massage is a kneading type and should be gentle at first, becoming more firm as the muscle tolerates the mechanical stimulation. Fifteen to twenty minutes of massage effects relaxation. Pressure should be directed slightly upward to relieve tension on the part of the muscle above. Downward stroking is irritating. A soft collar worn for days to weeks gives considerable relief if the symptoms have lasted for several weeks.

Good posture is not an end in itself but constitutes a major contribution to general well-being. Postural instruction and training are clearly part of the overall management of any disorder of the cervical spine and contribute very significantly to prevention of symptoms caused by poor posture rather than disease. Postural instruction and training are integral parts of a good program of health education generally as well as being essential in management of disorders of the cervical spine.

Since round or drooping shoulders causes compensatory hyperextension of the neck, one of the several types of shoulder brace may be used effectively. Remember, the brace is worn until the patient becomes posture conscious, that is, capable of holding the shoulders up and back with no outside assistance or reminder by a restrictive brace. With correction of the shoulder posture, the cervical spine is in a more normal position. Hyperextension is mechanically eliminated. This position does not obstruct the cervicothoracic outlet and, of course, is important in managing all of the thoracic outlet syndromes. Occasionally, shoulder braces obliterate pain associated with cervical nerve root irritation, with no other management necessary. Many people have overall poor posture while sitting, standing, walking, and lying, as if they are too tired or lazy to be aware of their destructive postural attitude. Such habits are correctable. However, remember that corrective exercises and bracing are like crutches in that they are to be used properly and discontinued as soon as possible.

Cervical Pillows

There are many sizes and types of cervical pillows available, varying from air pillows blown up to the thickness that raises the head to the most comfortable level, to a tubular-shaped contour pillow (Cervipillo), to a multipurpose pillow (Wal-Pil-O). The Wal-Pil-O provides four combinations of head and neck support, one of which is proper for almost all cervical spine problems. I recommend it highly. Another design is called "the shape of sleep." It features a neck support ridge that fits under the neck and is a physiologic, biomechanically sound model. A bolster-type pillow is available in several different diameters, and pillows with a contour cutout for the head are also obtainable. These pillows are available in a variety of thicknesses, firmnesses, and cutout sizes from surgical supply stores. A pillow made up of three baby pillows stitched together provides neck support for the patient lying on the back or on either side.

Night pain is a frequent complaint. Correction of poor sleeping posture is often successful in alleviating this discomfort. Most people sleep on one or more pillows, which promotes prolonged flexion of the neck and aggravation of or increase in pain due to muscle spasm. Sleeping with no pillow almost always makes symptoms worse. To sleep prone is to keep the neck rotated, strained, and laterally flexed for long periods.

The cervical contour pillow is 18 inches long and 8 inches in diameter. It is stuffed with feathers and down (or, more recently, Dacron) and smaller in the center than at the ends so that the neck rests with the proper amount of support for comfortable sleep. There is a bulge on either side that prevents excess rotation and lateral bending. While the patient sleeps on the side, the bulge at either end gives adequate support to keep the neck straight. The Wal-Pil-O cradles the head and supports the neck in both side-lying and back-lying postures; it comprises four pillows in one, with soft and medium centers for the head, and narrow and wide firmer borders for the neck. This pillow provides multiple combinations of head and neck support. Since sleep is the least controlled postural activity and poor sleeping posture does result in cervical spine and head pain, the use of the pillow is very effective. I find that placing the pillow on a foam rubber slant is also an effective therapeutic measure. Nocturnal chest pain, stiff neck in the morning, and pain in the cervical spine and shoulder girdle are often relieved through the use of the Wal-Pil-O.

MANAGEMENT OF PAIN

Pain reactions are caused by the arrival of abnormal volleys of nerve impulses in the brain. We do not completely understand the mechanisms of pain arising in the cervical spine. Rational, optimal therapy requires an understanding of mechanism. Thus we should, in each clinical instance, try to comprehend the pain mechanism involved. Wall[33] has asked all of the appropriate questions and dealt with possible answers having clinical application.

Which innervated structures are subject to damage?

Roots. An irritative lesion of dorsal roots, acute or chronic damage of normal nerve roots, pressure, compression, and twisting cause a severe volley of impulses at the moment of insult. It seems probable that chronic irritation results in chronic pain.

Are root signs caused by partial block?

Axons are blocked or destroyed, since we see muscle atrophy and anesthesias. Afferent nerve impulses arriving in the spinal cord cause both excitation and inhibition in the central nervous system, and the gate-control theory suggests that cells triggering pain reactions "balance" excitatory and inhibitory forces. Thus, root damage may block impulses that have an inhibitory central effect. Regional anesthetic block of a plexus distal to the root prevents the nerve impulses that arrive normally but does not affect nerve impulses generated by the presumed irritative lesion on the root. Validity of the partial block hypothesis is suggested if block abolishes the pain.

Is some pain from the root explained by partial deafferentation of spinal cord cells?

Denervation hypersensitivity occurs in the periphery in both muscle and autonomic cells. There is no secure evidence for a similar denervation hypersensitivity. Still, some cases do not become pain-free on root, bone, or disc surgery (which should abolish the peripheral source of pain-inducing impulses). The clinician must keep this in mind.

Is segmental distribution of pain referred pain rather than evidence of direct root involvement (Fig. 12–16)?

The clinician must inquire whether the pain could be referred from some deep focus. For example, a lesion in the head of the pancreas may cause pain radiating in the right side of the eighth thoracic segment.

Structures Other Than Roots Damaged by Cervical Spine Disorders. We refer here to capsules, joints, blood vessels, muscles, periosteum, bones, tendons, dura, and ligaments. Most such structures are heavily innervated. The capability of a tissue to fire off pain stimuli is not always necessarily correlated with density of innervation. Many dense connective tissue structures in the cervical spine are innervated by very fine fibers that are difficult to identify with our best histologic techniques. Once fired, nerve endings are sensitized such that even low-level stimuli later may generate nerve impulses and clinical pain. Metabolic tissue breakdown products may be the stimulating mechanism. Vascular damage can cause changes in tissues at a distance from the primary locus of pathology. Even noninnervated connective tissue can be invaded in a pathologic, connective tissue response, such as diffusion of pain-producing substances, local ischemia, or mechanical tension on distant structures by way of ligament and tendon inserting in bone.

On clinical examination, active and passive motion and motion against resistance can manipulate these structures, giving one clinical information regarding origin of pain stimuli. We can often determine which type of movement causes pain and, equally important, which type does not. Local anesthetic infiltration is diagnostically and therapeutically useful. The effect of position on pain and vasodilators may allow some insight into the circulatory role.

Do reflexes initiate pain stimuli?

Muscles. It is clear that pathologic damage in tissue results in afferent volleys of stimuli, causing prolonged reflex muscle contraction. There is associated ischemia, and such muscles clearly become painful, often at a site distant from the primary lesion. It is strange that electromyographic studies disclose muscles in spasm and in presumed pain, maintained at a low firing frequency, but such voluntary contraction in a normal subject produces no pain. Such muscles in spasm are tender to palpation, suggesting that these reflex contractions are contributing to at least some of the pain. Muscle in cramp is extremely painful, presumably because the magnitude of contraction is much greater and ischemia results.

Blood Vessels. Blood vessels are very pain-sensitive, particularly on vasodilation. Prolonged vasodilation leads to edema, stretching of tissues, and ultimate initiation of pain impulses.

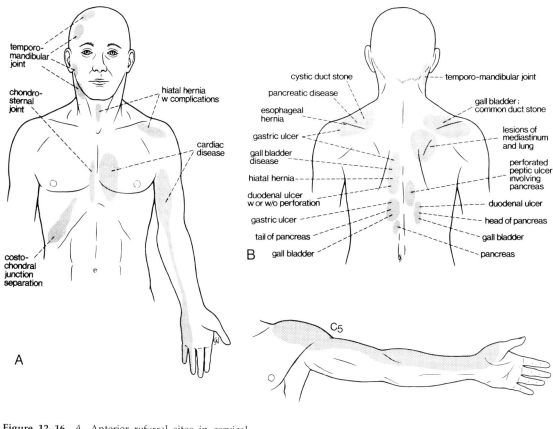

Figure 12–16. *A*, Anterior referral sites in cervical spine arising from distant visceral or somatic structures. *B*, Posterior referral sites. *C*, The dermatome distribution of C5. Only structures within the shoulder joint (exception, the acromioclavicular joint) can be perceived in this C5 pattern. Any pain pattern outside this C5 distribution cannot have arisen from structures within the shoulder.

Do distant structures contribute to the pain-producing mechanism?

The term "referred pain" describes a pain perception arising in one tissue but perceived at a distant site of apparently normal tissue. The area of pain perception is tender. Local anesthesia diminishes this pain to some degree. At its greatest severity, there may be extreme tenderness on just light touch of the skin or hair. Surrounding segments also become painful and tender. The pain pattern may not fit simple segmental distribution but involves distant areas, such as the head. The best explanation is that we are dealing with sclerotome, myotome, and dermatome distribution patterns of pain arising from a focus.

Over which peripheral pathways do sensory nerves travel?

We consider here two types of sensory afferent nerves; those that transmit impulses from an area of damaged tissue, and those from normal tissue converging on cells activated by the first. All afferents eventually run over dorsal roots and enter the spinal cord. Some afferents, probably most, pass to the dorsal root through the common mixed peripheral nerve. Others, the minority (perhaps a crucial minority of fine afferents), travel in the autonomic nervous system, passing through sympathetic ganglia and, from there, to dorsal roots. One explanation for referred pain in the head in cervical spine disease is that afferents from the diseased region traverse dorsal roots as afferents from the head that have traveled over the sympathetic chain and through the stellate ganglion to enter the dorsal roots. Sympathetic ganglia have cells that generate efferent nerve impulses as well as afferent nerve fibers. Surgical removal or local anesthesia abolishes both components. Ganglionic blocking agents may influence the efferent component, as may a peripheral blocking agent.

Which spinal cord mechanisms may relay the pain? Do *spinal cord neurons* respond to one or many types of peripheral afferent stimuli?

Consider the transmission of pain stimuli from cord to higher structures (brain). Arriving peripheral axons have an extraordinary specificity in regard to the type of stimulus that excites them and the location of the tissue the stimuli innervate. Do spinal cord neurons just collect, or do they organize interactions between incoming impulses? All cord interneurons show signs of intense interaction in their response to combinations of afferent inputs. Many afferent nerves cause a burst of excitation followed by inhibition. Very fine afferents may produce excitation followed by facilitation lasting at least 2 seconds so that slowly repeated stimuli raise the cell to higher and higher firing rates. Although we know relatively little of the pain mechanism within the spinal cord, such questions should remain in our clinical assessments.

Are spinal interneurons influenced by descending controls as well as by afferent nerve impulses?

Spinal interneurons are influenced by descending controls, including the cortex by way of the corticospinal tract and indirect pathway, the brain stem (including several undefined regions), and other segments of the cord itself.

OTHER THERAPEUTIC METHODS FOR PAIN RELIEF

Local Injection Therapy

Nonarticular rheumatism, fibrositis, and trigger areas are all terms designating pain and tenderness in localized areas throughout the body. We are concerned here with such areas in the cervical spine. These focal points and tender tissues are characterized by pain, tenderness, and stiffness, usually with spasm of neighboring muscles and impairment of function. The underlying pathophysiologic details are poorly understood. Pain may originate in structures below the deep fascia, myotomal and sclerotomal structures having a distribution other than the dermatomal pattern. Such trigger areas can be readily identified through careful palpation by a knowledgeable physician. Injections of local anesthetic in the trigger areas of tenderness and pain has gained wide acceptance and does have some therapeutic usefulness. This technique was applied utilizing only anesthetic solutions before the use of local steroid injections became popular. The efficacy of steroid injections is greater in myofascial, periarticular, and intra-articular disorders, but the procedure is widely used in injecting focal points with solutions containing both local anesthetic and corticosteroid for articular and extra-articular injection.

Best results are achieved by inserting the needle exactly into the painful point, which has been previously located by palpation. The patient can identify the exact point because contact is very painful. Some say that the physician can perceive increased resistance to advancement of the needle as it enters the trigger point. Local anesthetics include lidocaine hydrochloride (Xylocaine 1% and 2%), procaine 2%, and lignocaine 1%. They are usually in plain solutions, and the injections are 1 to 5 ml. Steroid preparations are hydrocortisone acetate, 50 to 100 mg, methylprednisolone acetate (Depo-Medrol), 40 to 80 mg, and triamcinolone hexacetonide (Aristospan), 10 to 20 mg. Because the steroid preparations are themselves crystalline—capable of initiating their own inflammatory response—they should be diluted with either saline or the local anesthetic in a 1:3:6 dilution.

These injections may be repeated a number of times before permanent relief is achieved. The clinical result should be used as a guide. If the pain relief is of short duration after 2 to 3 injections, it is unlikely that they will be successful in the long run.

Zygapophyseal joint facet involvement can be separated into two syndromes: upper cervical and lower cervical. In the upper cervical syndrome, the neck pain radiates to the occiput, temporal area, and retro-orbital region. The most prominent and constant finding is elicitation of the specific pain on pressure over the facet joints. Rotator cuff, tennis elbow, and carpal tunnel syndrome are commonly associated with these instances. In the lower cervical syndrome, usually one or two of the facet joints from C4 to T1 are very tender. The injection of combinations of anesthetics and steroids have been useful when the diagnosis is precise. If one cannot be secure regarding the clinical signs and radiologic evidence, the probability of improvement is not great. Nevertheless, the method is reasonably safe and worth a trial in severe pain problems.

Other anesthetic considerations—though not commonly used—are sympathetic blockade and epidural and subarachnoid block, again using the anesthetic in various combinations with corticosteroid. Such techniques may interrupt the vicious cycle and, in some cases, provide permanent relief of symptoms. Biofeedback as a mechanism of pain control arose from the general concept of the effect of anxiety on muscle tension in chronic, painful disorders. Control over motor unit function has lead to development of instrumentation, notably electromyographic monitoring of muscle tension, to aid patients in learning muscle relaxation by voluntary control. Patients with either acute or chronic pain in the neck and shoulder can assess their magnitude of muscle tension. The patient has the sole responsibility for the success of therapy after having been taught the technique. Controlled studies have not shown a clear advantage of biofeedback over placebo. Nevertheless, it is clearly worth a trial in complicated and difficult problems of pain control.

Operant Conditioning

The recognition that pain can be an all-encompassing psychophysiologic phenomenon that is culturally conditioned has resulted in the development of pain clinics and pain centers. The effort in these centers is utilization of an operant conditioning methodology for managing chronic pain. They are team-coordinated programs relying on reconditioning the patient's feeling states and attitude toward pain by rewarding the patient for non–pain-focused behavior. For long-standing, chronic pain not responsive to conventional measures, these centers have been very successful.

Acupuncture

For over a decade, acupuncture has been utilized in the West. Carefully controlled studies have not shown any specificity for acupuncture over placebo, and optimism and enthusiasm for comprehending a new neurophysiologic mechanism are certainly waning.

Nevertheless, acupuncture has been successful enough that it need not be rejected out-of-hand. Though acupuncture stimulation has a clear beneficial effect on pain in certain patients, there is no acceptable proof currently that acupuncture points exist. The acupuncturist's claim is that there are certain areas in the body where stimulation by an acupuncture needle has widespread effects at a distance from the area of stimulation. In general, the greater the stimulation, the more effective and prolonged the result is likely to be. The region most likely to be successfully stimulated is one in the dermatomal distribution of the part to be affected.

Manipulation Therapy

Manipulation and massage are generally considered together. Massage can induce muscle relaxation of spastic, tight, cramped muscle and is widely practiced and favorably viewed by nonmedical people. There is no firm and acceptable study of the long-term effectiveness of massage in cervical spine disease. Nevertheless, massage is comforting, has a significant, soothing effect, does result in muscle relaxation, and is symptomatically useful. Massage techniques include stroking (effleurage), which provides a general sense of well-being and deep muscle relaxation; compression (pétrissage), a kneading of tissues to stretch adhesions, increase removal of metabolic products, and produce muscle relaxation; and percussion (tapotement), which stimulates counterirritant vibration.

Manipulation, by definition, involves positioning the patient to achieve optimum comfort and promote relaxation such that muscles or joints can be placed at maximum stretch and the stretched muscles cannot effectively resist the manipulative maneuver. Usually the operator, having achieved this, applies an abrupt additional stretch, commonly called "thrust," resulting in a distraction of the joint or tissues being treated. The thrust is often associated with an audible cracking sound. If the cracking occurs, the maneuver is generally regarded as successful. The additional abrupt stretch on the maximally extended muscle is said to stimulate the muscle spindles and connective tissue proprioceptive organs, resulting in further, sudden relaxation and "overmovement" of the connective tissue structure. The most thoughtful, perceptive, and penetrating discussion of the subject is by Swezey.[34]

Manipulation is commonly the practice of chiropractic. Chiropractic dogma has it that all disease is a consequence of spinal subluxations and is cured by spinal adjustments. There is no acceptable scientific evidence to support this contention. Though manipulation is relatively safe when applied to the lumbar spine, there are certain significant risks, uncommon though they are, to manipulation in the cervical spine. Thus the physician must assess the question of risk versus benefit. There are many well-documented instances of cerebrovascular, cervicoarterial, and spinal cord damage secondary to manipulation. In recent years, serious consideration has been given to manipulative therapy[17] and has led to the formation of an organization, the North American Academy of Manipulative Medicine, which is a society of physicians with a scientific interest in the science and technology of manipulation.[35, 36, 37]

There are certain assumptions regarding what manipulation accomplishes. They depend upon whether the primary cause of pain is abnormality in the zygapophyseal joints or in the intervertebral disc or both! Movement of either it is assumed results in movement in the others as well as movement in the joints of Luschka. Certainly the zygapophyseal joints, the joints of Luschka, and the intervertebral discs are all involved in osteoarthritis, with varying degrees of pathologic change, malalignment, and mechanical instability. Furthermore, there are menisci in virtually all of the small joints in the cervical spine that have been indicted as causes of entrapment by disc-facet joint movement. Swezey asks, "What is the pathologic lesion that we are thrusting against, popping and 'adjusting'?"[34] Why is the loud associated pop or crack relied upon to give the manipulator assurance of success? We do not really know what the popping represents. We do know that cracking knuckles produces a similar popping. Knuckle cracking is benign, rarely if ever causes pain or pathologic change, and is a common experience normally. Osteopathic physicians believe the zygapophyseal joints are at fault. The cracking sound certainly may be a normal facet joint being cracked, achieving the same result as that obtained when knuckles are cracked—that is, the joint has a subatmospheric pressure normally, and on being distracted, the subatmospheric pressure falls, resulting in the gas (nitrogen) coming out of solution and into the joint space as a bubble, hence the pop.

If the disc is the cause of pain, a general assumption is that the cracking is due to anular tears, posterior movement of the viscous nuclear material, and relief of pain. This squeezing type of manipulation would reasonably apply to the intervertebral discs of young people, but discs usually become desiccated and fibrotic with age, and, being hard, anular inspissated fragments would seem less likely to move back into a position. A rather alarming recommendation of manipulators is that if manipulation to one side does not work, the patient can be "turned over" for manipulation of the other side—the "whatever works" policy.

There exists testimony of thousands of patients, chiropractors, osteopaths, physicians, and therapeutic manipulators supporting the efficacy of manipulative therapy; however, there remains little convincing scientific evidence of a cause and effect relationship between the use of manipulation and relief of symptoms. Some physicians have enormous confidence in the manipulative programs and ask, "Can we justify not manipulating?"[17]

Manipulation therapy is far from completely safe, yet it is widely practiced and catastrophic events are uncommon. It is certain that a manipulator should be highly trained, should have the knowledge and skills required for making an appropriate decision regarding manual therapy, and should be aware of the dangers involved. Most manipulative therapy is in the hands of chiropractors. Physical therapists usually lack sufficient sophistication in the pathophysiology involved and, by and large, are not extensively practicing manipulation.

It does seem reasonable that in the future physicians are going to become more interested in this area. Physical therapists and osteopaths will probably begin to develop standard criteria for the performance of manual therapies, including manipulation.

References

1. Spengler D, Loeser J, Murphy T: Orthopedic aspects of the chronic pain syndrome. *In* Brindley HH (ed): American Academy of Orthopedic Surgeons: AAOS Instructional Course Lectures, vol 29. St Louis: C.V. Mosby Co, 1980.
2. McMasters WC, Liddle S, Waugh TR: Laboratory evaluation of various cold therapy modalities. Am J Sports Med 6:291, 1978.
3. Stillwell JK: General principle of thermotherapy. *In* Licht S, Kamenetz H (eds): Therapeutic Heat and Cold, 2nd ed. New Haven, CT: Elizabeth Licht, Publisher, 1965.
4. Lehmann J, de Lateur B: Therapeutic heat. *In* Lehman J (ed): Therapeutic Heat and Cold, 3rd ed. Baltimore: Williams & Wilkins Co, 1982.
5. Doyle J, Smart B: Stimulation of bone growth by short wave diathermy. J Bone Joint Surg 45A:15, 1963.
6. Klafs C, Arnheim D: Modern Principles of Athletic Training, 5th ed. St Louis: C.V. Mosby Co, 1981.
7. Melzack R, Wall P: Pain mechanism, a new theory. Science 150:971, 1965.
8. Gersch M: Postoperative pain and transcutaneous electrical nerve stimulation. Phys Ther 58:1463, 1978.
9. Smith GE: The most ancient splints. B Med J 1:732, 1908.
10. Hartman JT: The cervical orthosis—does it immobilize? Orthop Rev 5:53, 1976.
11. Hartman JT, Palumbo F, Hill BJ: Cineradiography of the braced cervical spine. Clin Orthop 109:97, 1975.
12. Fisher SV, Bowar JF, Awad EA, et al: Cervical orthoses effect on cervical spine motion: roentgenographic and goniometric method of study. Arch Phys Med Rehabil 58:109, 1977.
13. Johnson RM, Hart DL, Simmons EF, et al: Cervical orthoses: A study comparing their effectiveness in restricting cervical motion in normal subjects. J Bone Joint Surg 59A:332, 1977.
14. Segal J: Biofeedback as a medical treatment. JAMA 232:2, 1975.
15. Jacobs B: The arthritic spine. *In* Ehrlich GE (ed): Total Management of the Arthritic Patient. Philadelphia: J.B. Lippincott Company, 1973, p 139.
16. Smith PH, Sharp J, Kellgren JH: Natural history of rheumatoid cervical subluxations. Ann Rheum Dis 31:222, 1972.
17. Cyriax JH, Cyriax PJ: Illustrated Manual of Orthopedic Medicine. London: Butterworth Publishers, 1984, pp 145–167.
18. McKenzie R: Treat Your Own Neck. New Zealand: Spinal Publications, 1983.
19. Stoddard A: Manual of Osteopathic Technique, 10th impression. London: Hutchinson Co, 1978.
20. Rath WW: Cervical traction, a clinical perspective. Orthop Rev 13:430, 1984.
21. Deets A, Hand RT, Hopp JB: Cervical traction, a comparison of sitting and supine position. Phys Ther 3:57, 1977.
22. White A, Panjabi M: Clinical biomechanics of the spine. Philadelphia: J.B. Lippincott Co, 1978.
23. Delacerda JE: Effect of angle of traction pull on upper trapezius muscle activity. J Orthop Phys Ther 1:205, 1980.
24. Judovich B: Herniated cervical disc: A new form of traction therapy. Am J Surg 84:646, 1952.
25. Colachis S, Strohm B: Cervical traction: Relationship of time to varied traction force with constant angle of pull. Arch Phys Med Rehabil 46:815, 1965.
26. Gupta RC, Ramarao SV: Epidurography in reduction of lumbar disc prolapse by traction. Arch Phys Med Rehabil 59:322, 1978.
27. Swezey RL: Arthritis: Rational Therapy and Rehabilitation. Philadelphia: W.B. Saunders Co, 1978, pp 140–141.
28. Farfan AF: Mechanical disorders of the low back. Philadelphia: Lea & Febiger, 1973, pp 206–207.
29. Ziebell B: Wellness: An Arthritis Reality. Dubuque, IA: Kendall/Hunt Publishing Co, 1981.
30. Benson H: The Relaxation Response. New York: Avon Books, 1980.

31. Smith EL, Serfass RC: Exercise and Aging. The Scientific Basis. Hillside, NJ: Enslow Publishing, 1981.

32. Kendall HO, Kendall FP, Boynton DX: Posture and Pain. Baltimore: Williams & Wilkins Co., 1977.

33. Wall PD: The mechanisms of pain associated with cervical vertebral disease. *In* Hirsch C, Zotterman Y (eds): Cervical Pain. New York: Pergamon Press, 1971, pp 201–221.

34. Swezey RL: The modern thrust of manipulation and traction therapy. Semin Arthritis Rheum 12:322, 1983.

35. Young RA: The spine. Low back. *In* Roberts GC (ed): Orthopedics Clinical Surgery, vol 13. London: Butterworth Publishers, 1967, p 345.

36. Pubek RA: Brain stem vascular accident following neck manipulation. Wis Med J 62:141, 1963.

37. Maigne R: Orthopedic Medicine. A New Approach to Vertebral Manipulation. Springfield, IL: Charles C Thomas Publisher, 1972.

Chapter 13

Emergency Management of Fractures, Subluxation, and Soft-Tissue Injury

Cervical spine injuries, increasingly common, are surely among the most serious injuries caused by falls, automobile accidents, athletic game participation, and industrial accidents. Neck injuries range in consequence for simple pain in the neck to quadriplegia to death. In the United States, about 5000 new quadriplegia patients are identified and enter our statistical records yearly. These cases are of great importance to doctors, patients' families and employers, insurance brokers, lawyers, and the federal government. Tax payers commonly are called upon to shoulder the financial burdens of the extreme disability, liability, and unemployment that is generated by such catastrophic illness. Cervical spine injury with spinal cord damage commonly occurs to otherwise strong, healthy people who, in an automobile crash, a diving accident, or a football game, are abruptly totally paralyzed—helpless for the rest of their lives. They are totally dependent on others for all bodily needs, yet they still have a keen and alert mind. Diagnosis is far from simple, and misdiagnosis as well as delayed diagnosis is common. *In one of the largest series of fracture dislocations of the cervical spine (300 in number), gross disability of one third of the patients resulted from either error or lack of suspicion on the part of the examining physician.*[1]

The moment of injury, the minutes to hours following the injury, and the events transpiring prior to arrival of the patient in a completely equipped medical center constitute the most critical period in the history of an acute cervical spine injury. Thus, it is the goal of this chapter to deal with the emergency management of the victim of cervical spine injury—the on-the-scene preparation for transport to an emergency room and

(optimally) to a center for the management of cervical spine and spinal cord injuries.

CLASSIFICATION

A number of classifications of cervical spine injuries have been described. One simple anatomic classification is as follows: (1) Fractures and dislocations at the base of the skull and the upper cervical spine, including atlanto-occipital and atlantoaxial and axial–C3 fractures and dislocations, Jefferson's fracture, odontoid fractures, vertebrobasilar injury, and traumatic spondylolisthesis of the axis (hangman's fracture). (2) Fractures and dislocations of the lower cervical spine, including posterior, anterior, and lateral vertebral element injury, fracture, and dislocation.

Another classification is one using anatomic criteria of the tissue mainly involved: (1) bony injury, (2) soft-tissue injury, (3) nerve root trauma, and (4) spinal cord trauma. Radiologic classification has been useful to identify the mechanism of injury and the forces applied to the spine by flexion, extension, and compression. In a flexion injury, complete dislocation of one or both inferior articulating facets of the zygapophyseal joints is required to produce spinal cord damage. Damage to the spinal cord caused by hyperextension of the neck requires posterior dislocation of the vertebrae. The term teardrop was coined to describe the radiologic appearance of compression fractures associated with hyperflexion injury. All of these mechanisms along with the well-known, acute, traumatic disc rupture are used to classify cervical spine injuries according to radiologic findings. The neurologist and neurosurgeon are more

279

concerned with injuries to the spinal cord and nerve roots, whereas the orthopedic surgeon focuses more on bone, joint, and ligamentous trauma. The pathologist is a student of gross and microscopic changes of all tissues of the cervical spine in trauma.

Radiologic, clinical, and pathologic findings do not always serve well for description and assessment of the nature and extent of cervical spine injuries. The patient may initially have none or only minor neurologic damage, progressing rapidly over minutes to an hour to total quadriplegia both with and without treatment, as in the case of intramedullary hemorrhage. Conversely, a person with a cervical spine injury may have gross, extensive, and immediate generalized neurologic loss below the level of the injury because of spinal shock. Within a short period after the administration of steroid drugs and skull traction, much if not all of this function may return. Severe damage to the spinal cord may occur with soft tissue injury only and with quite normal radiologic findings. Transient subluxation can occur at the instant of injury, severely damaging the spinal cord but spontaneously realigning itself, with resultant normal radiologic study. Soft-tissue injuries may include rupture and tear of intervertebral discs, contusion of nerve roots, and splitting of anterior and posterior longitudinal ligaments and the ligamentum flavum.

The clinical examination is more effective than any radiologic study in identifying damage to soft tissues of the neck, particularly damage to the nerve roots and spinal cord. The best single classification of cervical spine injuries brings together all available data, including the description, as much as is available of the dynamics of the trauma, the nature of the injury itself, and the direction of forces impacting the head and neck. It provides a more useful clinical framework for comprehending the damage sustained and for taking appropriate measures. There are four categories in this classification: (1) The hyperextension injury (whiplash); damage is confined to muscles and ligaments and, sometimes, the intervertebral discs; it does not involve the peripheral or central nervous system. (2) Paralysis without injury or dislocation of vertebrae as clinically and radiologically determined. (3) Injuries to the cervical vetebrae, without clinical involvement of nerve roots or spinal cord—dislocations and compression fractures of the cervical vertebrae. (4) Vertebral injury and dislocation associated with paralysis.

CLINICAL ASSESSMENT, MANAGEMENT, AND INITIAL CARE AT THE SITE OF THE ACCIDENT

The entire future of the injured patient is at risk at the site of the accident. Proper management of the patient with neck injury is critical. An unstable, cervicovertebral fracture is a dangerous trauma, and even minor movements may irreparably damage the spinal cord. Any shift causing loose bone fragments to compress the spinal cord or block its blood supply results in sudden paralysis. Ambulance attendants and people from the police and fire departments are usually the first to arrive at the scene. They are generally very well trained and, in most instances, are preferable to random physician attendants. In a large series of fatal cervical spine injuries, 25% of deaths were related to the period between the accident and the transport of the patient to the emergency room. The injured spine is an obvious emergency, with or without neurologic findings. Definitive management of spine injuries is best done only in medical centers that are set up for such emergencies and handle them daily. There is no other injury in which meticulous, correct handling and emergency care are more important.

The first person, most certainly the first physician, to examine the patient has a great responsibility. The precarious nature of the injury is due not only to the fracture or dislocation itself but also to the great risk of damage to delicate tissues of the spinal cord. *If the cord has been completely severed, the worst has happened, but anything less than that has the possibility of complete or varying degrees of recovery—a possibility that easily can be dashed by improper handling.* Even today, without expert emergency personnel, patients with cervical spine injury continue to suffer irreparable cord damage in a wild and rough ride in a car or ambulance driven by a well-meaning but poorly instructed Samaritan. The key is to move any badly injured patient as little as possible. Patients should be delivered to the emergency room in the same or better condition as when they left the site of the accident.

The following suggestions are of key importance:

1. Always suspect serious cervical spine injury, particularly damage to the nerve roots and spinal cord; assume that the spine has been injured and that any movement will increase the damage.

2. Be particularly alert in dealing with people injured through automobile crashes, diving, contact sports, or falls from a height and with people having any history of direct trauma to the head, neck, or upper chest. Any unconscious patient is automatically very suspect, since the trauma leading to loss of consciousness tends to parallel that leading to fracture and dislocation of the neck. Fifteen to twenty per cent of patients with significant head trauma have associated neck injury.

3. Immobilize the spine on a rigid surface, such as a cervical stabilization–traction board,[2] which is a rigid board with two detachable blocks rotating on three axes. The patient's trunk is immobilized by a strong waist strap and two shoulder straps, and the blocks are positioned

along both sides of the head to prevent lateral movement and rotation. A standard halter or traction sling placed under the mandibular and suboccipital areas provides traction and prevents flexion and extension movements of the head and neck. With the patient thus immobilized, all subsequent transfers are performed without risk to the cervical spine. Without such special equipment, one can improvise. Examples include using a removed door, moving the patient as if he were a log—one inflexible piece—paying special attention to the head and neck; placing sandbags along each side of the head; using a firm cervical collar, the so-called extrication collar, which immobilizes the head and neck very well and is easy to slip on in seconds without moving the patient; or using a head halter with weights (see Chapter 12, *General Management Methods*).

4. Carefully observe the patient while you are immobilizing them. Do they move arms and legs spontaneously? Are any limbs inert or flaccid? A lower cord lesion involves legs only, whereas the cervical cord lesion affects upper limbs as well. The legs will be motionless if a lower cord lesion has occurred. Look closely at the breathing pattern; is the chest rising with each inspiration? Is only the stomach rising? Intercostal muscles are supplied by motor outflow from the thoracic spine, but the diaphragm is innervated by C3–C4–C5. If intercostal muscles are not functioning, the patient breaths abdominally. This sign provides a virtual certainty that the injury is somewhere in the lower cervical area, since it has compromised the thoracic nerve supply but left the phrenic nerve supply (C3–C4–C5) intact.

5. Are there involuntary muscle contractions, twitching, fasciculations? A damaged cord evokes fasciculations in muscles innervated by the spinal cord segment above the level of denervation (Schiff-Sherrington phenomenon). If the cord is transected in the midthoracic region or lower, the stretch and other postural reflexes of the upper extremity are exaggerated; if the lesion is in the sacral cord, the same thing occurs in the lower limb.

6. *If the patient is conscious, talk to him! He will tell you the diagnosis!* The cardinal symptom of spinal injury is severe, acute, local pain radiating peripherally along the involved nerves. Commonly, the patient's great fear is that the neck is broken. Ask the patient how it happened. For instance, if the patient was in an automobile crash, where was he in the car? What can the patient remember? Diving off a bank? Tackling on a football field? Did the head hit the windshield? But it's the neck that hurts.

7. If patient is unconscious inquire of witnesses, ambulance crew, and other people involved in the accident.

8. Check size, equality, and reactivity of pupils.

9. Examine the spine. Look carefully. Do not allow the head and neck to rotate, that is, the head and neck must be rotated at exactly the same speed as the body, without deviation, flexion, or extension. Look for contusions, abrasions, open wounds, and ecchymoses. Examine the scalp. Identify by palpation the cervicovertebral spinous processes, feeling each one. Note any obvious deformity, local tenderness, muscle spasm, prominent spinous processes, and crepitus.

10. Quickly assess both motor and sensory responses. Remember they come off at the same spinal cord level but run in quite different areas in the columns of the cord itself. Only complete transection affects them equally, but a partial lesion injures only one type or the other of both motor and sensory end-organs in different degrees, that is, a posterior cord contusion is reflected by sensory symptoms, and an anterior cord lesion results in paralysis and has motor clinical reflection. *Check both patterns on both sides of the patient's body, rapidly!*

11. With complete transection, diagnosis is obvious. With transection at C4 and below, the patient is paralyzed from the chin down. Survival is rare if there is gross injury at C1–C2 and C3, owing to respiratory failure.

12. If time is on your hands do a more complete neurologic examination and keep accurate records for use by the neurologist, neurosurgeon, and orthopedic surgeon in the spine center. Test temperature, vibration, two-point discrimination, proprioception, and position sense. Remember, your primary job is to get a quick motor and sensory assessment. The other tests are simply ''fine tuning.''

13. *Some practical points*: Ask the patient to wiggle the toes and to lift the leg. If the patient cannot do either, ask him to move the hands and lift the arms. The hand and arm movement gives you information about nearly every level of the neck. Ask the patient to spread his fingers. If the patient can do this, the interosseous muscles are functioning, which indicates that any lesion present is below the C8–T1 level. If the patient cannot spread his fingers, ask him to squeeze your hand. If this is done well with all fingers, the patient's seventh cervical level is intact. While the patient extends his wrist, check the function of the biceps and triceps muscles, which are mediated through C6. If they are abnormal, check function of the deltoid muscle by asking the patient to shrug his shoulders (C5). Doing these tests on both sides requires little time, and accurate results are usual.[13] Ask the patient to close the eyes, and check responses to pain with a safety pin. Start at the toes and move up, always going from the anesthetic area to the normal area (all of us are more sensitive to the appearance of sensation than its disappearance). Observe the patient's facial expression. Ask the patient to tell you as soon as he feels the pin (the facial expression tells you more than the words).

14. *You may note sensory perception just above the*

nipple line and assume the neck is uninvolved; not so! The "shawl" area is really supplied by C4 and C5, and if you stop looking at the level of T3, you have missed the event in the lower cervical spine. That information comes when you check the arm pattern.

With motor and sensory function below a given level, spinal injury suppresses reflex response in the same area; thus, test deep tendon reflexes as you move up. Testing for Babinski's and Hoffmann's reflexes is very useful.

15. Drive the ambulance or automobile at a reasonable speed with as little jarring and turning as possible.

EMERGENCY ROOM CARE

1. Continue to stress the danger of movement; catastrophe can still occur as the patient goes from one set of hands to another. A certain degree of movement and manipulation is inevitable during transfer from the site of the trauma to the emergency room, the hospital, or another hospital; resuscitative pocedures may become necessary; physical examination will be done. Remember that an even slightly uninformed person can do great damage to a victim who does not have obvious paralysis or gross neurologic signs.

2. *Remove clothes very carefully! Never remove anything over the head* (no matter how careful you are you could cause a complete transection of the cord). Cut off any clothing not easily removed (a type of paramedic scissors invented during the Vietnam war and manufactured by Dyna-med will cut through anything, including shoes).

3. *Radiologic assessment*: Get a cross-table lateral view of the cervical spine, with the neck completely immobilized; pull the shoulders gently down so that they clear the C7–T1 junction; be sure the upper cervical spine is included, particularly the odontoid process. Then take an anteroposterior film—nothing more complex for the moment. Assess these two films; if there is no evidence of fracture or dislocation, consider flexion, extension, and oblique views. If in doubt, do not do it!

4. Since automobile crashes are associated with multiple injuries, obtain radiographs of the remainder of the spine—thoracic, lumbar, and lumbosacral areas—as well as suspicious looking extremities. Remember the mnemonic, the "ABC'S" of radiologic diagnostics: *A* for alignment, *B* for bony mineralization, *C* for cartilage space, and *S* for soft tissue.

5. Check alignment by drawing a line along the anterior and posterior margins of the vertebrae and along the anterior margins of the spinous processes. If the normally smooth and continuous arc that results is interrupted, a fracture probably exists. Anterior and posterior margins of each vertebra should be approximately—a wedge-shaped vertebra means compression fracture. (See Chapter 7, *Craniometry and Roentgenometry of the Skull and Cervical Spine* and Chapter 14, *Cervical Spine in Infancy and Childhood* for the possibilities of gross misinterpretation in children.) Pay special attention to the occipito-atlanto-axial region; look for areas of possible "bony" weakness, such as cervical osteoarthritis, rheumatoid arthritis, osteoporosis, and malacia; examine the intervertebral disc spaces; pay particular attention to soft-tissue shadows. Remember that a patient can sustain gross injury of the cervical spine and spinal cord with no radiologic abnormalities.

6. Start any patient with suspected cord or nerve root damage on corticosteroid therapy as early as possible. Methylprednisolone is usually administered for 10 days (without a tapering schedule), starting at the time of initial phone contact with the referring persons—paramedics, local physician, neurosurgeon. Many neurosurgeons use dexamethasone sodium phosphate, the loading dose for which has tended to increase over the years.

7. *Perform electrophysiologic studies (if equipment is available)*: Somatosensory-evoked cortical potentials and the H reflex may help one assess functional status of the cord. Sometimes the study detects residual sensory function not apparent on clinical examination. At the very least, somatosensory-evoked cortical potentials are a sensory indicator of spinal cord damage and serve as a baseline study in follow-up care.

8. Large doses of vitamin B1 and B12 once per day are said to be helpful in controlling the nerve swelling syndrome.

9. Re-examine the patient frequently—at least several times each day; the number of things you note on a second or third exam that you missed initially is striking. Also chart and follow changes taking place. It is hoped that changes for the better are occurring, nevertheless, the patient may regress and deteriorate in the motor or sensory level. Such regression and deterioration indicate developing cord compression or a cord hematoma that might be dealt with clinically.

10. Consider using a nasogastric tube, a Foley catheter, a running intravenous drip, or an intracatheter as well as endotracheal intubation. When using these instruments, take great care to maintain the airway without disturbing the cervical spine.

11. Consider using skeletal traction and rapid reduction alignment. Attempt these procedures without using any manipulative techniques.

12. Myelography usually is performed in all cases. Emulsified Pantopaque (iophendylate) or metrizamide is injected through a lateral C1–C2 puncture except in the case of C1–C2 fracture. An anesthesiologist, if available, should assess respiratory function.

13. Make decision regarding surgical decompression, stabilization, and ultimate fusion.

14. With the most expert advice, consider the

use of vasodilator therapy since there is so much vasospasm and constriction of central nervous system arterial supply in head trauma and spinal cord injury. In spinal cord injury, vessel caliber decreases in a manner similar to cerebral vasospasm, with blood in the subarachnoid space. Serotonin, catecholamine, and prostaglandins have all been implicated as causative agents. Naloxone hydrochloride has been used experimentally but has little clinical validation.

INJURIES
Hyperextension Cervical Spine Injury (Whiplash)

Definition. Classic hyperextension injury to the neck is caused by an indirect force, such as an automobile collision from the rear. *The patient's head is thrown backward in violent, unrestrained hyperextension of the neck.* Recoil follows, and the head projects forward in extreme flexion. Cervical, sternocleidomastoid, and scalene muscles and the long muscles of the neck are all stretched, with variable tearing. *The recoil flexion of the neck is limited by the chin's striking the chest or steering wheel.* With very severe extension, esophagus and larynx are stretched, resulting in dysphagia and hoarseness, difficulty in chewing, and limited opening of the mouth. Temporomandibular joint ligaments are sprained as head is jerked away from the mandible; muscle laceration with hematomata occurs; damage to sympathetic nerve fibers causes nausea, vertigo, visual and auditory symptoms, and unusually, a unilaterally dilated pupil (Horner's syndrome). Anterior fibers of the intervertebral disc and the anterior longitudinal ligament may be stretched and torn. Head injury may occur as brain is forced forward and backward in the skull by the extreme flexion-extension, with consequent cerebral concussion, contrecoup, cerebral contusion with petechial hemorrhages, and headache.

Symptoms and Signs. Initially, the victim is often unaware of the injury, but in 12 to 36 hours pain appears in the neck—increasing in severity and aggravated by neck movements. Limitation of motion occurs mostly in extension. Other symptoms include wryneck, tenderness of the muscles of the neck, hoarseness, dysphagia, and bizarre symptoms secondary to sympathetic fiber damage.

Treatment and Management. (1) Full radiographic studies, taking great care before they are accomplished to determine that there has been no spinal cord injury. (2) Soft cervical collar. (3) Physical therapy as heat and gentle stretching exercises; analgesia and anti-inflammatory agents; mild cervical traction with a halter, on outpatient or at-home basis; local anesthetic injections in trigger points of pain and tenderness.

With persistence of symptoms beyond 8 to 12 weeks, especially if litigation is in process, one must differentiate between compensation neurosis and an injury of greater magnitude than initially suspected. With scapular pain, paresthesias, or other neurologic signs, one may suspect a torn intervertebral disc. Note that muscles and ligaments heal within 2 to 4 weeks, whereas intervertebral discs, having no blood supply, heal much more slowly (see Chapter 20, *Disability Determinations*).

Hyperextension Injury with Paralysis

Definition. This is injury to the spinal cord and nerve roots or both, without detectable fracture or dislocation; the severe hyperextension is most commonly caused by a direct force. This injury occurs more frequently in older people, who tend to fall forward, striking face and forehead. Often, immediate paralysis of arms occurs, with a rapidly developing quadriplegia. Radiologic findings include cervical osteoarthritis with posterior osteophytes, hypertrophied ligamentum flavum, and zygapophyseal and Luschka joint involvement; accompanying osteoarthritis narrows the spinal canal, with the trauma narrowing it further. Edema of the cord may result in death. Venous as well as arterial circulation is compromised by the narrow spinal canal.

Treatment and Management. (1) Gentle traction with the neck slightly flexed, avoiding all hyperextension; neurologic and neurosurgical consultation with consideration for anterior surgical decompression; corticosteroid therapy, dexamethasone preferred; computed tomography and surgical removal of any torn fragments of the anulus fibrosus or detached cartilage pieces in the spinal canal.

Cervicovertebral Dislocation-Fracture or Dislocation and Fracture

Definition. If fracture or dislocation is remotely suspected, remember that it may occur without paralysis. Never delay proper assessment and medical examination. Occasionally, this diagnosis is made weeks or months after an accident. Types of lesions are dislocations, flexion injuries with vertebral malalignment, compression fracture, combinations of dislocation and fracture, anterior dislocation with posterior element fracture, flexion fractures of C2 (odontoid process), extension fractures (C2–C3 pedicles), compression fracture of C1 arch of the atlas, and Jefferson's fracture. Cervical spine fractures involve the vertebral bodies and are caused by a force that is supplied to the vertex of the head and transmitted to the spine in a vertical direction—dives into shallow water, falls from moving vehicles or high places, and athletic activity such as wrestling and football.

Treatment and Management. The severity of the lesion and degree of involvement of the nervous system constitute the deciding factors in treatment and management.

Cervicovertebral Injury without Paralysis

Definition. Dislocation, hyperflexion, or deceleration injuries are the reverse of the hyperextension injury, whiplash. This type accounts for about two thirds of neck injuries. The body is in forward motion and strikes an immovable object, as in a head-on automobile crash or falling backward, usually while intoxicated. With the violent throwing of the head forward, the interspinous ligaments, capsules of the zygapophyseal joints, and posterior fibers of the intervertebral discs may all be torn. Such structures maintain stability of the intervertebral joints in the upright position. Loss of continuity allows forward subluxation or dislocation at the level of the injury. Symptoms of plain anterior dislocation are pain, muscle spasm, limitation of cervical spine movements, and pain referral to the muscles of the neck, medioscapular border, shoulders, and upper arm. The pain may radiate into the forearm and hands, with associated numbness and paresthesia. Lateral films of the cervical spine often allow proper diagnosis; one may see only an increase in the distance between spinous processes and zygapophyseal articular facets at the level of injury.

Treatment and Management. If there is no cord compression, treatment is conservative. Dislocated spine is realigned by halter or skull traction, with subsequent immobilization in a brace. Usually, the brace is worn for about 3 months, the time necessary for ligaments to heal by scar and calcification. Gentle exercises (active and passive) should be performed almost from the beginning.

Compression Fracture

Definition. Compression fracture usually occurs without dislocation and with only slight malalignment. Spinal cord and nerve roots are not injured; intervertebral discs above and below the fracture usually are intact even though the bone is crushed. Symptoms are pain in the neck (especially on movement), muscle spasm, and decreased range of motion. Lateral radiographs allow proper diagnosis. Myelography may occasionally be indicated if there is question or doubt regarding protrusion into the spinal canal.

Treatment and Management. Treatment is conservative; prescribe brace or collar. If malalignment and anterior angulation exist, consider surgical management to prevent subsequent myelopathy.

Cervical Vertebral Injury with Paralysis

Definition. In this injury, nerve roots and spinal cord are damaged, and the methods of diagnosis and management are completely different from those of the previously discussed injuries of this classification. Management is urgent; patient must not be moved. Assessment of nerve root involvement and spinal cord injury as previously noted in the sections on management at the site of injury and in the emergency room should be performed. All of the urgent treatment and management considerations apply here.

DIAGNOSTIC PITFALLS IN CERVICAL SPINE INJURY

1. A confusing set of terms is used in characterizing neck injury. "Whiplash" really tells how the injury happened, not what it is. Such terms as sprain and strain of the cervical spine, disc syndrome, hyperextension or hyperflexion injury to the cervical spine, subluxations of the cervical spine, traumatic fibrositis, and craniocervical syndrome are all used, particularly when the issue comes into litigation. To avoid this terminological pitfall, base the diagnosis on as precise an analysis of anatomic, radiologic, and clinical findings as possible, avoiding the wastebasket terms.

2. Cervical spine injuries in automobile collisions from the rear are not usually "mild" sprains. The victim's head is violently thrown backward—even when the car is traveling at relatively slow speeds—then forward, usually tearing soft tissues in some degree and injuring the zygapophyseal joint ligaments. More damage is done than the patient, the family, and physician deem likely. Bizarre symptoms and signs are not unusual, and they may occur weeks to months or, occasionally, even a year after the incident. Thus, suspect neck injury in all rear-end or head-on collisions, pay very close attention to the patient, obtain complete historical data, and perform a thorough physical and radiologic examination. See the patient as early as possible after the accident and do a complete clinical study. Keep the patient in follow-up care and do not make light of the problem.

3. The results of the radiologic study may be negative even though definite and, sometimes, very serious injury has been done. This fact is too little appreciated by the average physician.

Thus, do complete historical elicitation and physical examination. Pay close attention to even a slight abnormality. Keep the patient in follow-up care. Do not hesitate to repeat films, obtaining all views, including flexion, neutral, extension, both oblique views, and AP and open-mouth views. Get expert radiologic assessment.

4. Symptoms may be bizarre—headache, dizziness, vertigo, blurring of vision, and visual and auditory hallucination—all of which may be valid. Herniation of the intervertebral discs may occur incidentally after a cervical spine injury. This may or may not be related to the injury.

To avoid this diagnostic pitfall, take the patient seriously, study the patient in follow-up care, and reinquire regarding all details of the injury. Determine whether the patient has ever had any clinical experience similar to the present one.

5. It is usual for the cervical spine to have a normal range of motion at the time and immediately after the injury. The range of motion becomes increasingly restricted, particularly in extension, lateral flexion, and rotation, much less so in flexion. Thus, be certain that the cervical spine range of motion rather than the shoulder range of motion is being examined. Pay close attention to the differences between active and passive motion and motion against resistance. Consider the possibility that the decreased range of motion, if truly present, may or may not be related to the accident.

References

1. Bohlman HH: Acute fracture and dislocation of the cervical spine. J Bone Joint Surg 61A:1119, 1979.
2. Prole DJ, Hanbery JW: Cervical stabilization–traction board. A new device for immediate stabilization of the injured cervical spine. JAMA 224:615, 1973.

Chapter 14

Cervical Spine in Infancy and Childhood

Because the anatomic characteristics of the cervical spine of the infant and the child differ significantly from those of the adult, a far different clinical and radiologic assessment is required. The joints, ligaments, tendons, and cervical muscles in the neonate are strikingly weak; the child cannot adequately support the head in a vertical posture until about age 3 months. The infant is thus incapable of protecting the cervical spine and cord in torsional or tractional trauma. Such forces may readily overcome the stretch capability of the neck; the normally lax ligaments of the neck of an infant or child cannot protect the less elastic spinal cord. *Rather severe cord injuries may occur, with no apparent skeletal or bony injury.* Because of immature muscle development in young infants, a reversal of the normally smooth anterior curve is seen in the lateral radiographic projection of the cervical spine. In lateral films of the adult cervical spine with the neck in mild flexion, there is some "step off" normally observed, that is, the body of each vertebra is displaced slightly anteriorly in relation to the vertebra below. Infants and children show the same normal finding when the neck is held in mild flexion, especially at the level of C2–C3, where the step off can be as great as 2 to 3 mm normally. The presence of unclosed epiphyseal plates, many synchondroses, and very active ossification centers renders interpretation of radiologic studies in children very difficult (Fig. 14–1). Open spaces are likely to be mistaken for fractures in the context of a history of trauma. The infant spine is extremely hypermobile. The hypermobility decreases gradually in childhood and adolescence. Nonetheless, knowledge of radiologic and anatomic characteristics of the cervical spine from birth to 25 years is a sine qua non of proper management of the clinical problems of the cervical spine in infancy and childhood. The spinal cord at birth has immature myelin development in the white matter, and the myelin is needed for protection against shearing or stretching forces. Breech presentation or prolonged labor may require manipulation of a baby's head and neck, causing spinal cord damage without any cervical spine dislocation.

The characteristics of the immature cervical spine—hypermobility, incomplete ossification, epiphyses, synchondroses, unique vertebral configuration, hyperlaxity of ligamentous and capsular structures—all contribute to the difficulty of interpretation of radiograms (Fig. 14–2). The literature contains many case reports of children with neck injuries whose radiographs reveal abnormalities that are initially interpreted as subluxations, dislocations, and fractures but are later regarded as normal variations. Cervical spine injuries are common, particularly in sports and automobile crashes. Examination of such an injured child often discloses pain on motion and muscle spasm, without evidence localizing the site of injury. This leads one to rely on radiologic evidence of the site injury. Physicians dealing with injuries of infants, children, and adolescents absolutely require a complete knowledge of normal variations to avoid misdiagnosis and the sometimes tragic application of improper therapy.

DEVELOPMENTAL ANATOMY OF THE CERVICAL SPINE

The anatomic development of the atlas, axis, and third cervical vertebra as it relates to functional anatomy in neonates, children, and adolescents is described in the subsequent sections.

First Cervical Vertebra, Atlas

The cervical vertebrae differ from thoracic and lumbar vetebrae in that they have a foramen in

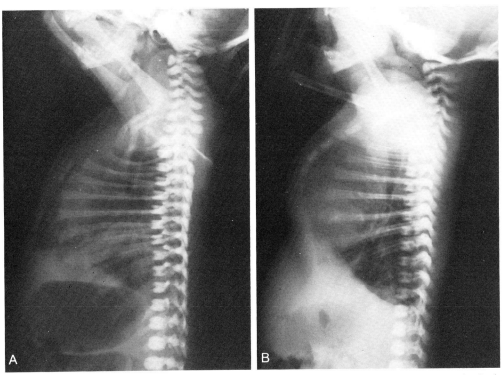

Figure 14–1. *A,* Radiograph of the entire spine of a normal infant girl being held up. Note incompletely formed vertebrae, very wide intervertebral disc spaces (fanlike), spreading of spinous processes, gross tipping of the atlas, and general sense of laxity and hypermobility. *B,* X-ray film of normal infant, showing very incompletely formed vertebrae, cervical spine kyphos with widely spread spinous processes, and visible scattered ossification centers. All bones vary widely in individual density, indicating the spectrum of developing cartilage template and bone.

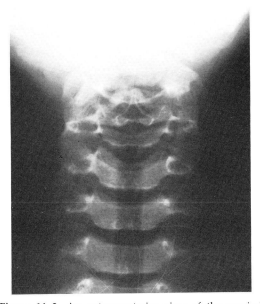

Figure 14–2. An anteroposterior view of the cervical spine in an 11-year-old boy. Note the relatively wide intervertebral discs, undeveloped uncinate processes (Luschka joints), marked slope of the upper facets of the axis, and lack of clear definition of joints.

each transverse process. The first and second cervical vertebrae are anatomically distinctive, differing from the other five vertebrae.

The atlas is normally formed from three primary ossification centers—one for each neural arch and one for the body. Variations in embryologic development are that (1) the bodies may arise from two centers that ultimately fuse with each other and with the neural arches; (2) an ossification center for the body may fail to appear, resulting in forward extension and fusion of the anterior portions of each neural arch; and (3) the ossification center for the body may be absent, and lateral masses may fail to fuse anteriorly, leaving a cleft (Fig. 14–3).

The ossification center for the vertebral body is normally not ossified at birth; it becomes visible only after the first year of life. Two neurocentral synchondroses (see Fig. 14–3) fuse at about the seventh year, and before this age, the fusion line can easily be mistaken for a fracture. Ligaments surrounding the superior vertebral notch are lax. The notch is not ossified in children and therefore is no problem—as it may be in adults. The normal atlanto-occipital joint is formed but does not appear ossified until age 2½ years. Also at about

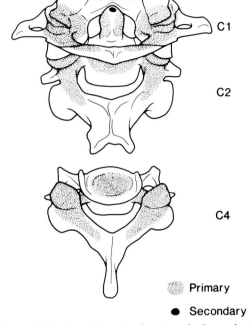

Primary

● **Secondary**

Figure 14–3. *Top,* Schematic drawing of atlas and axis with their ossification centers. Remember that the odontoid process is the "old" body of the atlas (phylogenetically) and that it has two ossification centers (one on each side). The odontoid process "shears out" of the atlas and unites below with the body of the axis to articulate with the anterior arch of the atlas. Dotted areas represent primary ossification centers, and the solid black areas are secondary centers. It is evident that the radiolucent areas between ossifying bone could appear as tears, shearing injuries, or fractures. Fusion of the centers (still incomplete bone) occurs between the ages of 3 and 6 years. *Bottom,* Schematic drawing of ossification centers of typical cervical vertebra (C3 to C7). The transverse process of C7, anterior or posterior, may persist as a separate process, become elongated, and present years later as a cervical rib.

age 2 years, the ossification of the primary center for the body of the atlas (the odontoid process) occurs later becoming firmly ossified to the body of the axis.

Second Cervical Vertebra, Axis

The complex developmental events in the axis make the differentiation of normal and abnormal changes difficult. There are four primary ossification centers in the axis, and all are present at birth. One is in the odontoid process, one in the body, and two are in the neural arches. Fusion of the centers occurs between the ages of 3 and 6 years, any of the synchondroses may be readily mistaken for a fracture, particularly the synchondrosis between the odontoid process and the body

of the axis (see Fig. 14–3). An ossification center at the summit of the odontoid process appears when the child is between the ages of 3 and 6 years and fuses with the odontoid process at the age of 12 years—also a source of interpretive error. A normal variant is that of two ossification centers in the odontoid process that have not fused at the midline. Fusion between the odontoid process and the body may also fail to occur. Likewise, the neural arches may fail to fuse, remaining unfused until about age 3.

Characteristics of Cervical Vertebrae C3 Through C7

The cervical vertebrae below C2 are very similar to each other, with the exception of C7, which has a long, strong, nonbifid spinous process. The vertebral artery and vein bypass the transverse process of C7, entering the transverse foramen of C6. The anterior part of the transverse process of C7 may persist as a separate process, becoming elongated and forming a cervical rib (see Fig. 14–3). In the lateral film, typical cervical bodies appear wedge-shaped, narrower anteriorly than posteriorly, with the degree of wedging decreasing with increasing age. Since laryngeal cartilage does not calcify in children, it does not block visualization of the child's spine in the anterior, posterior, and oblique projections. Figure 14–4 shows a characteristic lateral view of the cervical spine in a normal 5-year-old child (see also Fig. 14–5, p. 292).

BIRTH INJURIES

Neonatal trauma is unusual but does occur. Sherk et al[1] and Stern et al[2] studied spinal cords removed from neonates dying from obstetric trauma. They described pathologic changes over long segments of the cord, implying that longitudinal traction was the principal injuring force. In adults, cord injury occurs over a much shorter segment. The neonate's spinal cord is known to be less elastic than that of the adolescent or adult. Actual bony or skeletal trauma is very difficult to identify owing to the greater percentage of cartilage in the infantile spine. Radiologic assessment is difficult, if not impossible, particularly if the lesion is through cartilage or at a cartilage-bone interface.[3] Yates[4] emphasizes obstetric, traumatic injury to cervical cord, nerve roots, brain, and vertebral arteries, suggesting that vertebral artery trauma at birth may result later in cerebral palsy. The Yates study included dissection of 30 cervical spines randomly chosen from 78 stillbirths and 114 neonatal deaths. He reported extradural, dural, subdural, and subarachnoid hemorrhages as well as tears and hemorrhages in the nerve roots and the spinal ganglia. Spinal cord lesions were detected in two cases, cord contusion in one case, and bilateral necrosis of the bilateral columns in another. Nineteen cases showed evidence of hemorrhage around one or both vertebral arteries and crescentic adventitial hematomas or massive hemorrhage surrounding the vessel. Skeletal injury was not mentioned; nonetheless, such trauma had to have occurred to account for such extreme soft-tissue damage. The Yates study is very important and pertinent to clinical obstetric considerations.

Complete transection of the spinal cord can occur during a breech delivery, with consequent quadriplegia. Massive epidural hemorrhages have been reported in infants suffering birth trauma. Infants dropped, falling from a table or couch, or in auto crashes may sustain cervical spine injury along with frequently associated cerebral trauma. The increasing awareness of the battered child has brought cervical spine injuries into the open. The infant holding the neck rigidly should instantly alert the physician to cervical spine fracture, traumatic subluxation dislocation, or torticollis. A cautionary note: radiologic studies, very difficult in interpretation, may not show fracture, dislocation, or callus formation with partial healing.

Bresnam and Abrams[5] described and named the syndrome consequent to cervical hyperextension in utero—the "star gazing fetus." Breech presentation causes an approximate 25% cord transection in vaginal delivery. Cord transection does not occur in caesarean section.[5]

With increasingly occurring child abuse, the term "whiplash shaken infant syndrome" has arisen.[6] Violent shaking of a child whose weak cervical spine cannot even support the head results in intracranial and intraocular hemorrhages, latent cerebral injury, mental retardation, variable visual or hearing defects, fractures of the cervical spine, and spinal cord injury. Swischuck[6] reported that the incidence of spinal trauma is not as high as that of trauma in the extremities and skull. He described a cord injury in a 3-year-old girl caused by violent shaking—cervical fracture dislocation with apparent spontaneous reduction. Caffey[7] formulated the whiplash mechanism in severely shaken infants.

Presumably Painless Cervical Spine Disorders in Infancy

Cervical spine conditions and diseases in the adult are almost uniformly painful, whereas the infant presents with deformity, rarely pain, as a primary symptom.

Congenital Anomalies of the Cervical Spine

Chapter 15, *Congenital Anomalies*, deals with congenital disorders of the cervical spine in detail. Bony congenital anomalies develop during the first 6 to 7 weeks of early embryonic life. Congen-

ital anomalies of one organ system are usually associated with anomalies of others, such as clubfoot, cleft palate, harelip, and congenital cardiac and gastrointestinal lesions. Anomalies of the craniovertebral junction are likely to be associated with syringomyelia and intramedullary cavitation. Thirty per cent of patients with Klippel-Feil syndrome (fusion of the cervical vertebrae) have genitourinary tract anomaly. Such malformations are usually asymptomatic until adolescence or adulthood or even into middle age or early old age, when neurologic signs develop. The common congenital anomalies of infancy that may be recognized are basilar invagination or impression, dysplasia of the odontoid process, occipitalization of the atlas, fusion of the cervical vertebrae, and spinal dysraphism.

Basilar impression or invagination occurs when margins of the foramen magnum turn upward. Other anomalies of the atlas and axis are often associated. Clinical signs and symptoms include syringomyelia, with sensory loss to pain and temperature over the neck, shoulders, and upper extremities, and weakness and atrophy of the contralateral upper extremity. Radiologically, basilar invagination is identified as displacement of the lip of the foramen magnum above McGregor's line (see Chapter 6, *Radiologic Evaluation*, Chapter 7, *Craniometry and Roentgenometry of the Skull and Cervical Spine*, and Chapter 15, *Congenital Anomalies*). This congenital anomaly is asymptomatic and thus painless until later in life.

Dysplasia of the Odontoid Process and Atlanto-axial Instability. Malformation of the odontoid process may be congenital or associated with either Down's syndrome or the several forms of dwarfism. The odontoid process may be absent, aplastic, or simply hypermobile. Subluxation of the atlas on the axis is usual; torticollis may be a sign, but it generally appears later in childhood. Spinal cord compression may follow chronic and intermittent subluxation of the atlas on the axis, with consequent neurologic symptoms and signs. Flexion-extension radiograms and laminograms are required for proper diagnosis.

Occipitalization of the Atlas (Atlanto-occipital Fusion). The fusion of atlas to occiput varies from fusion all around to fusion of areas of contact. Basilar impression and odontoid dysplasia are often associated. Diagnosis cannot be made without carefully done laminograms and flexion-extension lateral view radiograms. There is no motion between the lateral masses of the atlas and the occiput (the atlanto-occipital joint). Neurologic symptoms are absent in neonates and infants but appear later during adolescence or late adult life. Fifty per cent of cases of occipitalization of the atlas are associated with fusion of the second and third cervical vertebrae also.

Fusion of Cervical Vertebrae. This lesion occurs in varying magnitude from as little as one block vertebra (two vertebra fused) to fusion of the entire cervical spine, a good example of failure of segmentation. The signs are short neck, low hairline, restricted neck movement, and a posture of the head similar to that seen in cases of torticollis. Radiologic study is required for precise diagnosis. The intervertebral disc spaces are either nonexistent or very narrow between the fused vertebrae, and anomalies of the central nervous system, such as meningomyelocele or Arnold-Chiari malformation, may be evident. Compensatory hypermobility of the unfused segments may lead to intervertebral disc disease (see Chapter 15, *Congenital Anomalies*, for details).

Spinal Dysraphism. This term describes failure of closure of the spinal canal, varying from simple, localized spina bifida to severe diastematomyelia, dermal cysts, and meningomyelocele. In the cervical spine, severe anomalies are usually fatal. Simple hairy nevus or radiologic but clinically insignificant bony changes may be seen.

See Chapter 2, *Anatomy and Biomechanics*; for a description of early embryologic development. See also Chapter 7, *Craniometry and Roentgenometry of the Skull and Cervical Spine*.

Congenital Torticollis. Torticollis, by definition, is a rotational deformity of the head and neck. Characteristically, the sternocleidomastoid muscle is contracted or at least spastic. The head tilts toward the side of the contracted muscle, and the chin is rotated in the opposite direction. There is a palpable, seemingly nontender, fibrous tissue mass in the middle part of the sternomastoid muscle, and growth there appears asymmetric, with striking changes caused by failure of development and hypertrophy and asymmetry of external facial features. Radiographic study is required to rule out other congenital bony anomalies of the cervical spine. This condition is potentially very serious and deforming and is discussed in more detail in Chapter 11, *Differential Diagnosis and Specific Treatment*.

Pseudosubluxation. Step formation, also termed step off or offset, along the posterior borders of the vertebral bodies in the flexed cervical spine is striking and evident in children. The greater mobility and offset is at the C2–C3 region. This phenomenon has frequently resulted in a diagnosis of subluxation or dislocation. The condition is now regarded as a normal variation called pseudosubluxation (Fig. 14–4).

All of these lesions may be quite asymptomatic during childhood, only to appear later in life (see Chapter 15, *Congenital Anomalies*).

THE NORMAL CHILD'S CERVICAL SPINE

In a study of 100 children, Bailey[8] examined the correlation of developmental anatomy of the cervical spine with the radiologic appearance. All subjects of the study were under 8 years of age.

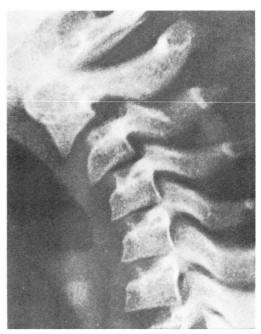

Figure 14–4. A normal 5-year-old's cervical spine in flexion. Note the seemingly gross subluxation of the axis on the C3 vertebra and, to lesser degree, of the atlas on the axis—a normal finding at this age, likely to be mistaken for a serious injury by individuals uninformed regarding the child's cervical spine.

He cited the difficulties of interpretation, the high frequency of anterior pseudosubluxation, and the step off seen in the majority of children in films taken in flexion, and he concluded that measuring portions of the cervical spine in normal children was not as useful clinically as paying careful attention to symmetry and normal anatomic development. Cattell and Filtzer[9] studied 160 randomly selected children who had no history or symptoms of neck injury or recent respiratory infection. Ten children representing each year of age from 1 to 16 were selected. The anterior displacement of the axis on C3 could not be measured, since there were no constant reference points in the young cervical spine. Differences in configuration, size, and the degree of ossification again made direct measurements of anterior displacement unreliable. Forty per cent of children under 8 years of age showed a clear tendency toward anterior displacement of both the atlas on the axis and the axis on C3. Thirty-two of seventy children under age 8 had posterior movement of the second cervical vertebra (axis) on C3. Two thirds of them had anterior displacement that was described as marked to moderate.

Among other normal findings were the following:

1. A measured distance of 5 mm or more between the odontoid process and the anterior arch of the atlas in flexion was regarded as pathologic.

2. In extension, the anterior arch of the atlas tended to ride up on top of the odontoid process, suggesting a threatened posterior subluxation.

3. In lateral radiograms of the neck in flexion, there was a consistent incidence of marked angulation at a single interspace in all groups studied. The degree of angulation was commonly so "severe" that with a history of trauma it would have been interpreted as injury to the interspinous or posterior longitudinal ligament. "Severe angulation was seen in 25 of the 160 subjects, 16%."

4. Absent lordosis in the neutral position was common.

5. In 25 (16%) of all flexion views, there was absence of the flexion curvature between C2 and C3—a normal variation that could be interpreted erroneously as splinting secondary to muscle spasm and trauma.

6. The basilar odontoid synchondrosis uniting the odontoid process with the body of the axis was a distinct radiolucent line in all children through the age of 3 years and present in 50% of those between the ages of 4 and 5 years. It was still visible in vestigial form in about one half of the subjects up to age 11. In the group from 5 to 11 years of age, the basilar odontoid plate was quite narrow and had sclerotic margins strikingly resembling an old fracture. Less commonly, it remained a single radiolucent line that again could be regarded erroneously as an undisplaced recent fracture.

7. The apical odontoid epiphysis was not seen with any reproducibility on lateral radiograms. It is thought to appear at age 2 and to unite with the odontoid process at about 12 years. In some children, this epiphysis was separated from the odontoid process by a narrow radiolucent line.

8. In the lower portions of the cervical spine, secondary centers of ossification of the spinous processes resembled avulsion fracture, and a secondary ossification center was demonstrated in one 16-year-old girl at the seventh cervical spinous process.

The variations described are reflections of four anatomic and physiologic characteristics of the immature skeleton: hypermobility, unique vertebral configuration, incomplete ossification, and the presence of synchondroses and epiphyses singly or in combination. Caffey[7] suggested that the anterior displacement could be a consequence of lack of development of the joints of Luschka in this age group; they do appear between ages 10 and 20 years. The hypermobility of atlas on axis and the wide separation of the anterior arch from the odontoid process are surely due to laxity of the anterior atlantoaxial ligaments, the check ligaments, and the transverse ligament of the axis. Incomplete ossification of the anterior arch, which begins in the first year of life, and incomplete ossification of the apical odontoid epiphysis contribute to this radiologic characteristic. These variations are easily mistaken for evidence of

ligamentous or bony injury and secondary subluxation of atlas on axis.

The basilar odontoid cartilaginous plate, closing usually at age 3, may persist beyond the age of 5 years in a vestigial form. Odontoid fractures often occur at this level, and the normal is readily confused with the abnormal. The interspinous, posterior, and anterior longitudinal ligaments and the ligamenta flava are surely lax in the children's age group, permitting marked angulation at a single intervertebral level and irregular as well as smooth subluxations in extension, with the irregular angulation being normal. The normal lordotic curve cannot be depended upon as clinical evidence of trauma. Secondary centers of ossification at the tips of the spinous processes seem not to be a diagnostic pitfall.

Since there is a tendency to rely on radiologic evidence of injury, we need to have a thorough knowledge of normal variation and to treat the patient symptomatically (in the presence of normal neurologic examination) and assess the initial response to treatment. *With the rapid disappearance of symptoms and persistence of the variation, a reasonable conclusion may be that the radiologic finding is normal for that child. However, patients with specific and persistent symptoms and signs—torticollis, limitation of motion, marked paraspinal muscle spasm—that are associated with a radiologic abnormality of marginal significance should receive treatment appropriate to the suspected diagnosis.* Surely fewer children will be overtreated for a neck injury, with the accompanying psychologic and economic consequences, if this procedure is followed. The more serious error of withholding treatment of a true fracture will also be avoided.

The stairstep appearance is characteristic for the flexed spine but not for the spine in a neutral position. However, if the patient is lying down and unconscious, the cervical spine sags, assuming a flexed position. Step formation in this circumstance at C2–C3, C3–C4, and even C4–C5 is normal. Furthermore, in torticollis in young adults in whom a cervical kyphosis is induced by severe reflex spasm of paraspinal muscles, the cervical spine in flexion can normally show the step appearance. Such may be the case in trivial injury of the neck, which is painful but not serious. The same is true in Grisel's syndrome, infection in and about the upper respiratory tract.

Cattell and Filtzer[9] cited variations in cervical spine curvature that resemble ligamentous injury—absence of uniform angulation between adjacent vertebrae and disappearance of the normal lordotic curve in the neutral position. Absence of a flexion curvature with normal step formation in the flexed position often leads to diagnostic errors and improper management. Juhl, Miller, and Roberts[10] noted that voluntary muscle contraction in normal children and young adults causes reversal or angulation of the cervical spine or both. Muscle spasm consequent to injury and pain in

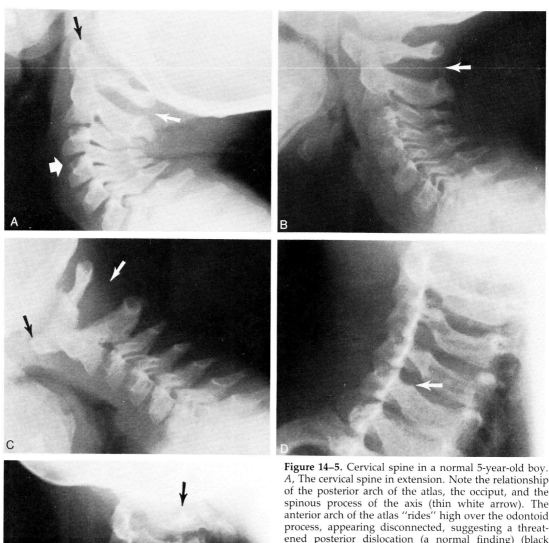

Figure 14–5. Cervical spine in a normal 5-year-old boy. *A,* The cervical spine in extension. Note the relationship of the posterior arch of the atlas, the occiput, and the spinous process of the axis (thin white arrow). The anterior arch of the atlas "rides" high over the odontoid process, appearing disconnected, suggesting a threatened posterior dislocation (a normal finding) (black arrow). Subaxial vertebrae subluxate dorsally on the vertebrae below. The vertebral bodies are incompletely formed, and the disc spaces are very wide (thick white arrow). Lastly, note the space between the anterior arch of the atlas and the pharynx. In flexion a gross bulging of the posterior pharynx becomes apparent as the atlas (normally) subluxates. *B,* Neutral position. Note the widening of spaces between the posterior arch of the atlas, the occiput, and the spinous process of the axis (arrow). Vertebral subluxations persist (normal). The atlas tips up and slides forward. *C,* Flexion. The atlas is grossly tipped, and anterior atlantoaxial subluxation has occurred (white arrow). The pharynx has bulged forward, pushed by the anterior arch of the atlas in its slide forward (black arrow). The atlas has now "settled" over the odontoid in a seemingly more anatomic position. Vertebrae now subluxate forward on the vertebrae below. Zygapophyseal joints are not fully formed, disc spaces are wide, and vertebrae are incompletely ossified. *D,* An anteroposterior view (partially oblique) to show absent (not yet developed) uncinate processes (arrow), wide intervertebral foramina, transverse processes, and zygapophyseal joints. *E,* Another anteroposterior (partially oblique) view to show the body of the axis (arrow) and the atlantoaxial joints (lateral masses).

the neck produces minor but impressive changes in the curves of the cervical spine. Such changes do not necessarily indicate weakening or rupture of ligamentous structures at the level of angulation.[11] In trauma cases, a diagnosis of rotational subluxation of the atlantoaxial joint has often been made on observation of deviation of the spinous process of C2 from the midline. Remember that in lateral flexion of the cervical spine, rotation in the atlantoaxial motor segment causes deviation of the spinous process of the axis to the side opposite to flexion. It is a normal physiologic, anatomic event. Arcual scoliosis (lateral scoliosis) is like simple lateral flexion (lateral bending), except that the head is held in the neutral position by a countermovement in the upper cervical spine. Thus, in arcual scoliosis, atlantoaxial rotation is normal, and in trauma cases, arcual scoliosis may be caused by unilateral muscle spasm in the area of injury.

Lateral subluxation of the atlas on the axis is a controversial subject in the literature. Brav[12] reported a patient who voluntarily could displace the atlas laterally on the axis, with apparent dislocation. He exploited this interesting phenomenon for financial gain. This "abduction" is not proof of traumatic change in the atlantoaxial region. Paul and Moir[13] noted lateral displacement of the atlas in normal subjects. Brocher[14] reported an asymmetric congenital implantation of the odontoid process in the body of the axis, simulating lateral subluxation of the atlas, clinically insignificant. Hohl[15] and Hohl and Baker[16] have clearly shown lateral atlantoaxial movement in normal subjects that is particularly exaggerated and evident in children. Such lateral displacement of the atlas on the axis has no certain diagnostic value. It should not seduce the pediatrician to a diagnosis of subluxation. In anatomic specimens at postmortem study, it is possible to produce all types of atlantoaxial offset, specifically, overriding of the lateral borders of the atlantoaxial joint as observed in AP views. Thus, it is theoretically possible to produce atlantoaxial offset in a normal subject, particularly in children. Figure 14–5 illustrates views of the cervical spine in a normal 5-year-old boy.

CERVICAL DISORDERS AND DISEASES IN CHILDHOOD AND ADOLESCENCE
Strain and Sprain

Cervical sprain occurs more commonly in the adult than in the child, as the supporting tissues of the adult are less elastic. Great mobility of the child's spine permits dissipation of forces over a larger number of segments. Sprain means microscopic tearing of tissues stretched beyond their elastic limit. The term rupture describes gross tear. Cervical soft-tissue trauma results from hyperflex-

ion, hyperextension, or over-rotation forces. The more severe the mechanical force, the more likely is the rupture of deep structures of high-tensile strength, such as anterior and posterior longitudinal ligaments, zygapophyseal joint capsules, and intervertebral discs.

A child injured by strain or sprain holds the head rigidly in one position, resisting movement by the examiner. Muscle spasm is prominent and readily palpable as hardened contractions of the posterior erector muscles of the spine. The patient prevents any effort to move the neck, particularly in flexion or extension. Pain is severe, becomes much worse on even slight movement, and is not referred (as occurs in cervical osteoarthritis in adults) to shoulder and scapular levels or to the upper extremity. Paresthesias are unusual but if they are present, it may be assumed that the brachial plexus is overstretched. Occipital headache is common. The child is usually neurologically intact. Pain and discomfort last days to weeks but generally disappear with rest, analgesic medication, and partial immobilization with collar. The epiphyseal plates of the axis-atlas-skull complex are vulnerable before fusion and may constitute a part of cervical sprain. Occasional shearing of the anterior apophyses of vertebrae occurs in hyperextension injury. Anteroposterior and lateral radiograms are useful, but one must keep in mind the wide range of normal findings.

In severe trauma, cartilage end plates may be sheared away from bony end plates. This cannot be diagnosed clinically but it may be a part of tentative clinicopathologic formulation. Any congenital abnormality, otherwise clinically insignificant, may predispose one to atlantoaxial dislocations in the case of trauma. Any injured child with apparent head injury and diminished level of consciousness requires cervical spine radiologic study to rule out fracture and dislocation.

The young child and adolescent are particularly prone to the consequences of trauma, which is usually related to auto crashes and sports injuries. The underlying mechanisms are the incompleteness of cervical spine growth; the immaturity of epiphyseal and apophyseal centers, with thickened cartilage end plates between the disc and the vertebral bodies; synchondroses; and the enormous mobility of the young cervical spine.

Torticollis

Acquired Torticollis. Relatively mild twisting or torsional trauma may cause torticollis in children. Rotatory subluxation of the atlas on the axis due to lax capsular ligaments in these joints is the etiology.[17] Clinically the head is tilted to the side of the subluxation, with the chin rotated in the opposite direction. This wryneck is associated with upper cervical spine pain that is usually quite disabling. Open-mouth, anteroposterior, and odontoid views and lateral radiograms demonstrate asymmetry of the atlantoaxial joints. The lateral masses of atlas and axis remain parallel, but the horizontal atlantoaxial joint spaces are asymmetric. Even slight tilt or rotation of the head on the neck causes change in the distance between the odontoid processes and the medial borders of the lateral masses. It is important to remember that this may be a normal variation.

Congenital Torticollis. Congenital torticollis, observed at or shortly after birth, may become progressive and much more intensely evident in later life. Most cases of childhood and adolescent torticollis are acquired. Torticollis may accompany an acute and severe upper respiratory infection, with consequent wryneck and acute cervical pain. The child may report a crepitant, snapping sound on suddenly turning the neck. Careful search for any seemingly mild or clinically unimportant congenital anomalies in the upper cervical spine is required. Children with tumors of the upper cervical cord or spinal canal or posterior fossa may present with acquired torticollis. Again, a careful search to rule out other possible diagnoses is always required.

Infections and Inflammation of the Cervical Spine

Grisel[18] described the phenomenon of atlantoaxial displacement that occurs in the absence of trauma and is due to chronic and acute inflammatory diseases of the neck and throat. Etiologies include upper respiratory and throat infections, tuberculosis, and rheumatoid arthritis. The pathophysiology is that of ligamentous laxity and softening, capsular distention, severe osteoporosis, and general loss of density of bony structures secondary to hyperemia and overall weakening of the fibro-osseous junction (enthesopathies).[19, 20] Torticollis may be secondary to a severe muscle spasm that holds the neck in flexion and aggravates the usual forward displacement of atlas on axis.

The clinical behavior is strange in that there is no perceivable relationship between the severity or intensity of the inflammatory process and the subluxation. The pathologic process may be primarily in the throat or due to drainage of the septic material into the lymph nodes of the throat from a remote focus. The clinical picture seemingly evolves following resolution of the original site, and the pain varies from a relatively mild degree to acute agony. Fortunately, the lesion heals following reduction and immobilization even if the causative inflammation continues, as in tuberculosis.[20] Clinical assessment is difficult because of the painful torticollis and rotatory atlantoaxial deformity. Radiograms are absolutely required. A true lateral view of C1–C2 is needed to measure the magnitude of anterior displacement of atlas on axis, and the open-mouth, anteroposterior view should be obtained.

It is probable that the route of entry is hematogenous, sometimes postsurgical, sometimes from contiguous infection, or possibly from some diagnostic procedure. Acute osteomyelitis is blood-borne, originating at distal sites. Dermatologic, pulmonary, and urinary tract infections may be the site of primary bacteremia. Bacteria in the blood stream may readily enter the very highly vascular cervical vertebrae. The most common organism in pyogenic osteomyelitis is *Staphylococcus aureus*, followed by *Streptococcus, Klebsiella* and *Pseudomonas* in that order of incidence. Tuberculous osteomyelitis generally arises from active pulmonary tuberculosis.

Clinically, the symptoms of pain and cervical rigidity precede any radiologic finding. Tenderness to posterior percussion of spinous processes is a useful diagnostic sign. Sometimes anterior palpation discloses an abscess. The neck pain is severe and constant, night and day; it improves somewhat when the patient is in a recumbent position. Radiation may occur to the occiput or the shoulders and rarely, down the arm. The child will support head in hands if the abscess is very painful, because that is the most comfortable position. If it has spread to the spinal canal with cord involvement, quadriplegia or upper extremity paralysis may occur, owing to gross anterior intraspinal pressure on the cord. The paralysis is upper motor neuron in type, with spasticity, hyperactive reflexes, positive Babinski's and Hoffman's signs, sustained clonus, and frequent inability to urinate. If it is a tuberculous infection, it may involve the vertebral body—central, anterior, or epiphyseal.

The osteoporosis occurs rapidly and is extreme, and the infectious process, if in bone, may involve the end plate and eventually break into the disc space. Vertebral collapse due to bone destruction results in a wedge-shaped vertebra, with increased density accompanying the marked decrease in density of the porosis.

An abscess may lie anterior to the posterior longitudinal ligament and protrude into the spinal canal, or it may even lie under the anterior longitudinal ligament or burst into the retroesophageal space. A paravertebral abscess rarely extends into the thorax. Reactive bone formation in pyogenic osteomyelitis produces radiologic evidence of sclerosis. The retroesophageal space in the lateral view may be 4 to 5 mm just anterior to the third cervical vertebra, along with bony destruction of the vertebral body and the more severe osteoporosis (see Chapter 7, *Craniometry and Roetgenometry of the Skull and Cervical Spine*). Tomograms are useful in delineating bone detail and differentiating the septic lesion from tumor. Cervical myelograms may be required in the case of paralysis to assess the level of the intraspinal abscess.

Tonsillitis, acute lymphadenitis, and dental abscesses may lead to retroesophageal sepsis unrelated to the vertebrae. An inhalation increases the space normally if the child is crying. The expected leukocytosis and septic fever of localized abscess increases mononuclear cells in tuberculosis and polymorphonuclear leukocytes in pyogenic infection. The sedimentation rate is elevated, and results of blood cultures are expected to be positive. Skin tests to identify tuberculosis or fungal infections are useful. The differentiation of osteomyelitis from tumor may be difficult, since gross destruction of bone is common to these diseases.

Management involves reduction by traction or cervical spine extension, followed by a halo brace or minerva jacket for 6 to 10 weeks. The diagnosis may be made eventually only by surgical drainage, cultures, and organism identification.

Juvenile Polyarthritis

Juvenile polyarthritis, occurring as early as age 1 year and as late as age 16 years, commonly involves the cervical spine. The lesions are more characteristic of ankylosing spondylitis than adult rheumatoid arthritis; however, atlantoaxial subluxation is common to both ankylosing spondylitis and juvenile polyarthritis. Monarticular arthritis or polyarthritis and cervical spine pain are clinical characteristics. In children, the sedimentation rate is elevated, but the rheumatoid factor is only rarely positive. A leukocyte count may be so high as to suggest leukemia (Still's disease). Bony ankylosis of the zygapophyseal joints, especially in the upper cervical spine, is common. Diminishing cervical spine motion occurs and is irreversible. Spontaneous fusion seems to occur posteriorly, becoming anterior as the years of disease go on. Physical examination of the cervical spine mobility and cervical spine radiograms are diagnostic in identifying fusion. Posterior facet joints are ossified, and the interspinous ligaments become so.

Ankylosing Spondylitis

Ankylosing spondylitis is far more likely to occur in late adolescence and early adulthood than in childhood. Nevertheless, it does occur. It is a progressive inflammatory disease of bone; the enthesopathy is the characteristic and primary lesion. Root joints are the main peripheral joints involved, and they also proceed to ankylosis, as occurs in the spine. Ninety-five per cent of patients with ankylosing spondylitis have the HLA-B27 antigen characteristic.

In any ankylosing spondylitic population in which all have the HLA-B27 antigen, there is no correlation between sex and incidence, though the female is far less intensely affected than the male. Vertebral segments become ossified and ankylosed, and ossification of the anterior and posterior longitudinal ligaments and multiple periarticular structures occurs. The erythrocyte sedimentation rate is elevated. Symptoms begin more commonly in the lower lumbar and sacroiliac regions, but the cervical pine may be the site of original symptomatology. Atlantoaxial subluxation and ligamentous laxity do occur despite the fundamental nature of the disease (ankylosing). The loss of motion is demonstrated clinically, and radiologic studies confirm the basic process. Disc spaces are not narrowed as occurs in characteristic osteoarthritis involving the intervertebral discs. Congenital fusion of the vertebrae (Klippel-Feil) syndrome, is readily differentiated from ankylosing spondylitis by the narrowing of vertebral bodies in the anteroposterior diameter, as seen on the lateral radiogram. Also, there is evidence of the very small discs never having really developed in the congenital defect.

Morquio's Disease, Spondyloepiphyseal Dysplasia, Diastrophic Dwarfism

These three dysplasias are occasionally associated with odontoid process dysplasia and atlantoaxial subluxation. Lower vertebral subluxations also occur. Morquio's disease is due to an autosomal recessive trait, resulting in excessive urinary excretion of keratosulfate. Corneal opacities and gross dental abnormalities are clinically evident. Vertebrae are strangely flattened, as seen on lateral radiograms, and the neck is short with a pectus chest deformity. Thoracolumbar kyphosis is also characteristic and is caused by upper lumbar wedging of the vertebrae. The most serious skeletal deformity is atlantoaxial subluxation due to odontoid hypoplasia and ligamentous laxity, with resultant cervical myelopathy. Neurologic deficit may occur slowly or rapidly, and stabilization attempts should be considered early.

Spondyloepiphyseal dysplasia manifests neither keratosulfate defect nor corneal opacities. There is platyspondylisis, flattened vertebrae.

These patients are neurologically intact grossly, but careful clinical study usually reveals leg weakness and muscle fatigue as the day goes on, secondary to early spinal cord compression. A separate or dysplastic odontoid process with atlantoaxial dislocation seen on flexion and extension views is diagnostic. Rarely, air myelography is the means of demonstrating spinal cord compression in the upper cervical spine. Tomograms with the child sedated are necessary.

Achondroplasia. Achondroplasia is a form of dwarfism characterized by short limbs. It is usually diagnosed at birth. It is transmitted as an autosomal dominant characteristic. There is seeming bulging of the forehead and relatively small face, with flattening of the bridge of the nose. The anteroposterior diameter of the spinal canal is narrow, leaving little space for the cervical cord. Even minor herniations of intervertebral disc can produce serious spinal cord compression. There is no compromise of intelligence, and there are no abnormal results of routine laboratory studies in this condition.

Tumors of the Cervical Spine

Both primary and metastatic bone tumors are extremely rare in childhood and adolescence. Tumors presenting with neck pain may be malignant or benign; the most common benign tumors are aneurysmal bone cysts, eosinophilic granuloma, osteochondroma, osteoblastoma, hemangioma, and histiocytosis. Diagnosis is usually made by radiologic techniques. Tomograms help in assessing the extent of tumor spread in the anterior and posterior elements of the vertebrae. Whether the tumor is osteoblastic or osteolytic is also radiologically determined. Ultimate diagnosis really requires open biopsy and histologic study. Rarely, primary cervical cord tumors present with neck pain both with and without paralysis. They may be extramedullary or intramedullary; onset of pain may be slow and insidious and without fever; abnormal gait and upper extremity pain may occur. These are all clues to the nature of the lesion. Very detailed neurologic examination is rewarding, and presence of clinical cervical myelopathy may define the lesion.

Specific Atlanto-Occipital Abnormality

Atlanto-occipital abnormalities are very unusual. When they do occur, the patient is likely to die immediately, owing to medullary cord compression and respiratory failure. Davis et al[21] noted that the atlanto-occipital junction is frequently grossly damaged in fatal craniospinal injuries in children; however, such lesions are identified post mortem in the presence of multiple other fatal traumata. Bohlman[22] described in a 14-year-old child an atlanto-occipital lesion not revealed by an angiogram that demonstrated vertebral artery stretching. Experimental investigation in primate animals shows that the head is catapulted forward, causing craniovertebral dislocation, but with immediate spontaneous reduction and thus normal radiologic findings. Autopsies of these experimental subjects disclosed rupture of the atlanto-occipital joints, spinal cord, and vertebral artery. Such injuries, rare though they are, should be reduced by traction, with ultimate atlanto-occipital fusion.

Specific Atlantoaxial Traumata[25]

The three most common abnormalities occurring in children are ligamentous laxity related to an inflammatory process (septic or nonspecific), odontoid epiphyseal separation, and traumatic ligamentous rupture.[26] In the atlantoaxial joints, odontoid process, and lateral masses, stability is dependent on ligaments that not only allow extensive motion but also protect the joint. Clearly, the

main motion is rotation, but extension, vertical stretch, and lateral slide also occur. Fifty per cent of cervical rotation occurs between the C1–C2 vertebrae around the eccentrically located, axle-like odontoid process. Hence, the lateral wall of the vertebral foramen of C1 rotates across the canal of C2, decreasing the opening of the spinal canal between the two segments (see Chapter 2, *Anatomy and Biomechanics*). The most spacious area of the cervical spinal canal is at C1, and it accommodates this rotation with no compromise. Steel[23] describes a "rule of thirds," that is, the spinal canal at C1 is occupied equally by spinal cord, odontoid process, and free space. The cord moves into the free space when C1 is displaced, hence forward displacement of the atlas on the axis beyond the anteroposterior thickness of the odontoid process puts that segment of the cord at risk to compression. The clinical point here is that trauma to this extremely mobile set of joints may damage the medulla oblongata. Injury to the respiratory center and other brain stem centers located in the medulla oblongata can lead to abrupt death. The vertebral arteries supplying the upper cervical cord, brain stem, and cerebellum are relatively fixed in the transverse foramina of C1 and C2 and can thus be stretched, pulled forward, and compressed by atlantoaxial shift, resulting in not only damage to spinal cord but also hemorrhage in varying degree from the vertebral artery branches, the anterior and posterior spinal artery, and any radicular arteries at that level or below.[24]

References

1. Sherk HH, Schaet L, Lane JM: Fractures and dislocations of the cervical spine in children. Orthop Clin North Am 7:593, 1976.
2. Stern WE, Rand RW: Birth injuries to the spinal cord: Report of 2 cases and review of the literature. Am J Obstet Gynecol 78:498, 1959.
3. Aufdermaur M: Spinal injuries in juvenile necropsy findings in twelve cases. J Bone Joint Surg 56B:513, 1971.
4. Yates PO: Birth trauma both vertebral arteries. Arch Dis Child 34:346, 1959.
5. Bresnam J, Abrams F: Neonatal cord transection secondary to intrauterine hyperextension of the neck in breech presentation. Fetal and Neonatal Med 84:734, 1979.
6. Swischuck LE: Spine and spinal cord trauma in the battered child syndrome. Radiology 92:733, 1969.
7. Caffey J: The whiplash shake infant syndrome. Pediatrics 54:396, 1974.
8. Bailey DK: The normal cervical spine in infants and children. Radiology 59:712, 1952.
9. Cattel HS, Filtzer DL: Pseudosubluxation and other normal variations in the cervical spine in children. J Bone Joint Surg 47A:1295, 1965.
10. Juhl HJ, Miller RM, Roberts GW: Roentgenographic variation in the normal cervical spine. Radiology 78:591, 1962.
11. Gaizler, G: Die Beurteilung der Ruhehaltung der H. W. S. Eine erledigte Frage? Fortschr Rontgenstr 103:566, 1965.
12. Brav EA: Voluntary dislocation of the neck, unilateral rotatory subluxation of the atlas. Am J Surg 32:144,

1964. (As cited by Hohl M, Baker HR: The atlanto-axial joint, roentgenographic and anatomical study of normal and abnormal motion. J Bone Joint Surg 46A:1739, 1964.)

13. Paul LW, Moir WM: Nonpathologic variations in the relationships of the upper cervical vertebrae. AJR 62:519, 1949.
14. Brocher JEW: Die occipito cervical Gegend. Stuttgart: Georg Thieme, 1955.
15. Hohl M: Normal motions of the cervical spine. J Bone Joint Surg 46A:1777, 1964.
16. Hohl M, Baker HR: The atlanto-axial joint, roentgenographic and anatomical study of normal and abnormal motion. J Bone Joint Surg 46A:1739, 1964.
17. El-Khoury GY, Clark CR, Bravett AW: Acute rotatory atlanto-axial dislocation in children. J Bone Joint Surg 66A:774, 1984.
18. Grisel P: Énucléation de l'atlas et torticollis nasopharyngien. Presse Med 38:50, 1930.
19. Watson-Jones R: Spontaneous hyperemic dislocation of the atlas. Proc R Soc Med 25:586, 1932.
20. Lippman RK: Arthropathy due to adjacent inflammation. J Bone Joint Surg 35A:4, 1953.
21. Davis D, Bohlman H, Walker AE, et al: The pathological findings in fatal cranio-spinal injuries. J Neurosurg 34:603, 1971.
22. Bohlman HH: Acute fractures and dislocation of the cervical spine. J Bone Joint Surg 61A:1119, 1979.
23. Steel HH: Anatomical and mechanical consideration of the atlanto-axial articulation. Proceedings of the American Orthopedic Association. J Bone Joint Surg 50A:1481, 1968.
24. Domisse GF: The Arteries and Veins of the Human Spinal Cord from Birth. New York: Churchill Livingstone, 1975.
25. Watson-Jones R: Fractures and Joint Injuries, vol 2, 4th ed. Baltimore: William & Wilkins Co, 1955.
26. Parke WW, Rothman RH, Brown MD: The pharyngovertebral veins. An anatomical rationale for Grisel's syndrome. J Bone Joint Surg 66A:568, 1984.

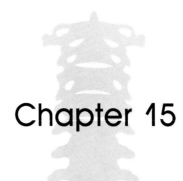

Chapter 15

Congenital Anomalies

Congenital defects of the cervical spine are common and vary from simple fusion of two vertebrae, discovered by chance radiogram and of no practical significance, to gross failures of development that are incompatible with life and clinically obvious. They may be single or multiple within the cervical spine and sometimes constitute only one of multiple congenital deformities affecting other systems. Many defects and deformities of the neck coexist, making classification difficult. Prompt radiologic study of the cervical spine is essential to ascertain available space for spinal cord or brain stem. Study of the rest of the body is also imperative, since many patients with congenital cervical spine anomalies may have congenital heart disease. Congenital heart disease is more common in patients with cervical spine congenital defects than in the general population.

Table 15–1 lists congenital bony anomalies of the cervical spine, and Table 15–2 lists congenital nervous system anomalies of the cervical spine. All can, and often do, coexist.

The upper portion of the cervical spine is transitional. Its development is unstable, causing many variants, anomalies, and malformations. The developmental errors are those of segmentation, aplasias, partial and complete dysplasias, and dysraphic lesions. Genetic transmission is increasingly identified as a major cause of many congenital anomalies, with environmental factors presumably responsible for the remainder. Relative genetic incidence versus environmental etiologies is indeterminate. It is estimated that 25% of developmental defects are genetic in origin, and the increasing sophistication of genetic studies will surely bring this percentage up.

The major susceptibility to teratogenesis occurs as the primitive germ layers differentiate into tissue systems and organs. In the neural axis, this occurs in the first 4 weeks of embryonic life. Environmental forces include drugs, irradiation, metabolic abnormalities, infections, and most probably the pollution of our environment.[1]

In order to understand congenital anomalies of the cervical spine, a brief review of the involved embryology is necessary.

EMBRYOLOGIC DEVELOPMENT

About the third week following fertilization, the notochord forms between the ectoderm and the endoderm. The ectoderm at the cephalic end of the embryo begins to thicken and differentiate into neuroectoderm, forming the neural plate. The

---

Table 15–1. CONGENITAL BONY ANOMALIES OF THE CERVICAL SPINE

Cranio-occipital Defects
  Occipital vertebrae
  Basilar impression
  Occipital dysplasias
  Condylar hypoplasia
  Assimilation of the atlas
Atlantoaxial Defects
  Aplasia of the arch of the atlas
  Aplasia of the odontoid process
  Variants of the above
Anomalies Below C2
  Primary failure of embryonic segmentation
    (Klippel-Feil syndrome and its variants)
  Failures of fusion
  Spina bifida
  Spondylolisthesis
  Cervical rib syndrome (scalenus syndrome)
Defects Associated with Multiple Congenital Deformities of Other Body Systems

---

Table 15–2. CONGENITAL NEUROLOGIC ANOMALIES OF THE CERVICAL SPINE

Arnold-Chiari malformations
Syringomyelia
Meningomyelocele (spina bifida)
Neurofibromatosis

neural plate then folds along its midline to shape the neural groove and the neural fold on each side (see Chapter 2, *Anatomy and Biomechanics*). Simultaneously, the loose aggregation of intraembryonic mesenchymal cells coalesces into three regions. The most medial is a solid mass, the paraxial mesoderm just lateral to the notochord and on either side of it. This mesoderm is the anlage of the somites that are to become myotome, sclerotome, and dermatome (muscle, bone, and skin). Toward the end of the third week, this undifferentiated mesoderm segments from a cephalic to a caudal direction. About the fourth or fifth week, a total of 42 to 44 somites is formed. There are 4 occipital, 8 cervical, 12 thoracic, 5 lumbar, 5 sacral, and 8 to 10 coccygeal somite pairs. Then each somite differentiates into its three parts, the ventromedial being the sclerotome programmed to form vertebral bodies. The bilateral, ventromedial cells migrate to the midline, surrounding the notochord. Each somite finally separates into a caudal and a cephalic portion, with the cells in the middle portion aggregating and condensing to become the intervertebral disc. The caudal half of one sclerotome unites with the cranial half of its neighbor, creating the earliest indication of a vertebral body.[2]

At this point, the second, third, and fourth somites follow this pattern, finally fusing to become the occipital bone and the posterior portion of the foramen magnum. The course of the first somite is still not well understood. At the cephalic end of the notochord, another mesenchymal cell collection condenses to become a plate-like mass between the notochord and the brain stem. This basal plate fuses with occipital somites and forms the basiocciput, which encircles the neural tube in the region of the foramen magnum (this occurs simultaneously with the somite division and the forming of vertebral bodies). The nervous system differentiation is proceeding in tandem with the cartilaginous skeleton. The neural plate assumes its tubular appearance at the end of the third week, and during the fourth week the neural folds forming the side walls begin to fuse in the midline to become the definitive neural tube. This occurs first in the region of the fourth and fifth somites, the location of the atlanto-occipital junction. The closure of the neural tube proceeds in a cephalad to caudad direction, closing its entire length by the end of the fourth week. Note here that both ends of the tube remain open.[3] The size of the neural tube is the determining factor in the diameter of the developing spinal canal.

In the fifth and sixth weeks, the cellular and tissue differentiation of the brain and spinal cord follow. The roof of the fourth ventricle develops, where the foramen of Magendie and the paired foramina of Luschka on either side will appear. They do not open until the seventh week, when a direct connection between the subarachnoid and the fourth ventricle is apparent.[3] Table 15–3 is a summary of developmental errors that can occur in the occipito-atlas-axis area.[4]

GENERAL CLINICAL SYMPTOMS AND SIGNS

The clinical symptoms and signs of congenital anomalies of the cervical spine are diverse and variable. There may be no signs or symptoms—or only minor ones—and some symptoms may arise only fairly late, that is, in the fourth to the fifth decade of life. Rarely, they may not allow survival for more than days or weeks after birth or may result in unexpected, abrupt death.

General and overall symptoms consist of pain in the occiput and neck, nonspecific dizziness, and true vertigo, often related to head movements; clinical signs as described in the literature depend on the specialty of the author. In one study by Deichmann,[5] signs and symptoms in decreasing frequency were as follows: pain in the occiput and neck, vertigo, unsteady gait, paresis of the limbs, paresthesia, speech disturbances, hoarseness, double vision, syncope, auditory noise, and dysphagia. A more general symptom that should attract attention is intermittent but

Table 15–3. PATTERN OF CONGENITAL ANOMALIES IN OCCIPITOCERVICAL REGION

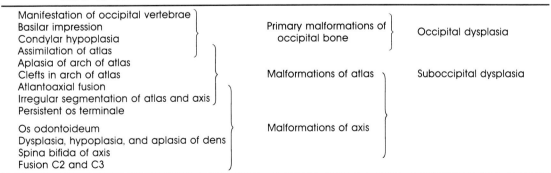

Manifestation of occipital vertebrae Basilar impression Condylar hypoplasia Assimilation of atlas	Primary malformations of occipital bone	Occipital dysplasia
Aplasia of arch of atlas Clefts in arch of atlas Atlantoaxial fusion Irregular segmentation of atlas and axis Persistent os terminale	Malformations of atlas	Suboccipital dysplasia
Os odontoideum Dysplasia, hypoplasia, and aplasia of dens Spina bifida of axis Fusion C2 and C3	Malformations of axis	

Adapted from Von Torklus D, Gehle W: The Upper Cervical Spine. New York: Grune & Stratton, 1972, p 21.

disabling neck stiffness, with no other specific diagnosis made.

One may suspect congenital anomaly if the patient has a very long or very short neck; a high or cleft palate; crooked teeth; or an asymmetric face, with peculiar formations of facial bones and muscles. Congenital anomaly of the cervical spine is also suggested in babies or children who are not well developed; a prominent or deformed mandible; a short, broad neck; a high scapula; an unusual head position; a hairline lying low on the neck; a deformed skull (tower or cone skull); or hydrocephalus. Also suggestive are kyphosis or scoliosis of the spine, dwarfism, funnel chest, pes cavus or equinovarus, partial syndactylism; localized gigantism, or malformations of the toes. Limitation of movement of the head is often striking but not specific.

It is puzzling and unexplained that symptoms may begin late and progress very slowly. Movement in the cervical spine is diminished with increasing age, and the congenital anomaly may be asymptomatic until cervical osteoarthritis becomes symptomatic.

Initial symptoms may appear following trauma or one of the rheumatic diseases involving the cervical spine, or they may appear at the menopause and, for poorly understood reasons, may become symptomatic during psychoneurotic or psychotic episodes. Malformations in the upper cervical spine become symptomatic owing to mechanical compression of nervous tissue, vascular disturbances involving the vertebral arteries, the posterior cervical sympathetic plexus, or occlusion of the venous or cerebrospinal fluid circulation, and the consequences of malalignment in the cervical spine.

Radiologic study is essential in the diagnosis of congenital anomalies of the cervical spine, and the earlier identification of the specific lesions is accomplished, the less likely are major complications to occur. Plain films of the upper cervical spine are difficult to interpret owing to the many overlying structures. Tomograms (both frontal and lateral projections) are often essential for adequate assessment. The goal of radiologic study is to determine the available space for the cord and the brain stem. Because this space varies with head position, dynamic studies may be required for proper evaluation. The cervical spine is examined in the lateral position in flexion, neutral position, and extension, with plain films and tomograms. Cineradiography or videotape recording may also be required if plain film studies are not diagnostic.

CONGENITAL ANOMALIES
Congenital Torticollis

Torticollis is a rotational deformity of the head and neck. The sternocleidomastoid muscle is spastic and shortened, with the head tilted toward the involved muscle and the chin rotated away to the opposite side. In the infant, there is a palpable fibrous tissue mass in the midportion of the affected muscle. As the patient grows older, growth asymmetry of the external facial features occurs. Early radiographic study is mandatory, and initiation of optimum management is best done on earliest identification.

Basilar Impression (Invagination)

Basilar impression, the most common congenital anomaly affecting the atlanto-occipital region, is an upward bulging of the margins of the foramen magnum, diminishing the volume of the posterior cranial fossa. If severe, the invagination can involve the petrous portions of the temporal bone. In plain lateral radiograms, it may be impossible to determine whether the anterior arch of the atlas is fused or separate from the base of the skull, or how much space there is available for the spinal cord.[6]

There is confusion regarding the terms basilar impression and platybasia. They are separate conditions (see Chapter 7, *Craniometry and Roentgenometry of the Skull and Cervical Spine*). Platybasia means an increase in the basal angle of the skull, determined by one line drawn along the plane of the sphenoid bone and another along the clivus on a lateral radiogram of the skull.[7] Platybasia is present when this angle exceeds 145 degrees. In 1939, Chamberlain[8] started this confusion in first describing Chamberlain's line, a line drawn between the posterior edge of the hard palate to the posterior lip of the foramen magnum. Chamberlain regarded basilar impression as present if the tip of the odontoid process was above this line. Other authors[9] have since considered intracranial projection of the odontoid process up to one third of its length to be within normal limits. McGregor's line is drawn from the upper surface of the posterior edge of the hard palate to the most caudal point of the occipital curve and is a commonly used measurement. Although the simultaneous occurrence of platybasia and basilar impression is possible, it is uncommon.

Acquired basilar impression, most commonly due to involvement by rheumatoid arthritis of the upper cervical spine, is consequent to the rheumatoid granuloma involving bone and joint, with softening and upward movement of the atlas, odontoid process, and axis into the foramen magnum. The measurements previously mentioned are very significant in assessment of acquired basilar impression, because the symptoms are due to the effects of pressure on the odontoid process. In the congenital variety, other anomalies are usually present, and it may not be possible to distinguish the primary reason for the symptom. When the anomaly presents at birth or in early

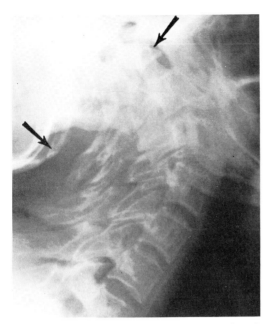

Figure 15–1. Severe basilar impression. Note the atlas and the odontoid process are in the foramen magnum, within the shadow of the skull. The posterior arrow points to the posterior arch of the atlas, the anterior arrow to the attenuated body of the axis.

childhood, there are likely to be cerebellar and brain stem signs. In the majority of patients, problems do not appear until the third to the fifth decade.[10] The Arnold-Chiari malformation and syringomyelia are common in basilar impression; less so is severe kyphoscoliosis.[11]

Clinical Picture. The symptoms and signs are consequent to neurologic structure involvement. Long tract symptoms, including all four extremities, are common, with consequent weakness with or without spasticity, depending on duration of symptoms. Sensory defects are frequent and variable, again depending on whether they arise from direct pressure on the cord or on a central spinal cord cavity, as in syringomyelia. Cerebellar ataxia and lower cranial nerve involvement may occur with dysarthria, dysphagia, nystagmus, and bizarre respiratory patterns due to respiratory center compression.[10] Altered states of consciousness and transient confusion are due to vertebral artery compromise and transient ischemia to the brain.

Management. Management requires surgical decompression, which is best done by laminectomy and suboccipital craniectomy, particularly if the Arnold-Chiari anomaly is present, with tonsillar herniation or a syrinx. Less commonly, the compression occurs anteriorly because the odontoid process occupies the foramen magnum. A transoral resection of the odontoid process is required.[12] Figure 15–1 illustrates severe basilar impression.

Occipitalization of the Atlas (Atlas Assimilation)

This lesion is a bony union between the skull and the atlas. Fusion usually occurs anteriorly between the anterior arch and the rim of the foramen magnum, with some segment of the posterior arch of the atlas present in most cases. This fragment can narrow the spinal canal, with intermittent symptoms depending on head position. Abnormal position or size of the odontoid process is usual, particularly if there are neurologic signs. The odontoid process may compress and indent the medulla oblongata. Posterior displacement of the odontoid process from the complex of the anterior foramen magnum and anterior arch is also common and may occur with no clinical findings, depending on the size of the canal at the foramen magnum level.

Other skeletal abnormalities are usual, particularly fusion of the second and third cervical vertebrae and hemivertebrae. Involvement at lower levels is less common. These fusions may represent a Klippel-Feil malformation though many such patients do not have the short neck and low hairline typical of this anomaly. Figure 15–2 is an excellent example of occipitalization of the atlas.

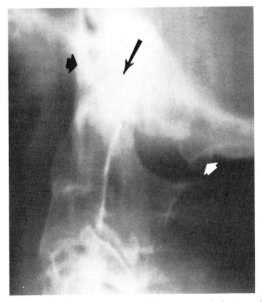

Figure 15–2. Occipitalization of the atlas, with fusion of the anterior arch to the anterior lip of the foramen magnum. The second and third cervical vertebrae are fused, and the fourth cervical vertebra is a hemivertebra. The odontoid process occupies the foramen magnum. The thin black arrow points to the odontoid process, the left one to the anterior arch of the atlas, and the white arrow to the posterior arch. The patient is a 56-year-old male with occipital headache of 2 years duration and severe neck stiffness. He has a short, asymmetric neck, a low hairline, and marked limitation of motion of the head and neck.

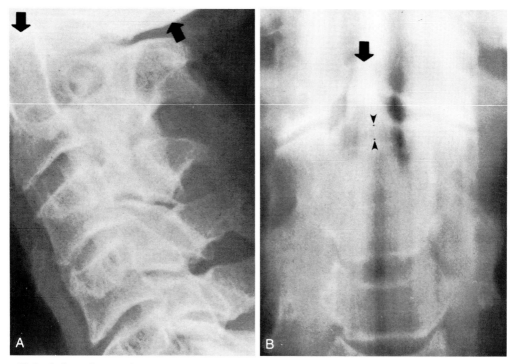

Figure 15–3. *A*, Lateral view of the cervical spine showing assimilation of the atlas. Note the posterior arch of the atlas is not visible and is fused to the occipital bone. Anterior fusion of the arch of the atlas to the foramen magnum was also present (not shown). The odontoid process projects well above Chamberlain's line, and there is invagination (basilar impression) of the posterior fossa into the normal cranial cavity. The right arrow points to the occiput, and the superior arrow to the odontoid process. *B*, Anteroposterior view showing a separate odontoid process of abnormal shape and size (upper arrow). Between the arrowheads is the separated (probably cartilaginous) area between the body of the axis and the odontoid process.

Clinical Picture. The majority of patients have signs or are symptomatic, though this is not necessarily the case. Clinical identification is usually confusing, with ataxia of the extremities, paresthesias, and limb pain, long tract signs, hyper-reflexia, positive Babinski's sign, weakness, and spasticity. Neck pain is usually present, as is a peculiar head posture.

Intracranial manifestations are headache, visual symptoms and signs, tinnitus, and lower cranial nerve pressure phenomena causing dysphagia and dysarthria. Horner's syndrome is unusual but has been reported. Downbeat nystagmus is common. Multiple sclerosis is a frequent mistaken diagnosis. Myelography is the definitive study to outline cord and brain stem, and computed tomography scanning techniques increasingly allow precise diagnosis.

Management. Upper cervical laminectomy and suboccipital craniectomy are done if compression is actively present posteriorly, with consequent anterior compression of the cord and brain stem. The transoral, surgical approach is to remove the odontoid process and the rim of the foramen magnum. Figure 15–3 depicts assimilation of the atlas, a separate odontoid process, and basilar impression.

Separate Odontoid Process

Agenesis or hypoplasia of the odontoid process implies failure of development. This may be recognizable at birth. In the case of multiple anomalies, usual radiographs are not reliable in identifying the presence or absence of the odontoid process. Os odontoideum implies a joint-like articulation between the odontoid and the body of the axis that suggests a wide radiolucent band. It may be associated with certain forms of dwarfism as well as Down's syndrome. Dislocation of the atlas on the axis anteriorly is the usual event. An infant may have torticollis as well. Spinal cord compressive syndromes with neurologic symptoms is the common clinical presentation. Odontoid abnormalities are more common in males than in females, but total absence of the odontoid process is quite rare.

Axis embryology is complex, because the axis is derived from three separate sclerotomes. The body and the arches of C2 are derived from the second cervical sclerotome, and the base of the odontoid process as well as the axis derives from the first cervical sclerotome. The apex of the odontoid process arises from the fourth occipital sclerotome. The occipital sclerotome also gives rise to the proatlas, which becomes a separate vertebra in reptiles. In man, it normally forms a portion of the occipital bone. Thus, the mechanism of failure of development, partial development, or a separate odontoid bone is caused by failure of normal embryologic events.

Clinical Picture. The clinical presentation of abnormalities of the odontoid is dependent upon whether there is spinal cord compression from the dislocation or whether multiple congenital anomalies in addition to the odontoid defect occur. Limitation of neck movement and the clinical reflections of spinal cord damage usually occur.

Management. Congenital anomalies of the odontoid process result in a precarious existence. A minor injury may be catastrophic. Transient myelopathy may occur. Optimum management remains controversial. The question of prophylactic atlantoaxial stabilization is unsettled, particularly in patients who have complete resolution of symptoms or in an asymptomatic patient whose diagnosis was made on routine radiologic examination.

Surgical therapy is associated with a high mortality rate and an increase in the neurologic clinical picture. The patient should avoid any and all activities that may cause trauma to the head and neck. Some feel such restrictions are unrealistic and impractical and propose that all patients with either absent odontoid process or os odontoideum should have elective stabilization. If there is neurologic involvement (even transient), surgical stabilization by posterior cervical fusion of C1 and C2, with wire fixation and an iliac bone graft, is clearly indicated. Figure 15–4 illustrates an os odontoideum, an ununited odontoid bone, and also platybasia. Incidentally, an arcuate foramen is readily seen. Figures 15–5 and 15–6 are further examples of congenital absence of the odontoid bone.

Klippel-Feil Syndrome

Use of the term Klippel-Feil syndrome is variable, but the words generally refer to any congenital fusion of the cervical spine. Whether the lesion is a fusion or a primary failure of segmentation is still under dispute. The lesion is present at birth, but the radiographic findings may be progressive. The original description was that of a short neck, low posterior hairline, and gross limitation of movement of the head and neck. It is usually painless. The anomaly has been seen in gorillas. Both sexes are affected equally. The severity of involvement is highly variable. There are three types described:[13] (1) Vertebrae massively fused into blocks, giving the patient a grossly abnormal appearance and severe disability in childhood; this type is often associated with other anomalies of other portions of the body. (2) Fusions involving

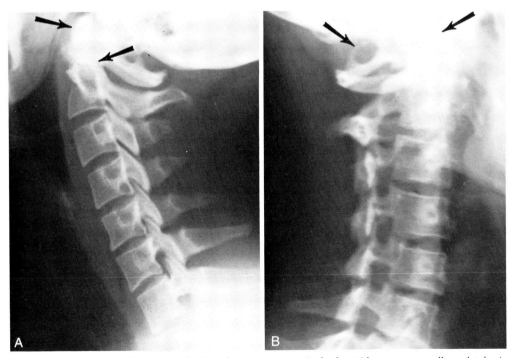

Figure 15–4. *A,* Lateral view of the cervical spine showing an ununited odontoid process as well as platybasia. The small, mobile odontoid process has slipped posteriorly (lower arrow), and the upper arrow (left) points to the anterior arch of the atlas. *B,* An oblique view showing the small ununited odontoid process in the shadow of the skull (right arrow). The arcuate foramen is in obvious profile (left arrow).

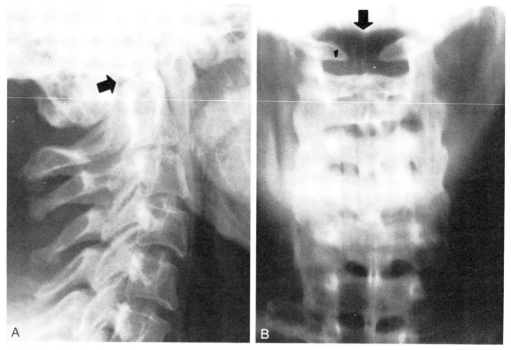

Figure 15–5. *A,* Lateral view of the cervical spine showing the absence of the odontoid process (arrow). The mastoid process overlies the posterior arch of the atlas. There is basilar impression. The styloid process is visualized just anterior to the body of the axis. *B,* An anteroposterior view of the same patient. The absence of the odontoid process is evident. Arrow points to the empty space and an open posterior arch of the atlas.

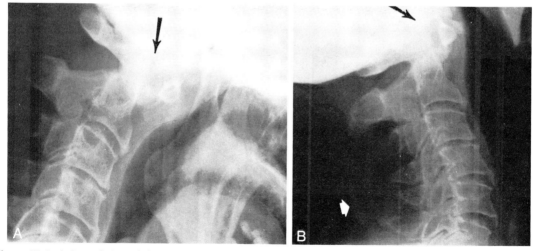

Figure 15–6. *A,* Lateral view of the cervical spine, with a massive dislocation of the atlas and skull on the axis in the absence of the normally restraining odontoid process and transverse ligament (arrow). Note the bulge of the pharynx caused by the pressure of the anterior arch of the atlas. The atlas itself has tipped severely, and clinically there were signs and symptoms of spinal cord compression. *B,* Cervical spine of same patient, with partial reduction of the subluxation on extension of the spine (black arrow). Note the incidental dense calcification of the nuchal ligament (white arrow).

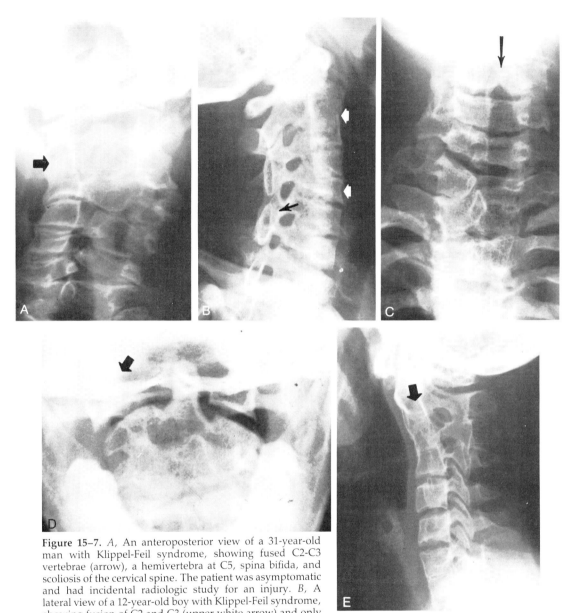

Figure 15–7. *A,* An anteroposterior view of a 31-year-old man with Klippel-Feil syndrome, showing fused C2-C3 vertebrae (arrow), a hemivertebra at C5, spina bifida, and scoliosis of the cervical spine. The patient was asymptomatic and had incidental radiologic study for an injury. *B,* A lateral view of a 12-year-old boy with Klippel-Feil syndrome, showing fusion of C2 and C3 (upper white arrow) and only partial fusion with poorly developed disc spaces at C3–C4, C4–C5, and C6–C7. A hemivertebra is seen at C5 (lower white arrow). The zygapophyseal joint is fused at C3–C4 and C5–C6 (black arrow). *C,* An anteroposterior view of *B,* showing a butterfly vertebra (C3 and C4, arrow), hemivertebrae (C7–T1), and T2 and spina bifida, seen just above level of first rib. In other views there is a surprising amount of remodeling and osteophytosis. *D,* Open-mouth view of *B,* showing deviation of the odontoid process to the right caused by having two sets of posterior elements in the left (arrow) and only one on the right. *E,* Lateral view of the cervical spine of a 15-year-old girl with Klippel-Feil syndrome, showing fusion of the C2–C3–C4 vertebrae (arrow), with a kyphotic deformity of the cervical spine. Fusion also occurred at C7 through T3, and a hemivertebra was seen at C7. The neck was not short, and there was no evidence of basilar impression or occipitalization of the atlas. The patient was asymptomatic.

only one or two interspaces; the patient is usually normal in appearance and is asymptomatic until later in life because the fusions are discovered incidentally in radiographs taken for trauma. (3) Deformity including cervical fusion, with coexisting fusion in or segmental failure in the lumbar or thoracic spine. These characteristics are inherited as an autosomal dominant trait.

Clinical Picture. The triad of short neck, low hairline, and limited range of neck motion occurs in only 50% of patients, many of whom have a normal appearance. Associated clinical findings may be facial asymmetry, torticollis, and webbing of the neck. Thus, limitation of neck motion is the most consistent and constant clinical manifestation. Examine all planes of motion—flexion, extension, lateral flexion, and rotation—paying particular attention to the atlantoaxial joint. Occasionally Sprengel's deformity and scoliosis are associated with Klippel-Feil syndrome. The radiologic findings include the pattern of congenital,

cervical, and vertebral fusion, with frequent coexistent occipitalization of the atlas; and instability of the atlantoaxial joint may be present. The lateral radiograph of a very young child may appear normal until ossification develops to disclose the congenital changes. Rudimentary disc spaces may be noted, and the vertebrae may appear smaller in width, suggesting a "wasp waist" appearance. The spinal canal is usually normal in width, and if it is enlarged, syringomyelia, hydromyelia, or Arnold-Chiari anomaly should be ruled out. Forty-five per cent of patients with Klippel-Feil syndrome have spina bifida occulta.

Associated congenital lesions may be cleft lip, cleft palate, high arched palate, ocular ptosis, coloboma, ocular muscle palsies, and deafness.

Management. Usually no treatment is necessary, but serial reassessment, with repeated radiographic study is needed. Physical therapy may be useful, and the maintenance of maximal range of motion is essential. With maturing and growth,

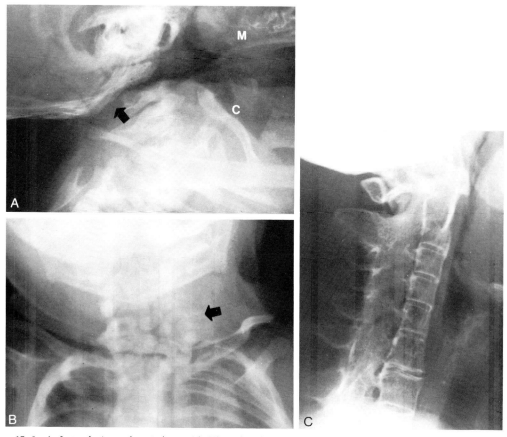

Figure 15–8. *A,* Lateral view of an infant with Klippel-Feil syndrome. The neck is scarcely visible. **M** marks the mandible, **C** the clavicle, and the arrow points to the space between the occiput and the thorax. The neck was very short. *B,* The anteroposterior view of *A,* showing the disrupted anatomy of the cervical spine. The child also had Arnold-Chiari syndrome and died. This is an example of the inability to diagnose a fusion of the spine in infancy. *C,* Lateral view of the spine of a 16-year-old girl with total, congenital fusion of the cervical spine, discs, and zygapophyseal joints. The disc spaces, however, are preserved. Clinically there was no motion of the neck, but the patient was otherwise well.

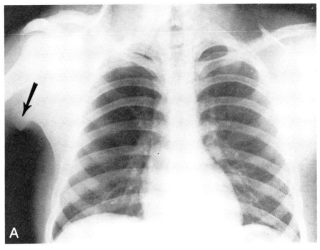

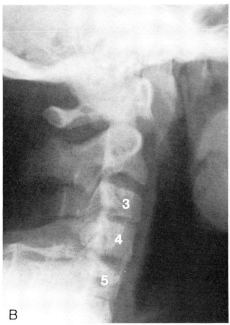

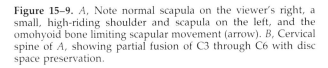

Figure 15–9. *A,* Note normal scapula on the viewer's right, a small, high-riding shoulder and scapula on the left, and the omohyoid bone limiting scapular movement (arrow). *B,* Cervical spine of *A,* showing partial fusion of C3 through C6 with disc space preservation.

the patient with Klippel-Feil syndrome should be assessed for intersegmental instability of the cervical spine, cervical osteoarthritis, and the development of radiculopathy or myelopathy. Pain syndromes may appear and may require surgical stabilization.

Cosmetic management has not been successful, and efforts to realign the cervical spine have usually failed and are sometimes associated with neurologic catastrophe. Bracing of the torticollis is not used extensively. If Sprengel's deformity is present, its correction may be useful. Figure 15–7 provides examples of the many manifestations of the Klippel-Feil syndrome. Figure 15–8 provides further examples.

Sprengel's Deformity (Undescended Scapula)

Sprengel's deformity is presented here because it is frequently associated with the Klippel-Feil syndrome. In Sprengel's deformity, the scapula remains small because it fails to descend. It is sometimes attached to the cervical spine by the omohyoid bone. The child has a small, palpable scapula, with an abnormal contour of the neck and limited abduction of the shoulder on the affected side. Radiographs show the abnormal position and shape of the scapula, disclosing an attachment to the cervical spine by the omohyoid bone. This anomaly results from failure of embryologic descent of the shoulder girdle.

Sprengel's deformity is of more cosmetic than functional concern, although the range of motion

of the shoulder may be significantly compromised. At 30 days, the mesodermal scapula is at the C4 level, and by 42 days it descends to a level below the first rib. The timing of scapular descent coincides with the most critical period in the development of the Klippel-Feil anomaly. Figure 15–9 shows films of a 13-year-old boy with Sprengel's deformity and elements of the Klippel-Feil syndrome.

Cervical Ribs

Anomalous ribs have been noted in both the lumbar and the cervical regions. Their size is variable, from tiny ossicles or even cartilaginous structures to fully formed ribs. The ribs have the same embryologic origin as the costal processes of the cervical vertebrae, from which they require differentiation. The costal processes have separate ossification centers anterior to the transverse process. They fuse with the remainder of the transverse process at about age 10. The costal processes may be just below the remainder of the transverse process, mimicking a cervical rib. Differentiation from cervical ribs can be made by assessing the course of the bone. Cervical ribs point downwards. They may be fused to the first rib or appear asymmetrical.

Most cervical ribs are probably asymptomatic. They may, of course, produce thoracic outlet syndromes by compression of the brachial plexus or the subclavian artery and vein. Symptoms include neck pain or pain along the part of the brachial plexus involved, or there may be evidence of vascular occlusion, venous or arterial. Paresthesia

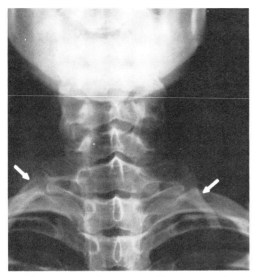

Figure 15–10. Film of a 36-year-old woman with pain, numbness, and tingling of the left hand and arm in the ulnar distribution. The arrows point to the well-developed cervical ribs at the C7 level. She was successfully treated conservatively.

and pain in the ulnar distribution are common manifestations. One can sometimes palpate the extra rib in the supraclavicular fossa at the base of the neck. Adson's sign is positive, with reproduction of the symptoms (see Chapter 4, *Clinical Methods*). Figure 15–10 shows a 36-year-old

woman with pain, numbness, and tingling in the ulnar distribution of her left arm. The well-developed cervical ribs are noted by the arrows. Figure 15–11 is an anteroposterior view of the cervical spine of a 21-year-old man, whose bilateral cervical ribs became symptomatic after an auto accident resulting in neck injury and reversal of the lordotic curve caused by severe muscle spasm. Figure 15–12 illustrates a rather large but asymptomatic cervical rib that was incidentally discovered in a 32-year-old woman.

The management of cervical rib syndromes is primarily that of education of the patient, specific exercises designed to lessen the compressive effect of a cervical rib, shrugging exercises, maintaining proper posture while sitting, walking, and running, occasionally bracing the shoulders, and putting the shoulders in an exaggerated military posture. Removal of the cervical rib is a simple procedure that is not frequently indicated because these congenital anomalies are usually asymptomatic.

Miscellaneous Congenital Anomalies of the Cervical Spine

1. *Synostosis of C5–C6, with preservation of small disc space.* Figure 15–13 illustrates a synostosis of C5–C6. Note the decreased size of the vertebrae, small osteophytes, and a small, contracted intervertebral disc space. This lesion was asymptomatic and was discovered incidentally in a cervical spine radiograph that was obtained for other reasons.

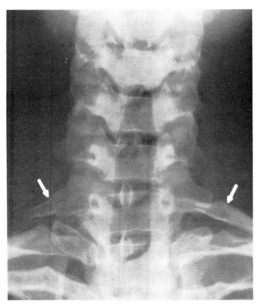

Figure 15–11. Anteroposterior view of the cervical spine of a 21-year-old man whose incidentally discovered cervical ribs became typically symptomatic after an automobile accident resulting in a neck injury (arrows).

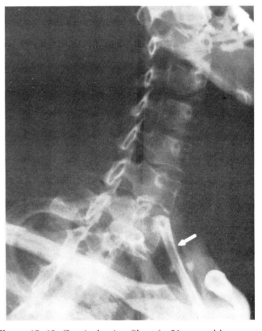

Figure 15–12. Cervical spine film of a 31-year-old woman showing a large asymptomatic cervical rib (arrow).

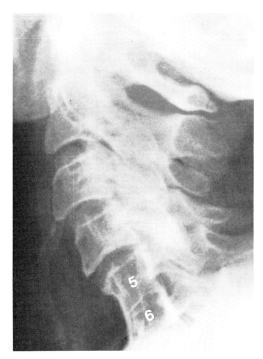

Figure 15–13. Synostosis of C5–C6 in a 52-year-old woman.

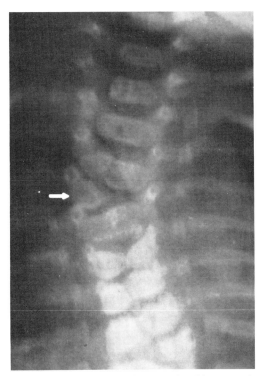

Figure 15–14. At the T4 level is an isolated hemivertebra in an infant. These may be seen in the cervical spine and are of little clinical consequence. A kyphoscoliosis may develop with growth. It is caused by lack or only partial fusion of the right and left halves of the vertebral bodies.

2. *Anomalous hemivertebra in an infant* (Fig. 15–14).

3. *Isolated cystic lesion of the right transverse process of C7* (Fig. 15–15).

4. *Neurofibromatosis with secondary changes in the cervical spine.* Figure 15–16 is the cervical spine of a 55-year-old man with neurofibromatosis. The lesion principally involved C5 and C6, with vertebral collapse and subluxation. A cervical spine fusion was done utilizing bone grafts, as is apparent in part *B* of the figure.

5. Figure 15–17 illustrates a congenital calcification in the C7–T1 intervertebral disc, resulting in left scapular pain and dysphagia.

Arnold-Chiari Anomaly

The Arnold-Chiari anomaly occurs in conjunction with most of the other congenital malformations of the upper cervical spine. Cleland[14] first appreciated the pathologic anatomy of the lesion, and Chiari[15] advanced the knowledge and formulated it into a more clinically recognized syndrome. In 1894, Arnold[16] published a subsequent definitive paper. The best modern review of the subject is by Bloch et al.[17] The most severe form of Arnold-Chiari anomaly is the infantile presentation. Hydrocephalus, spina bifida, and myelomeningocele are usually present. The adult syndrome lacks these features, representing a less severe form of the malformation. Many patients do not become clinically symptomatic until the third to the fifth decade. Basilar impression, atlanto-occipital fusion, Klippel-Feil syndrome, and spina bifida occulta are common accompaniments (most common however is syringomyelia or hydromyelia).

A point of great clinical importance in the Arnold-Chiari malformation is that since some lesions are not clinically manifest until adult life, they are easily misdiagnosed as an acquired progressive neurologic disease. They can present with early symptoms and signs, suggesting lower cervical spine disease, and be mistaken for spinal cord and brachial root lesions due to cervical osteoarthritis. Cerebellar tonsillar prolapse may persist asymptomatically or develop symptomatic manifestations when cervical osteoarthritis with its additional compressive forces bring the Arnold-Chiari lesions to light. The degree of caudal displacement ranges from simple prolapse of the cerebellar tonsils into the spinal canal to displacement of the brain stem such that the fourth ventricle extends through the foramen magnum. There may be herniation of the cerebellum into a cervical meningeal encephalocele.

Clinically, most patients present with headache, limb pain, ataxia, and evidence of sensory loss. About two thirds have clinical signs of cerebellar, brain stem, and high cervical spinal cord compression. Such patients are not commonly seen in orthopedic or rheumatologic clinics. About one half of the patients can be diagnosed by standard

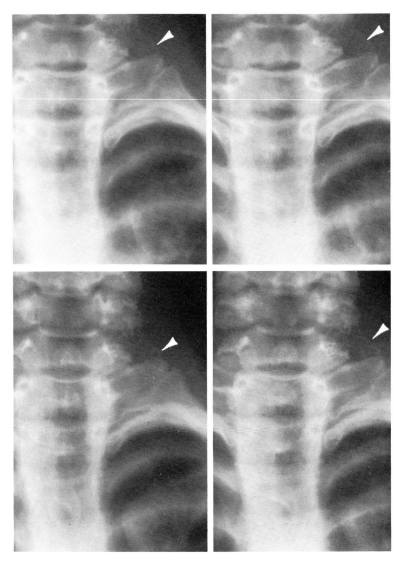

Figure 15–15. Tomograms (lower left to upper left) showing an isolated, large cystic lesion of the transverse process of C7, an incidental finding in an asymptomatic 24-year-old woman. Ten years follow-up has disclosed no clinical developments. (See arrows.)

radiographic study in demonstrating some craniovertebral abnormalities, such as basilar impression, leading to the suspicion of Arnold-Chiari syndrome.

Clinical Picture. The clinical picture in children is dominated by hydrocephalus and myelomeningocele, which overshadow spinal cord compression and abnormalities of the craniovertebral junction. If brain stem compression predominates secondary to severe tonsillar and fourth ventricle herniation into the cervical canal, lower cranial nerve symptoms and signs appear—dysarthria, dysphagia, and dysphonia.

In adults, the clinical picture develops much more slowly, and spinal cord abnormalities are accentuated. Hydrocephalus is rare. Unfortunately, many patients are initially diagnosed as having chronic osteoarthritis. An early symptom is loss of pain sensation in the cervical dermatomes due to central cavitation of the spinal cord. This is followed by atrophy and weakness of the upper extremities as the cavity extends into the anterior horn cell area, resulting in a central spinal cord syndrome. Foramen magnum compression, cerebellar ataxia, nystagmus, and lower cranial nerve abnormalities follow. Headaches are the rule when normal circulation of spinal fluid is compromised by medullary impaction; cerebellar tonsils and, sometimes, the vermis herniate into the foramen magnum and cervical canal.

Management. Management is surgical and highly individualized. Laminectomy to below the level of the tonsillar herniation and opening of the foramen magnum may be done in adults. In children, a myelomeningocele is repaired, and if hydrocephalus is present, a shunting procedure is required. The management is clearly neurosurgical.

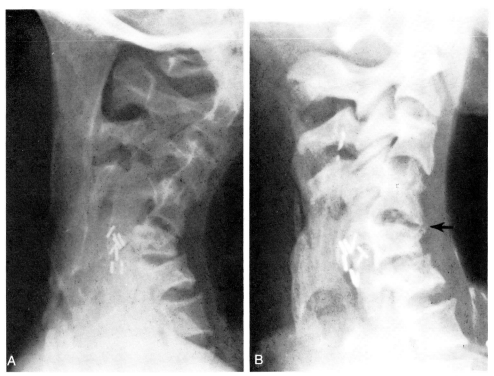

Figure 15–16. *A,* A lateral cervical spine film in a 54-year-old man with neurofibromatosis. The bony lesion involves C5 and C6 and causes vertebral collapse and subluxation. *B,* Patient shown in *A,* 8 years after bone graft and successful cervical spinal fusion. Lateral view of the cervical spine shows the vertebral lesion and the heavy overgrowth of bone graft stabilizing the cervical spine (arrow).

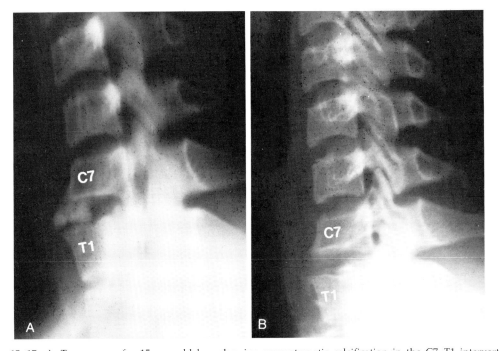

Figure 15–17. *A,* Tomogram of a 15-year-old boy showing asymptomatic calcification in the C7–T1 intervertebral disc. *B,* Lateral cervical spine film done postoperatively. The lesion was surgically removed and proved to be an embryonic "rest" containing bone, hyaline cartilage, fibrocartilage, and amorphous calcification. Cure followed surgical removal.

References

1. Wynn-Davis R: A review of genetics in orthopaedics. Acta Orthop Scand 46:338, 1975.
2. Truex RD, Johnson CH: Congenital anomalies of the upper cervical spine. Orthop Clin North Am 9:891, 1978.
3. Thomas JB: Introduction to Human Embryology. Philadelphia: Lea & Febiger, 1968, Chapters 9, 10, 13.
4. Von Torklus D, Gehle W: The Upper Cervical Spine. New York: Grune & Stratton, 1972, p 21.
5. Deichmann H: Chronisch zervicale Myelopathie. Deutsch Med Wochsch 92:1821, 1967.
6. Hinck VC, Hopkins CE, Savara BS: Diagnostic criteria of basilar impression. Radiology 76:572, 1961.
7. McRae DL, Barnum AS: Occipitalization of the atlas. AJR 70:23, 1953.
8. Chamberlain WE: Basilar impression (platybasia): A bizarre developmental anomaly of the occipital bone and upper cervical spine with striking and misleading neurological signs. Yale J Biol Med 11:487, 1939.
9. Taveras JM, Wood EH: Diagnostic Radiology. Baltimore: Williams & Wilkins Co, 1964, pp 64–66.
10. Scoville WB, Sherman IJ: Platybasia: Report of 10 cases. Ann Surg 133:496, 1951.
11. Spillane JD, Pallis C, Jones AM: Developmental abnormalities in the region of the foramen magnum. Brain 90:11, 1957.
12. Pasztor E, Vajda J, Piffko P, et al: Transoral surgery of basilar impression. Surg Neurol 14:473, 1980.
13. Gunderson CH, Greenspan RH, Glaser GH, et al: The Klippel-Feil syndrome: genetic and clinical re-evaluation of cervical fusion. Medicine 46:491, 1967.
14. Cleland J: Contribution to the study of spina bifida, encephalocele and anencephalus. J Anat Physiol 17:257, 1883.
15. Chiari H: Ueber Veränderungen des Kleinhirns infolge von Hydrocephalie des Grosshirns. Deutsche Med Wochsch 17:1172, 1891.
16. Arnold J: Myelocyste, Transposition von Gewebskeimen und Sympodie. Beitrage zur pathologischen Anatomie und zur allgemeinen Pathologie 16:1, 1894.
17. Bloch S, Van Reusbert MJ, Danziger J: The Arnold-Chiari malformation. Clin Radiol 25:335, 1974.

Chapter 16

Dislocations and Subluxations

The cervical spine, with its relatively great mobility and wide clinical range of motion compared with other joint systems, is equally at relative risk to dislocations and subluxations. Though rarely occurring in the normal spine, subluxations are commonly associated with rheumatoid arthritis. They are frequent events in trauma, with fracture-dislocation or just dislocation. There are fixed subluxations in cervical osteoarthritis and in certain congenital lesions.[1, 2] Subluxations, over a period of years, follow single laminectomy as well as multiple laminectomies. Laminectomy is a relatively little appreciated cause of subluxation. Severe infections of the throat result in ligamentous laxity and dislocation. In children, rotatory dislocation of both atlantoaxial joints is not rare; it is rare in adults. Congenital basilar invagination (upward translocation of the odontoid process) may be associated with subluxation.

Each of these types has its peculiar and characteristic clinical history, physical signs, and radiologic characteristics. Cervical spine dislocations, fracture-dislocations, and subluxations and dislocations due to gross inflammatory involvement or congenital underlying mechanisms all potentially result in such striking, severe, painful, very disabling, and fatal consequences that it behooves us to study and understand these syndromes. Table 16–1 is a classification of dislocations and subluxations of the cervical spine. Table 16–2 lists the types of fracture-dislocations of the cervical spine.

Table 16–1. DISLOCATIONS AND SUBLUXATIONS OF THE CERVICAL SPINE

Atlanto-Occipital (base of skull at C1) Trauma
Jefferson's fracture[1]
Atanto-occipital anterior dislocation
Atlanto-occipital posterior dislocation
Odontoid fracture
Atlantoaxial Subluxation
Hangman's fracture[2]
Traumatic spondylolisthesis of the axis
Fracture pars interarticularis axis
Atlantoaxial anterior subluxation
Atlantoaxial posterior subluxation
Transverse (lateral) atlantoaxial subluxation
Atlantoaxial rotation and subluxation
Upward atlantoaxial subluxation[4, 5, 6, 7] ("cranial settling," superior "migration")
Nonreducible rotational head tilt and lateral mass collapse[10]
Rotary dislocation atlantoaxial joints[11]
Subaxial Dislocations and Subluxations
Stairstep vertebral subluxation of rheumatoid arthritis
Fixed subluxation of cervical osteoarthritis
Fracture dislocation of the ankylosed cervical spine (ankylosing spondylitis)
Traumatic subluxation without fracture
Traumatic fracture dislocation
    Automobile crashes
    Sports injuries

Table 16–2. FRACTURE-DISLOCATIONS OF THE CERVICAL SPINE

Anterior Spinal Elements
Compression fracture vertebral body with displacement
Compression fracture vertebral body without displacement
Avulsion fracture
Disc space fracture
Posterior Spinal Elements
Unilateral zygapophyseal dislocation
Bilateral
Bilateral perched facets ("locking")
Fractured facets
Fractured spinous processes
Laminal fractures
Lateral Spinal Elements
Lateral mass fracture

313

ETIOLOGY AND PATHOGENESIS

Since fractures, fracture-dislocations, and subluxations of the cervical spine occur with a variety of etiologic and pathogenetic mechanisms, each is treated separately in this section. The diagnosis and management of these cervical spine disorders and diseases is detailed in Chapter 7, *Craniometry and Roentgenometry of the Skull and Cervical Spine*, Chapter 11, *Differential Diagnosis and Specific Treatment*, and Chapter 15, *Congenital Anomalies*.

Congenital Mechanisms Leading to Dislocations and Subluxations

Congenital Malformations of the Cervical Spine—Basilar Impression. In basilar impression, there is an upward movement of the base of the skull in the area of the foramen magnum. People with severe basilar impression usually present to physicians in childhood or early adult life as they develop brain stem and cerebellar symptoms and signs caused by upward and anterior displacement of the odontoid bone into the cranial cavity. The majority of patients are not recognized until the third to the fifth decade of life.

Congenital Defects of the Atlantoaxial Joints. The atlantoaxial joints are the most mobile joints in the vertebral column, hence they have the least stability. The defect may be an abnormal odontoid process, atlanto-occipital fusion, or simple laxity of the transverse ligament. In any event the consequence is compromise of the anteroposterior diameter of the spinal canal and impingement on the spinal cord or nerve roots. Atlantoaxial instability is usually associated with other anomalies, most of which are etiologic in developing scoliosis. Down's syndrome, Morquio's syndrome, osteogenesis imperfecta, spondyloepiphyseal dysplasia, and neurofibromatosis may be associated with atlantoaxial laxity. Os odontoideum, complete congenital absence of the odontoid process, or a traumatic nonunion will result in atlantoaxial subluxation. Other congenital defects are presented in Chapter 15, *Congenital Anomalies*.

Rheumatoid Arthritis

In rheumatoid arthritis, virtually all tissues in the upper cervical spine undergo changes—bone, ligament, tendon, capsule, and cartilage. Osteoporosis with some element of osteomalacia occurs. There is strikingly diminished motor power in muscle, and rheumatoid granulomatous synovitis destroys facet joints and erodes and deforms the odontoid bone, compromising insertions of ligaments, tendons, and capsule into bone. Virtually all types of subluxation and dislocation may occur in rheumatoid arthritis.[3, 4, 5] The most serious lesion occurs in the upper cervical spine, involving the occipito-atlanto-axial complex and permitting anterior, lateral, and vertical dislocation and translocation of the odontoid process.[6, 7] There are both anterior and posterior true synovial joints in the atlanto-odontoid area. Continuing movement and physical activity accelerate the process of the disease, as does the atrophy of disuse.[8]

Ranawat et al[9] studied 33 patients with rheumatoid arthritis, who were treated surgically for their subluxations. Seventy per cent had atlantoaxial subluxation; 16% had upward translocation of the odontoid process, and 60% had subaxial subluxations.

Figure 16–1 illustrates a grossly subluxated atlas on the axis, with more space anteriorly than posteriorly, where the spinal cord lies.[10, 11] Note also forward subluxation of the body of the axis on C3. Figure 16–2 illustrates a very loose atlas, with subluxation forward, compressing and bulging the posterior pharynx. There is destruction of the C3, C4, and C5 vertebrae, with subluxations

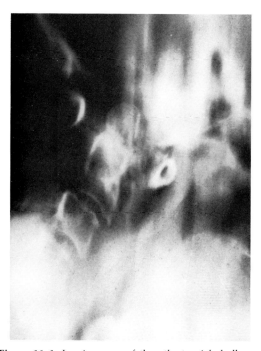

Figure 16–1. Laminogram of the atlantoaxial skull area in a patient with rheumatoid arthritis. Note the posterior lip of the foramen magnum to the left, the eroded posterior and anterior odontoid process, and a subluxation compressing the spinal cord. Note that the space between the anterior arch of the atlas and the anterior surface of the odontoid process is greater than the space between the posterior arch of the atlas and the posterior surface of the odontoid process. The body of the axis has also slid forward on C3, and there are erosions of the vertebral end plate. Note that the odontoid process is situated squarely in the foramen magnum, abutting against the anterior lip of the foramen.

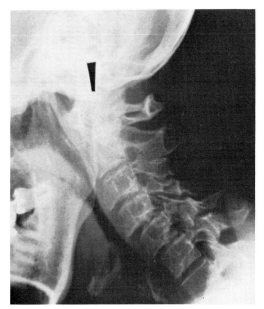

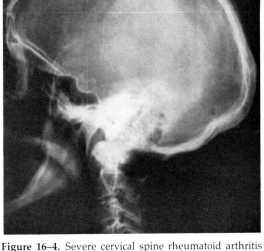

Figure 16–2. Cervical spine subluxation in rheumatoid arthritis. The atlas has "settled" over the odontoid process, which is migrating superiorly, not yet reaching the foramen magnum. There is a very loose connection between the atlas and the odontoid process. Note the narrow discs without osteophytes in the vertebrae below and the gross erosions of the vertebral bodies and end plates. At C3–C4, C4–C5, and C5–C6 there are gross stairstep subluxations forward.

Figure 16–4. Severe cervical spine rheumatoid arthritis with destruction of the posterior arch of the atlas. There is involvement of the odontoid process but no subluxation. The vertebrae at C2 and C3 are grossly involved with erosive disease.

forward in a stairstep array. Figure 16–3 illustrates an 11-mm subluxation of the atlas on the axis-odontoid. The subluxation is reduced completely in extension and grossly evident on flexion. Apart from osteoporosis and narrowing of C3–C4 and C4–C5, the cervical spine appears nearly normal. Figure 16–4 shows a rheumatoid spine in which

the posterior arch of the atlas has been destroyed. There is granulomatous disease of the apophyseal joints, the intervertebral discs, and the cartilage plates. There was subluxation on flexion. Figure 16–5 illustrates a tipping of the atlas, with relatively little subluxation. Note on the left the relationship between the posterior arch of the atlas and the spinous process of the axis, which "tips" on flexion secondary to gross ligamentous laxity. Figure 16–6 illustrates lateral subluxation, which, again is secondary to capsular and ligamentous instability, although a relatively normal odontoid process is retained. Figure 16–7 illustrates upward migration of the odontoid process, which is im-

Figure 16–3. Atlantoaxial subluxation in rheumatoid arthritis. This subluxation measures 11 mm. The patient has relatively little disease below that level, though he has seropositive, nodular rheumatoid arthritis. The subluxation is reduced completely in extension of the cervical spine. The atlas tips up as well as slides forward. There is no upward migration as yet.

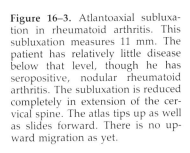

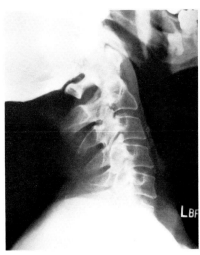

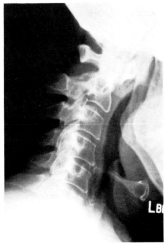

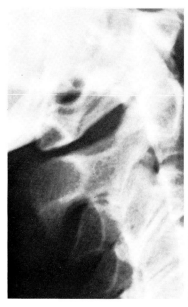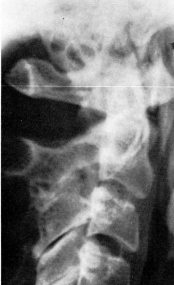

Figure 16–5. Rheumatoid arthritis of the cervical spine to illustrate "tipping" of the atlas. Note the space on the left between the posterior arch of the atlas and the spinous process of the axis, approximately 3 mm. With even slight flexion of the spine, the atlas tips to 13 mm—clearly pathologic. Also the space between the occiput and the posterior arch of the atlas widens to about 7 mm. There is anterior subluxation (sliding), with a triangular space between the odontoid process and the anterior arch of the atlas.

pinging upon the anterior lip of the foramen magnum. Figure 16–8 illustrates the characteristic stairstep subluxations in rheumatoid arthritis, with additional atlantoaxial subluxation.

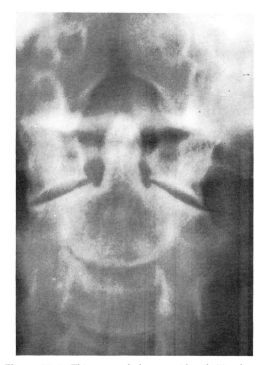

Figure 16–6. This case of rheumatoid arthritis shows lateral subluxation (in the illustration from right to left). Note that the apophyseal joint is narrower on the right side. The atlanto-occipital joint is seen, and there is clear erosion on the right side.

Fracture and Fracture-Dislocation Caused by Trauma

Fractures and dislocations secondary to trauma, which is usually due to automobile crashes and sports activity, may be divided into two general anatomic areas: (1) the base of the skull and the upper cervical spine (C1 and C2 joints and vertebrae) and (2) fractures and dislocations from C3 and T1. The first group includes the Jefferson fractures;[1] the odontoid fractures, with atlas subluxation due to rupture of the transverse ligament; and fractures of the odontoid process primarily. The hangman's fracture, or traumatic spondylolisthesis of the axis, also falls into the first category. Fractures and dislocations of the lower cervical spine may be divided into three major areas; (1) soft-tissue damage without actual bony fracture, (2) bone and joint lesions, and (3) fractures and dislocations with central nervous system involvement. Since these lesions are virtually always treated surgically, they will not be dealt with here.

Subluxations and Dislocations Secondary to Laminectomy

Not widely appreciated is the fact that laminectomy is frequently followed months or years later by dislocation in the cervical spine, which may result in severe and crippling neurologic events. There are few reports in the literature on this subject.[12] Laminectomy done for any reason may result in subluxation and dislocation many years after the operation. Because of the time lapse, one is not likely to suspect the surgery as the cause of such an event. The greater the number of laminae removed, the more likely the occurrence of increased mobility leading to instability from pro-

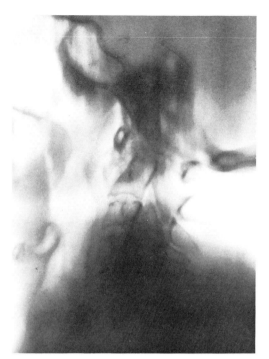

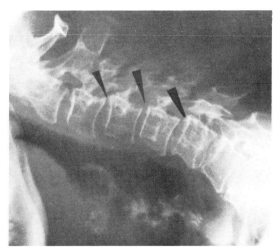

Figure 16–8. Rheumatoid arthritis of the cervical spine with characteristic stairstep subluxations, narrow discs without osteophytes, erosions of the vertebral end plates, and an atlantoaxial subluxation above. There is no superior migration. Note the space between the anterior arch of the atlas and the anterior surface of the odontoid process.

Figure 16–7. A case of rheumatoid arthritis of the cervical spine, with upward migration and severe erosion of the odontoid process, with an area of radiolucency between the body of the axis and the odontoid process itself. This case was histologically studied post mortem. There was gross, space-occupying granuloma completely surrounding the odontoid process. The anterior lip of the foramen magnum was grossly eroded—note the anterior arch of the atlas has slipped forward anterior to the foramen magnum lip. The relationhip between the posterior arch of the atlas and the posterior lip of the foramen magnum is apparent. The odontoid process is occupying the foramen magnum. Interestingly, there were few and trivial neurologic signs. The available space at the foramen magnum–atlas level is often sufficient to preclude cervical myelopathy.

study should be done until full growth is reached. If zygapophyseal joint function has been compromised at operation, early anterior fusion of the spine is a consideration. It is important to take great surgical care in the removal of the laminae, so that the zygapophyseal joints and their ligaments are not inadvertently removed. Dislocations have occurred as many as 25 years after discharge of the patient from postlaminectomy follow-up care. Laminectomy and excision of discs for cervical spine pain with few objective findings should be condemned.

gressive loss of function of the intervertebral disc bond. Such instability follows removal of the ligamenta flava, which is necessary to the laminectomy. If the zygapophyseal joints are damaged or their integrity is disrupted, with the intervertebral disc bond broken, dislocation may follow, even with prolonged immobilization. It is impossible to determine the point at which a laminectomy becomes too extensive because of the widely varying pathology for which the surgery is done in the first place—spasmodic torticollis, operation for trauma with cord compression, ankylosing spondylitis, osteoarthritis and intervertebral disc disease, and traumatic fracture dislocation.

In children, laminectomy done as management of kyphoscoliosis may result in subsequent subluxations; growth of the child constitutes a major consideration in this regard. Follow-up radiologic

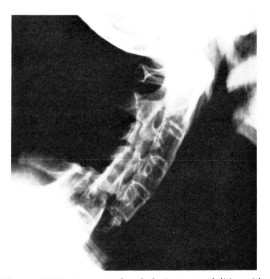

Figure 16–9. A case of ankylosing spondylitis with complete transection of the cord and through-and-through fracture of the cervical spine at the C5–C6 level.

Ankylosing Spondylitis

Ankylosing spondylitis, because of the ankylosis itself, renders the patient at risk to any fall or trauma. Fractures through the ankylosed spine are uncommon but not rare. Figure 16–9 illustrates a through-and-through fracture of the cervical spine in a patient with a completely ankylosed cervical spine. There was complete transection of the spinal cord. Figure 16–10 illustrates a fracture in the lower cervical spine through an intervertebral disc space following a fall. This patient was successfully treated, though there were severe neurologic signs initially. Figure 16–11 illustrates the severity of ankylosis, with preservation of the disc space. This patient had a fall, with consequent neurologic syndrome; however, the injury proved to be to the soft tissues and spinal cord. It was presumably vascular in origin, without bony fracture. Figure 16–12 illustrates the ankylosing spondylitic lesion, with destruction of the posterior elements of the atlas. In this case, there was no subluxation of the atlas; thus, the transverse ligament remained intact.

Cervical Osteoarthritis (Spondylosis)

Fixed subluxations are common in osteoarthritis involving intervertebral discs, zygapophyseal joints, and the joints of Luschka. Depending on the magnitude of osteophyte formation, bony remodeling, and specific lesions at the zygapophy-

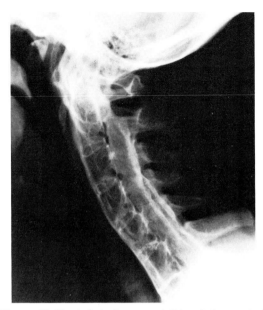

Figure 16–11. Ankylosing spondylitis of the cervical spine. A fall and trauma to soft tissues occurred, but no bony fracture or dislocation was seen on the films. The anterior arch of the atlas is visible above. Note that the entire cervical spine, C1–C7, is one continuous bone. The risk to fall, with consequent fracture or dislocation, is great.

seal and Luschka joints, neurologic syndromes are common. Figure 16–13 illustrates a subluxation at C4–C5, with lesser subluxations at C3–C4 and C5–C6. Note the remodeling and enlargement of

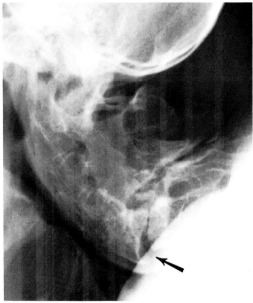

Figure 16–10. A case of ankylosing spondylitis with through-and-through fracture (arrow) and relatively little subluxation. There was spinal cord damage and hematomyelia, but the patient recovered sufficiently to remain functional.

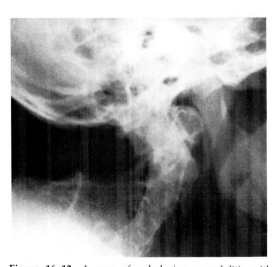

Figure 16–12. A case of ankylosing spondylitis with extreme bone atrophy, complete ankylosis, and continuous bone, with destruction of the posterior elements of the atlas and part of the spinous process of the axis. Note there is no subluxation and the space between the anterior arch of the atlas and the odontoid process is normal.

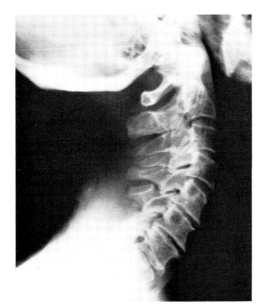

Figure 16–13. Cervical osteoarthritis with narrow discs, marked chondro-osteophytosis, zygapophyseal joint involvement, and marked remodeling of C5–C6–C7. Note the subluxations at C4–C5 and C5–C6; they are fixed subluxations with little movement of either the discs or zygapophyseal joints.

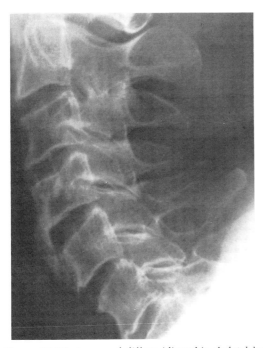

Figure 16–14. A case of diffuse idiopathic skeletal hyperostosis (DISH). Although much more apparent in the thoracic spine, it is still clear-cut DISH here. Note that the intervertebral disc spaces are preserved. The laminar bone is at the C4–C5 level; the posterior elements are normal, and there are small subluxations between C3–C4 and C5–C6. Again, the subluxations are fixed, not mobile.

the vertebrae beginning at C5, C6, and C7—all a part of cervical osteoarthritis. Figure 16–14, from a patient with diffuse idiopathic skeletal hyperostosis (DISH), also shows small, fixed subluxations at C3–C4 and C4–C5. Note that the intervertebral discs are intact and the posterior elements are normal—characteristic of the DISH syndrome.

Severe Infection

Children with severe pharyngeal infection, tonsillitis, and peritonsillar abscess—diseases in which the spread of the infectious process via lymphatic vessels occurs—may have gross atlantoaxial subluxation secondary to extreme swelling, with ligamentous and capsular laxity (Grisel's syndrome).[13] The clinical diagnosis is made on the basis of fever, dysphagia, tonsillitis, or peritonsillar abscess. The child frequently shows wryneck, atlantoaxial dislocation, and stairstep dislocations (C2–C3, C3–C4, and C4–C5). The atlas is often tilted, as noted in atlantoaxial subluxations of rheumatoid arthritis. There is widening of the prevertebral space, because the bulge of the soft-tissue shadow is secondary to the space-taking pharyngeal infection, which is usually an abscess.

References

1. Jefferson G: Fracture of the atlas vertebra. Br J Surg 7:407, 1920.
2. Bohlman HH: Acute fractures and dislocations of the cervical spine. J Bone Joint Surg 61A:1119, 1979.
3. Weiner S, Bassett L, Spiegel T: Superior, posterior and lateral displacement of C1 in rheumatoid arthritis. Arthritis Rheum 25:1378, 1982.
4. Bland JH: Rheumatoid arthritis of the cervical spine. J Rheumatol 3:319, 1974.
5. Pelliccii PM, Ranawat CS, Tsaris P, et al: A prospective study of the progression of rheumatoid arthritis of the cervical spine. J Bone Joint Surg 63A:342, 1981.
6. Meijers KAE, Van Beusekom G TH, Luyendijk W, et al: Dislocation of the cervical spine with cord compression in rheumatoid arthritis. J Bone Joint Surg 56B:668, 1974.
7. Rana NA, Hancock DO, Taylor AR: Upward translocation of the dens in rheumatoid arthritis. J Bone Joint Surg 55B:471, 1973.
8. Frigard E: Posterior atlanto-axial subluxation in rheumatoid arthritis. Scand J Rheumatol 7:65, 1978.
9. Ranawat CS, O'Leary P, Pellicci P, et al: Cervical spine fusion in rheumatoid arthritis. J Bone Joint Surg 61A:100, 1979.
10. Halla JT, Fallahi S, Hardin JG: Nonreducible rotational head tilt and lateral mass collapse. Arthritis Rheum 25:1316, 1982.
11. Jones RN: Rotatory dislocation of both atlanto-axial joints. J Bone Joint Surg 66B:6, 1984.
12. Bailey RW: The Cervical Spine. Philadelphia: Lea & Febiger, 1974, p 187.
13. Von Torklus D, Gehle W: The Upper Cervical Spine. New York: Grune & Stratton, 1972, p 61.

Chapter 17

Indications for Surgery: Trauma, Rheumatoid Arthritis, and Osteoarthritis

Though the vast majority of patients with disorders of the cervical spine are quite successfully treated and managed conservatively and without surgery, there is clearly a small, identifiable group of patients in each category of cervical spine disorder and disease for whom surgery is clearly indicated and enjoys significant, predictable success in alleviation of symptoms, and, in certain instances, provides cure. The problem is that of identification of this group of patients by clinical, radiologic, computed tomographic, and magnetic resonance imaging techniques in order to select those most likely to benefit from surgery and to avoid surgical treatment in those in whom the disease either will not be influenced or will possibly become worse. In general, the bony and soft-tissue changes do not require surgical management unless they have a significant functional effect on all adjacent structures. Cervical osteoarthritis is very commonly associated with brachial neuralgia and cervical myelopathy, though the incidence of the latter is low. The symptoms and signs, though present, are often trivial and functionally unimportant. The radiologically evident bony changes appear obvious and often severe by radiographic examination, but clinically the disease may be mild and functionally insignificant. In such cases, surgery should never be performed. Thus the prognosis is good in general for the great majority of cervical spine disorders. Even with full use of conservative management, there has been a clear, increasing tendency over the past two to three decades to attempt surgical procedures in severely afflicted patients. In the main, indications and criteria for surgical intervention are directly related to neurologic compromise, central and peripheral.

The principal clinical disorders requiring surgical management include rheumatoid arthritis, with its occipito-atlanto-axial subluxations and subaxial subluxation; cervical osteoarthritis, including intervertebral disc disease, and zygapophyseal and Luschka joint osteoarthritis; trauma (fractures and subluxations); tumors; and, rarely, infections. It is the goal of this chapter to present indications for and supply reliable criteria for the selection of patients for surgical management in each instance previously noted.

The lack of basic knowledge of cervical spine physiology, anatomy, and pathology and the failure to use what basic knowledge we have, plus having a serviceable understanding of the etiology and pathogenesis of clinical symptoms and signs have led to the development of many different surgical procedures designed to affect favorably or eliminate presumed causative factors. The main surgical approaches have been the decompression of nerve and vascular elements at the foramen by laminectomy; resection of osteophytes and protruding intervertebral disc material; and hemifacetectomy and fusion of the vertebral bodies, with or without resection of intervertebral disc material, eliminating motion and presumed abnormal mechanical influence upon neural structures.

This chapter deals not with the type of surgery, surgical techniques, or anterior or posterior approaches, but rather with the criteria for considering surgical therapy at all.

CERVICAL OSTEOARTHRITIS OF ALL THREE TYPES—INTERVERTEBRAL DISCS, ZYGAPOPHYSEAL JOINTS, AND JOINTS OF LUSCHKA

The most important surgical consideration in cervical osteoarthritis is a knowledge of the natural history of cervical osteoarthritis.[1, 2, 3] Patients both

320

with and without radiculopathy and myelopathy tend to have a very prolonged course. There are lengthy periods of nonprogressive—sometimes only annoying, sometimes more severe—disability. A progressively deteriorating course is unusual and exceptional. Few deaths can be attributed to cervical osteoarthritis.

Cervical Osteoarthritic Myelopathy

Cervical myelopathy of osteoarthritis rarely develops in any patient who does not have the symptoms and signs during the first visit to the physician.[1] In this very chronic and long-term disease, it is difficult to assess the effectiveness of conservative versus surgical treatment, since the condition itself is relatively benign and has a good prognosis without treatment. Treatment and management may alleviate symptoms without influencing the natural history of the disease. Consideration of cervical laminectomy should be most cautiously and conservatively approached in patients with cervical osteoarthritic myelopathy. We need the results of prospective studies, performed over decades before we can precisely define the indications and criteria for operation and the relative value of the many forms of treatment and management used today. We must always remember that cervical osteoarthritis is ubiquitous and universal. Hunt[4] has said that "numerically, at least, the skilled neurosurgeon can probably relieve more patients of suffering by the avoidance of unnecessary surgery than by the most skillful application of necessary surgery." Remember that the osteoarthritic process itself is glacially slow and largely asymptomatic. Even so, onset of symptoms can be abrupt and it may be characterized by intractable pain, compromise of peripheral nerve function, nerve root disease, interference with cervical arteries (carotid and vertebral), and spinal cord compressive phenomenon. It is the latter symptoms that often put the surgeon in the position of sitting at the final court of appeal. That surgeon should remember that cervical osteoarthritis generally tends to improve gradually with age, even though the radiologic findings are progressively "more severe." These findings are clinically unimportant. In more recent years, cervical osteophytosis in all three of the sites of osteoarthritic involvement in the cervical spine has been shown to diminish and even disappear, presumably in the process of remodeling according to Wolff's law. The best management program for all except for a tiny percentage of cases of osteoarthritis includes exercise to maintain muscle and ligamentous tone, education concerning optimal posture, judicious rest, short periods of partial immobilization, analgesic and anti-inflammatory drugs, and symptomatic therapy, including heat, traction, massage, and the many other means of treatment at our disposal. Such is clearly the management of choice (see Chapter 11, *Differential*

Diagnosis and Specific Treatment and Chapter 12, *General Management Methods*).

A further surgical consideration is that myelopathy unrelated to any direct spinal cord compression may occur. Compression of important blood vessels supplying the spinal cord has not been sufficiently stressed as a primary cause of myelopathy associated with cervical osteoarthritis. Only one to three cervical radicular arteries from the vertebral artery contribute to the anterior spinal artery, and three to five lesser branches contribute to the posterior spinal arteries. At surgery, the spinal cord in most patients with spinal cervical osteoarthritis is not compressed. Furthermore, the neurologic level usually does not correspond to the level of radiologic change. This suggests that cervical osteoarthritic myelopathy is not always caused by direct cord compression but by vascular insufficiency, ischemia, and cord infarction. Spinal cord syndromes of compression and ischemia are substantially similar, or both processes may be causative. Important radicular arteries entering at the C5–C6 and C7 levels may be compressed, resulting in ischemic areas of the spinal cord. The compression, then, is to these arteries in the narrowed foramina and to the fibrotic root sleeves. If this can be diagnosed, then partial laminectomy and foraminotomy may be the operations of choice.

What are the indications for surgical intervention? Intractable pain, total failure of conservative therapy over a period of 9 to 12 months, and significant neurologic deficit, objectively determined by clinical, radiologic, electrophysiologic, and computer tomographic techniques. Often unappreciated is the fact that the anteroposterior diameter of the bony spinal canal may be narrowed as a constitutional or congenital consequence, with further narrowing by osteophytes of osteoarthritis, fibrotic processes, and ligamentous hypertrophy. Bulgings into the spinal canal put such patients at much greater risk. The threat of acute myelopathy from relatively minor trauma in such a patient should be a surgical consideration.

Intractable pain is the most controversial of the indications previously mentioned. *Disabling pain with no neurologic deficit does not constitute an indication for surgical intervention.* The surgeon should be slow indeed to accept the term intractable. Certainly the patient who recovers with a spine that has not been operated on is far better off than one who has had spinal fusion. The interaction of the personalities of surgeon and patient is an important factor here. Patients should not be encouraged to regard their pain as intolerable, and they should be treated with as much honest reassurance as possible to get them through the critical period. Since the anterior approach to intervertebral disc disease has become so feasible technically and anesthesiology is at a level of competence to allow such surgery safely, many operations are done. Fusion may be followed by immediate success, but long-term osteoarthritis continues or is made worse by the postural consequences of the surgery, leading to accelerated osteoarthritis of adjacent discs and recurrence of symptoms. The less interference with physiologic, anatomic, and biomechanical factors the surgeon induces, the better. Remember that since everyone has cervical intervertebral disc disease, patients with abnormal radiograms, discograms, and even computed tomographic studies still should not be operated on. Objective clinical factors are the most important single category of evidence in surgical decision making.

Nevertheless, in very skilled hands, the results of anterior diskectomy and interbody fusion are often dramatic and permanently curative. Recurrence rate should be very low, but it should be remembered that the osteoarthritic process also involves adjacent vertebrae, zygapophyseal joints, and Luschka joints.

Be cautious and analytic about the pain-prone patient. Collins[5] has said that "98% relief is unacceptable." Such patients may continue to have occipital headaches, vertigo, blurring of vision, skin hypersensitivity of neck and scalp and focal areas of muscle, and ligamentous and capsular tenderness in the suboccipital and trapezius areas.

Radiculopathy

The obvious syndrome requiring immediate and aggressive surgery is the acute monoradiculopathy due to the protrusion of a herniated nucleus pulposus into the spinal canal or foramen. There are sensory, motor, and reflex changes referable to one or more of the cervical roots. If there is no immediate improvement or disappearance of clinical symptoms and signs on conservative management within 10 days, aggressive surgery is clearly indicated. Surgical therapy may be better applied sooner (i.e., in 2 to 3 days) if there is rapid progression of neurologic signs. Remember that a C7–C8 syndrome threatens many people with severe or even total disability because of the consequent failure of pronation, extension, interosseous, and lumbrical muscle function. The possibility of permanent weakness is very real, even when pain has been controlled. Surgical results are excellent; criteria are clear cut.

Indications are not so clear when the cervical osteoarthritic process involves several levels of the spine, usually C4–C5, C5–C6, and C7–T1, with protrusions into intervertebral foramina, into the spinal canal, or anteriorly compressing the esophagus and hypopharynx. As this pathophysiologic process is evolving there is pressure and stretching of anterior and posterior longitudinal ligaments, joint capsules, ligamenta flava, and the fibrotic process in the dural root sleeve. This results in symptoms of neck and arm pain, occipital headache, chest pain, various paresthesias, dysesthesias, and, rarely anesthesias. Generally,

there are few or no objective clinical findings, and the results of the radiologic studies may be normal or similar to those of a sample population of individuals the same age as the patient. The "soft" disc previously noted occurs in the younger patient, whereas the "hard" disc, gradual in development and evolution, occurs in the older patient.

Surgical intervention is considered for those patients experiencing truly intractable pain over a period of 8 to 12 weeks during which maximal therapeutic and management programs (including hospitalization) are carried on.

With no relief, such patients should be operated upon (remembering that one cannot operate on three levels), and often a free disc fragment is found compressing a cervical root. Removal of the fragment relieves the pain. The surgical timing is of great importance in order that the patient not be left with a compromising functional deficit that could have been avoided by early surgical management.

Myelopathy

Acute myelopathy caused by a midline, herniated, soft nucleus pulposus is rare. When it happens, surgical indications are obvious. With a congenitally narrow bony canal, the possibility of myelopathy is enhanced. Such implies that the surgeon should obtain on standard radiographs the measurements of transverse and anteroposterior diameters throughout the spine, relating them to the mean and standard deviation figures available (see Chapter 7, *Craniometry and Roentgenometry of the Skull and Cervical Spine*). Some authors have thought that spondylotic myelopathy occurs mainly in patients who have a congenitally narrow spinal canal upon which is superimposed the osteoarthritic process. The pathophysiologic etiology is multiple, that is, it involves intervertebral disc osteoarthritis, bony vertebral proliferation, foraminal encroachment, zygapophyseal and Luschka joint osteoarthritis, impaired circulation to the spinal cord from compressive forces involving the anterior and posterior spinal arteries, and finally the compression of radicular arteries branching from the vertebral artery. Obviously, abnormal motion, trauma, and accidents may transform the syndrome from an asymptomatic to a very symptomatic state. The clinical presentation is commonly that of vague complaints of pain in the arms, legs, and cervical spine; however, the manifestations occur mainly in the lower extremity. Gradually progressive, painless, spastic gait is characteristic when the myelopathy is progressive. A set of neurologic findings, some trivial, some very serious, allow formulation of the pattern of cervical cord compression. (1) Such clinical divisions are a transverse myelitic lesion, with corticospinal, spinothalamic, and dorsal column involvement, primarily of the motor system, with corticospinal tract and anterior horn cell compromise (requires differentiation from amyotrophic lateral sclerosis); (2) a mixed syndrome with radicular and spinal cord dysfunction; and (3) a partial Brown-Séquard syndrome, with ipsilateral proprioceptive loss, contralateral weakness, and a syringomyelia-like picture of dissociated pain and temperature loss in the upper extremities, but with amyotrophy and hyporeflexia and hyperactive reflexes in the legs.

The natural history of myelopathy is not one (in the majority of cases) of progressive, neurologic defect. Thus decision making is most difficult in this category. One should not wait until the symptoms and signs have progressed to permanent disabling magnitude. On the other hand, one also should not accelerate the course of what might be a benign process with only trivial symptom development. The presence of known congenital stenosis of the cervical spinal canal along with documented, increasingly progressive cervical osteoarthritis constitutes the main data on which a decision is made. Such patients probably can enjoy delay or prevention of the development of myelopathy to the point of neurologic deficits compromising function. With unequivocal progression, surgical decompression is required. A cautionary note: radiologic findings, too often, do not correlate with symptoms and signs.

Cervical Osteoarthritis with Dysphagia

In osteoarthritis, the occurrence of chondro-osteophytes sufficient in size to compress the esophagus and hypopharynx is uncommon. Nonetheless, difficulty in swallowing, throat discomfort, hoarseness, decreased neck motion, and nasal regurgitation of fluid are symptoms that can become intolerable. An important set of differential diagnostic factors are those of hiatal hernia, esophageal tumors, Zenker's diverticulum, and mediastinal and lung tumor, all of which could occur in the presence of expected cervical osteoarthritis. The point is that, prior to considering surgical intervention, the physician should be very secure that the osteoarthritic lesions are etiologic and pathogenetic. In most cases, the clinical symptoms and signs are caused by an osteophyte at a single level rather than at multiple levels. Surgical intervention is more likely to be successful if the osteophyte is at a single level.

Obstruction of Cervical Arteries

Both the carotid and the vertebral arteries may be obstructed in cervical osteoarthritis. The primary reason for obstruction, however, is atherosclerosis—very common and almost universal—leading to ischemia of the territory of the carotid artery as well as that of the vertebral artery. In the past, strokes were regarded as being caused by vascular lesions, hemorrhage, or thrombosis within the brain, but clinical and pathologic correlation is usually poor. Modern angiographic studies have shown that a great proportion of these presumed intracranial lesions are abnormalities of vessels in the neck. Abnormalities of the carotid arteries affect mainly the cerebral hemispheres, and those of the vertebral arteries lead to brain stem ischemia. Ischemia of the carotid territory causes weakness or disturbance of sensation of one limb or one side of the face, sometimes with dysphasia. Angiography can demonstrate the vascular abnormality in about two thirds of patients with such ischemic clinical signs, and the primary lesion of the "stroke" is found in the neck twice as often as it is in the skull. The major obstructive site in the carotid artery is the proximal 2 cm of the internal carotid artery. The obstruction is atheromatous, a plaque with stenosis or superimposed thrombosis. The clinical picture is that of recurrent ischemic attacks lasting less than an hour, with many lasting only seconds to minutes. Another possibility is that recurrent emboli are discharged from the atheromatous lesion.

The symptoms of vertebral artery obstruction are headache (perhaps due to secondary dilation of collateral vessels), vertigo, visual changes, facial dysesthesia, evidence of ischemia of the long tracts, drop attacks, and rarely, tetraplegia. Angiography usually shows the lesions to lie at the origins of the subclavian or vertebral arteries. The narrowing may be more apparent if films are taken with the neck in rotation, because such narrowing is a common, normal event on rotating the head.

When it is documented that symptoms are clearly related to vascular stenosis, attacks may be relieved by operation. Remember that the operation does nothing for the underlying disease (nor does triple bypass do anything for atherosclerosis involving the coronary arteries) and that the disease goes on after the operation. Thus, with multiple lesions or postoperative thrombosis, results may be disappointing. Nevertheless, a single, well-localized stenosis demonstrated by angiography should indicate surgical assessment and therapy.

Remember, anticoagulants have been found to abolish or reduce the frequency of transient ischemic attacks in many patients, consequently reducing the number of emboli released from the lesion. Treatment with anticoagulants is the best management for most patients because it does relieve the attacks.[6] Hypertension seems to be a contraindication to anticoagulants. The prognosis for surgery is worse in hypertensive patients. Vasodilator therapy has not been effective.

Chondro-osteophytes forming about the joints of Luschka may project into the foramina, compressing the vertebral artery and compromising blood flow to the brain stem. Symptoms may occur on rotation of the head and cervical spine or they may occur spontaneously for reasons little understood. Vertebral angiograms aid in identifying these unusual and rare instances.

In summary it should be remembered that a single cervical spinal root innervates its corresponding segmental cutaneous area of dermatome as well as the myotome and sclerotome—muscles, bones, joints, ligaments and viscera. All of these tissues may be remote from the corresponding dermatome and, hence, may be symptomatic.

The symptoms of cervical osteoarthritis may precisely simulate those of other disorders, such as visceral, cardiac, diaphragmatic, and gall bladder disorders. Cervical osteoarthritis is ubiquitous and universal and may coexist with some other condition that is the real cause of symptoms. Other diseases of the cervical spine may simulate cervical osteoarthritis and are particularly liable to cause difficulty if they are primary diseases of the nervous system.

Those of use old enough to remember are aware of the various "fashions" that the brachial neuropathies have passed through—C7 large transverse process, cervical rib, high first rib, narrow costoclavicular space, tight scalene muscles, and many others! Thus, let us not always put the blame on cervical osteoarthritis.

Carpal Tunnel Syndrome, "Tennis Elbow," and Rotator Cuff Tendonitis

These are all closely associated with cervical osteoarthritis. Symptoms of brachial neuropathy often are not those expected from pressure on the nerve or nerve root. The pain often is not referred like a root pain to the limb periphery; rather it is most severe in the proximal portion of the limb and is associated with tenderness of muscles and nerve trunks, particularly of the large nerves. Ischemic cuff tests on the affected limb result in almost instant development of a sense of numbness in the fingers. These characteristics suggest that there is some abnormality of the nerve sheath rather than the nerve fiber—root sleeve fibrosis, adhesions, or development of rigidity with loss of nerve root elasticity. This cautionary note is to suggest that pressure on nerves in the spinal canal and the foramina may not always be the cause of the painful neuropathy. The pain depends on a neuritis or radiculitis in which the changes are probably in the nerve sheath, and management may be directed more appropriately to the neuritis rather than to the cervical arthritis directly.

One must constantly be aware that cervical osteoarthritis is too often a radiologic diagnosis only, a diagnosis based on physical signs seen on the radiogram. Such radiographic findings are the rule, not the exception, in all middle-aged and elderly patients, and their significance is limited. Many such patients have intermittent torticollis that lasts weeks to months and disappears. A considerable proportion have asymptomatic, trivial neurologic signs, indicating either minor lesions of nerve roots or possibly involvement of the long tracts of the spinal cord. It may be that the pendulum has swung too far in one direction, and that we are attributing too many clinical syndromes to cervical osteoarthritis. Many neurologic diseases may be attributed to osteoarthritic changes, since they are so universal. The most important single mistake in medical practice is to overlook something readily treatable.

Finally, surgery plays only a very small part in the management of cervical osteoarthritis and should be reserved for cases in which conservative measures have truly failed over a sufficient period of time. One weakness of surgical management is that there are often multiple levels of involvement, and chondro-osteophytic bars crossing the spinal canal cannot be removed without unacceptable risk of increasing the patient's disability. The risks of anesthesia and of surgery are great. The already injured spinal cord is narrow, and procedures to remove dense bone in the extremely limited space anterior to the spinal cord are likely to exceed the limit of tolerance. Since we now know there are clearly vascular factors involved in the myelopathy of cervical osteoarthritis, compression may play but a minor role in the production of myelopathy, rendering surgical management inadequate.

RHEUMATOID ARTHRITIS OF THE CERVICAL SPINE

The pathologic mechanisms by which the cervical spine becomes unstable in rheumatoid arthritis are the same as mechanisms elsewhere: synovitis in the zygapophyseal joints and Luschka joints, with spread of the granulomatous process and inflammatory and enzymatic digestion and destruction of the surrounding tissues and intervertebral discs, erosions of ligaments, the anulus, the intervertebral discs themselves, and capsular tissue; and the process may spread, further eroding bone, resulting in an unstable cervical spine. Patterns of abnormality are varied, but the most common is anterior subluxation of the atlas on the axis. Subaxial multiple subluxations occur, as does vertical subluxation in which the axis telescopes into the atlas, and the odontoid occupies the foramen magnum. These abnormalities may result in rheumatoid cervical myelopathy, radiculopathy, medullary compression, and compromise of blood flow to the spinal cord via either the radicular arteries or the anterior and posterior spinal artery. Relationships between radiologic changes and neurologic features are not consistent and often difficult to explain. Studies of the natural history of rheumatoid arthritis of the cervical spine suggest that the life expectancy of such patients is not shorter than that of other patients with rheumatoid arthritis.[7]

The comparison of conservative with surgical management is fraught with difficulty, since the selection of cases is limited and different surgical techniques have not been well standardized. Conaty and Mongan[8] reported improvement in two thirds of patients with atlantoaxial fusions. Marks and Sharp[9] concluded that their surgically treated patients probably had a better prognosis, but they also pointed out that this group of patients has a bad prognosis independent of their neurologic state. Ranawat et al[10] reported a high mortality rate (27%) in the 2 postoperative years, but many of these deaths "were not obviously related to surgery." Though clinicians disagree on specific indications for surgery, the most recent reported results are encouraging enough to warrant a more aggressive attitude for surgical management. At the very least, a surgical consultation should be sought for patients who have symptomatic atlantoaxial, vertical, and subaxial subluxations; a displacement greater than 30% of the sagittal diameter of the cervical canal; progressive subluxations; myelopathy, progressive or otherwise; or evidence of brain stem ischemia.

Meijers et al[11] identified a series of symptoms indicative of an imminent transverse spinal cord lesion. These symptoms are called "alarm signs," and they serve very well in decision making for surgical intervention:

1. Severe occipitocervical pain suggestive of subluxation of the atlas.

2. Disorders of urination—retention, incontinence, urgency—these symptoms have always suggested severe abnormality of the spinal cord.

3. Paresis of the arm or legs or both.

4. So-called jumping legs, suggesting spinal automatism and experienced as painful.

5. Paresthesia of fingers or feet, described as an "emery paper sensation," suggesting mixed disorder of sensory perception.

6. A striking finding was called a "stone or marble sensation" in the limbs, interpreted as evidence of abnormality of deep perception and proprioception.

These symptoms were not seen in severe cases of rheumatoid arthritis without cervical subluxation and spinal cord compression. Neurologic examination may be difficult in cases with severe pain; abnormalities of muscle strength may occur because of peripheral neuropathy as well as radiculopathy and myelopathy. A detailed sensory perception clinical study is the single most reliable method of identifying cord compression. Partial monolateral or bilateral paresis as well as total loss of gnostic sensitivity may be seen.

Of course, one would like to anticipate and prevent the development of such clinical events. The published papers of Meijers et al,[11] Stevens et al,[12] Eulderdink and Meijers,[13] and Bland[14] constitute the overall best sources of information upon which to base decisions regarding surgical intervention.

TRAUMA, FRACTURE, FRACTURE-DISLOCATION

Surgical decisions in trauma of the spine and spinal cord are associated with variable opinion. Kahn[15] proposes that the following criteria be used in decision making:

1. If paralysis occurs promptly following injury and is complete (sensory and motor) and lasts at least 24 hours (indicating permanence), it is rarely associated with any useful return of function. Nevertheless, no such case should be viewed as hopeless, and careful, clinical, serial study should be pursued.

2. Any closed type of fracture-dislocation should have immediate application of skeletal traction.

3. With progressive neurological lesions, immediate laminectomy is indicated even in the presence of an abnormal alignment of the vertebral bodies not readily corrected by skeletal traction.

4. In acute central cervical cord injury with no evidence of fracture dislocation, but with paralysis of the upper extremity and some remaining function of the lower extremities, laminectomy is ordinarily contraindicated. A myelogram should be obtained if improvement is not occurring; rule out herniated disc.

5. If after reduction or partial reduction of a fracture-dislocation, paralysis is absent and instability persists, surgical management should be directed at preventing late or further cord damage by stabilizing the cervical spine via internal fixation and fusion. If a cervical dislocation is easily reduced, it can as easily redislocate.

Bailey's[16] indications for laminectomy in the cervical spine are as follows: (1) compound or open fracture or a fracture-dislocation caused by a penetrating wound; (2) bone fragments present in the spinal canal; (3) when the neurologic lesion is progressive (acute, anterior spinal cord injury syndrome), immediate laminectomy is mandatory; (4) psychologic factors.

Contraindications for laminectomy are as follows: (1) total and immediate paralysis lasting 24 hours, with little hope of improvement except at the C5–C6 level, where foraminotomy might affect root decompression; (2) acute central cervical spinal cord injury; (3) fracture dislocation at or above C4, with or without evidence of cervico-medullary syndrome; (4) the patient's general condition will not allow surgery; (5) hospital facilities or personnel are inadequately equipped for such surgery.

Cervical Spinal Cord Injury

The most precise, predictable treatment of traumatic lesions of the cervical spinal cord is cervical decompression at the site of the lesion followed by cervical spine stabilization as indicated. Perhaps even more important may be the appropriate and timely use of large doses of adrenal corticosteroid therapy.[17, 18, 19] Sometimes traumatic damage in the long spinal tracts requires several hours to develop and can be blocked completely or in varying degree by steroid hormone and antifibrinolytic therapy.

There are little available data on which to base criteria and indications for surgical management of the traumatized cervical spinal cord. Surgical decompression of the cord remains controversial, more so than criteria for stabilization. Rapid and progressive loss of function, though very uncommon, is a certain indication for surgical intervention and acute decompression. A cautionary note is that laminectomy carried out in the hours to days after trauma, without proper stabilization, has been associated with a poor prognosis. Some patients with clinically measureable residual cord function have developed permanent paralysis after laminectomy. It is not clear why laminectomy may accelerate the consequence of the injury, unless it is related to operative damage. It may be that decreased spinal cord blood flow is a factor.

Spinal cord function above the level of C3 includes regulation of respiration. Transection above C3 is only rarely associated with survival. Spinal cord function above the level of C4 to C7 includes anterior horn cells for the upper extremities and the long pathways serving the trunk, lower extremities, and sphincters. Below the level of the cervical spine, flexibility is lost; the thoracic spine is relatively fixed.

The following recommendations are made: (1) extensive and frequent neurologic assessment by neurosurgeons and neurologists; (2) immediate radiologic studies on admission; application of skeletal traction and achievement of prompt reduction and alignment of the cervical spine without manipulative techniques; (3) myelographic assessment in all patients; (4) electrophysiologic assessment; (5) surgical intervention in patients who have clear evidence of cervical spinal cord compression documented on myelography; (6) with complete areflexic loss of neurologic function and cord compression, surgery can be done reasonably up to 48 hours after injury; patients with a total lesion, whose surgical management is initiated 48 hours after injury, have no chance of neurologic recovery.

TUMORS OF THE CERVICAL SPINE

Infections and tumors of the cervical spine are discussed in Chapter 18, *Infections and Tumors of the Cervical Spine*. Benign tumors of the cervical spine are rare and include neurofibromatosis, aneurysmal bone cyst, benign giant cell tumor, solitary eosinophilic granuloma, solitary plasmacytoma, desmoid tumor, and chondromyxoid fibroma. Malignant tumors include the chordoma, chondrosarcoma, osteosarcoma, Ewing's sarcoma, and aggressive solitary plasmacytoma.

Precise diagnosis is of the greatest importance. When a cervical tumor has been diagnosed, with definite tissue diagnosis included, one considers and assesses the effects of the tumor, both im-

mediate and long-term, on neurologic function and the effects of surgery on mechanical stability of the spine. Histologic diagnosis guides therapy, aids in prognosis, and assesses how aggressive the surgical procedures must be (curative, reconstructive, or palliative). Considerations following tissue diagnosis are those of complete removal of the tumor; pain relief; prevention, arrest, and reversal of the neurologic deficit; and the achievement of as much mechanical stability as possible.

References

1. Lees F, Turner JWA: Natural history and prognosis of cervical spondylosis. Br Med J 2:1607, 1963.
2. Nurick S: The natural history and the results of surgical treatment of the spinal cord disorder associated with cervical spondylosis. Brain 95:101, 1972.
3. Nurick S: The pathogenesis of the cervical spine disorder associated with cervical spondylosis. Brain 95:87, 1972.
4. Hunt WE, Paul S: Herniated cervical and lumbar disc. A discussion of clinical findings and diagnosis procedures. Ohio State Med J 65:6, 1969.
5. Collins WF. (As cited by Hunt WE, Paul S: Herniated cervical and lumbar discs. A discussion of clinical findings and diagnostic procedures. Ohio State Med J 65:6, 1969.)
6. Baker RN, Schwartz WS, Rose AS: Transient ischemic stroke. Neurology 16:841, 1966.
7. Smith PH, Benn RT, Sharp J: Natural history of rheumatoid cervical subluxations. Ann Rheum Dis 31:431, 1972.
8. Conaty JP, Mongan ES: Cervical fusion in rheumatoid arthritis. J Bone Joint Surg 63A:1218, 1981.
9. Marks JS, Sharp J: Rheumatoid cervical myelopathy. Q J Med 199:307, 1981.
10. Ranawat CS, O'Leary P, Pellicci P, et al: Cervical spine fusion in rheumatoid arthritis. J Bone Joint Surg 61A:1003, 1979.
11. Meijers KAE, Van Beusekom GT, Luyendijk W, et al: Dislocation of the cervical spine with cord compression in rheumatoid arthritis. J Bone Joint Surg 56B:668, 1974.
12. Stevens JC, Cartlidge NEF, Saunders M, et al: Atlanto-axial subluxation and cervical myelopathy in rheumatoid arthritis. Q J Med 40:391, 1971.
13. Eulerdink F, Meijers KAE: Pathology of the cervical spine in rheumatoid arthritis: A controlled study of 44 spines. J Pathol 120:91, 1975.
14. Bland JH: Rheumatoid arthritis of the cervical spine. J Rheumatol 3:319, 1974.
15. Kahn EA: Neurosurgical aspects of spinal injuries. *In* Bailey RW (ed): The Cervical Spine. Philadelphia: Lea & Febiger, 1974.
16. Bailey RW: Fracture and dislocation in the cervical spine. *In* Bailey RW (ed): The Cervical Spine. Philadelphia: Lea & Febiger, 1974.
17. Campbell JB, DeCrescito V, Tomasula J, et al: Effects of antifibrinolytic and steroid therapy on the contused spinal cord of cats. J Neurosurg 40:726, 1974.
18. Demopoulos H, Flavin E, Seligman M, et al: Molecular pathology of lipids in CNS membranes. *In* Jobsis F (ed): Oxygen and Physiologic Function. Dallas: Dallas Professional Information Library, 1976, p 491.
19. Koenig C, Dohrman GJ: Histological variability in "standardized" spinal cord trauma. J Neurol Neurosurg Psychiatry 40:1203, 1977.

Chapter 18

Infections and Tumors of the Cervical Spine

Fortunately infections and tumors, benign and malignant, are rare occurrences in the cervical spine. However, the cervical spine is so unique anatomically and physiologically, having such a concentration of crowded critical structures, that rapid clinical catastrophe is a constant threat unless early diagnosis and optimum management of tumor and infection are instituted. Neurologic structures have little tolerance to mechanical compression, and the possibilities of quadriplegia, spinal cord stroke, and death are always in the background. The close anatomic and physiologic relationships between the spinal cord, nerve roots, and peripheral nervous system and the structurally confining implications of the skeletal and soft tissues make early diagnosis mandatory in these rare cervical spine disorders. Space-taking lesions in or around the spinal canal cause a broad spectrum of clinical syndromes from pain in the neck, radiculitis, and paresthesia to quadriparesis and death. Cervical cord compression can be caused by the gross space occupation of an expanding abscess or a rapidly growing vertebral, medullary, or extramedullary tumor or by the fracture, collapse, and dislocation of the supporting structures themselves—bones, joints, ligaments, and tendons. Therapeutic choices require identification of either or both of these destructive pathologic processes. Critical structures at risk in tumors and infections of the cervical spine are the lower brain stem, cervical spinal cord, nerve rootlets, roots, ganglia and common spinal nerves, vertebral arteries, carotid arteries, trachea, and esophagus.

Thus, though their incidence is low, cervical infections and tumors are very significant, owing to their potential for causing extreme morbidity and death.

TUMORS OF THE CERVICAL SPINE

Tumors, both primary and malignant, though rare, are seen 2 to 3 times yearly in a rheumato-

logic practice. This incidence is surely greater in an orthopedic or neurologic or neurosurgical practice. Metastatic carcinoma is by far the most common malignant tumor of the vertebral column. Geschickter and Copeland reported on 291 tumors of the spine, of which 172 were metastatic carcinomas.[1] Carcinoma of the breast was the most common metastasis in women, and carcinoma of the prostate was the most common metastasis in men. Since that time, the striking increase in lung cancer has been clearly associated with a concomitant increase in pulmonary malignant metastases to the vertebral column. Such metastases are multiple, and radiologic study of the whole skeleton is required. Symptomatic vertebral involvement often precedes any radiologic capability of diagnosis, particularly with a lesion in the midbody of the vertebra, as is usual. Serial radiologic study is necessary in tumor identification (Table 18–1).

Tumors arising primarily in tissues of the cervical spine constitute the next largest group of bone tumors. The most common benign tumors are giant cell tumors and benign bone cysts. Benign tumors occur much more frequently than primary, unicentric malignant tumors.[2] Table 18–2

Table 18–1. SITE OF PRIMARY CARCINOMA IN VERTEBRAL METASTASES

Primary Site	Number of Cases
Prostate	86
Breast	60
Unidentified	14
Gastrointestinal tract	5
Kidney	4
Thyroid	1
Lung	1
Nasopharynx	1
Total	172

Adapted from Geschickter CF, Copeland MM: Tumors of Bone, 3rd ed. Philadelphia: J. B. Lippincott Co, 1949.

Table 18–2. PRIMARY TUMORS OF THE VERTEBRAL COLUMN

Tumor Type	Number of Cases
Benign	
Giant cell	15
Osteochondroma	10
Bone cysts	7
Chondroma	3
Hemangioma	2
Total	37
Malignant	
Osteogenic sarcoma	
Chondrosarcoma	8
Osteolytic sarcoma	4
Sclerosing sarcoma	4
Chordoma	5
Total	21

Data from Geschickter CF, Copeland MM: Tumors of Bone, 3rd ed. Philadelphia: J. B. Lippincott Co, 1949.

lists benign and malignant tumors in order of incidence according to Geschickter and Copeland.[1] Table 18–3 represents an update in tumor types experienced in a neurosurgical practice.[2]

Table 18–3. PRIMARY AND MALIGNANT TUMORS OF THE CERVICAL SPINE

Tumor Type	Number of Cases
Benign	
Neurofibroma	7
Aneurysmal bone cyst	5
Benign giant cell tumor	3
Benign osteoblastoma	2
Solitary eosinophilic granuloma	2
Solitary plasmacytoma	1
Chondromyxoid fibroma	1
Desmoid tumor	2
Hemangioma	1
Osteocartilaginous exostosis	3
Tumor-sized rheumatoid synovitis around the odontoid process	1
Total	28
Malignant	
Chordoma	2
Mesenchymal chondrosarcoma	1
Chondrosarcoma	3
Osteosarcoma	1
Ewing's sarcoma	1
Aggressive solitary plasmacytoma	1
Hemangiopericytoma	1
Total	10

Adapted from Verbiest H: Tumors involving the cervical spine. *In* Bailey RW, Sherk HH (eds): The Cervical Spine. Philadelphia: J. B. Lippincott Co, 1984.

Multiple Myeloma, Hodgkin's Disease, Lymphoma, Xanthomatous Disease, and Hyperparathyroidism

Multiple myeloma is the most important generalized neoplastic disease to be considered in clinical study for metastatic disease. The multiple punched-out areas seen radiologically and severe osteopenia are characteristic. Multiple myeloma, sometimes initially solitary, usually is ultimately multiple. The peak age of onset and diagnosis of multiple myeloma is the sixth decade, making multiple myeloma a parallel consideration with metastatic carcinoma. Clinical, radiologic, and pathologic characteristics of multiple myeloma are presented in Table 18–4. In the vast majority of instances, multiple myeloma allows precise diagnosis and hence therapeutic initiation.

Diagnostic Methods in Cervical Spine Tumors

As elsewhere in medicine, clinical examination stands primary. The most frequent symptom in cervical tumors is localized pain. Pain experienced while resting and at night is common and ominous. The most common error made in assessing the patient presenting with neck pain is to diagnose osteoarthritis or intervertebral disc disease

Table 18–4. MULTIPLE MYELOMA

Clinical Characteristics
Between 20 and 80 years of age (average 64)
Sex predilection for men (2:1)
Bone pain
Anemia
Pathologic fractures (especially vertebral) in two thirds of patients
Neurologic involvement
Hypercalcemia
Renal failure
Para-amyloidosis
Bence Jones proteinuria
Hyperuricemia
Bleeding tendencies
Hyperglobulinemia, macroglobulinemia (by serum electrophoresis)
Polyarthropathy
Hyperviscosity syndrome
Radiologic Characteristics
"Punched-out" osteolytic areas
Severe generalized osteoporosis
Pathologic fractures
"Moth-eaten" bone
Pathologic Characteristics
Proliferation of abnormal plasma cells in the bone marrow
Invasive destruction of skeleton
Hemopoietic depression
One or more distinctive immunoglobulins

without first performing a complete clinical and radiologic study. Pain in the cervical spine, shoulder, and arm radiating variously and in multiple directions, tenderness, muscle spasm, and decreased cervical spine movement may be the only clinical manifestations of benign tumor. Torticollis is much more common in tumors of the upper cervical spine. Tumor enlargement or bony displacement may cause clinical symptoms and signs of radiculitis or spinal cord compression. Spinal stroke occurs by constriction of radicular arteries or of the end-arteries in the cord itself or of anterior and posterior spinal arteries. Loss of power is uncommon but rarely may occur primarily.

Clinical assessment of localized pain, range of motion, external deformity, function of roots, ganglia, and spinal nerves, and long tract signs should be made. A very early sign of tumors in the atlanto-axial-occipital complex is loss of rotatory motion.[3] Tenderness and pain on pressure palpation of spinous processes are common and early localizing signs of involvement of posterior elements and lateral masses. Pain elicitation on palpation of and pressure on the lateral transverse processes is likewise an identifying characteristic.

Complete neurologic and rheumatologic examination is mandatory to elicit the earliest neurologic characteristics. Early diagnosis allows realization of the ultimate goal, which is prevention or elimination of central or peripheral nervous system damage. Rapid progression from paresthesia and posterior root symptomatology to motor root and Brown-Séquard syndrome with quadriparesis is not rare. Detailed clinical study will identify the earliest signs, permitting effective medical or surgical therapy before onset of quadriparesis. Identification of gross neurologic signs provides evidence of a departed opportunity!

Radiologic Study. Complete plain radiographic study is the next step in the diagnostic process, as outlined in Chapter 6, *Radiologic Evaluation*. Remember that 30% to 60% of bone density is gone before the radiologist can identify definite change, that is, a normal radiologic study does not rule out tumor, and strong clinical awareness promotes intensive investigation. Benign tumors can be identified when they become clinically manifest. This is not true of the primary or metastatic malignancy. The technetium bone scan is the most sensitive single diagnostic procedure for identifying occult cervical spine malignancy. Plain radiograph reading requires differentiating lytic and blastic processes to permit recognition of very slowly advancing and rapidly expanding bone-destroying disease and to offer some insight into the rate at which bony support may be lost.

The clinician can usually localize the disease process to the anterior or posterior cervical spine elements. This does not mean that both may not be involved; they may be!

Anatomic structures essential to cervical stability have been identified by White.[4] Functional understanding of these anatomic characteristics, considered with the radiologic evidence of which bone, ligament, and joint structures have been or will be damaged, allows some prediction of the duration of cervical stability and, hence, of the necessity for urgent management.

Plain tomography and computed tomography (CAT scan) aid in assessing spinal skeletal function and precise location of expanding compressive lesions. CAT scan is the most important current method of identifying extent of bony tumors in the cervical spine. Myelography is often necessary to proper evaluation; indeed, it is mandatory if there are neurologic symptoms and signs. An intradural cord lesion may be diagnostically separated from bone tumor that is extending into the spinal canal and compressing the cord. Also, asymptomatic extradural tumors, not yet observable on plain films, are identifiable through myelography. Angiography allows assessment of vascularization and provides evidence of vertebral artery obstruction, tortuosity, or arterial deflection by bony lesion.

The diagnostic methods previously discussed permit projection of the best means of obtaining tissue biopsy, the ultimate necessity in diagnosis. These methods are also useful in operative planning, radiologic therapy of a tumor, and educated guessing of the type of tumor, which further identifies degree of urgency.

Histologic Identification. Unfortunately, some physicians are still willing to treat patients with tumors of the cervical spine without first making a precise histologic and pathologic diagnosis of the tumor type. Both radiotherapy and surgical management require tissue diagnosis and virtually always should be pursued.

Data Useful in Clinical Projection of Probable Tumor Type. Metastatic tumor disease of the cervical spine is far more common than primary malignancy. Bony metastatic tumors coexist at different levels. Benign tumors are more common than malignant tumors. Benign tumors of the cervical spine can cause far more severe damage, morbidity, and even death because of their location, the mechanical difficulty of excision, and the damage to spinal cord, rootlets, nerve roots, ganglia, or peripheral nerves secondary to their expansile growth.

One can be secure about metastatic disease in the presence of identified, primary malignant disease or multiple bony metastases elsewhere in the skeleton. Malignant disease may appear first as a spinal metastasis. The most common primary sites for vertebral metastases are breast, lung, prostate, thyroid, and colon, in that order of frequency. Cohen et al[5] reports that one half of vertebral metastases originate from those primary sites. A child with a cervical spine tumor is far more likely to have a benign disease, but an adult is more likely to have metastatic lesions from a primary malignancy. Primary cervical tumors in adults are likely to be malignant. Thoracic and lumbar spine metastases are more common than cervical spine metastases.

Spinal Cord Tumors

Spinal cord tumors, rare though they are, are always a part of the differential diagnosis of neck pain. They arise from cell types within the spinal cord or may be metastatic. Such tumors can be primary or secondary, extradural or intradural, and intradural tumors require further sorting into extramedullary or intramedullary. Extradural tumors can be primary or metastatic and can involve vertebral bodies or the extradural space or both. Tumor types are lymphoma, carcinoma, sarcoma, or multiple myeloma, which by bony encroachment may compress the spinal cord. Intradural but extramedullary tumors (neurofibromas, lipomas, dermoids, hemangiomas, and even metastatic tumors) come from nerve roots, meninges, and possibly blood vessels or other nervous system connective tissue. Onset of symptoms and signs is slow and only very gradually progressive; onset is rarely abrupt. Pain and paresthesias are the most common symptoms. Motor and reflex signs are also important but usually not primary in onset.

Pain is gradual in onset and may be sharply localized or radicular in character. Change in position, cough, sneeze, or rise in cerebrospinal fluid pressure results in increased pain. Loss of ascending and descending neural pathways is so gradual that motor and sensory functional changes are very slow in appearance. A Brown-Séquard syndrome is frequent, with contralateral loss of pain and temperature and ipsilateral loss of proprioceptive perception.

With anteroposterior pressure by the tumor, proprioceptive sensation symptoms are more striking; with lateral compression, the lateral spinothalamic tracts are involved, and more sensory loss occurs at distal sites in the body. Motor changes are spastic in type in the lower extremity, with little atrophy. There is root involvement with a lower motor neuron deficit in the area of the involved root. Spasm and hyper-reflexia are common, as paramedial tract function is compromised. Useful diagnostic clinical tests include Babinski's sign, Gordon's sign, and Hoffmann's sign.

Intramedullary tumors, of neural origin and of glial, ependymal, or vascular cell type, arise in the gray matter of the cord, near the central canal, and later extend into the white matter. Pain is poorly localized and is rarely radicular; sensory changes are only vaguely described, with segmental loss of pain and temperature and little change in proprioception or tactile perception. Spotty sensation changes may occur, and with lower motor neuron involvement, motor signs are focal and widespread, with paralysis, atrophy, and fasciculations—sometimes simulating multiple sclerosis. Changes in deep tendon reflexes (paramedial tract signs) are late. Syringomyelia is a part of the differential diagnosis.

Detailed clinical examination, radiologic study, electromyography, cerebrospinal fluid analysis, and myelography are all properly applied in diagnosis. Results of Queckenstedt's test may be positive, and the test is always important to do. A finding of xanthochromic spinal fluid with increase in cerebrospinal fluid protein concentration is diagnostically useful, and the electromyogram may localize the area of root involvement, especially in extramedullary tumors. Myelography is required for differentiation of extra- and intramedullary tumors and their localization. The common herniation of intervertebral cervical discs may produce a clinical syndrome similar to that of extramedullary tumors, particularly in the cervical spine. Table 18–5, adapted from DeJong,[6] lists differential points in diagnosis of extramedullary and intramedullary spinal cord tumors.

Neurofibromatosis. The cervical spine has received little attention in the literature on neurofibromatosis. Abnormal curvatures in the thoracic and lumbar spine are often reported. Yong-Hing[7] noted that 17 of 56 patients with neurofibromatosis had cervical spine abnormalities. Scalloping of vertebral bodies, foraminal enlargement, and radicular symptoms occur. There may be limited or very painful cervical spine motion. There are more deformities of the anterior portion of the cervical spine than of the posterior. Kyphosis and atlanto-occipital subluxation have occurred, and neurologic deficit, tetraparesis, hemiparesis, and radicular symptoms may occur. The neurofibromatosis process may occur in the ligaments, particularly anteriorly and around the anterior bony structures, with varying magnitudes of bony involvement. Parts A and B of Figure 18–1 illustrate radiologic lesions of cervical neurofibromatosis in a 52-year-old man. Part C shows early neurofibromatosis in a 58-year-old man. The neurofibromatosis involves C5 and C6 and is superimposed on cervical osteoarthritis. There was a large defect on the right side at C5–C6. The lesion would not have been suspected had he not had neurofibromatosis in skin, café au lait spots, kyphosis due to lesions in the thoracic spine, and mental deficiency.

Desmoid Tumors. Desmoid tumors result from fibromatosis. They are benign, nonencapsulated, fibroblastic tissues, without mitoses or other malignant characteristics. They may be mono- or multifocal, even generalized, and they infiltrate surrounding tissues but do not have metastases. The etiology of these lesions is unkown. In children, they may be self-limiting or even disappear or develop into benign fibromas that can be excised. Recurrence will follow incomplete excision.

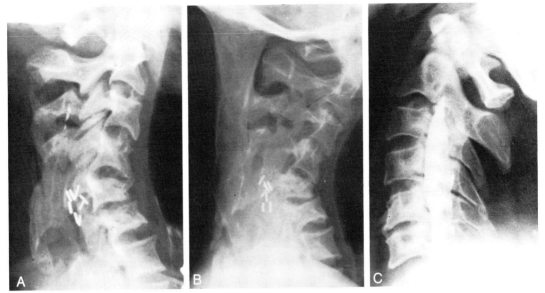

Figure 18–1. *A,* Neurofibromatosis involving C3 and C4 in minimal degree and in marked degree, the collapse of C5 and C6 with consequent kyphosis in the cervical spine. *B,* Neurofibromatosis 7 years after cervical spine fusion, showing the solid bone from the occiput throughout the cervical spine. *C,* Early neurofibromatosis at C5 and C6 in a 58-year-old man.

The tumor is thought to arise from muscular aponeurosis and other connective tissues of skeletal muscle.[2]

Multiple Myeloma. The most common cervical tumor in the adult spine is multiple myeloma. Two thirds of the patients with multiple myeloma have vertebral involvement, and one third have vertebral pain. Occasionally, a single vertebral body with solitary plasmacytoma may appear. Such patients have an improved prognosis and longer survival over those with multiple myeloma (Figs. 18–2 and 18–3). The tumor is well encapsulated, and complete excision is a possibility.

Giant Cell Tumors. Giant cell tumors in the cervical spine may be characterized by local pain as well as spinal cord compression symptomatology. The symptoms vary with the level of the vertebra involved. The majority of these tumors have a benign course and only rarely metastasize. Spastic tetraparesis, tetraplegia, and a whole spec-

Table 18–5. EXTRAMEDULLARY AND INTRAMEDULLARY TUMORS OF THE SPINAL CORD

	Extramedullary Tumor	Intramedullary Tumor
Spontaneous pain	Radicular in type and distribution; early and important symptom	Burning in type; poorly localized
Sensory changes	Contralateral loss of pain and temperature sensation; ipsilateral loss of proprioception	Dissociation of sensation; spotty changes
Change in pain and temperature perception in saddle area	More marked than at level of lesion	Less marked than at level of lesion
Lower motor neuron involvement	Segmental	Marked and widespread with atrophy and fasciculation
Pyramidal paresis	Prominent	Late and minimal
Deep reflexes	Increased early	Change minimal and late
Pyramidal responses	Early	Late
Trophic changes	Usually not marked	Marked
Spinal subarachnoid block and spinal fluid changes	Early and marked	Late and less marked

Adapted from DeJong RN: The Neurologic Examination, 3rd ed. New York: Harper & Row, 1967.

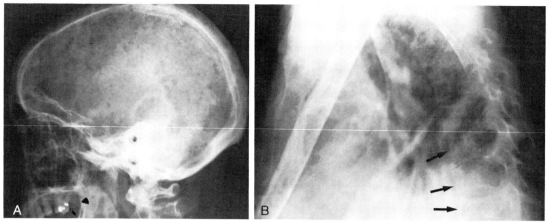

Figure 18–2. *A,* Multiple myeloma. Note the many "punched out" areas in the skull, a very commonly involved site that is diagnostic. There are some lesions in the mandible. *B,* The cervical spine in this case was quite symptomatic, and although the characteristic and extreme osteopenia was noted, there were no lesions detected with certainty. There were clearly myelomatous lesions with collapse of vertebra, as shown by the arrows in the thoracic spine. Note that the humerus in the illustration also had large myelomatous lesions.

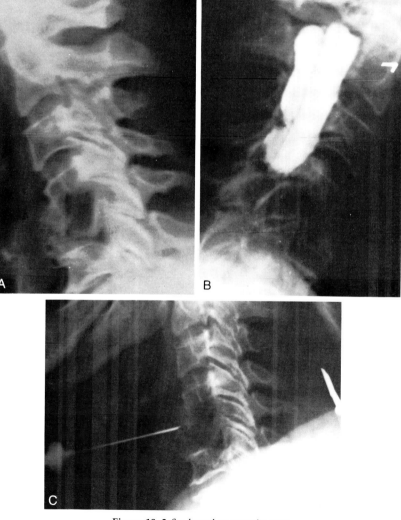

Figure 18–3 *See legend on opposite page*

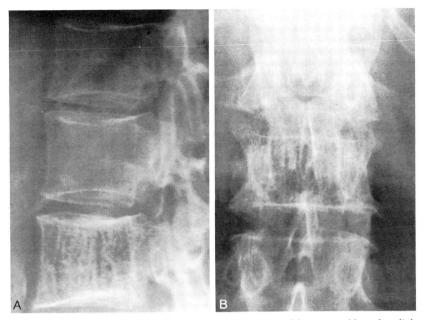

Figure 18–4. *A*, Vertebral hemangioma of L2; lateral view in a 44-year-old woman. Note the slight articular plate depression, marked coarsening of the trabeculae, and a very coarse medullary pattern involving all of the major part of a vertebral body, sometimes extending into the pedicle. Vertical striations within the vertebral body represent residual trabeculae. Hemangiomas do not result in either vertebral enlargement or cortical thickening, as is seen in Paget's disease. The differential diagnosis includes solitary metastases and solitary plasmacytoma. Hemangiomas are usually benign with no malignant degeneration and, as in his case, are asymptomatic, discovered by chance. The incidence increases with increasing age, and there is a female preponderance. *B*, Anteroposterior view of the lesion in *A*. This illustration is characteristic of the same lesion in a cervical vertebra.

trum of neurologic and rheumatologic symptoms and signs may occur. Incomplete excision of a vertebral giant cell tumor leaves the possibility of malignant transformation. Radiation therapy likewise may contribute to this unfortunate event. Giant cell tumors usually involve the vertebral body rather than the posterior elements, and they commonly present with neural compression as their primary clinical sign.

Eosinophilic Granuloma. Eosinophilic granuloma occurs in both children and adults and results in neurologic signs and symptoms, depending on the site and level of the lesion. A lytic lesion with erosion and collapse of the vertebra may be the initial radiographic appearance.

Aneurysmal Bone Cysts. These benign lesions occur frequently in the cervical spine. Expansile destruction of bone is a possibility and may involve two or more vertebral bodies, usually serially. The extension through the disc space is characteristic of a malignant lesion.

Osteoid Osteoma. Osteoid osteoma occurs primarily in the pedicle and the posterior elements, not in the vertebral body.[8] It may become symptomatic before becoming apparent on the plain radiogram. Technetium bone scan nearly always identifies the lesion.

Osteochondroma. This lesion results in a very large mass that is usually benign and well delineated on the radiograph. If the radiologist diagnoses a benign osteoblastoma, one must be aware of the possibility that the lesion could represent primary osteogenic sarcoma.

Vertebral Hemangioma. The most common types of vertebral hemangioma are venous and cavernous hemangiomas. Characteristic vertical trabeculation of the body of the vertebra is diagnostic. Transosseous phlebography shows the massive staining of the body of the involved vertebra, with considerable venous outflow. Figure 18–4 shows a typical vertebral hemangioma in a lumbar vertebra.

Figure 18–3. *A*, Multiple myeloma involving C1–C5 with major lesions and C6 with a smaller one. There is vertebral collapse, with the greatest severity in C5, almost obliterating the vertebra. *B*, The same patient's myelogram shows complete obstruction, with no flow of dye past the multiple myeloma lesion. *C*, The placing of a needle for diagnostic purposes and aspiration from the anterior approach, penetrating the approximate level of the upper border of C5 near the intervertebral disc. Successful aspiration was achieved and histologic diagnosis confirmed. Strangely, in this case there were no neurologic symptoms.

Cartilaginous Exostoses (Osteochondromas, Osteochondral Exostoses). The clinical symptoms are usually of long duration, are characterized by paresthesia, and often are located in the ulnar nerve distribution, with brachialgia and weakness of the involved side. Pain is worse with movements of the head, particularly flexion and extension. Weakness of most muscles on the involved side and depressed tendon reflexes occur.

The clinical syndrome may be intermittent, involving weakness of one arm and hand for weeks to months, with a return of power that is eventually replaced by a recurrence of the syndrome. Atrophy of the hand muscles occurs, particularly if the lesion is at the C7–T1 level.

The exostoses are usually seen on plain films and may be in unusual places on the vertebra (on the pedicles as well as the body). They are not necessarily in the usual distribution of chondro-osteophytes of osteoarthritis. Clinically, the hard swellings may be felt at the site of the radiologic lesion. There may be no neurologic disturbances; vertebral angiograms may be indicated.

Metastatic Carcinoma. Any malignant tumor can metastasize to bone, but the most common sites of primary carcinoma are the breast, prostate gland, kidney, thyroid, and lung. Primary malignant tumors in the spine are rare, but metastatic tumors are common, particularly in patients over age 50. In some large series metastatic bone cancer is the most common malignancy of bone. In fact, it is estimated that 50% to 70% of cancer patients have metastases of the spine.[9] The first evidence of malignant disease is commonly the appearance of a spinal metastasis, and spread to the thoracic and lumbar portions of the spine is more frequent than spread to the cervical area.

The two pathways by which tumor cells reach the vertebral column are the venous system and the arterial system. The lymphatic channels serve as a third but less probable pathway. Bone destruction occurs owing to tumor cell proliferation and reactive bone formation stimulated to combat the tumor's destructive forces. Thus, both osteolytic and osteoblastic activity can be seen in any one tumor. Most tumors are osteolytic, but prostatic carcinoma is predominantly osteoblastic. Pain is a predominant complaint and in nature, severity, and distribution may mimic that caused by any of the other tumors, sepsis, osteoarthritis, and herniated intervertebral disc. Pain usually precedes any radiologic signs, and thus normal radiologic study does not rule out metastatic carcinoma. An extensive history and physical examination are required, particularly since the surgeon tends to gloss over examination of thyroid, breast, and prostate gland. A high index of suspicion should be maintained regarding patients over 50 years of age who are experiencing even slightly obscure spinal pain. Serum alkaline phosphatase level may be elevated in patients with metastatic carcinoma of the cervical spine, and acid phosphatase level is elevated if the primary source is prostatic carcinoma. The sedimentation rate is usually elevated in patients who have any malignant tumor. Bone, thyroid, and liver scans are useful in more precise diagnosis. Figure 18–5 illustrates metastatic carcinoma from a primary source in the breast to the upper cervical spine.

Ependymoma. Ependymomas are intramedullary tumors of two major histologic types: 28% are ependymomas, and 34% are astrocytomas. No other type of tumor has a significant percentage, but almost any other glioma type may be intramedullary.

Pain is common at the level of the lesion but is

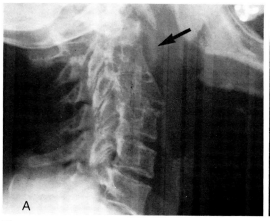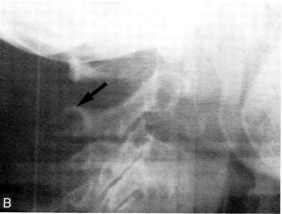

Figure 18–5. *A*, Metastatic carcinoma from a primary source in the breast to the cervical spine. Note the extreme softening and partial collapse of C2 and C3, with some remodeling of the second and third vertebral bodies. *B*, The softening of bone about the foramen magnum, and projection of the odontoid process into the foramen magnum. The base of the body of the axis is grossly eroded and extremely thin. There is a mottled appearance to C2–C3, with "holes" in the vertebra as well as in the intervertebral disc.

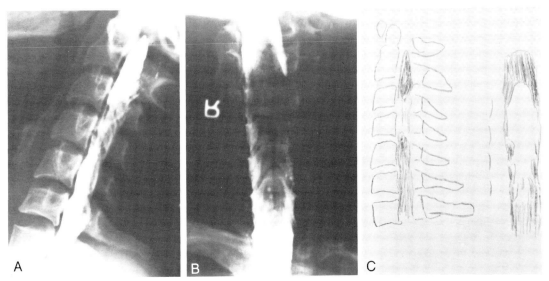

Figure 18–6. *A,* Myelogram in the case of a 40-year-old woman with an ependymoma at the level of C3–C4. Note the large ovoid defect surrounding the radiopaque myelographic dye. Satisfactory filling of the spinal canal occurred, but the oil passed slowly along the periphery of the spinal cord in this area. There is no abnormality above or below this level. The radiologist strongly suspected an intramedullary expanding lesion, tumor, or syringomyelia. The tumor was successfully removed and there was histologic confirmation of the ependymoma. *B,* Anteroposterior view of the same lesion. *C,* Drawing of the lateral film as perceived by the radiologist, and on the right the anteroposterior view is drawn in. Planograms failed to show any erosive lesions of the pedicles; the interpedicular distances were normal, as was the sagittal diameter of the spinal canal. There was no evidence of local bony changes noted in the myelogram at the site of the bulge in the spinal cord.

not radicular in type. A local band of hyperesthesia occurs. Sensory and motor changes normally are worse at the level of the lesion than distally (the reverse of the extramedullary tumor). Perianal sensory sparing is common. With this anterior horn cell involvement, segmental fasciculations are seen. Quadriparesis and spasticity occur late in the disease, as does bowel and bladder dysfunction. Plain cervical spine films may show widening of the spinal canal, with pedicle erosion and an increase in the transverse diameter (interpedicular distance). The myelogram, sometimes combined with the CAT scan, is usually diagnostic. A symmetric widening of the spinal cord, fusiform, is characteristic. There are no diagnostic differential characteristics between astrocytoma and ependymoma; surgical exploration is necessary for precise identification.

It is possible to remove an ependymoma, with complete preservation of neurologic function. This was first accomplished in 1954 by Greenwood.[10] With microsurgical techniques, an ependymoma is a curable tumor. It is readily separable from the enclosing spinal cord and can usually be removed with no neurologic catastrophe. This is not true of the astrocytoma. Figure 18–6 illustrates an ependymoma.

Meningioma. Seventy-one per cent of the intradural tumors are extramedullary. Of these, 32% are meningiomas, and 38% are schwannomas.

Other rare tumors occurring intradurally are sarcomas, angiomas, cordomas, lymphomas, lipomas, epidermoids, melanomas, and neuroblastomas. Meningiomas are benign tumors and are usually curable. They are first suspected with the symptom of radicular pain and paresthesia. The pain is distinctively continuous, exaggerated by cough, sneeze, or straining, and very typically worse at night.[11] Muscle atrophy, diminished reflexes, and sensory loss are characteristic. If there is anterior horn cell compression, focal fasciculations may follow. Spinal cord compression signs, though uncommon, are rarely symmetric. Motor function is usually compromised on the side of the tumor, and pain and temperature loss occurs on the opposite side. The motor loss is spastic, and it is exaggerated in the flexors rather than the extensors. Sense of touch is diminished in a patchy distribution. Sweating may be decreased below the level of the lesion, and bowel and bladder dysfunction is common. Results of the plain radiographic study may be normal. Bone erosions may occur. Both CAT scan and myelography are necessary for proper diagnostic security. Intradural, extramedullary tumors are sharply circumscribed and clearly separate from the spinal cord. A lumbar puncture no longer aids in the diagnosis, and electromyelography is rarely indicated. If hemangioma or arterial venous fistula is suspected, spinal cord angiography is indicated.

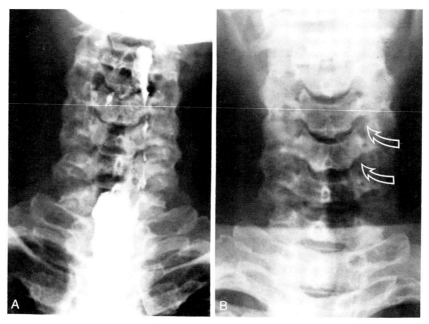

Figure 18–7. *A,* Meningioma. A myelogram of a 45-year-old woman with 2 years of paresis and unsteady gait. Note the almost complete obstruction of the pantopaque column by the tumor at the level of C6–C7. The tumor was intradural and extramedullary and was successfully removed, with the patient achieving an asymptomatic state. It was a histologically proven meningioma. *B,* The anteroposterior view shows some bony erosion at the C5–C6 and C6–C7 levels.

The only available therapy is surgical removal through a standard laminectomy. Figure 18–7 illustrates radiologic diagnosis of a meningioma in a 45-year-old woman. The tumor was successfully removed.

Osteochondroma. Osteocartilaginous exostoses are really the manifestations of osteoarthritis, and they may show gross radiologic evidence of huge exostoses, with no clinical symptoms or signs. Or the reverse situation may occur, in which there is only moderate evidence of osteochondromas, with extensive disability and objective as well as subjective symptoms and signs. Figure 18–8 illustrates the cervical film of a patient with moderate radiologic changes and gross clinical changes. Surgical removal of these osteochondral exostoses was successful; some residua were left, but the patient was fully functional.

INFECTIONS OF THE CERVICAL SPINE

Though infections in the cervical spine are rare, the consequence of failure of diagnosis is so ominous as to make infection a necessary consideration in instances of even slightly aberrant cervical spine syndromes. About 15% of bone infections involve the spine, but it is the most common site of tuberculosis of bone. Of the entire spine—cervical, thoracic, lumbar, and sacral—the cervical spine is the most uncommon site for infection. Though all age groups may have infections in the spine, the two heights of incidence are in the second and after the fifth decade.

Only 1% of all cases of skeletal infections occur in the spine; only 4% of these occur in the cervical spine.[12, 13] Spinal tuberculosis is more frequent than pyogenic infections of the spine. The prevalence and incidence of tuberculosis of the cervical spine are a function of the prevalence and incidence of the disease in the geographic area. Thus, the greater the disease prevalence, the greater the incidence of cervical spine involvement.

Certain population groups may be more susceptible to cervical spine infection. These groups include very young children, hemodialysis patients, and the elderly, with such diseases as diabetes, severe osteoarthritis, and renal failure. Persons being operated upon for cervical osteoarthritis and those having angiograms or discograms are also at risk. The commonest organisms found in all series are the staphylococcus, with gram-negative bacilli infections increasing, and the streptococcus, which is more common in children. Involvement by fungi and parasites is extremely rare. The route of entry of organisms is usually hematogenous, but the organisms may spread from such areas as the nasopharynx or tonsils, or they may enter via intervertebral disc surgery or procedures such as enzyme treatment of discs or discography. Infection following interbody vertebral fusion may occur, and it sometimes remains undiagnosed for long periods.

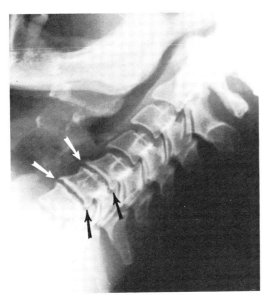

Figure 18–8. At the C5–C6 level are large anterior and posterior osteocartilaginous exostoses (osteochondromas) compressing the spinal cord (white arrows anterior, black, posterior). This lesion was neurologically symptomatic and was successfully removed. Clinically there were marked paresthesias and atrophy of muscles of the thenar eminence, the hypothenar eminence, and the dorsal interosseous muscles. Ring fingers and little fingers were in flexion, and there was weakness of the abductor muscles of the little finger, the interosseous, lumbrical muscles, and the muscles of the thumb. Light-touch and pin-prick and vibration sense were absent over the little finger and the medial half of the ring finger. The objective clinical evidence takes precedence over radiologic characteristics.

Pathologic Events

Owing to the lush vascular supply to vertebral bone, the bacterial entry is hematogenous. It is more likely arterial than venous because of the pressure gradient phenomenon. The valveless internal venous system promotes interspinal spread once infection is established.[14]

Organisms may accumulate and localize in the vertebral metaphysis, where an abscess may begin in the hairpin-loop, capillary sinusoidal space of cancellous bone. Success of the spread of the organism can lead to bone destruction and spread to adjacent vertebrae or into the intervertebral discs. Increased blood flow as hyperemia results in the loss of bone density and ultimate bony collapse and deformity. Pyogenic abscesses develop more rapidly than tuberculous abscesses. Hypertrophic changes occur in the area, with excess bone production and sclerosis. Sequestra of bone and disc may isolate and compress roots and ganglia. The balance between organism virulence and immunologic competence of the host is the deciding factor regarding degree of disease development.

In children, atlantoaxial subluxation occurs in response to infectious processes without direct bony involvement. This is known as Grisel's syndrome (see Chapter 14, *Cervical Spine in Infancy and Childhood*). This sepsis produces torticollis secondary to atlantoaxial subluxation. The mechanisms are hyperemia and osteopenia, which induce joint effusion and ligamentous laxity, culminating in instability. Management is usually satisfactory.

Clinical Symptoms and Signs

Cervical spine sepsis may have relatively little systemic or immunologic response. Neck pain, with radiation to the shoulders and sometimes into the arms, and occipital headache are more likely early symptoms, that is, the symptoms are not very impressive. Dysphagia may occur. Radicular signs or even myelopathy may appear later. Other signs include restricted range of motion, rather striking muscle spasm, and occipital tenderness. Attention to examination of tenderness of the cervical spinous processes is clinically rewarding. The Spurling test result may be positive (head compression). Sometimes an abscess may be palpable anteriorly. Neurologic signs, paresthesia, pain, and radiculitis are likely to occur late.

Cervical spine infection usually has been present 3 weeks before diagnosis is made, and even then a high index of suspicion is required. Radiographic changes occur in 3 to 6 weeks. Leukocytosis and anemia occur in the presence of a vigorous immunologic response, and the erythrocyte sedimentation rate is commonly elevated early, raising a red flag to the clinician. Blood culture should always be done but may not be helpful. Tomographic evidence will appear after 2 weeks at the earliest, and radiographic changes appear at least 4 weeks following onset of disease. Bone scan with technetium or gallium is the most important diagnostic test apart from clinical examination and careful re-examination. The appearance of osteopenia secondary to reactive hyperemia and consequent osteolysis is diagnostically useful though not an early sign. Retropharyngeal space enlargement may provide the first definitive clue. Pyogenic lesions are associated with reactive new bone formation, which occurs within 2 to 3 months or even later in tuberculosis.

Bacteriologic confirmation is necessary in order to select appropriate antibiotic. Trocar aspiration from bone or even open vertebral biopsy may be done; the latter procedure is safer. Differentiation from tumor is a part of the differential diagnosis. Chills, fever, and malaise of varying intensity and frequency occur.

Management

All general measures are required—rest, proper diet, treatment of the underlying general medical problem, external cervical support, and specific

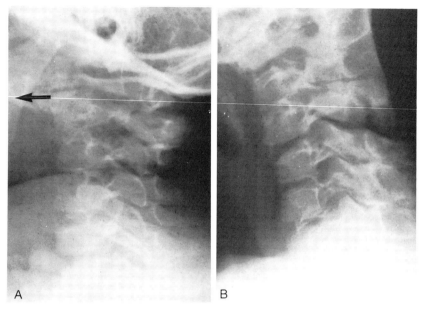

Figure 18–9. *A*, A 3½-year-old boy with severe tuberculosis of the cervical spine. Note bone destruction, marked subluxation of the atlas on the axis. (See arrow for anterior arch of the atlas, extensive bony erosion, and loss of bone substance.) *B*, One year later, after fusion of the cervical spine, a pseudoarthrosis at C4–C5 was noted. The radiologic evidence for activity of the tuberculosis was gone. Incidentally, films 20 years later disclosed a completely fused cervical spine (pseudoarthrosis repaired in 1973). The patient had had a very functional existence, and the cervical spine tuberculosis was cured.

antibiotic therapy for pyogenic infection. Tuberculosis requires triple therapy—streptomycin, 2 g per week, para-aminosalicylic acid (PAS), 12 g per day, and isoniazid, 300 mg daily.

The role of surgery is not clear, but one should always have surgical consultation, particularly if the disease is progressing rapidly. Indications for surgery include the establishment of a diagnosis (i.e., open biopsy), moderate to severe uncontrolled infection, rapidly developing neurologic deficits, cervical spine instability, abscess or sequestrum, and clear-cut definite lack of response to medical management.

In the case of tuberculosis, vertebral material must be obtained and the primary focus identified (Fig. 18–9). Histologic confirmation is desirable, but culture and sensitivity studies require 4 to 6 weeks, and triple-drug therapy should be initiated as soon as bacterial diagnosis is made. In general, the prevention of instability and deformity is required, and the principles of management for cervical spine trauma apply. Complete immobilization should almost never be done. The cervical spine tends to stabilize itself if given proper and continuing management. Surgery is indicated relatively rarely in tuberculosis nowadays. In the Western World, pyogenic bacteria from an iatrogenic source are more often responsible for tuberculosis than the tubercle bacillus. In the remaining three quarters of the world's population that is not true, and tuberculosis remains an endemic scourge.

References

1. Geschickter CF, Copeland MM: Tumors of Bone, 3rd ed. Philadelphia: J. B. Lippincott Co, 1949.
2. Verbiest H: Tumors involving the cervical spine. *In* Bailey RW, Sherk HH (eds): The Cervical Spine. Philadelphia: J. B. Lippincott Co, 1984, ch 12, p 430.
3. Hastings D, McNab I, Lawson V: Neoplasms of the atlas and axis. Can J Surg 11:290, 1968.
4. White A: Biomechanical stability of the cervical spine. Clin Orthop 109:85, 1975.
5. Cohen D, Dohlin D, McCarty C: Apparently solitary tumors of the vertebral column. Mayo Clin Proc 39:509, 1964.
6. DeJong RN: The Neurologic Examination, 3rd ed. New York: Harper & Row, 1967.
7. Yong-Hing K, Kalamchi A, MacEwen G: Cervical spine abnormalities in neurofibromatosis. J Bone Joint Surg 61A:695, 1979.
8. MacLellan D, Wilson F Jr: Osteoid osteoma of the spine. J Bone Joint Surg 49A:111, 1967.
9. Fornasier V, Horne J: Metastases to the vertebral column. Cancer 36:590, 1975.
10. Greenwood J: Total removal of intramedullary tumors. J Neurosurg 11:616, 1954.
11. Austin GM: The significance and nature of pain in tumors of the spinal cord. Surg Forum 10:782, 1959.
12. Stone DB, Bonfiglio M: Pyogenic vertebral osteomyelitis. Arch Intern Med 112:491, 1963.
13. Forsythe M, Rothman RH: New concepts in the diagnosis and treatment of infections of the cervical spine. Orthop Clin North Am 9:1039, 1978.
14. Wiley AM, Trueta J: The vascular anatomy of the spine and its relationship to pyogenic vertebral osteomyelitis. J Bone Joint Surg 41B:796, 1959.

Part III ○ SPECIAL CONSIDERATIONS

Chapter 19

Consultation for Disease and Trauma of the Cervical Spine: Who? When? Why? Where? How?

Since one in every six visits by a patient to a health professional is for a musculoskeletal complaint[1] and at any given time 9% of the adult male population and 12% of the adult female population has some discomfort in the neck with and without associated arm pain and 35% of the population can recall having pain in the neck, it is obvious that these complaints are commonplace indeed.[2] Rheumatology is surely the most complicated subspecialty in all of medicine. In terms of sound basic science understructure it is also the youngest. Beginning about 1948, basic knowledge in immunology, biochemistry, physical chemistry, biomechanics, basic physiology of connective tissue structures (particularly joints), and pharmacology has grown enormously. Many rheumatic diseases are now understandable as major clinical expressions of these basic sciences, i.e., pathophysiology. Orthopedic surgeons have become exceedingly capable in reconstructive surgery, with metal and plastic prostheses solving problems in pain relief and mobility. Many other health care professionals, including nurses, physical and occupational therapists, social workers, clinical psychologists, and physiatrists, have become very involved in the field of rheumatology.

Unfortunately, the word *arthritis* is regarded by the public at large and by a surprising number of physicians in practice as a single disease about which little can be done and for which aspirin is the best, and perhaps the only, medication—a sad but true commentary today. Thus, a great deal of public education as well as physician and other health care professional education remains to be done. Since there are officially 109 different diseases in the field of rheumatology, making the most precise diagnosis and identification possible is an important issue.[3] Having said that, one can still state that the great majority of patients with musculoskeletal complaints can be well and properly managed by the primary care physician, requiring no consultation. This is true of virtually all musculoskeletal complaints, including those concerning the cervical spine. Rheumatic reasons for visits to health care professionals turn out to be focal conditions, with little or no threat to the health, performance, and continuing activity of the patient. The great majority of these conditions can be readily identified as self-limiting. The physician's job is to rule out more significant diseases, to teach the patient the mechanism of production of symptoms, to advise the patient regarding alternating physical activity and rest, to reassure the patient, sometimes to prescribe symptomatic therapy with pharmacologic agents, and always to teach that natural healing processes will solve the clinical problem. In general, such lesions require 2 to 6 weeks to heal. The time is a function of how serious the problem is; how symptomatic it is; if it resulted from an injury, what the magnitude of injury was, and whether reinjury may occur during the waiting period. An important issue is that at a basic science level there is no evidence to suggest that any pharmacologic agent will favorably affect the healing process in clinical disorders discussed here. The clinical problems should not be raised to a degree of concern unrelated to their magnitude. Excessive investigative efforts are costly and sometimes damaging, and the side effects of drugs may prolong the simple problem. Of great importance is that the rheumatic disease patient be managed as an individual (not as a disease); decisions in management must be based on individual characteristics and circumstances.[4] Any management and therapeutic decisions are made and modified on the basis of continual assessment of the interaction between application of treatment and response to treatment. Such serial decision making is the key to optimum management. Management changes and new decisions are made, and the old ones are discarded, altering with time, clinical response, rapidity of progress of the disease, and what favorable responses have been obtained in the past in a specific patient.

An important and critical clinical decision is whether further investigation (outside consultation) and management action are required initially or later in the course of the disorder—in other words, whether it is better to postpone further investigation until after the course of the disorder unfolds and the response to initial management is assessed. Fries has designed an excellent algorithm that is useful in determining the need for more than initial clinical investigation. Chronicity or duration of the clinical syndrome is the usual indication for more elaborate investigation, consultation, and changes in management. He proposes that in the great majority of clinical disorders an observation period of 6 weeks is proper. Figure 19–1 shows the Fries algorithm.[5] Four exceptions are made: (1) severe condition involving a single joint or a few joints; (2) febrile, systemically ill patient, with indications of major disease of multiple organs; (3) syndrome associated with major significant trauma; and (4) associated neurologic problem. Application of this algorithm to the great majority of patients with cervical spine complaints constitutes an effective guide to additional clinical and laboratory investigation and the seeking of consultation.

Although the great majority of patients with disease and disorder of the cervical spine are appropriately and properly managed by the pri-

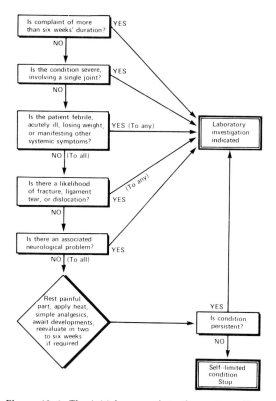

Figure 19–1. The initial approach to the patient. (From Fries JF: General approach to the rheumatic disease patient. *In* Kelley WN, Harris ED, Ruddy S, et al (eds): Textbook of Rheumatology, 2nd ed. Philadelphia: W. B. Saunders Co, 1985, p. 363.)

mary care physician, there are still instances in the course of the clinical syndrome when the ongoing feedback between application of treatment and clinical response clearly indicates consultation by specialists who are more skilled and better informed. In such circumstances, the course of the patient's illness may be favorably altered by such consultation. Some of the rheumatic diseases are highly variable, with remissions and exacerbations of unpredictable duration. The pathologic events proceeding as chronic disease can subtly impair function. The now extremely complicated immunologic events, physicochemical changes, biochemistry, and pharmacology result in the occasional requirement for interpretation and change of decision making. Among the factors affecting decisions concerning how to manage the problem are the highly variable clinical and immunologic response to a specific treatment, the too rapid loss of critical tissue to erosion, and, lastly and frequently most importantly, the innumerable and subtle ways in which some rheumatic diseases compromise the patient's lifestyle, marriage, other family relationships, employability, and self image. At critical times, the consultant may contribute to the prevention, rehabilitation,

Table 19–1. CONSULTANTS FOR PATIENTS WITH DISEASES OF THE CERVICAL SPINE

Rheumatologist
Neurologist
Physiatrist (rehabilitation specialist)
Neurosurgeon
Orthopedic surgeon
Psychiatrist
Clinical psychologist
Pain clinic
Radiologist
Pathologist
Physical therapist
Rehabilitation nurse
Occupational therapist
Social worker
Vocational counselor
Prosthetist, orthotist, and brace maker
Kinesiologist
Sexual counselor
Nutritionist
Visiting nurse
Recreational therapist

and arrest of the disease process and occasionally may even contribute to its reversal and the patient's cure. The goal of this chapter is to cite the consultants that may be sought, the reasons for selecting them, whom to select, when, why, where, and how. The decision to seek consultation requires considerable experience, clinical judgment, skill, sympathy, empathy, and humanity on the part of the managing physician.[6, 7] Table 19–1 provides a list of the consultants discussed in this chapter.

CONSULTANTS
Rheumatologist

The rheumatologist is the only physician devoting all professional effort to the rheumatic diseases. Rheumatology is surely the broadest of the subspecialties. The training and preparation to be a rheumatologist include years of study in the general field of internal medicine and successful completion of the examination for certification in the field of internal medicine by the American Board of Internal Medicine. Also included are several years of specific training in the field of rheumatology and successful completion of the examination for certification in the field of rheumatology by the American Subspecialty Board of Rheumatology. Because of the rheumatologist's broad education and special interest and focus on the diseases included in the field of rheumatology, it is his or her responsibility to apply the most recent scientific information to the direct care of patients with rheumatic diseases. Rheumatologic specialists, whether they are academics or practitioners, translate scientific knowledge into clinical

rheumatologic practice. They are consultants for patients, referring physicians, orthopedic surgeons, physical therapists, occupational therapists, and, most notably, primary care physicians. In general, the rheumatologist remains a consultant, extending care to patients through their primary care physician. Nowadays there are practicing rheumatologists who successfully deliver primary care in the field of rheumatology and serve as the primary care physician. There are several degrees of overlapping interest between internal medicine and rheumatology, and properly so.

As noted in Chapter 11, *Differential Diagnosis and Specific Treatment*, the syndromes involving the cervical spine are legion. The great majority can be managed properly without specific consultation. If, however, symptoms persist beyond 6 weeks, physical signs appear, and a secure and satisfactory diagnosis by the primary care physician or internist has not been made, a rheumatologist should be consulted. The rheumatologist, more and more, has become the physician to consult in the case of undiagnosed disease, ranging from fever of undetermined origin to drop attacks to amnesia and convulsions. Because cervical spine osteoarthritis is associated with so many bizarre, likely to be misunderstood syndromes, rheumatologic consultation is advised. Because the great majority of patients with rheumatoid arthritis of the cervical spine (a very common manifestation) do not develop disability or life-threatening symptoms or signs, consultation is not necessary until the physician either suspects or clearly diagnoses such disability. Since the evidence strongly suggests that most patients get along very well, with the subluxations in the upper cervical spine and subaxially strongly tending to stabilize over a decade, rheumatologic consultation seems a sound clinical move that allows the practicing physician to take maximum advantage of all available data. Such patients are fairly likely to be operated on unnecessarily because the natural history of that particular aspect of rheumatoid arthritis is, even now, insufficiently appreciated. Surgical management of subluxations in rheumatoid arthritis and in cervical osteoarthritis is experiencing a striking increase in understanding of the pathophysiology; hence, both diagnoses in a symptomatic patient indicate the need for rheumatologic consultation. More specifically, such clinical diagnoses as drop attacks, fainting, loss of speech, visual and auditory hallucinations, and transient amnesia in the clinical setting of cervical osteoarthritis call for rheumatologic consultation. Enthusiasm for and predictability of surgical intervention are diminishing presently, and conservative treatment of such patients has become increasingly successful.

Patients with ankylosing spondylitis and a completely or partially ankylosed cervical spine should also have the advantage of rheumatologic consultation. They are at risk of sustaining fracture in relatively minor injuries and falls. As our understanding of the pathophysiology of the enthesopathic lesion increases, more support in primary management can be offered. Also, both carotid and vertebral artery syndromes are in the province of the rheumatologic specialist. Special rheumatologic knowledge is needed in peripheral neuropathy, radiculopathy, and myelopathy of both rheumatoid arthritis and cervical osteoarthritis if management is not successful and symptoms and signs are either persistent or increasing. It is virtually always wise to seek rheumatologic, orthopedic surgical, or neurosurgical consultation; ideally, the two consultants should agree. Criteria are fairly well established for surgical intervention, and agreement is common and usual. Dysphagia occurring in the course of either diffuse idiopathic skeletal hyperostosis or the osteophytosis of osteoarthritis frequently calls for rheumatologic focus. By and large, consultation is indicated in female patients with rheumatoid arthritis of very insidious onset, who have high-titer rheumatoid factor; subcutaneous rheumatoid nodules; known cartilage and bone erosions, with severe and dense cellular infiltrate; high white polymorphonuclear cell counts (50,000 to 60,000 per mm³); eosinophilia; thrombocytosis; and striking elevation of C-reactive protein concentration and of Westergren sedimentation rate. All of the previously mentioned characteristics imply severe immunologic and inflammatory disease. The rheumatologist is well informed in this very complex immunologic storm and can provide the best advice in both short- and long-term management.

Neurologist

Neurologic consultation is indicated in the following general clinical circumstances: (1) The patient has rheumatoid arthritis of the cervical spine with subluxations that are associated with definite neurologic symptoms and signs. If the neurologic signs are progressive, the indication becomes urgent. A neurologic consultation may also be indicated for the purpose of identifying neurologic symptoms and signs that may not be apparent to the primary care physician. (2) Consideration for neurologic consultation should be given in instances of peripheral neuropathy of unidentified type, entrapment neuropathies at the thoracic outlet, at the elbow, and associated with carpal tunnel syndrome at the wrist; they may be symptoms and signs of cervical myelopathy. (3) Neurosurgical or orthopedic surgical operation is being contemplated for treatment and management of a patient with cervical osteoarthritis—facetectomy, laminectomy, or chondro-osteophyte removal. (4) The patient has severe and progressive inflammatory disease of muscle—polymyositis and dermatomyositis. One would like agreement between the primary care physician, the neurosurgeon, and the neurologist.

Neurosurgeon

Neurosurgical consultation may be required in cervical spine subluxations in rheumatoid arthritis in which surgical stabilization of the spine is considered. The following clinical circumstances may require neurosurgical consultation: (1) rheumatoid arthritis of the cervical spine, with subluxations, signs and symptoms of myelopathy, radiculopathy, and peripheral neuropathy; (2) osteoarthritis of the Luschka joints, zygapophyseal joints, or vertebral chondro-osteophytes, with progressive symptoms and signs; (3) cervical spine fractures, particularly fracture in ankylosing spondylitis, rheumatoid arthritis with fracture-subluxation, or juvenile polyarthritis with soft-tissue injury or fracture; (4) any circumstance of trauma with fracture, dislocation, or both. Virtually all instances of very significant trauma require neurosurgical consultation and sometimes surgical intervention.

Orthopedic Surgeon

There is overlap in the scope of consultative services provided by the orthopedic surgeon and the neurosurgeon. In general, orthopedic consultation is especially indicated when reconstructive surgery is being considered: (1) reconstructive surgery and rehabilitation of the hand (extremely active synovitis, evidence of progressive erosion and subluxation); (2) surgery of the hip in circumstances in which there is little probability of arrest or reversal, with pain and limitation of motion being the principal considerations; (3) reconstructive surgery in ankylosing spondylitis, hip, lumbar spine, and cervical spine; (4) reconstructive surgery and rehabilitation of the knee (rheumatoid arthritis, osteoarthritis), including total knee replacement and various prostheses; (5) reconstructive surgery of the ankle and foot, including resections of the metatarsal heads and various fusions in the hindfoot—talus, calcaneus, and navicular bone; (6) surgical subluxations of the cervical spine in rheumatoid arthritis (various fusions and wiring techniques to stabilize the cervical spine); (7) correction of shoulder destruction in secondary osteoarthritis and rheumatoid arthritis.

Physiatrist

The physiatrist, or rehabilitation expert, plays a major role in problems involving the cervical spine as well as in the rheumatic diseases generally, particularly rheumatoid arthritis and osteoarthritis. Rehabilitation implies a management program designed to prevent, minimize, arrest, or reverse threatened, permanent, or protracted disability. The methods are quite different from those of usual medical care, which concentrates on curing the patient's pathology and assumes function will not be compromised. Too often, lack of cure is accepted, and the patient is left to deal with the consequences. Curative medicine focuses on reversing the primary disease process, whereas rehabilitation concentrates on preventing loss of function, restoring function, preventing contractures, maintaining muscle strength, stimulating latent control, training the patient to utilize all residual function maximally and effectively, providing assistive devices, and counseling patient and family in, when necessary, accepting an altered lifestyle.

Both curative and rehabilitation medicine should go hand in hand. The management continuum gradually shifts its emphasis from control or reversal of the pathologic lesion in the tissues to restoration of function. The physiatrist best knows the methods of preventing the terrible, debilitating consequences of uninterrupted bed rest, a frequent problem in the most severe instances of rheumatoid arthritis. Rehabilitation medicine is a multidisciplinary program as well as a multispecialty, and it blends physical therapy, occupational therapy, social work, psychology, vocational counseling, prosthetics, recreational therapy, communication education, reconstructive surgery, and rehabilitation nursing. Thus at various points in the course of disorders and diseases of the cervical spine, the physiatrist's skills and advice are required.

Radiologist

The interpretation of radiologic studies is of great importance, and consultation in unusual circumstances is indicated. In particular, the following indications exist: (1) undiagnosed clinical symptoms and signs in the cervical spine; (2) computed tomography in circumstances of soft-tissue lesions, inflammatory synovitis, metabolic bone disease, tumors, and suspected intervertebral disc herniation; (3) metrizamide-enhanced computed tomography and myelography; (4) scintigraphy and selected angiography (often critical diagnostic methods); (5) radiologic assessment of congenital malformations, particularly of the occiput-atlas-axis complex; (6) problems in clinical symptoms and signs of myelopathy, without known pathologic mechanism; (7) diagnostic ultrasonography (occasionally useful); (8) bone imaging by radonuclide methods (helpful in inflammation, tumor growth); (9) occasional needle biopsy of bone under fluoroscopic control; (10) xeroradiography (indicated uncommonly).

Pathologist

Consultation with a pathologist is indicated in the following circumstances: (1) biopsy tissue interpretation, synovium, bone biopsy, tumors of the cervical spine, spinal fluid analysis, culture of aspirated material in the case of suspected sepsis, osteomyelitis, small joint infection in the cervical spine; (2) hematologic diagnosis in rheumatic syndromes associated with hematologic diseases, hemophilia, sickle cell disease, and other hemoglobinopathies; (3) biochemical and endocrine studies in arthropathies of endocrine disorders and arthritis associated with hyperlipidemia and hypercholesterolemia; (4) musculoskeletal syndromes. Musculoskeletal syndromes are associated with malignancy often, and such diagnosis is usually a tissue diagnosis.

Psychiatrist

Though the primary care physician and rheumatologist successfully deal with the intense psychologic pressures under which patients with arthritis labor, psychiatric consultation and methods are occasionally of great importance. Crippling and employment-threatening diseases compromise or even destroy self image; having to accept dependence upon others is a further threat; the patient's view of the future (if uninformed by his or her physicians) will be drawn from the most severely involved patients the patient has known. Recognition of such threats is mandatory in good management. Only 15% of patients with rheumatoid arthritis actually experience crippling and deformity, and most of these instances are probably preventable. Never should a patient with rheumatoid arthritis be told to prepare for ongoing progression of the disease, a bed–wheelchair existence, and removal from society. Most cases subside to acceptable levels of disease.

The psychiatrist is best equipped to deal with mental mechanisms that the primary care physician or rheumatologist may not sufficiently understand. Compromised function in osteoarthritis or rheumatoid arthritis of the cervical spine causes the psychologic reactions to rheumatic disease. In some people good health and self respect are intimately related, and loss of good health may result in damage to self image, a sense of continuing loss, a feeling of "wearing out" and getting old. Change in physical appearance is damaging. Pain has a powerful influence on personality and emotion. The senses of weakness, fatigue, and lack of energy are most discouraging and may require specific psychologic care.

Clinics Specializing in the Management of Chronic Pain

There are now many clinics staffed by multidisciplinary health professionals who deal with the problem of chronic pain. When this occurs in an individual patient and is unsuccessfully managed, consultation, usually over several days, may be very effective.

Physical Therapist

The physical therapist plays a most important role in the management of rheumatic disease specifically and in assessing the magnitude of the patient's disability (or, stated more positively, the patient's remaining ability); preventing pain, deformity, and further disability; maintaining and improving muscle power and motor skills; and restoring maximal functional capability. The practicing physical therapist also works on alteration of the settings in which the patient functions.

The physical therapist is a thorough professional, and when a consultation is sought, one may expect the physical therapist to evaluate the patient individually and to establish a baseline from which immediate priorities and short-term goals are defined. The tests, measurements, and assessments the physical therapist carries out are many and varied; some are unique to physical therapy and require special training. More specifically, the physical therapist's consultation and evaluation include tests of range of motion, muscle function, manual muscles, and motor control; electroneuromyography; sensation and proprioception tests; and evaluation of perceptual and functional capacity, neurodevelopment, and gait. The physical therapist selects plans, and teaches a management program.

Physicians, by and large, are not capable of prescribing the most effective programs, and such matters as gait training, stretching exercises, exercises to restore function, and improving muscle strength and motor skills constitute the province of the physical therapist. Too often, proper consultation is delayed, not allowing the physical therapists maximal application of their preventive skills.

Occupational Therapist

The occupational therapist's range of skills is broad, including functional evaluation and management to arrest, reverse, or minimize consequences of rheumatic disease, trauma, psychologic and social disability, even poverty and cultural differences. In the case of the cervical spine, the occupational therapist's goals are to identify areas of loss and to restore them to the maximum functional ability for optimum use in activities of daily living. Like physical therapists, occupational therapists are trained to perform as independent practitioners. Occupational therapists contribute knowledge and skills, making independent decisions within the spectrum of occupational therapy practice. In general, the consultation in occupational therapy includes an assessment of the patient's diagnosis, current functional compromise, present or future complications, and precautions to be taken. The occupational therapist recommends appropriate testing procedures; assists the rehabilitation team, patients, and families in establishing attainable goals; estimates the time required for accomplishment of the goals and monitors them; educates patient and family concerning progress and lack of it; plans and carries out a management program in the total context of treatment; identifies, prescribes, and makes specialized equipment (splints, casts) to enhance the patient's abilities; works continually with rehabilitation team members; and maintains optimum records. The occupational therapist's role in the case of cervical spine diseases may be related to the total disease and to the cervical spine involvement itself.

Social Worker

The role of the social worker, also a highly trained, independent professional, is that of diagnosing and managing the social and emotional problems that render patients less able to realize maximum benefit from medical and surgical care. The social worker helps patients and families deal with personal problems; psychosocial aspects of illness and disability are as profound as their physical symptoms. The job of the social worker is that of application of all support systems—friends, family, community, leisure, work, education, economics, and religion.

A social service consultation may include a report of the patient's adjustment capability before the illness; social, emotional, and economic problems created or increased by the illness (mechanisms of management are suggested); the patient's goals in life and any necessary redirection; assessment of people important to the patient; nature of interpersonal relationships (usual social roles and necessitated changes in those roles); emotional reactions to the illness; capability of coping (coping mechanisms); overall expectations of a rehabilitation program; social resources and personal strengths; and attitudes and behaviors suggesting mental illness, severe anxiety, depression, grief, or suicidal intent.

Rehabilitation Nurse

The concept of rehabilitation nursing has emerged as a specialty nowadays and is indeed a subspecialty in the broad field of nursing. A consultation with a rehabilitation nurse should reveal an assessment of the patient's comprehension of his or her health; the patient's capability of communication; limitations of the patient's nutritional status; expectations of hospitalization or outpatient management, as assessed by the rehabilitation team; general appearance and behavior of the patient; pulmonary function; skin condition; motor and sensory function; general ability; knowledge; motivation and attitude of patient to accept and meet self-care requirements; current and future medications, with some insight into their pharmacologic action; and available resources (work, family, friends, religion).

Sexual Counselor

Sexual health is commonly compromised in several rheumatic diseases, specifically rheumatoid arthritis involving cervical spine, hips, and knees. Libido is decreased owing to the overall weakness and depression likely to occur in this disease. Thus, the patient is vulnerable, and sexuality in such cases requires overall assessment. One determines whether drugs used in the management of the patient are affecting sexuality, a very common and unrecognized circumstance. Alteration of physical appearance and the unhappy feeling of having lost attractiveness, sexual interest, and energy are problems. Though sexuality is somewhat widely regarded as an area to be managed by health care professionals, resources to deal with sexuality are not widely available. Physicians are not comfortable in dealing with sexuality and in general find it difficult to commit themselves to handle such matters. Hence, consultation with a sexual counselor may be very critical to the patient's health and best interest. Thus to deal predictably and effectively with sexuality requires that the counselor be a good listener and know how to elicit a sexual history. The counselor must manifest concern for the patient's feelings, be sensitive and not sexist, judge whether the sexual problem is one the counselor can help the patient manage, and be free and comfortable with sexual topics. If the physician feels insecure in handling these matters, referral to a sexual counselor is indicated. In general, the problems arise because of pain, depression, fatigue, lack of interest, limited range of motion, lack of lubrication, erectile difficulties, pregnancy, feelings of unattractiveness, problems with a partner, and lack of a partner.

Nutritionist

Though not commonly regarded as a consultative service, the field of nutrition is increasingly recognized. However, there is great folklore and quackery concerning the relationship of rheumatic diseases and nutrition. A broad segment of the population believes that nutrition has something to do with the primary cause of several forms of arthritis. Many people, without any scientific evidence or confirmation, believe that diet is important in the cure of these conditions.

Nevertheless, since nutrition is poorly taught in our medical schools and it is only the unusual physician who is really knowledgeable concerning nutrition, and since there have been major advances in the science of nutrition, nutritional consultation can be of major importance. Anorexia and weight loss are frequent constitutional symptoms. Pain itself can result in loss of appetite. Anorexia, weight loss, and loss of appetite may be caused by the various drugs used. Considerations for consultation are the possible interference with food consumption caused by anorexia, fever, pain, and drugs; gastrointestinal disease associated with arthritis; difficulty swallowing, compromising self-feeding; oral disease; xerostomia (Sjögren's syndrome) causing anorexia; compromise of absorption; absent normal digestive secretions; decreased intestinal motility; reduction of absorbing surface; liver dysfunction; metabolic changes; and increased nutritive requirements. Nutrition is almost always a consideration. Competent nutritionists can make assessments and specific recommendations in rheumatoid arthritis, osteoarthritis, osteopenia, and gout.

Vocational Consultation

To most human beings, work is as important to psychologic and social function as it is to economic survival. The perception of being powerless results in much human suffering, depression, suicide, failure to recover from illness and trauma, and inability to rebuild a life even with rehabilitative care. Persons unable to work are deprived not only of their most effective survival tool but also of their major available source of self-esteem. Work occupies about one half of one's life, and even more than that for some people, including a good number of physicians. In a materialistically oriented society, a person without earnings loses access to a great variety of comforts and pleasures that others enjoy, a depressing experience. To become involved in a welfare system is to receive the least possible support to survive and to sustain the psychologic catastrophe of losing privacy, pride, and motivation in the "mortification process."[8] The mainstream of life means work. The vocational counselor deals with barriers to work performance, changing occupation, and employer's apathy and fear of hiring and presents and works out all available solutions.

Clinical Psychologist

The clinical psychologist's role overlaps to some degree with that of the psychiatric consultant. The clinical psychologist understands the patient's emotional reaction to the disability while also having knowledge of the characteristic tissue pathology. The patient's physical and psychologic responses are monitored; the interpersonal dynamics among family members is appreciated, and close contact is maintained with the patient and other members of the rehabilitation team—primary care physician and other health professionals. A clinical psychologist's job also includes communicating psychologic information to the patient's physician and to all other professionals in clear and comprehensible terms, not in psychologic terms that are vague, esoteric, and inconclusive.

Too many doctors still expect and demand precise obedience from patients and assume patients understand such explanations as, "You were born with it," or "You've slipped a disc," or "You have a little arthritis in your zygapophyseal joints," or, worse yet, "You have rusty pipes." The sensitive clinical psychologist can correct and explain these defective communications. The patient always nods in seeming understanding, but this head-nodding correlates highly with complete lack of understanding.

A common occurrence among the chronically ill who do not respond to management in the magnitude expected is that they are labeled, usually by attending doctors and housestaff, as kooks, cranks, crocks, flaky, manipulative, combative, and uncooperative. These labels are accurate only occasionally, and their use commonly simply reflects poor understanding by medical attendants of the patient's needs—a problem solvable by the clinical psychologist.

Other Consultants

Other professionals occasionally serving as consultants include visiting nurses, prosthetists, or- thotists, brace makers, kinesiologists, engineers, and recreational therapists.

References

1. Fries JF, Mitchell DM: Joint pain or arthritis. JAMA 235:199, 1976.
2. Lawrence JS: Disc degeneration: Its frequency and relationship to symptoms. Ann Rheum Dis 28:121, 1969.
3. Hollander JL: Introduction to arthritis and rheumatic diseases. *In* McCarty DJ (ed): Arthritis and Allied Conditions: A Textbook of Rheumatology, 9th ed. Philadelphia: Lea & Febiger, 1979, p 45.
4. Urowitz MB: SLE subsets—divide and conquer. J Rheumatol 4:332, 1977.
5. Fries JF: General approach to the rheumatic disease patient. *In* Kelley WN, Harris ED, Ruddy S, et al (eds): Textbook of Rheumatology, 2nd ed. Philadelphia: W. B. Saunders Co, 1985, p 363.
6. Feinstein AR: Clinical Judgment. Baltimore: Waverly Press, 1967.
7. Tumulty PA: The Effective Clinician. Philadelphia: W. B. Saunders Co, 1973.
8. Goffman E: The Mortification Process. Chicago: Asylum Adline Publishing, 1961.

Chapter 20

Disability Determinations

A major problem in disability determination is a lack of agreement by radiologists on normality, abnormality, compensable, and noncompensable radiologic findings. In examination of the cervical spine to award compensation for job-related complaints, radiographic interpretation is often held as the major factor in decision making. This is especially true in the Veterans' Administration system.

Three thoroughly certified senior radiologists reviewed 200 consecutive cervical and lumbar spine examinations and put each case in one of three categories: normal, normal for age (not compensable), and degenerative disease (osteoarthritis) (compensable). A critical disagreement in which at least one radiologist considered a case compensable and another considered the same case not compensable occurred in the interpretation of 31% of the cervical and 46% of the lumbar spine examinations. Although detection of radiographic findings was similar among all three radiologists, diagnostic interpretation of the findings varied greatly.[1]

Most radiologists and orthopedists agree that the use of plain radiographic films of the spine as a deciding factor in awarding compensation is inappropriate and unjustified. However, unless the regulations are changed, there is a pressing need for strict objective radiographic criteria for determining the "normal aging" of the cervical spine such that interpretation can be more uniform. I have no solution for this problem currently.

Disorders of the cervical spine constitute a common and major source of litigation and the need for disability determination. The incidence of neck trauma and the cost of liability insurance have increased enormously in the past few decades, with ever-increasing prevalence. One distinguished author suggests categorizing patients with cervical spine injury who are covered by insurance as medico-legal cases and those who are not as private patients.[2] Short of fracture or

fracture-dislocation, the supporting ligaments, muscles, tendons, and capsules of the cervical spine can be damaged by injury, resulting in both brief and extremely prolonged clinical syndromes. Such patients are seen daily in our emergency rooms, orthopedic clinics, emergency medicine units, and physicians' offices. Without the frightening neurologic signs of spinal cord damage or the radiologic evidence of fracture or vertebral displacement, such cases early on are likely to be treated superficially. Once bone, joint, and malalignment injuries have been ruled out, initial management is usually perfunctory, and return visits and ongoing complaints are pushed aside. Such attitudes of medical attendants are perceived by patients with resentment, a sense of guilt, consequent aggressive behavior, and a worsening of the so-called traumatic cervical syndrome. When litigation (as is usual) begins, the combined physician-patient resentment results in a relationship in which proper clinical assessment cannot occur, treatment is unsuccessful, and the outlook is frustrating and gloomy.

Three terms—whiplash, slipped disc, and "my back went out"—which are presently in common use, may be blamed for some such problems. The worst of these terms is whiplash. This cliché eliminates the probability and seeming necessity for thought and proper assessment. Nevertheless, this grossly inaccurate term, with its emotional ripples of meaning, is used in official medical records describing almost any neck injury (other than fracture-dislocation) and is enormously misused by lawyer and client alike. Most of these injuries are a consequence of automobile crashes. The mechanism of injury has been extensively studied.[3, 4, 5, 6]

Another common circumstance requiring disability assessment is the ubiquitous and universal osteoarthritis of the cervical spine, including intervertebral discs, zygapophyseal joints, and the joints of Luschka. A flier published by the Arthritis Foundation titled "One out of Every Seven of

Your Employees Probably Has Arthritis," contains the following statements:

> Arthritis afflicts every age and can be costing your company many dollars unnecessarily. Arthritis ranks first as the cause of absenteeism. Twenty-seven million working days were lost last year because of it. No one knows how many costly industrial accidents and production line breakdowns occurred daily because of workers who have become weakened or crippled due to arthritis. Accidents and breakdowns mean untold dollars lost in down time, defective products and damaged equipment. Arthritis means higher workman's compensation and other health insurance premiums. Every day, thousands of American wage earners are forced to quit their jobs prematurely. They can no longer cope with the pain and crippling. Too often, these are highly skilled employees who have had years of experience and training. Another great loss to business.[7]

Obviously, the most common, indeed the universal, rheumatic disease is osteoarthritis, and the preceding statements apply clearly to that disease and especially to the cervical spine. Thus, sufficient involvement of the soft tissues, joints, intervertebral discs, nerve roots, and spinal cord—even the trachea and esophagus—can compromise function enough to result in disability and require disability determination. The problem of osteoarthritis in industry is unresolved. The evidence that osteoarthritis is caused by what one does at the job is anecdotal, though in some instances there clearly is a cause and effect relationship. Osteoarthritis in the cervical spine raises the issues of compensation, retirement, and disability. Industry is reluctant to accept this responsibility, because the disease is universal, and if osteoarthritis were to come under compensation laws, it would be extremely costly to industry. Employers far prefer to identify osteoarthritis as an intercurrent event that is common to all humans and unrelated to the job.

An important point concerning the injuries noted above is that the consequence of the trauma is much greater in patients with arthritis of the cervical spine, osteoarthritis (cervical spondylosis), ankylosing spondylitis, or rheumatoid arthritis. Obviously, the injuries in normal spines are quite different from those in spines in which there is definite disease.

DEFINITIONS AND CLASSIFICATION

A perception of the differences between the terms *impairment*, *handicap*, and *disability* is important to anyone who determines disability. An *impairment* is a damaged, deteriorated, or injured organ or extremity. A *handicap* is a consequent disadvantage in function caused by the impairment. *Disability* is the inability to function effectively due to an excessive handicap resulting from an impairment. According to the Social Security Administration of the United States, disability is

Table 20–1. COMPREHENSIVE CLASSIFICATION OF NECK INJURIES

Hyperextension strains
Acceleration extension injuries
Disruptive hyperextension in
  Normal spine
  Osteoarthritic spine
  Ankylosing spondylitis
  Rheumatoid arthritis
Hyperflexion sprains
Accleration flexion injuries
Disruptive hyperflexion in
  Normal spine
  Ankylosing spondylitic spine
  Children
Lateral flexion injuries (never quite pure, always some rotation)

Data from Babcock JL: Cervical spine injuries. Arch Surg 111:646, 1976.

determined by whether the person is unable to engage in any substantial gainful activity by reason of his or her physical or mental impairment, taking into account age, education, and previous work experience. Awards are made on the presumption that at least 12 months will elapse before the person will be able to work effectively.[8]

An occupational definition (Veterans' Administration) used by many pension plans is the determination of lack of capability to perform a previous occupation or the percentage of disability as judged against schedules of disability, based on a presumed effect of a given condition on the "average man."[9, 10]

Table 20–1 is a comprehensive classification of neck injuries.[11] Clinical correlates of cervical spine injuries are as follows:[3, 4, 5, 6]

1. Hyperextension injuries alone do not damage the spinal cord in the normal spine; they may injure nerve roots.

2. In full, normal cervical spine extension, the ligamentum flavum bulges anteriorly into the spinal canal, rarely, if ever, producing injury in acceleration extension.

3. Zygapophyseal joints may be fractured by compression, and in the experimental animal, damage to articular cartilage and subchondral bone occurs.

4. The anterior and posterior longitudinal ligaments are stretched (anterior more severely than posterior). Anterior longitudinal ligament may be torn from the anulus of the intervertebral disc, with hemorrhage beneath the prevertebral fascia.

5. The scalene and sternomastoid muscles and the long muscles of the neck and head may be torn and thus swollen by hematoma. The nerve supply to the rhomboid muscles runs through the middle scalene muscle, and nerve damage here may explain persistent periscapular pain (of which many patients complain).

6. The vertebral arteries may be stretched, causing transient ischemia of the medulla oblongata and brain stem.

7. Horner's syndrome may occur owing to stretching of and trauma to the sympathetic trunk.

8. Small bony fragments may be avulsed from the anterior margins of the vertebral bodies (anterior longitudinal ligament tears from bony attachment). This radiologic evidence is only significant if there is no further sign of cervical osteoarthritis.

9. Anular tearing as well as osteochondrophytes may result much later in intervertebral disc degeneration and prolapse.

10. The previous observations are pertinent to the normal spine. In acceleration extension injury in an osteoarthritic spine, limits of elasticity are reached much sooner, and the damage is accordingly more severe.

The clinical characteristics of the victim of cervical spine injury due to automobile crash follow:

1. The victim is usually a front-seat passenger, wearing a seat belt; the vehicle is stationary or moving slowly and is struck from the rear by another car. The struck car and occupants are accelerated forward, with unsupported heads thrown back, possibly striking the posterior chest in extreme extension. There is no immediate pain. The driver of the struck car usually gets out of the car to discuss the matter with the other driver. Examination at that time discloses no restriction of neck movement.

2. From within minutes to 3 hours, neck pain begins. The pain is probably secondary to the development of bleeding and hematoma and the edema of trauma. Duration of delay of onset of pain is not an accurate guide to the severity of the lesion and is of no prognostic significance.

3. Protective muscle spasm follows, and when the patient is in the emergency room, neck stiffness is obvious; symptoms include headache, radiation of pain to shoulders, paresthesia, arm or hand pain, interscapular pain, and even low back pain.

Objective physical signs follow:

1. Early on, neck movement is restricted in all directions. As time passes, restriction is decreased to one or two arcs of movement. All spheres of cervical spine movement are rarely if ever compromised. Extension nearly always is restricted. Rotation to one or the other side is very slow to improve. Flexion and lateral flexion may be normal.

2. Radiation of pain, paresthesia, or hypesthesia in the hand only is a symptom correlated with a poor prognosis. Age and sex are insignificant. Pain in both shoulders and in the back of the head is almost universal in patients who ultimately come to hospital and clinic; the symptoms frequently continue for a long time.

3. Average duration of symptoms is 10 months in the normal cervical spine. With osteoarthritis of the spine plus trauma, average duration of symptoms is 17 months.[12]

Radiologic Examination. Radiographic study is mandatory in assessing fracture and fracture-dislocation. Acceleration extension injury is associated with no pathognomonic radiologic finding. A "straight" cervical spine with loss of normal lordosis is common owing to muscle spasm. Small bony fragments at the anteroinferior margins of vertebral bodies are significant of avulsion fracture of the anterior longitudinal ligament. Anterior soft-tissue swelling may indicate hematoma. The measurement between the shadow of the pharynx and the lower margin of the anterior body of C3 should not be more than 5 mm[11] (see Chapter 7, *Craniometry and Roentgenometry of the Skull and Cervical Spine*).

With subsidence of muscle spasm, flexion, extension, and rotation films can be taken. In cervical osteoarthritis, the restrictions to movement are taken into consideration.

EVALUATION OF FUNCTION OF THE CERVICAL SPINE—ASSESSMENT OF DEGREE OF DISABILITY

Physical disability has three components: physical, psychologic, and socioeconomic. To measure physical disability, one must determine the amount of total normal function present. Conversely, one must determine the degree of lack of function. This is different from the measurement of pain; it is also different from loss of motion or loss of strength—that is, one may have 100% function for a given performance and still have pain, loss of motion, and loss of strength. The goal of evaluation of function is to determine levels of functional impairment and independent performance in various activities. Such quantitative assessment is required for the best assignment of work levels. The measure of function is useful to appreciate effectiveness of treatment. Functional improvement is second only to relief of pain, particularly in the patient's view. The investment made in increasing range of motion in the cervical spine in terms of expense, time, and discomfort to the patient should be justifiable in terms of improvement in function and relief of pain.

Functional evaluation for rheumatic diseases (in this instance the cervical spine) must be as objective as possible, reproducible, concise, and inexpensive. Such a measurement is affected by pain, psychologic factors, and level of intelligence. Functional testing cannot replace tests of range of motion or power, anatomic or radiographic assessments, or the estimation of magnitudes of pain and inflammation. Such testing should reflect the usual and ordinary functions of the cervical spine in normal daily activity so that inability to perform a given function (i.e., extend the cervical

Table 20–2. CRITERIA OF FUNCTION

American Rheumatism Association (United States)[13]
1. Performs all usual activities without handicap
2. Performs adequately for normal activities, despite discomfort occasionally in one or more joints
3. Limited to little or no activities or usual occupation or self-care
4. Largely or wholly incapacitated, bedridden, or confined to wheelchair; little or no self-care

Joint Committee (Great Britain)[14]
Grade I. Fully employed or employable in the usual work and able to undertake normal physical recreation
Grade II. Doing light or part-time work and only limited physical recreation; for housewives, all except the heaviest housework
Grade III. Not employed and not employable; no physical recreation; for housewives, only light housework and limited shopping
Grade IV. Confined to house or wheelchair, but able to look after oneself and essentials of life; hospital patients confined to bed
Grade V. Completely bedridden

spine or look behind) will identify some physical defect, thus letting no physical or functional deficit go undetected.

Though there are many schemes and systems of functional classification, none has emerged as refined and sensitive to describing, in brief, levels of functional impairment while still identifying important changes in function. Table 20–2 lists the two most widely used short functional classifications for rheumatic diseases. Both have received wide acceptance because of their brevity, conciseness, and ease of application. The criticism of these criteria is lack of refinement; however, they remain the best of a poor set of functional criteria.

INCIDENCE, CAUSES, AND DURATION

The National Health Survey of the United States Public Health Service showed that a 5-year average of cases of chronic stiffness and nonparalytic limitations of motion of the neck and cervical spine is 480,000 individuals. About 50% of these cases are due to previous injury. Motor vehicle crashes account for a very significant number of total neck injuries occurring in the United States. Braunstein[15] reported a study of 1678 persons injured as automobile passengers; 6.8% of these victims suffered injuries to the cervical spine, with a 1.1% fatality rate. Kulowski[16] reported that 28% of 215 consecutive automobile crash patients with chronic musculoskeletal complaints had residual cervical disability. In 1961, the National Safety Council reported 1,400,000 motor vehicle injuries that were disabling beyond the day of the accident. One can reasonably assume that 70,000 to

100,000 of these injuries involved the neck. The number of injuries restricting activity or requiring medical attention would triple these figures. Motor vehicle cervical injuries also have a high mortality rate; that in Braunstein's analysis is 16.7%—by far the highest of all body areas listed.

In contradistinction, neck injuries in workers' compensation cases accounted for only 0.2% of the workers' compensation injuries. The remainder of the back was responsible for nearly 10% of the injuries. This is not surprising when one considers the probability of neck injury in automobile crashes compared with that in occupational injuries. In fact, the average person seems more likely to sustain cervical injury in an automobile crash than in any other circumstance.

A survey of football fatalities disclosed that 15% followed injuries to the neck. Among professional and semiprofessional players, such injuries accounted for 35% of deaths; among college players, 39%; among high school players, 14%.

PREVENTION OF LEGAL AND DISABILITY CLAIMS

The best preventive measures occur in the first hours to days and weeks after injury to the cervical spine. These preventive measures are reassurance, temporary splinting, analgesia, and patient education—nonspecific psychotherapy. Reassurance must be firm and authoritative, with no hint of lack of sympathy or understanding. Patients should be told initially that they have no broken bones, that the neck is not broken, that all of the joints are intact; and that sprain, strain, bruising, and possible minor bleeding in the ligaments, tendons, and muscles of the neck have occurred. Any suggestion that it is "all in your head" or that there is nothing wrong constitutes the beginnings of a trauma-induced neurosis and sets the stage for mutual distrust, resulting in a very complicated long-term management. One cannot give such assurance in patient education except after thorough historical elicitation, physical examination, and radiologic survey. Other injuries more apparent at the time should not interfere with proper neurologic examination. The cervical spine will be stiff and painful long after the abrasions and sutured lacerations have healed.

Optimum management consists in regular follow-up visits to assess progress or lack of it; application of a properly fitting soft collar, without complete immobilization; physical therapy; gentle cervical spine traction; heat; massage; cervical spine pillows; rest alternating with activity; analgesic drugs, such as indomethacin (Indocin), phenylbutazone (Butazolidin), and aspirin; and general efforts to get the patient back to work and to avoid chronic, overly prolonged preoccupation with health. A common and usually justified complaint of such patients is that the doctor does not tell them what is wrong. Perfunctory management for patients whose symptoms are out of proportion to their physical signs is not reassuring, and it suggests a physician's attitude and plan to dismiss the patient, which brings on further fear and anxiety. The doctor, too busy to explain in plain terms what he or she thinks the diagnosis is and how the management fits the pathophysiology present, should not be practicing medicine. Prognosis may be nearly impossible. Litigation is a real factor in persistence of symptoms, and it seems no coincidence that the duration of the disorder equals the time to legal settlement in a significant number of patients.

Certain clinical features suggest a poor prognostic outlook—severe initial trauma, history of loss of consciousness, pain radiation to the head and shoulders, paresthesia in the fingers and hands, and pain persisting over 6 months. Radiologic features suggesting a long-term management problem are pre-existing osteoarthritis, persistent reversal of normal lordosis, and restricted movement at one level in the flexion-extension lateral radiograph of the cervical spine. Lastly, pending litigation is a force prolonging the clinical course.

DISABILITY DETERMINATIONS—PRACTICAL APPLICATION

The measurement and quantification of disability are determined by proper authorities, insurance carriers, and local, regional, and federal government health agencies, with the aid of a physician. The physician's problem of arriving at a scientifically sound diagnosis following an automobile crash injury is difficult, because too often a traumatic cervical syndrome involving soft tissues evolves over a period of months into what is popularly called *whiplash*. Usually, the physician can make an accurate diagnosis and communicate to an attorney or to responsible organizations the pathophysiologic processes involved.

The immediate disability generally lasts a few days to 3 weeks, with pain, tenderness, headache, and dizziness lasting for 2 to 3 months. Most people, though partially disabled, continue their regular duties. Eighty-five per cent have returned to their jobs at the end of three months.[17] Six months or beyond is the time arbitrarily set for chronic disability. The patient, physician, family, employer, attorneys, and insurance carrier must satisfy themselves that this has occurred—that the disability, particularly pain, has not changed over the 6-month time period. Reconsideration of the diagnosis is carried out. The possibility of surgical management is brought up (excise a causative, herniated intervertebral disc, relieve posterior root compressions, or fuse the cervical spine by interbody bone graft). *Cooperation of patient and family is required, and the probability of cure must be very high if a surgical approach is taken.* If it is determined that surgery is not indicated, very vigorous,

sound, and predictable medical forms of management should be continued and increased in intensity. The physical therapeutic forms of treatment—exercises, heat, and cold—and perhaps beginning psychotherapy should be carried out vigorously and with a projected rationale for their use, that is, they should not be done casually.

Disability Assessment

Finally, disability is determined by measurement of range of motion of head, neck, and both shoulders; power in muscles of hand, wrist, shoulders, and neck; neurologic examination for any objective evidence of deficit; study of any possible alterations in vertebral artery function as it relates to posture; and search for objective evidence of compromise of brain stem function. The two best sources of disability evaluation are Goff, Alden, and Aldes[17] and McBride.[18] From these references, it is estimated that about 25% of patients with cervical spine syndrome following automobile crashes and continuing beyond 6 months have cases in litigation. Basic underlying mechanisms of traffic crash injuries are seldom considered, such as the psychosomatic make-up of the drivers, tension, unwillingness to drive carefully, habitually driving fast and "taking chances," hoping to get away with it. Such pre-accident emotional make-up clearly influences recovery and surely accounts for some who develop the post-traumatic neuroses. An ongoing problem is that, in some areas, subjective complaints are considered ratable as objective functional impairment. For example, in California, subjective disability is assessed by (1) the description of the activity producing the disability, (2) the duration of the disability, (3) the activities that cannot be accomplished and those that can be done in spite of the disability, and (4) the management to result in relief of the disability.

Another problem lies in the cncept of activating or aggravating a pre-existing condition—activating a condition that was asymptomatic prior to the accident or increasing (aggravating) the condition's clinical symptoms and signs after the accident. Thurbert[19] believes that the concept of aggravation is beyond any reasonable scientific usefulness, that is, the physician's responsibility is to cure or alleviate the pre-existing condition and to reduce or relieve symptoms of the immediate physical impairment.

To rate magnitude of functional impairment, the McBride system is preferable.[18] Neck function is measured by observing movement at all ranges and including any functional compromise of shoulder, scapular area, proximal arm, elbow, wrist, and hand, including all of the small joints and any neurologic manifestation. Each part is described and measured separately—hand, forearm, arm, shoulder, and neck. Per cent impairment of each component is computed, and the sum of per cent loss of function is divided by the number of units of impairment. The final figure reflects the loss of function of the entire extremity plus that of the neck. McBride further rates this percentage as a part of the whole body, since one cannot separate impairments in different parts of the body. The arm, shoulder, and neck cannot stand alone in terms of disability.

Impairment involving any pre-existing disability is considered. Thus, osteoarthritis is included. Often, pre-existent disability requires determinations and apportionments of contribution to the disability, that is, what degree of impairment existed before the injury. Thus, past history is an integral part of the examination, necessitates factual verification, is difficult to obtain during litigation, and requires discussion with the injured person, the family, and sometimes the fellow workers. The American Medical Association's committee on the rating of physical impairment states that the function of the physician is not the rating of the disability but the reporting of physical impairment. The rating is a function of other qualified authorities.

Most post-traumatic symptoms are successfully eliminated with optimum management. The settlement of litigation claims is thought by most authorities to be the major element in recovery. Goff et al[17] suggest that the clinical findings and characteristics of the individual patient in post-traumatic disorders should correlate with usual and understood traumatic lesions. Symptoms should show reliable correlation with known conditions; familiar patterns should be present, and objective physical evidence is associated. If this is not so, post-traumatic neurosis is assumed. Measurements and assessments in this case are much more difficult, but when the diagnosis of post-traumatic neurosis is made, psychologic and psychiatric management is in order.

Post-traumatic Neurosis—The Concept

The term *whiplash* has generated much more heat than light, presumably related to litigation. Still one must consider the 75% of patients with whiplash who never become litigants. One asks, What is post-traumatic neurosis, and is the "whiplash" its etiology? Studies are available on the outcome of patients in litigation after settlement of their medical and legal problems. In one report, 88% recovered from their neck disability, leaving 12% who presumably did not recover. Why? The emotional factors often compromise proper medical care and result in distortion and confusion, and physician assessments are not predictable. In Gotten's series of 100 cases, 54 had no further complaints related to head and neck injury; 34 continued to have minor complaints but were finally functional; 12 complained severely; and 2 required surgery, with benefit.[20] Forty-nine were

satisfied with settlement of their claims, and 41 lost an average of 3 months from their employment and returned to their jobs after financial settlement. The personal reaction of the patient to the injury complicated evaluation of symptoms, management, and cure by compromising the physician's objective. Anxiety, apprehension, and nervous tension contribute to the patient's insecurity regarding his or her health. Gotten called this reaction post-traumatic neurosis.[20] Once the neurotic symptoms appeared, the case was much more complicated and became very refractory to further management. A financial settlement resolved many cases but not all. With trauma, not only physical but psychologic changes occur. The latter sometimes exceed the physical damage and after months may be the only remaining aspect of the trauma. All humans have roughly quantifiable emotional resources, and in a given instance, trauma may absorb and exceed all of those resources, resulting in the neurotic behavior. This may occur over weeks and presumably within 6 months to 1 year of the trauma. The previous behavior of the patient and his or her capability of dealing with other life situations are key to these assessments. Life situations, including many pressures, employment, interpersonal relationships in the family, children, and problems with behavior and the law prior to an automobile crash, may render the person very susceptible to traumatic neurosis. A diagnosis of traumatic neurosis requires the kind of clinical data previously noted. Observation of personality changes over weeks to months, inappropriate responses to questions, irritability, resentment, anger and hostility, overall nervous behavior, excessive drinking, insomnia, and moodiness or violent temper display contrary to the disposition of the patient prior to the accident can be elicited and assessed during the recording of a history. Bizarre symptoms are often early evidence of neurosis. Increase in complaints concerning a part of the body distant from that originally affected is to be appreciated. Fits of anger and antagonism to physician, attorney, and social workers are all evident. The doctor shopper is characteristic. If the physician does not find physical reasons for the patient's complaint, the patient commonly seeks another doctor who will.

A history of accident-proneness and garrulousness, suggesting an effort to prove something, can be identified by the commonly made statement, "I'm not interested in a settlement or any money really—I only want to get well." This is fantasy to warrant the patient's continued disability. Precipitating factors of the neurosis include the occurrence of the trauma to adolescents, during a divorce, after recent childbirth, during a marital separation, or resulting in the death of a relative or friend, the loss of job, or forced retirement. Finally, what is called *symbolic injury* is a consideration. There are parts of the body that have particular emotional significance, such as the eye, hand, heart, and abdomen. The patient may perceive injury to such parts as disfiguring, compromising his or her future. Amputated lower extremity or loss of an eye causes great emotional disruption. Neurotic behavior is frequently associated with gastrointestinal functional disorders, migraine headache, hypertension, and certain skin disorders. Any record of institutionalization or criminal records are useful in diagnosis.

The neurotic, traumatic cervical syndrome patient frequently arrives at the physician's or attorney's office with extensive written records of symptoms, episodes, and description—most of which turns out to be irrelevant and aids in identifying neurosis. A member of a minority group, cultural or ethnic, should be appreciated as susceptible to post-traumatic neurosis. Antagonism, suspicion, and hostility suggest a person who wants to "get even" against another individual, society, fate, or some family member. A classic example[17] is that of a working person who has cervical spine injury; treatment is begun and continued and seems to be gradually successful. After several follow-up visits, the physician decides that it is time for the patient to return to work. The person does so. The patient goes to work and, in a few hours or days, is given a lay-off slip, precipitating a severe emotional disturbance. The patient's world collapses; complete economic compromise is in the immediate future; income, happiness, and personal interrelationships are destroyed; the patient's life seems a failure, and a post-traumatic neurosis begins.

References

1. Isenberg RL, Hedsock MW, Gooding GA, et al: Compensation examination of the cervical and lumbar spine: Critical disagreement in radiographic interpretation. AJR 134:519, 1980.
2. Jackson R: The Cervical Syndrome, 4th ed. Springfield, IL: Charles C Thomas Publisher, 1977, p 169.
3. Wickstrom J, Rodriguez R, Martinez J: Experimental production of acceleration injuries of the head and neck in accident pathology. Washington D.C.: U.S. Government Printing Office, 1968.
4. Wickstrom J, LaRocca H: Management of cervical spine injuries from acceleration force. Curr Prac Orthop Surg 83:98, 1974.
5. MacNab I: Acceleration injuries of the cervical spine. J Bone Joint Surg 2:389, 1964.
6. MacNab I: The whiplash syndrome. Orthop Clin North Am 2:389, 1971.
7. Arthritis Foundation: One Out of Every Seven of Your Employees Probably Has Arthritis. 1979.
8. U.S. House of Representatives, Subcommittee on Social Security of the Committee on Ways and Means: Disability Insurance—Legislative Issue Paper. Washington D.C.: U.S. Government Printing Office, May 17, 1976, WMCP 94–132.
9. Wood WPM: Classification of impairments and handicaps. Geneva: World Health Organization, International Conference for the 9th Revision of the International Classification of Diseases, September–October 1975.
10. The Committee on Medical Rating of Physical Impairment: A guide to the evaluation of permanent impairment of the extremities and back. JAMA (special ed.), February 15, 1958.
11. Babcock JL: Cervical spine injuries. Arch Surg 111:646, 1976.
12. Jeffreys E: Disorders of the Cervical Spine. London: Butterworth Publishers, 1980, pp 83–84.
13. Steinbrocker O, Traeger CH, Batterman RC: Therapeutic criteria in rheumatoid arthritis. JAMA 140:659, 1949.
14. The Joint Committee of the Medical Research Council and Nuffield Trials of Cortisone, ACTH and Other Therapeutic Measures in Chronic Rheumatic Diseases: A comparison of cortisone and aspirin in the treatment of early cases of rheumatoid arthritis. Br Med J 1:1223, 1954.
15. Braunstein PW: Medical aspects of automotive crash injury research. JAMA 163:249, 1957.
16. Kulowski J: Motorist injuries and motorist safety. Clinical aspect. Clin Orthop 7:241, 1956.
17. Goff CW, Alden JO, Aldes JH: Traumatic Cervical Syndrome and Whiplash. Philadelphia: J. B. Lippincott Co, 1964, p 106.
18. McBride ED: Disability Evaluation, 6th ed. Philadelphia: J. B. Lippincott Co, 1963.
19. Thurbert P: Disability evaluation in California. Clin Orthop 32:24, 1964.
20. Gotten N: Survey of 100 cases of whiplash injury after settlement of litigation. JAMA 162:865, 1956.

Chapter 21

Malingering, Psychoneurosis, Hysteria, and "Compensationitis"

Interestingly enough, disorders of the cervical spine are rather frequently associated with psychologic and psychiatric symptoms and signs, and sometimes the basic diagnosis is psychiatric though the clinical syndrome is reflected in the cervical spine. This may be related to symbolism and conceptualization of the neck. The phrase *pain in the neck* is commonly used as an invective and seems to enjoy universal human comprehension. The syndrome of fibrositis (fibromyalgia) is characterized by symptoms of diffuse aching, sleep disturbance, and localized sites of deep myofascial tenderness occurring in tense, anxious patients. The term *fibrositis* is a misnomer, since pathologic studies have shown no inflammation of fibrous tissue. The syndrome is associated now with several measured personality characteristics, differing thresholds of pain perception, and a variety of psychologic disturbances. Personality measurements now serve as discriminators in the classification of fibromyalgia syndrome. Psychogenic musculoskeletal syndromes are characterized by symptoms presumably produced by psychologic stress or neurosis—vague, nonspecific problems, far out of proportion to objective findings. A proper history often reveals a stressful situation involving occupation, marriage, or other personal relationships. It has been estimated that about 15% of patients seeking rheumatologic diagnosis and management have one of the fibromyalgia syndromes.

The term *traumatic cervical syndrome* is a better description than the commoner term *whiplash*. Whiplash, a cliché, is generally understood by everyone, and, like other clichés, it eliminates any need for thought. I suggest the term be reserved for instances of cervical spine disorder in which litigation is planned or in process. It is an unsatisfactory term that is nevertheless meaningful and here to stay. The word *whip* suggests infliction of pain or fear of pain, and when *lash* is added, the ripples of meaning expand rapidly, creating a very striking, impressive, and "meaningful" word.

Thus in soft-tissue injuries of the cervical spine, we are often faced with the problem of assessing what fraction of a given patient's symptoms and signs is a consequence of psychologic and psychiatric mechanism, whether the entire spectrum of clinical manifestations is primarily psychologic or psychiatric, whether the patient, prior to injury or development of cervical spine symptoms, had unrecognized, undiagnosed hysteria, conversion neurosis, was always or has become a malingerer, or has developed the "compensationitis" syndrome.

The goal of this chapter is to present historical and physical methods of identifying and quantifying psychologic and psychiatric diagnoses and of making more precise identification of the malingerer, the true hysteric, and the spectrum of psychoneuroses and neuroses falling in the category of clinical cervical spine disorders. A list of clinical methods is included. The aim of these methods is not to reach a position allowing accusation but to develop a relationship of rapport with a patient such that he or she can communicate freely and prepare a sound basis for an alliance in further investigation and treatment, that is, problem solving. Too many doctors are totally put off by psychologic and psychiatric mechanisms, and such physicians predictably usually expand and perpetuate the problem and block true clinical problem solving.

PSYCHOLOGIC AND PSYCHIATRIC ASSESSMENT

Since at least one in three patients who consult their primary care physicians have significant psychologic problems, it is not unexpected that such will be the case to an even greater extent in patients with cervical spine disorders. Many present not with major psychiatric diseases but with a mixture of bodily and mental symptoms in a setting of personality weaknesses, social difficulties, and stressful interpersonal relationships. The clinical interview is by far the most important aspect of achieving precise diagnosis and hence proper continuing management. Through the interview, one must construct a comprehensive, longitudinal, cross-sectional picture of the patient's life and mental functioning. Perhaps strangely, the patient will supply only a limited amount of the necessary information. Thus one must obtain biographic data and details of the onset of the illness from other informants, such as family, other physicians, social worker, hospital records, and friends. The novice in this area tends to accept the patient's own account overcredulously and soon learns how misleading an impression can be that is based on data obtained from the patient only and not on information sought from others directly or indirectly.

Broad Categories of Disorder

A cautionary note suggests that socially deviant individuals or just the people one fears or disapproves of are often condemned as being sick, crazy, or inadequate. One should not equate behavioral deviations from the social norms with psychiatric illness. The lines drawn between normality and psychiatric and psychologic disorder are broad and varying. Some practical guidelines are useful.

Diagnosis of true psychiatric disease is properly used only if the patient has had such disabling alteration from his or her usual behavior by the development of clear-cut, unequivocal signs and symptoms of illness and morbid abnormalities of psychologic or psychophysiologic function. The clinical characteristics, severity, and personal lack of voluntary control by the patient are not explained by alterations of the environment. The symptoms should not be regarded as psychiatric if they constitute a rapid, transient response to a specific situation. True psychiatric categories include dementias, organic psychoses, schizophrenia, manic depressive psychoses, paranoid state and the severe neuroses, marked anxiety, hysteria, phobic obsessive-compulsive behavior, and phobic depressive behavior.

Personality Disorders. This term refers to a long-standing maladaptive lifestyle and to degree of deviation from usual behavior that results in suffering of the patient and society. Some categories of personality disorder are descriptively named according to the predominant characteristics—psychothymic, schizoid, obsessive-compulsive, hysteric, paranoid.

Gross deviations from social norms include sexual and behavioral disorders, pathologic indulgence, physical and psychologic dependency, alcoholism, and drug addiction. Psychologic problems characterized by marked physiologic dysfunction are generally regarded as psychosomatic disorders. Mental retardation, states of arrested or incomplete development of the mind, subnormal intelligence, and incapability of living an independent life are generally readily identified and are unusual in cervical spine disorders.

The Interview

The following suggestions are made to ensure success in the interview:

1. Conduct the interview in a private, quiet, comfortable surrounding. A desk between the doctor and the patient may hinder free communication.

2. Convey sincere interest, calm receptivity, and an understanding respect for the patient's views. Avoid excessive formality, casualness, or any hint of disingenuousness.

3. Allow full opportunity for the patient's questions; let the patient tell his or her own story.

4. Proceed from the general to the specific and from emotionally neutral, factual, and impersonal areas to more sensitive points of investigation. Open-ended questions or suggestions are preferred to direct questions early on.

5. Provide empathic understanding of the patient's position; seem passive and view some current circumstance as the patient views it. A common error is to empathize with a depressed patient to the degree of accepting the patient's view and mood, sympathizing and justifying the patient's behavior on that basis.

6. Continue to be alert to interactional processes between physician and patient.

7. Assess the patient's personality prior to the illness, capacity for interpersonal relationships, attitude to self, strengths, weaknesses, future ambition, moral attitudes and standards, mood and temperament, and reactions to stress, disappointment, and frustration.

8. Look for evidence of personality disorders: recurrent failures and conflicts in interpersonal relationships, marked overdependence on others, frequent changes of employment, repeated brushes with the law or other authorities, recurrent episodes of aggressive or impulsive behavior, multiple drug abuse incidents, repeated self-injury or overdoses, repeated medical or surgical treat-

ment for unexplained physical symptoms, long duration mood instability, tendencies to perfectionism or obsession, excessive introspection and aloofness, recurrent behavioral disorder, and minor neurotic symptoms in response to usual and normal life stresses.

Differentiation Between Personality Disorder and Psychiatric Illness

True psychiatric illness primarily discloses itself by a new occurrence of a syndrome, with recognizable onset that may be acute over hours or days or may occur gradually over weeks or months.

Personality disorders, on the other hand, represent a lifelong abnormality of personality, with a tendency to develop symptoms or behavioral disturbances at stress periods in life. The personality disorder appears to have emerged during the patient's early years, childhood, and adolescence, without precise identifiable time of onset. It tends to improve with increasing age. There are clear areas of overlap between psychiatric illness and personality disorder, but in general these distinctions are clinically useful.

Likewise, neurotic symptoms, often having some specific designated syndrome, also disclose themselves early in life, with recurrent neurotic disorders. The maxim that hysteric symptoms of neurotic origin do not occur for the first time in middle age or beyond is valid; there will have been previous hysteric episodes or anxiety symptoms during periods of personal stress.

Signs and Symptoms Reflecting the Mental State

Signs and symptoms reflecting the mental state include (1) appearance and general behavior; demeanor; style of dress; attitude to the physician, relatives, and other patients; lifestyle; gross abnormalities; and violent, embarrassing, incongruous, or uninhibited behavior; (2) level of consciousness; any suggestion of clouding of consciousness, semistupor, fluctuation of consciousness; (3) facial expression; patient looks generally ill; tension, misery, elation, or euphoria is readily recognized; anxiety, perplexity, suspiciousness; smile may occur but lacks warmth or conviction.

Motor Activity. Signs and symptoms related to motor activity are evidence of anxiety, sweaty palms, fine tremor, motor restlessness, and fidgeting; agitation; psychomotor retardation (general slowing of motor activity, speech, and cerebration); tics (blinking, facial grimacing); abnormalities of movement, posture, and gait; and catatonic phenomena.

Dress and Hygiene. Signs include self-neglect, slovenly dress, unkempt hair, unshaven beard (when occurring in spite of opportunity for self-care); exhibitionistic, provocative, seductive dress and behavior; self-display, histrionic personality; poor eye contact, vague or empty facial expression, gesturing; old scars of self-injury (mainline drug abuse), tattoos; red, abraded hands (compulsive hand washer); loose clothing from recent weight loss.

Vegetative Functions. Sleep, appetite, sexual performance, sexual drive, and excretory function are poor. Sleep pattern is a very common reflection of psychologic or psychiatric disorders. Loss of appetite may occur in any psychiatric disorder, mental distress and anxiety, or depressive illness. Loss or absence of sexual drive can be distinguished from failure of sexual performance, such as impotence, premature ejaculation, frigidity, and vaginismus, all of which can result from psychiatric disorder. Constipation is a feature of severe depression. Urinary retention can be a symptom of hysteria, but it is also a common side effect of antidepressant medication.

Hysteric Personality Traits. Histrionic, immature, egocentric, emotionally shallow and labile, extroverted, suggestible, manipulative, and seductive are all adjectives used to characterize the hysteric personality. Such patients have a greater tendency to develop symptoms of conversion and dissociation.

Psychoneuroses. These are minor psychiatric illnesses. Only a portion of the personality is involved, and most psychoneurotic patients can carry out their regular duties. With psychoneuroses, insight is not impaired, whereas it is impaired with psychoses. The illness follows a particular psychologic stress—in this instance, an injury or disorder associated with the cervical spine. The patient may not plainly state recognition of this setback, but it becomes apparent to the physician who, after detailed study, can identify it for the patient.

The essential clinical feature of psychoneurotic syndromes is a characteristic constellation of symptoms and signs typical of each type of psychoneurosis—anxiety, neurosis, hysterical neurosis, conversion or disassociative neurosis, phobic neurosis, reactive depressive illness, and obsessional neurosis.

Psychogenic Gait. Hysteria may be suspected if the gait is bizarre or if the patient is peculiarly unmoved by the disability. The malingerer is much more likely to mimic a painful gait but fails to display the normal rhythm, lingering on the painful neck, arm, or leg, and creating an impression of great agony in the process.

Identification of the Malingerer

A malingerer, by definition, is a person who consciously fakes disease or illness for personal gain or to avoid an adverse situation. Hysteria is induced by the same ultimate gains but at a subconscious level, that is, the patient is unaware of his or her motivation. Both malingering and hysteria have one thing in common: disability with no recognizable cause. One sees these disorders of the mind most commonly in industrial settings in which injury has occurred and compensation claims are pending. Although diagnosis of this disorder requires a great deal of experience, complaints may be so bizarre as to be readily recognized for what they are.

The malingerer's symptoms have an inconsistent pattern; the main complaint is pain that is constant and unrelieved by any factor (most pain is relieved by rest, except pain caused by advanced disease, which is usually obvious). Precise symmetric distribution of pain is rare in organic disease and usual in malingering. Absolute symmetry is strong evidence of a functional disorder.

The malingerer is defensive and often aggressive in attitude, whereas the hysteric patient is oddly indifferent or even cheerful about the disability. If the pain is in the leg, gait rhythm is atypical, that is, weight is not taken off the allegedly painful limb quickly; instead, the drama is increased by the patient's standing on it for even longer than usual. Conscious or subconscious perpetuation or exaggeration of disability is especially common if compensation is involved, making assessment difficult. Commonly enough, inconsistencies in movement of the cervical spine, upper or lower extremity, or trunk confirm the diagnosis. For example, the patient complains of severe neck pain and is unable to reach to point out the location of pain when standing, but when lying down, the patient has no limitation of movement. The patient with severe backache may, when standing, be unable to reach anywhere near the toes with the leg straight, but when lying down, straight-leg raising is not limited to a similar degree. If at the extreme of straight-leg raising the knee is flexed, the patient with genuine sciatic root tension will have pain relief and allow further hip flexion to occur, but the malingerer will not.

Neurologic defects, taking the form of sensory loss or paralysis, may be claimed, particularly after trauma. If anesthesia is claimed, the distribution does not follow an anatomic pattern and is usually of a glove or stocking configuration, affecting only one limb. At the same time, there may be symmetric loss of sensation affecting all four limbs—hardly anatomically possible—glove and stocking distribution configuration is characteristic of polyneuritis.

When paralysis is being faked, it is usually detected through gross inconsistencies—a consequence of the patient's lack of anatomic knowledge. For example, the patient with a "dropped" wrist is unable to extend the fingers or wrist, but when asked to clench the fingers, will, if malingering, show a normal fist, unaware that the wrist extensors are playing a part in which the patient thinks is purely flexion of the fingers. Also, passive movement through the range of paralysis

may be actively resisted by the patient, though the patient is unaware of this resistance.

Lower motor neuron paralysis or lack of muscle use causes wasting, which is best judged in the early stages by simple observation. Measurement is useful in assessing and should be recorded as objective evidence. Gross apparent weakness without wasting is always suspect. Malingering patients, when asked how far they used to be able to lift an arm or a leg or what it is that they cannot do as a consequence of the accident, may actually perform the movement that they claim is impossible. It is always worth asking this question and requesting performance casually at the end of the examination.

Throughout the clinical study, the examiner should remain impersonal but friendly. Hostility and intellectual browbeating of the patient magnify the problem. Precise records of the findings at the time are essential, since litigation may be in progress or a legal issue may arise.

Sometimes the grossly exaggerated way in which patients describe their symptoms enhances the likelihood of an hysteric, malingering, or other psychologic cause. Cervical spine pain may be described as an "iron vice constricting my neck," or as "red-hot nails driven into my cervical spine," or as "screws boring into my head like a red-hot poker," or the pain may be compared to being hit by a bolt of lightning or being hit over the head with a hammer. On the other hand, emotional under-reaction may occur (belle indifférence—inappropriate lack of concern for the magnitude of disability).

Hysteria—A Conceptual Update

Separating organic disease from hysteric conversion reactions is one of the most common yet most difficult diagnostic challenges. The symptoms are so extensive that the syndrome of hysteria can simulate nearly any physical disease, more commonly, disorders of the nervous system. All physicians, specialists and primary care alike, must deal with hysteria. Clinical studies, historical elicitation, and physical examination constitute the basis of diagnosis. Thus, knowledge of neuroanatomy and autonomic nervous system function is a requirement for formulating the diagnosis.

The word *hysteria* comes from the Greek word *hystera*, which means uterus. In ancient Greece, Egypt, and Rome hysteric syndromes were explained in terms of bodily alterations, that is, hysteria was a woman's disease caused by a frustrated, discontented, and wandering uterus. The clinical symptoms resulted as a function of where the "uterus" settled. In the middle ages, such illness was regarded as demonic possession, which in the United States culminated in the Salem witch trials. Freud was the first to define hysteria in psychologic terms and to define mechanism and the clinical syndromes. He thought that his hysteric patients were expressing fantasies of childhood seduction. He suggested that the memory of childhood sexual feelings for the parent (Oedipus complex) was painful and suppressed and that to prevent its resurfacing, the energy of the sexual drive was converted into a symptom; the conversion permitted relief from fear of such unacceptable impulses—primary gain. Modern psychiatrists now include far more than sexual conflicts, including any provocation that threatens the individual's integrity. The spectrum of hysteric conversion reactions is enormous, occurring at all ages and at all economic and social levels. Some studies report an incidence as high as 50%. With the maturing of an industrial society and the extremely rapid growth of the insurance industry, we see many more hysteric conversion reactions following unimportant injuries and focused on financial gain.

Definitions. Conversion hysteria is a neurosis with subconscious (patient unaware of it) change in sensory systems or motor systems or both, resulting in bodily dysfunction. Symptoms and signs reflect the conversion, often in the terms in which the patient perceives his or her own body. The severity of the symptoms and signs and their resultant production of disability are functions of the patient's intelligence, sophistication in terms of biology and medicine, and emotional resources to deal with ordinary life stresses. The patients seek gain subconsciously, and physicians should regard the symptoms as problem-solving cries for help. The great majority of hysteric conversion reactions occur abruptly in the setting of some intolerable life situation.

Psychosomatic illness and malingering are two similar illnesses readily confused with hysteria. Psychosomatic illness basically is the channeling of emotional energy into the nervous system. Clearly, anger, fear, anxiety, hate, and frustration result in physiologic responses—an over-reaction taking the form of visceral, gastrointestinal, pulmonary, and cardiovascular symptoms, such as palpitation, sweating, hyperpnea, diarrhea, abdominal pain, and dysphagia, all secondary to suppression of emotions.

Malingering is the conscious (patient is well aware) faking of illness or disability for primary gain. Contrary to hysteria, malingering is mainly a male disorder. The symptoms of both disorders are closely related, though the malingerer is not as grossly suggestible or as cooperative as the patient with hysteria. The malingerer is much more often resentful and hostile. The diagnosis of malingering is far more difficult from a medicolegal point of view. Incontrovertible evidence such as photographs may be the only secure mechanism of precise diagnosis.

The idea of an hysteric personality remains extant. The words and phrases, emotional lability, sexual frigidity, egocentricity, exhibitionism, emo-

Table 21–1. PERLEY AND GUZE CRITERIA FOR RETROSPECTIVE DIAGNOSIS OF HYSTERIA

Group 1	Group 7
Headache	Dysmenorrhea
Sickly most of life	Menstrual irregularity
Group 2	Amenorrhea for at least 2 months
Blindness	Excessive menstrual bleeding
Paralysis	
Anesthesia	**Group 8**
Aphoria	Sexual indifference
Fits or convulsions	Frigidity
Unconsciousness	Dyspareunia
Amnesia	Other sexual difficulties
Deafness	Vomiting for all 9 months of pregnancy or being hospitalized for hyperemesis gravidarum
Hallucination	
Urinary retention	
Ataxia	
Other conversion symptoms	
	Group 9
Group 3	Back pain
Fatigue	Joint pain
Lump in throat	Extremity pain
Fainting spells	Burning pain of sexual organs, mouth, or rectum
Visual blurring	
Weakness	Other body pains
Dysuria	
	Group 10
Group 4	Nervousness
Breathing difficulty	Fears
Anxiety attacks	Depressed feelings
Palpitation	Need to quit working or inability to carry on regular duties because of feeling sick
Chest pain	
Dizziness	
	Crying easily
Group 5	Feeling life is hopeless
Anorexia	Thinking a good deal about dying
Weight loss	
Marked fluctuation in weight	Wanting to die
	Thinking of suicide
Nausea	Suicide attempts
Abdominal bloating	
Food intolerance	
Diarrhea	
Constipation	
Group 6	
Abdominal pain	
Vomiting	

Data from Perley M, Guze SB: Hysteria—The stability and usefulness of clinical criteria. N Engl J Med 266:421, 1962.

tional shallowness, and sexual provocativeness are all said to be basic structural elements of the hysteric personality.

Perley and Guze (Table 21–1) worked out a list of ten categories of symptoms they regarded as characteristic features of the clinical history of hysteria. They used this list retrospectively to identify the hysteric patient. They were accurate to a 90% degree. Nevertheless, these criteria cannot properly be used as the basis for a medical diagnosis of hysteria.

The term *belle indifférence* has become connected to hysteric patients as a diagnostic behavior symptom. This sign of bizarre, unconcerned, withdrawn, indifferent attitude is depended upon by too many physicians for making a diagnosis. The stoic patient may behave in the same way toward pain. Furthermore, the patient with "compensationitis" displays enormous concern for the disability, certainly not indifference.

Another frequent error is the notion that the diagnosis of hysteria is made by exclusion. The symptoms and signs are labile, continually changing with the forces of suggestion and repeated clinical study. The occurrence of seeming autonomic or functional symptoms does not at all exclude even classic disease. The diagnostic label *hysteria* should only be used when the diagnosis is secure and unmistakable. Physicians, on seeing a patient they "know" to have "hysteria," are sorely tempted to carry out only a superficial study. The making of that diagnosis is a medical challenge in itself. Not only clinical but objective neurologic screening tests are of major importance—CAT scans, electromyograms, electroencephalograms, and study of spinal fluid should be done. Negative test results allow the doctor an excellent screen for conventional disease and also support the unusual and difficult diagnosis. Psychologic testing has not been useful in the diagnosis of hysteria.

Clinical Methods and Symptoms and Signs Useful in the Diagnosis of Hysteria, Malingering, Psychoneuroses, and More Obvious Psychiatric Diseases

1. Apply a vibrating, 128-frequency tuning fork to the skull, sternum, and tibia in two places each. If the patient perceives the vibratory sense in one place on the same bone and not in another, or if the test discloses a much different perception in the two sites, the test result is positive. Since the tuning fork has been placed on continuous bone, the patient normally must perceive the vibratory sense in both places. The test result can be positive only in cases of hysteria.

2. Ask the patient to lie down supine on the examining table. With knees extended, carry out the straight-leg raising maneuver and determine the point at which pain appears and the location of the pain (pain may not appear, but it commonly does). Note this and ask the patient to sit up. Then ask the patient to take off shoes and socks, examine the patient's heart, and auscultate the lungs. While the patient is sitting up with the knees straight or only slightly flexed, determine whether the patient has pain. The angle of the trunk and the lower leg will be from 65 to 90 degrees. The patient's experiencing pain at something less than this angle on straight-leg raising is evidence of hysteria or malingering.

3. Ask the patient to stand and touch the toes. If the patient cannot do this, ask the patient to bend forward as far as possible with the knees locked. The spine is flexed as maximally as possible and held there. If flexion of the spine is decreased or regarded as limited, ask the patient to sit on the examining table upright and touch the toes. Many patients with hysteria are able to touch their toes without pain, and this occurs even if the pain is not organic.

4. Magnuson's test. Ask the patient to place a hand or finger on the site of pain. Mark the site with a magic marker. Divert the patient's attention by examining other sites, and later ask the patient to point to the site of pain. If the pain is organic, the site is constant. In the other case, the pain is migratory, and localization of the maximum site of pain is never the same.

5. Ask the patient to kick up one leg as far as possible, like a football punt, steadying himself if necessary. The patient with a true herniated intervertebral disc has no difficulty kicking with the painful leg, but does experience pain when kicking with the healthy leg because the side tilt of the pelvis narrows the intervertebral foramen on the side opposite the kicking leg. The malingerer will complain bitterly after kicking with the painful leg. Though we deal here with disorders of the cervical spine, this test may be useful since both low back pain and cervical spine pain are so common in people with hysteria or malingering.

6. The patient with hysteria, psychoneurosis, or malingering is often very agitated, complaining of extremely severe pain—pain "all over," "all my joints hurt," "completely paralyzed, neck in a vice, burning nails driven through my head"—and still, in this distressing condition, the patient is often seemingly unconcerned (belle indifférence). The pain symptoms are continuous but do not disturb sleep. Patients demand to be seen immediately, often insisting that an ambulance take them to the doctor. They have a "touch me not" attitude—the lightest touch elicits a maximum response to this minimal stimulus.

7. The patient has a bizarre reaction to pinprick testing, that is, it is not felt until the midline of the body precisely is reached. At this point, extreme pain on pinprick, hyperesthesia, is felt; one half of the body may be numb (anesthetic)—a stocking-glove type anesthesia, with sharp demarcation between the areas of perception of the pinprick and those lacking that perception.

8. Deep tendon reflexes are hyperactive throughout and are out of proportion to the magnitude of the stimulus.

9. Cogwheel rigidity on forward bending or straight-leg raising; patient bends forward, flexing the spine, but comes back up in a "cogwheel" manner, groaning and crying out, complaining of severe pain, and climbing up the thighs with the hands to reattain an upright posture.

10. Pain complaints are out of proportion to the maneuvers of the examination.

11. The patient has a bizarre reaction to placebo

shot or pill and is very suggestible, changing the clinical symptoms and signs.

12. Such patients frequently flatter doctors about their reputations, degrade all previous physicians, and dare the doctor to effect a cure. They often tell the physicians that they are the last resort and that it is because of their reputation for curing everybody that they came to them.

13. Patients almost always have seen a lawyer before they see a doctor. They are reluctant to disclose the fact that they are involved in litigation—"I'm not really interested in any financial settlement, all I want is to get rid of my pain."

14. Such patients often have a history of unrest with employer, boss, wife, foreman, or fellow workers, or they have been laid off, especially if injured on the job.

15. Injuries often follow an automobile accident. "Whiplash" syndrome occurs after a collision from the rear. Such patients have many cervical spine complaints, with no organic basis for the pain, or they have a ridiculous disability after minor injury.

16. Patient recites a litany of symptoms and signs taught by the unscrupulous lawyer, such as frequent impairment of vision and hearing, loss of bowel or bladder function, and frequent loss of sexual capability.

17. Patient has a bizarre gait and often "postures" increased lumbar lordosis (patients with organic back disease usually have flattening or straightening of the lumbar spine, lumbar kyphosis). They have a marked decrease in range of motion in all directions of the spine. Their gait is likely to be steppage in type, as though they are walking on broken glass.

Sensory Changes. Areas of claimed sensory disturbance have sharply defined margins—usually the borders occurring at joints, the skin creases, or the midline—in a stocking-glove pattern. The patient is unaware that in true neural loss the gradations of perception of skin sensation are gradual because of the interdigitations of peripheral nerves. The patient is also unaware that paramedial sparing occurs for the same reason. Boundaries of the area of sensory change vary from one examination to the next. Sensory disturbances range from paresthesia, hypesthesia, dysesthesia, hyperesthesia, and anesthesia, and these may be interchangeable from one examination to the next. Sensory disturbances are usually much more widespread than those in true neurologic disease, and they tend to involve all modalities—touch, pain, temperature, pressure, proprioception, and vibration—a rare occurrence in true neurologic disease.

A common complaint is that of loss of sensation in precisely one half of the body, usually on the side of the dominant arm. This is commonly associated with alteration in taste, smell, hearing, and vision on the same side. Sensory loss is noted down the anterior portion of the body but sparing the back. Vibratory sense is usually reported as at least less responsive on the "bad side."

If a patient complains of anesthesia of an entire extremity, such as complete loss of perception of touch and pain in an arm or leg, ask the patient to perform the finger-to-nose or heel-to-shin test, with eyes closed. In true sensory damage, there is pseudoathetosis of the fingers or feet, as the patient does not apprehend the position of the extremities in space. Thus, the patient cannot accurately perform the test. The patient with hysteria is able to bring finger to nose and heel to shin successfully with the eyes closed.

Occasionally, patients with hysteria sustain thermal burn without evidence of pain. Yet, if one retests the patient while the patient sleeps, sensory perception can be demonstrated by the patient's appropriate withdrawal from the stimulus. A dichotomy in reaction discloses the power and protective function of the conversion symptoms.

Pain Complaints. The patient describes the pain in vivid, sensational terms. The pain is continuous but does permit sleep; it is not influenced by narcotics (though many such patients are addicted to narcotics). The patient frequently has multiple surgical scars, indicating previous treatment for various pain experiences. The patient has a single level of loss of all sensory modalities—an impossible neurologic achievement! True neurologic pain is almost always accompanied by some change in cutaneous perception (herpes zoster with anesthetic and dysesthetic sites on the skin). Other signs of organic disease are useful. In women, pain tends to involve the vaginal area, abdomen, face, and head; men more frequently describe pain in the back and chest; children have a high incidence of recurrent abdominal pains associated with attendance at school, midterm examination, or some personal crisis at school. Too often, laminectomy, appendectomy, or laparotomy is done by the sympathetic physician in response to the patient's long-term pain symptom.

In cervical spine syndrome, the physician should always rule out a constitutionally narrow cervical canal as a source of pain induced by the nerve roots or the cord. Even the whiplash-injured patient may have a small cervical canal; spinal stenosis is an occasional contributor to leg pain, a valid complaint.

Litigation that is pending or in process augments and increases the frequency of attacks of pain, particularly in the event of delay of trial or determination of the magnitude of the injury. Authorities now urge prompt settlement in the interest of shortening the period of disability. The financial gain in compensation cases is usually less than the amount the patient could earn by returning to work. If the patient continues to pursue a lawsuit, a detailed history generally discloses dissatisfaction at work, frustrating relationships with superiors, or unwillingness of a spouse to support and pamper the patient.

Motor Disturbances, Weakness, and Paralysis.
Fortunately, the diagnosis of true neurologic loss of power or weakness is simple. A stroke results in unilateral, initially flaccid paralysis of the extremities, followed by spastic paralysis. The lower two thirds of the face may be involved, and there are usually changes in sensation, speech, or vision; Babinski's and Hoffmann's responses are present. In hysterical paralysis, the patient appears to be deliberately withholding power; weakness fluctuates with recurrent examination and suggestion, and the paralysis does not conform to known anatomy.

Contraction of agonistic and antagonistic muscles should be tested for, and the response when resistance is suddenly withdrawn or increased can be observed. Hysteric weakness includes equal and simultaneous contraction of agonistic and antagonistic muscles. The arm will transiently hold its position after support has been removed. The test is to hold the arm above the patient's head, release it suddenly, and note that the extremity hovers for a few seconds before falling; this is not true in the case of real loss of motor power or diminished strength. Power of contraction can also be tested by putting sudden pressure on the hysterically contracted muscles; this force causes a protective unloading of those muscles, with a very strong counter-response. This is especially useful in weakness of biceps, triceps, or brachioradial muscles. Hysteric weakness may also be presented as an inability to make a special movement, such as extension of the wrist. Ask the patient to make a fist (a way of performing the movement synergistically). The examiner will note that the patient does have the strength that he or she claims not to have.

Place the patient in a supine position on the examining table. Move the arm over the patient's face, then release the arm. The arm falls to the face in true neurologic disease, but in the hysteric patient, the arm hovers and then falls safely to the side of the head, with no injury. Such patients subconsciously do not want to hurt themselves.

Hysteric patients, while eating, dressing, or performing activities of daily living, may show use of the arms, legs, hands, and feet in a way that would be impossible if they were truly paralyzed. Observation of patients while they sleep leads to identifying paralysis caused by hysteria. They may be observed to move "paralyzed limbs" in their sleep either spontaneously or in response to a pain stimulus. In testing the claim of weakness of the thigh adductor muscle, the examiner places one hand against the inner thigh of the "weak" leg and the other hand against the inner thigh of the "good" leg. As the examiner exerts pressure against the good thigh and the patient tries to resist it, the physician will note that adductor muscles of the "weak" leg contract as a normal, associated, involuntary movement.

Hoover Test. This test is based on the principle that when a person in a supine position attempts to lift one leg against resistance, a normal, associated, downward thrust of the other leg occurs. The physician places one hand under the heel of the "weak" leg and presses the other hand down on the "good" leg. When the patient tries to raise the "good" leg, the examiner's hand under the heel of the other leg perceives pressure. The associated pressure occurs if the paralysis is caused by hysteria but not if it is of true neurologic origin.

Normal tendon reflexes may be noted in association with complaints of severe weakness. Myasthenia gravis, thyroid myopathy, and polymyositis may also show this finding however. Creatine phosphokinase assay, thyroid hormone study, and electromyography may clarify the picture.

Gait Changes. Bizarre is the word for hysteric gait; it conforms to whatever motor disability the patient claims to have. For example, the patient may drag one leg as though it is paralyzed, showing no circumduction movements, spasticity, or Babinski's sign, as will occur following stroke. The patient may have a stiff gait or may walk only with assistance or the support of furniture, a nurse, or a physician. Patients often attempt to walk but fall toward the side of support, never away from it! Lurching, stylized, posturing, and zigzag motions and gyrations without reasonable physiologic explanation illustrate the noteworthy capability of the hysteric to make extremely rapid and appropriate postural adjustments; the hysteric patient rarely is injured.

Look for the characteristic disturbance of neurologic, rheumatologic, or orthopedic disorders: circumduction movements (stroke); festination (peculiar acceleration of gait noted in paralysis agitans and in some other extrapyramidal tract syndromes—parkinsonism); wide-based movements in walking (peripheral neuropathy); wide-based reeling (cerebellar ataxia); slapping gait (footdrop). The disparity between inability to walk and power in the leg does occur in two valid syndromes: midline cerebellar (vermis) lesions and frontal lobe ataxia. Proper neurologic examination brings out other clinical abnormalities to confirm the diagnosis of such neurologic diseases.

It is useful to test strength of the legs while the patient is supine in bed. The patient may refuse to bear weight, claiming weakness, and on standing may fall promptly to the floor. If power in the legs in bed is noted to be normal, the astasia-abasia diagnosis is confirmed (a state in which the patient is unable either to walk or to stand). Astasia-abasia is a clear manifestation of conversion hysteria.

Loss of coordination in the upper extremities may be claimed; the finger-to-nose test identifies hysteric incoordination. Rather than accurately reaching the nose (normal) or not getting the finger there at all (dysmetria), the hysteric patient's finger takes a circuitous route but accurately arrives on target or reaches an incorrect target (ear or eye) consistently.

Hysteric tremor is fairly common and bizarrely restricted to one limb. Oscillations are gross and may appear in the opposite limb if the physician restrains the affected arm.

Visual Disturbances. One visual manifestation of hysteria is narrowing of peripheral fields, or tunnel vision. It is identifiable by measuring visual fields, increasing by 2- to 3-fold the testing distance, and measuring the field again. If the visual field is just the same at these different distances, the patient is showing hysteric loss of vision (the size of the field increases as the distance of the target from the retina increases).

Another visual manifestation is abrupt unilateral blindness, sometimes with orbital pain. Funduscopic examination findings are normal in hysteria but are sometimes also normal in optic neuritis or other intraocular diseases. The pupillary response to light is the differentiating factor. In optic neuritis, direct pupillary light reflex is decreased or absent, and the consensual response is retained. In hysteria, both direct and consensual reactions are intact. In optic neuritis, the pupil may show the Marcus Gunn escape sign, that is, the involved pupil constricts in response to initial application of bright light in a dim room but then abruptly springs back and dilates. The pupils of normal and hysteric patients maintain constriction.

Another test involves the use of a highly refractive magnifying lens or a prism placed over the patient's "good" eye. The lens or prism actually distorts and reduces visual acuity, but the patient interprets that the piece is supposed to improve vision. The patient identifies numbers and objects at a distance using the affected eye, unknowingly demonstrating the true vision of this eye.

The red glass test detects unilateral loss of vision. The patient reads a line of alternating black and red letters with a red glass placed over the "good" eye. Since red letters are invisible when viewed through the red glass, proper identification of the letters means that the patient is reading with the "blind" eye.

Blepharospasm, photophobia, and convergent spasm are common visual disturbances in the patient with hysteria. Convergent spasm can look like bilateral abducent (VI) nerve paralysis caused by a brain tumor and thus trigger an extensive and expensive clinical work-up. The demonstration of miosis on attempted lateral gaze is an excellent and dependable clinical sign, distinguishing convergent spasm as hysteric.

Monocular diplopia is a common complaint of the patient with hysteria and requires ruling out dislocated lens or other monocular disease. Monocular diplopia is, of course, impossible except in the rare case of dislocated lens syndrome. Binocular diplopia, homonymous hemianopia, and central scotoma are always symptoms of real disease.

Cortical blindness is bilateral, with sparing of pupillary response because of extensive visual cortex and occipital lobe infarction in the vascular territory of the posterior cerebral artery. The most common etiologic forces are carbon monoxide poisoning, extreme basilar artery infarction, and hypoxia. Anton's syndrome is a neurologic variant of cortical blindness; the patient denies blindness but is noted to stumble over objects in walking and to handle objects as the blind do. Inconsistent perception of objects is the rule, and it is not unusual for such patients to confabulate about things they "see." To document Anton's syndrome, the ophthalmologist tests optokinetic nystagmus. The patient is presented with a slowly rotating, vertically striped drum. The ophthalmologist watches the patient's eyes for involuntary tracking movements (optokinetic nystagmus). The sign is absent because of posterior cortex damage. Such patients regard disease and illness as a weakness or imperfection and are unwilling to admit to any loss of bodily function. Again, the protective power in these mind-body relationships is illustrated; in Anton's syndrome, physical rather than psychologic illness is the source.

Deafness. Deafness is rare but does occur. It has been reported in times of war or very extreme stress. Formal audiometric testing is usually necessary. Deafness caused by hysteria disappears during sleep, and the patient's response to a loud noise may reveal his or her normal hearing level. The demonstration of K complexes in the sleep electroencephalogram confirms the presence of an intact neural pathway.

Dizziness and Vertigo. True vertigo is rare indeed. The etiology for dizziness is usually hyperventilation, and the patient can reproduce dizziness easily by voluntarily hyperventilating. Dizziness is such a common symptom in many other conditions, such as multiple sclerosis, labyrinthitis, brain tumor, cerebral ischemia, and temporal lobe epilepsy, that it requires more clinical study.

Speech Disturbances. Speech disturbances are rarely observed in the patient with hysteria, but they may appear as mutism or whispering speech. Ask the patient with whispering speech to cough. If the cough is loud, vocal cords can be approximated and vagus (X) nerve function is normal. These findings are corroborated by direct visualization of vocal cords (in vocal cord paralysis, coughing results in a loud, booming, cowlike sound). The simple cough test quickly and clearly distinguishes between whispering speech caused by hysteria and that resulting from other causes.

Loss of Sense of Smell. Loss of sense of smell rarely occurs after head injury, severe colds, heavy smoking, or an olfactory groove meningioma. It is rarely a symptom of functional disease. Differentiation is made by having the patient smell spirits of ammonia. Hysteric patients misinterpret the irritating odor as an olfactory stimulus, but it is really a trigeminal (V) nerve irritant. The patient with hysteria denies the stimulus, whereas the patient with true anosmia identifies it.

Fainting and Seizures. Hysteric patients have episodes, usually spectacular, before large groups of people. The episodes involve a bizarre series of contortions, convulsions, and odd movements, with no relation to tonic, clonic movements of grand mal epilepsy. Movements may resemble the sex act; these "seizures" last minutes to hours and are readily influenced by suggestion. Patients are never injured, nor do they bite their tongues or have urinary incontinence or any postictal stupor (also characteristic of epilepsy). Examination during the seizure shows no loss of consciousness; corneal reflexes are intact, and Babinski's response is absent. Electroencephalogram does not demonstrate epileptiform activity. Nevertheless, a true convulsive disorder can show the symptoms previously noted. An effective way to separate valid central nervous system seizures from hysteria is to use sternal massage during the spell. Deep, sustained pressure does not alter a true grand mal seizure, but this unpleasant sensation disturbs the patient with hysteria, who will attempt to push the hand away or grab it to decrease the pressure.

Fainting is common and usually occurs under dramatic circumstances. There is a conspicuous lack of alteration in blood pressure, pulse, or skin color—signs distinguishing hysteric fainting from vasovagal syncope.

Coma of Hysteric Origin. The coma of hysteric origin is an extension of syncope and resembles akinetic mutism. Pupils and corneal reflexes are active, with no evidence of either Babinski's sign or Hoffmann's sign. There is active resistance by the patient during examination.

Amnesia of Hysteric Origin. Amnesia of hysteric origin is common and widely variable. Diagnosis is made easily if the patient retains the capability of eating, dressing, speaking, and reading yet denies his or her personal identity. Acquired functions are lost before primitive functions in organic disease; the opposite is true in hysteria.

Such presentations in a person suggest psychopathology, commonly in association with crime. Some patients manifest a fugue state, wandering about for hours or days, engaging in complex activity of psychogenic origin. It is important to remember that a small percentage of cases represent temporal lobe or petit mal epilepsy; the electroencephalogram is an extremely important aid in making this distinction.

Dysphagia. Difficulty swallowing is common—"lump in the throat," so-called globus hystericus. The difficulty is intermittent and does not preclude easy swallowing of solids or liquids. Pain is usually present. Organic diseases compromising glossopharyngeal and vagus nerve functions rarely produce dysphagia.

Hysteric Vomiting. Hysteric vomiting is common and is accompanied by tenderness and pain in the lower abdominal region (rather than in the upper region). Symptom and sign persistence results in frequent, unnecessary surgery. Atypical features include occurrence after a meal, persistent hunger, variable frequency of occurrence, severe weight loss (often), dehydration, and electrolyte imbalance.

Pseudocyesis. Pseudocyesis, or false pregnancy, is seen in hysteric women who have an enormous desire to become pregnant. Signs of pseudocyesis are abdominal protuberance precisely mimicking pregnancy, with relaxation of abdominal muscles; lordosis of the lumbar spine; morning sickness; and breast enlargement. Diagnosis is made by noting a small uterus.

Other. Hysteric conversion is unusual in children, but it does occur. Clinical reflection is less refined. Signs include a high incidence of recurrent abdominal pains in association with school, aerophagia, and abdominal distention; oral mechanisms are also related. Criterion is the same as in adults, that is, obtaining positive evidence from clinical examination that the symptom does not conform to the anatomic and physiologic principles.

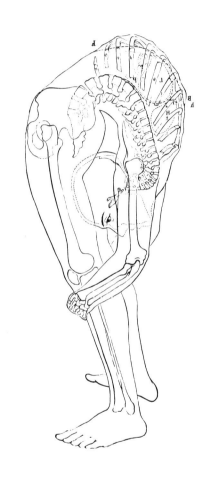

Index

Page numbers in *italics* indicate illustrations;
page numbers followed by t refer to tables.